Current
Clinical Trials
for
Colon
Cancer

2018 Edition

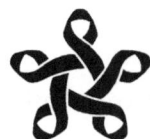

CUREBOUND
PUBLISHING

CureBound Publishing
70 Main Street, #11
Warrenton, VA 20186
www.curebound.com

Ordering Information:
Quantity sales. Special discounts are available on quantity purchases by corporations, associations, and others. For details, contact the publisher at the address above.
Printed in the United States of America

Introduction

This book contains information about every interventional clinical trial in the United States that is actively recruiting colon cancer patients, as of the date this book was published. The information inside this book was originally compiled by the National Institutes of Health (NIH) but not every clinical trial in this book has been evaluated by the NIH or other branch of the Federal Government. Before participating in a study, talk to your health care provider and learn about the risks and potential benefits.

What is a Clinical Trial?

An interventional clinical trial involves research using human volunteers (also called participants) that is intended to add to medical knowledge. In a clinical trial, participants receive specific interventions according to the research plan or protocol created by the investigators. These interventions may be medical products, such as drugs or devices; procedures; or changes to participants' behavior, such as diet. Clinical trials may compare a new medical approach to a standard one that is already available, to a placebo that contains no active ingredients, or to no intervention. Some clinical trials compare interventions that are already available to each other. When a new product or approach is being studied, it is not usually known whether it will be helpful, harmful, or no different than available alternatives (including no intervention). The investigators try to determine the safety and efficacy of the intervention by measuring certain outcomes in the participants. For example, investigators may give a drug or treatment to participants who have high blood pressure to see whether their blood pressure decreases. Clinical trials used in drug development are sometimes described by phase. These phases are defined by the Food and Drug Administration (FDA). Some people who are not eligible to participate in a clinical trial may be able to get experimental drugs or devices outside of a clinical trial through expanded access.

Who Conducts Clinical Trials?

Every clinical study is led by a principal investigator, who is often a medical doctor. Clinical studies also have a research team that may include doctors, nurses, social workers, and other health care professionals. Clinical studies can be sponsored, or funded, by pharmaceutical companies, academic medical centers, voluntary groups, and other organizations, in addition to Federal agencies such as the National Institutes of Health, the U.S. Department of Defense, and the U.S. Department of Veterans Affairs. Doctors, other health care providers, and other individuals can also sponsor clinical research.

Where are Clinical Studies Conducted?

Clinical studies can take place in many locations, including hospitals, universities, doctors' offices, and community clinics. The location depends on who is conducting the study.

How Long Do Clinical Studies Last?

The length of a clinical study varies, depending on what is being studied. Participants are told how long the study will last before they enroll.

Reasons for Conducting Clinical Studies:

In general, clinical studies are designed to add to medical knowledge related to the treatment, diagnosis, and prevention of diseases or conditions. Some common reasons for conducting clinical studies include:

- Evaluating one or more interventions (for example, drugs, medical devices, approaches to surgery or radiation therapy) for treating a disease, syndrome, or condition

- Finding ways to prevent the initial development or recurrence of a disease or condition. These can include medicines, vaccines, or lifestyle changes, among other approaches.

- Evaluating one or more interventions aimed at identifying or diagnosing a particular disease or condition

- Examining methods for identifying a condition or the risk factors for that condition

- Exploring and measuring ways to improve the comfort and quality of life through supportive care for people with a chronic illness

Participating in Clinical Studies:

A clinical study is conducted according to a research plan known as the protocol. The protocol is designed to answer specific research questions and safeguard the health of participants. It contains the following information:

- The reason for conducting the study
- Who may participate in the study (the eligibility criteria)
- The number of participants needed
- The schedule of tests, procedures, or drugs and their dosages
- The length of the study
- What information will be gathered about the participants

Who Can Participate in a Clinical Study?

Clinical studies have standards outlining who can participate. These standards are called eligibility criteria and are listed in the protocol. Some research studies seek participants who have the illnesses or conditions that will be studied, other studies are looking for healthy participants, and some studies are limited to a predetermined group of people who are asked by researchers to enroll.

Eligibility. The factors that allow someone to participate in a clinical study are called inclusion criteria, and the factors that disqualify someone from participating are called exclusion criteria. They are based on characteristics such as age, gender, the type and stage of a disease, previous treatment history, and other medical conditions.

How are Participants Protected?

Informed consent is a process used by researchers to provide potential and enrolled participants with information about a clinical study. This information helps people decide whether they want to enroll or continue to participate in the study. The informed consent process is intended to protect participants and should provide enough information for a person to understand the risks of, potential benefits of, and alternatives to the study. In addition to the informed consent document, the process may involve recruitment materials, verbal instructions, question-and-answer sessions, and activities to measure participant understanding. In general, a person must sign an informed consent document before joining a study to show that he or she was given information on the risks, potential benefits, and alternatives and that he or she understands it. Signing the document and providing consent is not a contract. Participants may withdraw from a study at any time, even if the study is not over. See the Questions to Ask section on this page for questions to ask a health care provider or researcher about participating in a clinical study. Institutional review boards. Each federally supported or conducted clinical study and each study of a drug, biological product, or medical device regulated by FDA must be reviewed, approved, and monitored by an institutional review board (IRB). An IRB is made up of doctors, researchers, and members of the community. Its role is to make sure that the study is ethical and that the rights and welfare of participants are protected. This includes making sure that research risks are minimized and are reasonable in relation to any potential benefits, among other responsibilities. The IRB also reviews the informed consent document. In addition to being monitored by an IRB, some clinical studies are also monitored by data monitoring committees (also called data safety and monitoring boards). Various Federal agencies, including the Office of Human Subjects Research Protection and FDA, have the authority to determine whether sponsors of certain clinical studies are adequately protecting research participants.

Relationship to Usual Health Care

Typically, participants continue to see their usual health care providers while enrolled in a clinical study. While most clinical studies provide participants with medical products or interventions related to the illness or condition being studied, they do not provide extended or complete health care. By having his or her usual health care provider work with the research team, a participant can make sure that the study protocol will not conflict with other medications or treatments that he or she receives.

Considerations for Participation

Participating in a clinical study contributes to medical knowledge. The results of these studies can make a difference in the care of future patients by providing information about the benefits and risks of therapeutic, preventative, or diagnostic products or interventions.

Clinical trials provide the basis for the development and marketing of new drugs, biological products, and medical devices. Sometimes, the safety and the effectiveness of the experimental approach or use may not be fully known at the time of the trial. Some trials may provide participants with the prospect of receiving direct medical benefits, while others do not. Most trials involve some risk of harm or injury to the participant, although it may not be greater than the risks related to routine medical care or disease progression. (For trials approved by IRBs, the IRB has decided that the risks of participation have been minimized and are reasonable in relation to anticipated benefits.) Many trials require participants to undergo additional procedures, tests, and assessments based on the study protocol. These requirements will be described in the informed consent document. A potential participant should also discuss these issues with members of the research team and with his or her usual health care provider.

Questions to Ask

Anyone interested in participating in a clinical study should know as much as possible about the study and feel comfortable asking the research team questions about the study, the related procedures, and any expenses. The following questions may be helpful during such a discussion. Answers to some of these questions are provided in theinformed consent document. Many of the questions are specific to clinical trials, but some also apply to observational studies.

- What is being studied?
- Why do researchers believe the intervention being tested might be effective? Why might it not be effective? Has it been tested before?
- What are the possible interventions that I might receive during the trial?
- How will it be determined which interventions I receive (for example, by chance)?
- Who will know which intervention I receive during the trial? Will I know? Will members of the research team know?
- How do the possible risks, side effects, and benefits of this trial compare with those of my current treatment?
- What will I have to do?
- What tests and procedures are involved?
- How often will I have to visit the hospital or clinic?
- Will hospitalization be required?
- How long will the study last?
- Who will pay for my participation?
- Will I be reimbursed for other expenses?
- What type of long-term follow-up care is part of this trial?
- If I benefit from the intervention, will I be allowed to continue receiving it after the trial ends?
- Will results of the study be provided to me?
- Who will oversee my medical care while I am participating in the trial?
- What are my options if I am injured during the study

How to Use This Book

This is a large book with lots of complicated medical and scientific information. Some of the language may only be easily understood by medical professionals. We recommend to patients, they seek out others to help them work through and understand the information. The information about each clinical trial in this book is divided into 7 categories: Study Description, Study Design, Arms and Interventions, Outcome Measures, Eligibility Criteria, Contacts and Locations, and Other Information. These categories are described below.

If you have questions about a specific clinical trial, you should contact the Clinical Trial directly. To enroll in a trial, you should also contact the Clinical Trial directly.

Study Description

This section explains what the researchers will do during the clinical study and why they are conducting the study, and it specifies what condition or disease is being studied and the questions that the researchers want to answer.

Study Design

This section explains the investigative methods or strategies used in the clinical study. It also provides other Information, such as study type, estimated or actual enrollment,study start and completion dates, and official study title.

Arms and Interventions

This section explains the type of intervention/treatment participants receive, what the dosage is for drugs, and how long the participants receive the intervention.

Outcome Measures

This section describes the measurements planned in the study protocol that are used to determine the effects of intervention or treatment on participants. Types of outcome measures include primary outcome measures, secondary outcome measures, and other pre-specified measures.

Eligibility Criteria

This section explains who can participate in the study. The most common criteria are listed first: ages eligible for the study, sexes eligible for study, and whether the study accepts healthy volunteers. A list of additional inclusion and exclusion criteria is also provided in this section.

Contacts and Locations

This section contains the study's ClinicalTrials.gov Identifier (NCT Number) and contact information for the study investigators when the study is recruiting participants. The study location is shown below the study sponsor's contact information. If the study is being conducted in many locations, you should contact the Clinical Trial directly for information.

More Information

This section contains information on references and links to Web sites that are relevant to the study. The study sponsor or investigator may provide citations for publications that are related to the background or results of the study.

Disclaimer

The information in this book was compiled from sources found in the public domain and is believed to be up-to-date and accurate. We cannot, however, guarantee it's accuracy and the organizers of each clinical study may add, delete, or change information at any time.

Colon Cancer Clinical Trials

Study Using Fluorine-18-Labeled Fluoro-Misonidazole Positron Emission Tomography to Detect Hypoxia in Locally Advanced (T3-T4 and./or N1)Primary Rectal Cancer Patients

Study ID:

NCT00574353

Sponsor:

Memorial Sloan Kettering Cancer Center

Information provided by (Responsible Party):

Memorial Sloan Kettering Cancer Center (Memorial Sloan Kettering Cancer Center)

Tracking Information

▨ **First Submitted Date**

December 13, 2007

▨ **Start Date**

December 2007

▨ **Primary Completion Date**

December 2018

▨ **Last Update Posted Date**

October 26, 2017

▨ **Current Primary Outcome Measures**

the feasibility of a non-invasive method of detecting hypoxia, using F-FMISO-PET imaging in colorectal cancer patients.[Time Frame: three times on the same day.]

▨ **Current Secondary Outcome Measures**

- determine volume of hypoxic tumor ROIs as a proportion of the entire tumor volume by this non-invasive imaging technique. ROIs are defined as those voxels, within the tumor volume defined on FDG PET/CT, for which the 18F-F-FMISO radioactivity concent[Time Frame: prior to F-FMISO injection, btw 2-40 min post injection, (ii) btw 80-100 min post injection & (iii) btw 110140 min post injection. Btw 1 & 3 cc of blood will be taken at each time point (making the max volume of blood withdrawn during this study < 9 cc]

Descriptive Information

▨ **Offical Title**

A Feasibility Study Using Fluorine-18-Labeled Fluoro-Misonidazole Positron Emission Tomography to Detect Hypoxia in Locally Advanced (T3-T4 and./or N1)Primary Rectal Cancer Patients

▨ **Brief Summary**

When used with a different radioactive tracer called FMISO, a PET scan can find areas of low oxygen in the tumor. We think that having areas of low oxygen is a reason why some tumors are hard to treat with radiation.

In a past study, FMISO PET scans were performed in 6 patients with rectal cancer that could not be operated on and that had spread to other areas. In this group of patients, FMISO PET scans were able to find the low oxygen areas in their tumors. But this study included only a few patients. In the present study, we want to use FMISO PET scans in patients who have tumors that can be operated on. This group of patients will have radiation, chemotherapy or both before they have their surgery. We want to see if FMISO PET can find low oxygen areas in this distinct group of patients.

▨ **Detailed Description**

Hypoxia is a characteristic feature of malignant solid tumors associated with poor prognosis and resistance to chemotherapy and radiation. It has also been shown (6) that the presence of hypoxia may reduce long-term survival post surgery. Hypoxia renders tumor cells up to three times more resistant to ionizing radiation than aerobic cells. The presence of hypoxic regions within tumors may be one factor leading to local failure after treatment with standard pre-operative radiotherapy doses. If these regions could be identified and verified using a non-invasive imaging technique prior to surgery, they could be specifically targeted using sophisticated planning techniques such as intensity modulated radiation therapy (IMRT) to deliver higher doses ionizing radiation with preoperative radiotherapy. Future studies using IMRT to "dose paint" areas of hypoxia within tumors will build upon the results of this feasibility study. Ultimately, by the delivery of differential dose of radiation to the tumor, in combination with surgery, the local control rates of rectal cancer patients may further be improved.

▨ **Study Type**

Interventional

▨ **Study Phase**

Phase 2

Condition

- Colorectal Cancer

Intervention

Radiation: Fluorine-18-Labeled Fluoro-Misonidazole Positron Emission

You will be scanned 2 to 3 times on the same day, but you will only be administered one dose of the FMISO tracer. The first scan will last about 30 minutes. Then you will have 1 to 3 hours to wait before you are scanned again. Some patients will undergo a second scan approximately one-and-a-half hours after the start of the first scan. This scan will last about 10 minutes. The final scan will occur between 2-4 hours after the start of the first scan. This final scan will also last about 10 minutes. During the PET scan, you may have a separate i.v. line put into your other arm so that we can take 2 to 3 blood samples. These samples will be less than half a teaspoon each. We are taking these blood samples to see how quickly FMISO leaves your blood stream. The first sample will be taken between 2 and 40 minutes after the FMISO is injected. The other two blood samples will be taken with each subsequent scan.

Study Arms

Experimental: 1

FMISO PET study.

Recruitment Information

Recruitment Status

Recruiting

Estimated Enrollment

50

Eligibility Criteria

Inclusion Criteria:

- Able to provide written informed consent
- Histologically confirmed diagnosis of Stage 2 or Stage 3 rectal carcinoma requiring preoperative radiation, chemotherapy or both, per treating physician
- 18 years of age or older
- Karnofsky performance status ≥ or = to 70

Exclusion Criteria:

- Women who are pregnant (confirmed by serum b-HCG in women of reproductive age) or breast feeding

Sex/Gender

All

Ages

18 Years to N/A

Accepts Healthy Volunteers

No

Contacts

Jose Guillem, MD   212-639-8278
John Humm, PhD   212-639-7367

Completion Date

December 2018

Primary Completion Date

December 2018

Veliparib and Irinotecan Hydrochloride in Treating Patients With Cancer That Is Metastatic or Cannot Be Removed by Surgery

Study ID:

NCT00576654

Sponsor:

National Cancer Institute (NCI)

Information provided by (Responsible Party):

National Cancer Institute (NCI) (National Cancer Institute (NCI))

Tracking Information

First Submitted Date

December 18, 2007

Start Date

December 5, 2007

Primary Completion Date

August 1, 2018

Last Update Posted Date

November 21, 2017

Current Primary Outcome Measures

Maximally tolerated dose (MTD) of study drugs[Time Frame: Up to 21 days]

Defined as the dose at which no more than 1 patient of 6 develops DLT as graded by the NCI CTCAE version 4.0.

Maximum administered dose of study drugs[Time Frame: Up to 21 days]

Defined as the dose level at which at least 2 of 6 patients develop dose-limiting toxicity (DLT) as graded by the National Cancer Institute (NCI) Common Terminology Criteria for Adverse Events (CTCAE) version 4.0.

Optimal biologic dose (OBD)[Time Frame: Up to day 9 of course 1]

Defined as the dose level at which no greater inhibition of poly(ADP-ribose) (PAR) levels in tumor cells is identified, relative to the next lower dose.

Recommended phase II dose (RP2D) of study drugs[Time Frame: Up to 21 days]

Defined as the MTD if DLTs are observed before achieving the OBD, or the OBD if DLTs are not observed before reaching the OBD as graded by the NCI CTCAE version 4.0.

Current Secondary Outcome Measures

Incidence of adverse events (AEs), graded using the National Cancer Institute (NCI) Common Terminology Criteria for Adverse Events (CTCAE) version 4.0[Time Frame: Up to 30 days]

Described by point estimates and exact 90% confidence intervals.

Tumor response[Time Frame: Up to 30 days]

Evaluated using Response Evaluation Criteria in Solid Tumors (RECIST) version 1.1.

Descriptive Information

Offical Title

A Phase I Dose-Escalation Study of Oral ABT-888 (NSC #737664) Plus Intravenous Irinotecan (CPT-11, NSC#616348) Administered in Patients With Advanced Solid Tumors

Brief Summary

This phase I trial studies the side effects and best dose of veliparib when given together with irinotecan hydrochloride in treating patients with cancer that has spread to other parts of the body or that cannot be removed by surgery. Irinotecan hydrochloride can kill cancer cells by damaging the deoxyribonucleic acid (DNA) that is needed for cancer cell survival and growth. Veliparib may block proteins that repair the damaged DNA and may help irinotecan hydrochloride to kill more tumor cells. Giving irinotecan hydrochloride together with veliparib may kill more cancer cells.

Detailed Description

PRIMARY OBJECTIVES:

I. To determine the optimal biologic dose (OBD) for poly (adenosine diphosphate [ADP]-ribose) polymerase (PARP) inhibition using irinotecan (irinotecan hydrochloride) (once weekly intravenously in 2 of 3 weeks), in combination with ABT-888 (veliparib) (twice daily orally for 2 of 3 weeks). (ORIGINAL DOSE ESCALATION PORTION) II. To determine the recommended phase II dose (RP2D) for irinotecan (once weekly intravenously in 2 of 3 weeks), in combination with ABT-888 (twice daily orally for 2 of 3 weeks), determined by evaluating the feasibility, safety, dose limiting toxicities and the maximally tolerated dose. (ORIGINAL DOSE ESCALATION PORTION) III. To determine the safety profile of irinotecan in combination with ABT-888: the incidence of adverse events (AEs) and clinically significant changes in laboratory tests, electrocardiograms (ECGs), and vital signs. (ORIGINAL DOSE ESCALATION PORTION) IV. To determine the safety profile of irinotecan in combination with ABT-888 at the recommended phase II dose: the incidence of adverse events (AEs) and clinically significant changes in laboratory tests, ECGs, and vital signs. (ORIGINAL DOSE ESCALATION PORTION) V. To determine the recommended phase II dose (RP2D) of each drug for irinotecan (once weekly intravenously in 2 of 3 weeks), in combination with ABT-888 (twice daily orally for intermittent dosing days 1 to 4 and days 8 to 11 of each cycle), determined by evaluating the feasibility, safety, dose limiting toxicities and the maximally tolerated dose (MTD). (DOSE ESCALATION FOR INTERMITTENT ABT-888 PORTION) VI. To determine the safety profile of irinotecan in combination with ABT-888: the incidence of adverse events (AEs) and clinically significant changes in laboratory tests, and vital signs. (DOSE ESCALATION FOR INTERMITTENT ABT-888 PORTION) VII. To determine the safety profile of irinotecan in combination with ABT-888 at the recommended phase II dose: the incidence of adverse events (AEs) and clinically significant changes in laboratory tests, and vital signs. (DOSE ESCALATION FOR INTERMITTENT ABT-888 PORTION)

SECONDARY OBJECTIVES:

I. To determine the pharmacokinetic (PK) profile of ABT-888. II. To determine the PK profile of irinotecan (CPT-11) both as a single agent and in combination with ABT-888.

III. To determine the tumor response as assessed by the Response Evaluation Criteria in Solid Tumors (RECIST).

IV. To determine the tumor response as assessed by the Response Evaluation Criteria in Solid Tumors (RECIST). (DOSE ESCALATION FOR INTERMITTENT ABT-888 PORTION) V. To determine response rate (RR) in patients. (DOSE ESCALATION FOR INTERMITTENT ABT-888 PORTION)

TERTIARY OBJECTIVES:

I. Pharmacodynamic (PD) biomarker response: PARP inhibition in peripheral blood mononuclear cells (PBMC) by measurement of PAR levels. (ORIGINAL DOSE ESCALATION PORTION) II. DNA damaging effects of irinotecan and the combination of irinotecan with ABT-888: levels of gamma H2A histone family, member X (gamma-H2AX) and RAD51 recombinase (Rad51) formation in tumor tissue. (ORIGINAL DOSE ESCALATION PORTION) III. Relevance of cytochrome P450 family 2, subfamily C, polypeptide 9 (CYP2C9) and 2C19 polymorphisms, uridine 5'-diphosphosphate (UDP) glucuronosyltransferase 1 family, polypeptide A1 (UGT1A1) polymorphism, and ATP-binding cassette, sub-family G (WHITE), member 2 (ABCG2) polymorphism to the pharmacokinetics of irinotecan and/or ABT-888. (ORIGINAL DOSE ESCALATION PORTION) IV. To explore whether a positive gamma-H2AX response in tumor tissue at 4-6 hours (hrs) is reflected in circulating tumor cells (CTCs) between 8-24 hrs but not at 4-6 hrs, as predicted. (EXPANSION PORTION) V. To explore whether PARP inhibition increases gamma-H2AX response of CTCs to plasma drug by 4-6 hrs after CPT-11 administration. (EXPANSION PORTION) VI. To explore whether PARP inhibition increases gamma-H2AX response of tumor cells to tissue drug level, as indicated by CTCs at 8-24 hrs after CPT-11. (EXPANSION PORTION) VII. To explore when the gamma-H2AX response peak in CTCs occurs, indicating a response in tumor. (EXPANSION PORTION) VIII. To explore whether there is a tumor switch between gamma-H2AX and excision repair cross-complementation group 1 (ERCC1)-mediated repair in the presence of PARP inhibition, (i.e., repeat initial PBMC and tumor findings). (EXPANSION PORTION) IX. To perform analysis of CTCs at day 15 to help guide alteration in ABT-888 drug administration schedule (continuous administration). (EXPANSION PORTION) X. To sequence the genome and transcriptome from both normal and tumor tissue from each study patient in the expansion cohort to evaluate point mutations, structural changes and copy number events. (EXPANSION PORTION) XI. To evaluate the damaging effects of irinotecan and the combination of irinotecan with ABT-888 by examining levels of Rad51 formation in tumors. (EXPANSION PORTION) XII. To evaluate the percentage of breast cancer stem cells (BCSC) in serial breast tumor biopsies before and after irinotecan alone and after 1 cycle of treatment with the combination of irinotecan and ABT-888. (EXPANSION PORTION) XIII. To perform molecular profiling of the tumor cell and BCSC populations before and after irinotecan alone and after 1 cycle of treatment with the combination of irinotecan and ABT-888. (EXPANSION PORTION) XIV. To compare Rad51 foci in aldehyde dehydrogenase-positive (ALDH+) stem cell populations to the bulk tumor cells. (EXPANSION PORTION) XV. To develop assays to detect trapping of PARP1 and 2 in tumor biopsy tissue in response to treatment with irinotecan plus a PARP inhibitor, in this case ABT-888. (DOSE ESCALATION FOR INTERMITTENT ABT-888 PORTION) XVI. Additional exploratory assay to be named later. (DOSE ESCALATION FOR INTERMITTENT ABT-888 PORTION) XVII. To determine the tumor response as assessed by the Response Evaluation Criteria in Solid Tumors (RECIST) in an expansion cohort of 12 triple-negative breast cancer (BRCA)-mutant breast cancer patients.

OUTLINE: This is a dose-escalation study of veliparib. Patients are assigned to 1 of 3 cohorts.

DOSE ESCALATION: Patients receive irinotecan hydrochloride intravenously (IV) over 90 minutes on days 1 and 8 and veliparib orally (PO) twice daily (BID) on days -1 to 14 (days 3-14 of course 1 only). Courses repeat every 21 days in the absence of disease progression or unacceptable toxicity.

EXPANSION PORTION: Patients receive irinotecan hydrochloride IV over 90 minutes on days 1 and 8 and veliparib PO BID on days 1-15 (days 2-15 of course 1 only). Courses repeat every 21 days in the absence of disease progression or unacceptable toxicity.

INTERMITTENT DOSE ESCALATION: Patients receive irinotecan hydrochloride IV over 90 minutes on days 3 and 10 and veliparib PO BID on days 1 to 4 and 8-11. Courses repeat every 21 days in the absence of disease progression or unacceptable toxicity.

After completion of study treatment, patients are followed up for 30 days.

Study Type

Interventional

Study Phase

Phase 1

Condition

- Advanced Malignant Solid Neoplasm
- Breast Carcinoma
- Colon Carcinoma
- Deleterious BRCA1 Gene Mutation
- Estrogen Receptor Negative
- HER2/Neu Negative
- Hodgkin Lymphoma
- Lung Carcinoma
- Metastatic Malignant Neoplasm

- Metastatic Malignant Solid Neoplasm
- Non-Hodgkin Lymphoma
- Ovarian Carcinoma
- Pancreatic Carcinoma
- Progesterone Receptor Negative
- Stage III Breast Cancer AJCC v7
- Stage III Colon Cancer AJCC v7
- Stage III Lung Cancer AJCC v7
- Stage III Ovarian Cancer AJCC v6 and v7
- Stage III Pancreatic Cancer AJCC v6 and v7
- Stage IIIA Breast Cancer AJCC v7
- Stage IIIA Colon Cancer AJCC v7
- Stage IIIA Ovarian Cancer AJCC v6 and v7
- Stage IIIB Breast Cancer AJCC v7
- Stage IIIB Colon Cancer AJCC v7
- Stage IIIB Ovarian Cancer AJCC v6 and v7
- Stage IIIC Breast Cancer AJCC v7
- Stage IIIC Colon Cancer AJCC v7
- Stage IIIC Ovarian Cancer AJCC v6 and v7
- Stage IV Breast Cancer AJCC v6 and v7
- Stage IV Colon Cancer AJCC v7
- Stage IV Lung Cancer AJCC v7
- Stage IV Ovarian Cancer AJCC v6 and v7
- Stage IV Pancreatic Cancer AJCC v6 and v7
- Stage IVA Colon Cancer AJCC v7
- Stage IVB Colon Cancer AJCC v7
- Triple-Negative Breast Carcinoma
- Unresectable Malignant Neoplasm
- Unresectable Solid Neoplasm

Intervention

Drug: Irinotecan Hydrochloride
Given IV

Other Names:

Campto

Camptosar

Camptothecin 11

Camptothecin-11

CPT 11

CPT-11

Irinomedac

U-101440E

Other: Laboratory Biomarker Analysis
Correlative studies

Other: Pharmacological Study
Correlative studies

Drug: Veliparib
Given PO

Other Names:

ABT-888

PARP-1 inhibitor ABT-888

Study Arms

Experimental: Dose escalation (irinotecan hydrochloride and veliparib)

Patients receive irinotecan hydrochloride IV over 90 minutes on days 1 and 8 and veliparib PO BID on days -1 to 14 (days 3-14 of course 1 only). Courses repeat every 21 days in the absence of disease progression or unacceptable toxicity.

Experimental: Expansion portion (irinotecan hydrochloride and veliparib)

Patients receive irinotecan hydrochloride IV over 90 minutes on days 1 and 8 and veliparib PO BID on days 1-15 (days 2-15 of course 1 only). Courses repeat every 21 days in the absence of disease progression or unacceptable toxicity.

Experimental: Intermittent dose escalation (irinotecan, ABT-888)

Patients receive irinotecan hydrochloride IV over 90 minutes on days 3 and 10 and veliparib PO BID on days 1 to 4 and 8-11. Courses repeat every 21 days in the absence of disease progression or unacceptable toxicity.

Recruitment Information

Recruitment Status

Recruiting

Estimated Enrollment

48

Completion Date

N/A

Primary Completion Date

August 1, 2018

Eligibility Criteria

Inclusion Criteria:

- Patients must have histologically or cytologically confirmed diagnosis of malignancy that is metastatic or unresectable and for which standard curative or palliative measures do not exist or are no longer effective or for whom CPT-11 treatment would be a viable therapy regimen; patients with solid hematologic malignancies (Hodgkin's and non-Hodgkin's lymphomas) may be included as long as a bone marrow has been performed within 6 weeks of treatment
- Patients enrolled on the expansion portion of the study will consist of two cohorts: those patients who are triple-negative, BRCA-mutant positive and those patients who have triple-negative, non-BRCA mutated breast cancer
- Patients enrolled on the dose escalation for intermittent ABT-888 portion of the study must histologically or cytologically confirmed diagnosis of malignancy that is metastatic or unresectable and for which standard curative or palliative measures do not exist or are no longer effective or for whom CPT-11 treatment would be a viable therapy regimen; patients with solid hematologic malignancies (Hodgkin's and non-Hodgkin's lymphomas) may be included as long as a bone marrow has been performed within 6 weeks of treatment; once the recommended phase 2 dose is determined, additional patients will be enrolled who MUST have a deleterious mutation in BRCA and have human epidermal growth factor receptor 2 (Her-2) negative, estrogen receptor (ER) negative (defined as less than 1% ER by immunohistochemistry [IHC]) and progesterone receptor (PR) negative breast cancer (defined as less than 1% PR staining by IHC)
- Patient must have measurable disease per Response Evaluation Criteria in Solid Tumors (RECIST) guidelines
- Patients must have tumors determined to be easily accessible for biopsy (e.g. pleural-based lesions, peripheral lymph nodes, soft tissue metastases, large liver metastases, etc)
- Prior chemotherapy is allowed; patients must not have received chemotherapy for 4 weeks prior to the initiation of study treatment and must have full recovery from any acute effects of any prior chemotherapy; patients must not have had nitrosoureas or mitomycin C for 6 weeks prior to the initiation of study treatment
- Prior radiation therapy is allowed; patients must not have received minimal radiation therapy (=< 5% of their total marrow volume) within 3 weeks prior to the initiation of study treatment; otherwise, patients must not have received radiation therapy (> 5% of their total marrow volume) within 4 weeks prior to the initiation of study treatment; patients who have received prior radiation to 50% or more of their total marrow volume will be excluded
- Prior experimental (non-Food and Drug Administration [FDA] approved) therapies and immunotherapies are allowed; patients must not have received these therapies for 4 weeks prior to the initiation of study treatment and must have full recovery from any acute effects of these therapies
- Eastern Cooperative Oncology Group (ECOG) performance status =< 2 (Karnofsky >= 60%)
- Life expectancy of greater than 12 weeks
- Absolute neutrophil count (ANC) >= 1,500/mcL
- Platelets (PLT) >= 100,000/mcL
- Aspartate aminotransferase (AST) and alanine aminotransferase (ALT) =< 2.5 x upper limit of normal (ULN); if liver metastases are present, =< 5 x ULN
- Bilirubin =< 1.5 x ULN
- Creatinine =< 1.5 x ULN OR calculated or measured creatinine clearance >= 60 mL/min/1.73 m^2 for patients with creatinine above institutional normal
- Women of child-bearing potential and men must agree to use adequate contraception (hormonal or barrier method of birth control; abstinence) prior to study entry, for the duration of study participation, and for three months following completion of study therapy; should a woman become pregnant or suspect she is pregnant while participating in this study, she should inform her treating physician immediately
- Ability to understand and the willingness to sign a written informed consent document

- All patients must provide archival tissue block or paraffin sample from archival tissue block (approximately 10 sections) for use in pharmacodynamic correlative studies (NOT required for patients enrolled on the dose escalation for intermittent ABT-888 portion of the study)

Exclusion Criteria:

- Patients who have had chemotherapy or radiotherapy within 4 weeks (6 weeks for nitrosoureas or mitomycin C) prior to entering the study or those who have not recovered from adverse events due to agents administered more than 4 weeks earlier; patients who have been administered ABT-888 as part of a single or limited dosing study, such as a phase 0 study, should not necessarily be excluded from participating in this study solely because of receiving prior ABT-888
- Patients may not have received any other investigational agents within 4 weeks of study entry
- **History of allergic reactions attributed to the following:**
- Camptothecin derivatives (e.g., topotecan [topotecan hydrochloride], irinotecan, or exatecan [exatecan mesylate])
- Any ingredients contained within the liquid irinotecan solution (e.g., sorbitol) or
- Any antiemetics or antidiarrheals appropriate for administration with study therapy (e.g., loperamide or dexamethasone)
- Patients must not receive any other anti-cancer therapy (cytotoxic, biologic, radiation, or hormonal other than for replacement) while on this study except for medications that are prescribed for supportive care but may potentially have an anti-cancer effect (i.e. megestrol acetate, bisphosphonates); these medications must have been started 1 month prior to enrollment on this study; in addition, men receiving treatment for prostate cancer will be maintained at castrate levels of testosterone by continuation of luteinizing-releasing hormone agonists
- Patients with active seizure or a history of seizure
- Patients with known active brain metastases should be excluded from this clinical trial; patients with prior treated brain metastases are allowed, providing that they were not accompanied by seizures and that a baseline brain magnetic resonance imaging (MRI) scan prior to study entry demonstrates no current evidence of brain metastases; all patients with central nervous system (CNS) metastases must be stable for > 3 months after treatment and off steroid treatment prior to study enrollment
- Any patient requiring chronic maintenance of white blood cell counts or granulocyte counts through the use of growth factor support (e.g. Neulasta, Neupogen)
- Any patient requiring cytochrome P450 family 3, subfamily A, polypeptide 4 (CYP3A4) isoform-inducing drugs (e.g. phenytoin, phenobarbital, carbamazepine, rifampin, rifabutin, ketoconazole, St. John's wort) will be excluded; CYP3A4-inducing drugs should be discontinued at least 2 weeks prior to the first cycle of irinotecan
- **Uncontrolled intercurrent illness including, but not limited to:**
- Ongoing or active infection
- Symptomatic congestive heart failure
- Unstable angina pectoris
- Cardiac arrhythmia or
- Psychiatric illness or social situations that would limit compliance with study requirements
- Pregnant women are excluded from this study; breastfeeding should be discontinued if the mother is treated with ABT-888
- Patients who are unable to reliably tolerate and/or receive oral medications

▨ Sex/Gender

All

▨ Ages

18 Years to N/A

▨ Accepts Healthy Volunteers

No

Natural Killer Cells and Bortezomib to Treat Cancer

Study ID:
NCT00720785

Sponsor:
National Heart, Lung, and Blood Institute (NHLBI)

Information provided by (Responsible Party):
National Institutes of Health Clinical Center (CC) (National Heart, Lung, and Blood Institute (NHLBI))

Tracking Information

First Submitted Date

July 22, 2008

Start Date

July 21, 2008

Primary Completion Date

January 1, 2020

Last Update Posted Date

January 12, 2018

Current Primary Outcome Measures

Safety of escalating NK cell doses[Time Frame:]

Current Secondary Outcome Measures

The anti-neoplastic effects of this treatment regimen (assessed using standard disease specific response criteria) and the toxicity profile associated with extended cycles of protocol therapy.[Time Frame:]

Descriptive Information

Offical Title

Safety and the Anti-Tumor Effects of Escalating Doses of Adoptively Infused Ex Vivo Expanded Autologous Natural Killer (NK) Cells Against Metastatic Cancers or Hematological Malignancies Sensitized to NK TRAIL Cytotoxicity With Bortezomib

Brief Summary

Natural killer (NK) cells are white blood cells that have a limited ability to kill cancer cells. This ability might be enhanced if they are given 24 hours after an injection of the drug bortezomib. This study will determine the following:

- What dose of NK cells can be given safely to subjects with metastatic solid tumors or leukemia.
- The effectiveness and side effects of NK cell therapy
- How the body handles NK cells.

People between 18 and 70 years of age who have a solid tumor or leukemia, and for whom standard treatments are not effective, may be eligible for this study. Participants undergo the following procedures:

Apheresis to collect NK cells. For this procedure, a catheter (plastic tube) is placed in a vein in the subject s arm. Blood flows from the vein into a cell separator machine, which separates the white cells from the other blood components. The white cells are extracted and the rest of the blood is returned to the body through a second tube placed in a vein in the other arm.

Chemotherapy with the drug pentostatin to suppress the immune system and prevent it from attacking the NK cells that will be infused.

Chemotherapy with bortezomib to increase NK cell function.

Infusion of the NK cells. In this dose-escalating study, successive groups of patients entering the study receive increasingly higher numbers of cells to determine the highest safe dose level. Up to ten dose levels may be studied.

Interleukin-2 drug therapy to maintain NK cell activity.

Evaluations during therapy including:

- Clinical assessment, history and review of medications
- Blood draws for routine and research tests.
- Pharmacokinetics study after the NK infusion to see how the body handles the cells. For this test, the number of NK cells in the blood are measured over time. This requires drawing about 1 teaspoon of blood at 15 minutes, 30 minutes, 1, 2, 4, 8, 12, and 24 hours after the infusion (day 1); then every 24 hours on days 2 through 7, then once on days 10, 14, and 21.
- Bone marrow biopsy (subjects with leukemia only).
- Chest x-ray.
- CT scan, bone scan and PET scan, if indicated, for disease evaluation.

Subjects who respond well after one treatment cycle may be eligible to continue NK cell therapy.

Detailed Description

Natural killer (NK) cells are innate immune lymphocytes that are identified by the expression of the CD56 surface antigen and the lack of CD3. Unlike antigen specific T cells, NK cells do not require the presence of a specific tumor antigen for the recognition and killing of cancer cells. Our in vitro studies have demonstrated that pretreatment of malignant cells with bortezomib significantly enhances NK-mediated tumor cytotoxicity by sensitizing cells to TNF-related apoptosis-inducing ligand (TRAIL). TRAIL is a member of tumor necrosis factor family of cytokines that promotes apoptosis. Importantly, in our laboratory, in vitro expanded NK cells isolated from patients with metastatic cancers or hematological malignancies exhibited significantly more cytotoxicity against their tumor cells when tumors were pre-treated with bortezomib compared with untreated tumor controls. These findings suggest that drug-induced sensitization to TRAIL could be used as a novel strategy to potentiate anticancer effects of autologous adoptively infused NK cells in patients with cancer.

Murine studies conducted in our laboratory have also established that bortezomib treatment sensitizes tumors in vivo to killing by adoptively infused syngeneic NK cells; murine renal cell carcinoma line (RENCA) tumors in BALB/c mice grew significantly slower and survival was prolonged when syngeneic NK cell infusions were given following bortezomib treatment compared to mice receiving NK cell infusions alone or bortezomib alone. This anti-tumor effect was further potentiated by eradicating

T-regulatory cells prior to adoptive NK cell infusion and by administering interleukin-2 after adoptive NK cell infusion.

Recently, our laboratory has developed techniques for the in vitro isolation and expansion of NK cells to levels suitable for the treatment of cancer patients. Furthermore, we have also established good viability and sterility of these expanded NK cells which, compared to fresh NK cells, have increased surface expression of TRAIL and have enhanced cytotoxicity against tumor cells.

- We therefore propose this non-randomized, Phase I, dose escalating study designed to evaluate the safety and the antitumor effects of escalating doses of adoptively infused ex vivo expanded autologous natural killer (NK) cells against metastatic cancers or hematological malignancies sensitized to NK TRAIL cytotoxicity with Bortezomib.

The primary study objective is to determine the safety (maximum tolerated dose) of escalating NK cell doses of adoptively infused ex vivo expanded autologous NK cells in subjects with treatment refractory metastatic tumors or hematological malignancies that are sensitized to NK cell cytotoxicity using bortezomib. Secondary objectives will include the anti-neoplastic effects of this treatment regimen (assessed using standard disease specific response criteria) and the toxicity profile associated with extended cycles of protocol therapy.

The primary endpoint will be assessed at day 21 (3 weeks after the Day 0 NK cell infusion).

Study Type

Interventional

Study Phase

Phase 1

Condition

- Lung or Prostatic Neoplasms
- Colorectal or Kidney Neoplasms
- Pancreatic Neoplasms
- Leukemia, Myelogenous, Chronic Lymphocytic Leukemia, BCR-ABL Positive
- Melanoma
- CLL

Intervention

Drug: NK cells +CliniMACs CD3 and CD56 systems

Publications

(Includes publications given by the data provider as well as publications identified by ClinicalTrials.gov Identifier (NCT Number) in Medline.)Farag SS, Fehniger TA, Becknell B, Blaser BW, Caligiuri MA. New directions in natural killer cell-based immunotherapy of human cancer. Expert Opin Biol Ther. 2003 Apr;3(2):237-50. Review. (https://www.ncbi.nlm.nih.gov/pubmed/12662139)

Farag SS, Caligiuri MA. Human natural killer cell development and biology. Blood Rev. 2006 May;20(3):123-37. Epub 2005 Dec 20. Review. (https://www.ncbi.nlm.nih.gov/pubmed/16364519)

Goy A, Younes A, McLaughlin P, Pro B, Romaguera JE, Hagemeister F, Fayad L, Dang NH, Samaniego F, Wang M, Broglio K, Samuels B, Gilles F, Sarris AH, Hart S, Trehu E, Schenkein D, Cabanillas F, Rodriguez AM. Phase II study of proteasome inhibitor bortezomib in relapsed or refractory B-cell non-Hodgkin's lymphoma. J Clin Oncol. 2005 Feb 1;23(4):667-75. Epub 2004 Dec 21. (https://www.ncbi.nlm.nih.gov/pubmed/15613697)

Recruitment Information

Recruitment Status

Recruiting

Estimated Enrollment

61

Completion Date

January 1, 2020

Primary Completion Date

January 1, 2020

Eligibility Criteria

- INCLUSION CRITERIA:
- 1. Diagnosed with histologically confirmed metastatic solid tumor cancer of the lung (small cell or non small cell), prostate (adenocarcinoma), colorectum, kidney (renal cell carcinoma), pancreas (adenocarcinoma),or malignant melanoma, metastatic Ewing's sarcoma, or metastatic epithelial neoplasms and adenocarcinoma of unknown primary, and disease confirmed to be metastatic and unresectable for which standard curative or beneficial treatments are no longer effective

OR

Diagnosed with a hematological malignancy (multiple myeloma, [MM] chronic myelogenous leukemia [CML] or chronic lymphocytic leukemia [CLL] or small lymphocytic lymphoma [SLL]) and disease resistant or refractory to standard therapy and CLL/SLL patients are required to have failed prior treatment with at least one nucleoside analogue. Myeloma patients are required to have disease which has progressed following treatment with bortezomib.

2. At least 4 weeks since any prior systemic therapy (excluding corticosteroid therapy) to treat the underlying malignancy

(standard or investigational). NOTE: subjects on FDA-approved tyrosine kinase inhibitors or other targeted therapies for RCC such as mTOR inhibitors that have evidence of disease progression on therapy may continue these medicines until the time of study enrollment (as accelerated disease progression following discontinuation of these drugs has been described).

3. At least 2 weeks since prior palliative radiotherapy.

4. Ages greater than or equal to 18 years and less than or equal to 70 years.

5. Evidence of progressive disease over a 3-month interval.

6. RBC transfusion independent (solid tumor patients only).

EXCLUSION CRITERIA:

1. Disease not evaluable radiographically (applies to solid tumor patients only).

2. Disease involving greater than 25% of the liver radiographically (estimated based on review of liver lesions seen on CT scan).

3. History of an allogeneic hematopoietic stem cell transplant.

4. Brain metastases (with the exception of patients with a single brain metastasis less than 1cm treated with either sterotactic or gamma knife radiotherapy) due to poor prognosis and potential for neurological dysfunction that would confound evaluation of neurological and other adverse events).

5. Peripheral neuropathy of grade greater than 1, which would require reduction of bortezomib dose.

6. Acute diffuse infiltrative pulmonary disease.

7. Acute pericardial disease.

8. Life expectancy less than 3 months.

9. ECOG performance status 2, 3 or 4.

10. Uncontrolled concurrent illness including, but not limited to, symptomatic congestive heart failure, unstable angina pectoris, life threatening cardiac arrhythmia. Patients with symptoms of coronary artery disease, cardiac arrhythmias or an abnormal thallium stress test must be evaluated and cleared by cardiology prior to enrollment.

11. Ongoing or active infection

12. Contraindication for administration of pentostatin, bortezomib, and/or interleukin-2.

13. Allergy or hypersensitivity to bortezomib, boron or mannitol by history.

14. Concurrent use of corticosteroids.

15. **For all tumor types:**

Marrow function characterized by

-Absolute neutrophil count less than 500/mcL (must be present off growth factors)

Organ function characterized by

- Total bilirubin greater than 3 times upper limit of normal
- AST (SGOT)/ALT (SGPT) greater than 4 times upper limit of normal
- Creatinine clearance less than 50 cc/min based on a 24 hour urine collection
- Left ventricular ejection fraction less than 40% by echocardiogram (ECHO)
- Hypercalcemia greater than 2.5 mmol/L

For all Hematologic malignancies:

Marrow function characterized by

- Neutrophil count less than or equal to 500/mcl
- Platelets less than or equal to 20,000/mcl

16. HIV-positive patients

17. Hepatitis C positive patients (Hep C PCR positive)

18. Active Hepatitis B infection (Hep B surface antigen positive)

19. Pregnant or nursing

20. Psychiatric illness/social situations that would limit compliance with study requirements and ability to comprehend the investigational nature of the study and provide informed consent.

■ Sex/Gender

All

■ Ages

18 Years to 70 Years

■ Accepts Healthy Volunteers

No

■ Contacts

Tatyana Worthy, R.N.   (301) 594-8013   worthyt@mail.nih.gov

Augmentation of Screening Colonoscopy With Fecal Immunochemical Testing

Study ID:

NCT00892593

Sponsor:

Forsyth Medical Center

Information provided by (Responsible Party):

Forsyth Medical Center (Forsyth Medical Center)

Tracking Information

▨ **First Submitted Date**

May 1, 2009

▨ **Start Date**

May 2009

▨ **Primary Completion Date**

May 2019

▨ **Last Update Posted Date**

July 21, 2014

▨ **Current Primary Outcome Measures**

rate of significant colon neoplasia among those who enter a screening or surveillance program with FIT testing added at yearly intervals vs. that of "usual care" patients in the same patient population.[Time Frame: yearly]

▨ **Current Secondary Outcome Measures**

the pathology found at repeat colonoscopy in each group.[Time Frame: Yearly]

Descriptive Information

▨ **Offical Title**

Augmentation of Screening Colonoscopy With Fecal Immunochemical Testing

▨ **Brief Summary**

The study will determine if adding fecal immunochemical testing (FIT) at yearly intervals to a colonoscopy screening program will improve colon cancer detection rates.

▨ **Detailed Description**

This study will evaluate the benefit of augmenting a compliant College of Gastroenterology colorectal cancer screening program with the addition of yearly FIT testing at two critical points in the current recommended follow up: 1. In patients found to have adenomatous polyps for the first time after colonoscopy, the addition of FIT in yearly intervals following index colonoscopy and 2. For subjects with "clean" colonoscopies (no polyps found), the addition of FIT at yearly intervals starting in year 6 and continuing to year 10 or subsequent colonoscopies. Current screening guidelines do not recommend the combination of colonoscopy and FOBT.

Two factors plague an effective colon cancer screening program: 1) a less than 100% sensitivity (95%) for optical colonoscopy to detect colon cancer, and 2) Limitations of guaiac based stool testing: low sensitivity (5% in single use) for detection of colon cancer and the traditional gFOBT is cumbersome for patients to perform, impeding patient acceptance and adherence.

FIT offers a FOBT with improved sensitivity (65% for invasive colon cancer) and improved specificity and better patient compliance. The addition of FIT after initial colonoscopy could be applied to a screening program and thereby salvage "missed" lesions by increased detection rates

▨ **Study Type**

Interventional

▨ **Study Phase**

N/A

▨ **Condition**

- Colon Cancer

▨ **Intervention**

Device: Fecal Immunochemical Testing

Fecal Immunochemical Testing is a stool test specific for human hemoglobin.

Other Names:

FIT

Device: Fecal Immunochemical Testing

Fecal Immunochemical Testing is a stool test specific for human hemoglobin.

Other Names:
FIT

Study Arms

Experimental: 1 Fecal Immunochemical Testing-Surveillance
Fecal Immunochemical Testing performed at yearly intervals.

- No Intervention: 2 Usual Care Surveillance
- No Intervention: 3 Usual Care Screening

Experimental: 4 Fecal Immunochemical Testing-Screening
Fecal Immunochemical Testing yearly, beginning at year 6.

Recruitment Information

Recruitment Status

Recruiting

Estimated Enrollment

4100

Completion Date

May 2020

Primary Completion Date

May 2019

Eligibility Criteria

Inclusion Criteria:

Group I (positive colonoscopy)

- 18 to 75 years of age
- male or female
- willing to provide written informed consent
- In the event that the colonoscopy is incomplete, or polypectomy is partial, the above patients are eligible if a successful examination is completed within 6 months of the inadequate exam.

Group II (negative colonoscopy)

- 50 to 69 years of age
- Male or female
- Willing to provide written informed consent
- In the event that the colonoscopy is incomplete, the patient is eligible if a successful examination is completed within 6 months of the inadequate exam.

Exclusion Criteria:

Group I (positive colonoscopy)

- chronic use of coumadin
- history of previous GI malignancy, inflammatory bowel disease (Crohns disease, ulcerative colitis)
- age or health status contraindicates repeat colonoscopy
- history of Familial Polyposis or Hereditary Nonpolyposis Colon Cancer Syndrome
- The index colonoscopy resulted in a perforation requiring surgical repair
- An otherwise qualifying colonoscopy is followed by a recommendation for repeat colonoscopy in ≤ 1 yr.

Group II (negative colonoscopy)

- chronic use of coumadin
- history of previous GI malignancy, inflammatory bowel disease (Crohns disease, ulcerative colitis)
- age or health status contraindicates repeat colonoscopy
- history of Familial Polyposis or Hereditary Nonpolyposis Colon Cancer Syndrome
- The index colonoscopy resulted in a perforation requiring surgical repair
- Significant family history resulting in a recommendation for repeat colonoscopy in 5 years or less

Sex/Gender

All

Ages

18 Years to N/A

- **Accepts Healthy Volunteers**

  No

- **Contacts**

  Debra W Norwood   336-718-6045   dwnorwood@novanthealth.org

  Wendy L Hobbs   336-718-5808   wlhobbs@novanthealth.org

177Lu-J591 Antibody in Patients With Nonprostate Metastatic Solid Tumors

Study ID:

NCT00967577

Sponsor:

Weill Medical College of Cornell University

Information provided by (Responsible Party):

Weill Medical College of Cornell University (Weill Medical College of Cornell University)

Tracking Information

- **First Submitted Date**

  August 26, 2009

- **Start Date**

  July 2009

- **Primary Completion Date**

  June 2019

- **Last Update Posted Date**

  January 30, 2018

- **Current Primary Outcome Measures**

  Change in tumor perfusion as based on DCE-MRI study as well as changes in cellularity as assessed using DWI.[Time Frame: Performed after administration of 177LuJ591 between Day 6-9 and on Day 29.]

- **Current Secondary Outcome Measures**

  Progression free survival[Time Frame: Day 58 after administration with 177Lu-J591 and repeated every 3 months until radiographic progression of disease.]

Descriptive Information

- **Offical Title**

  177Lu Radiolabeled Monoclonal Antibody HuJ591-GS (177Lu-J591) in Patients With Nonprostate Metastatic Solid Tumors: A Pilot Study

- **Brief Summary**

  The purpose of this study is to evaluate changes in tumor blood flow and disease response to the investigation agent, 177Lu-J591.

- **Detailed Description**

  177Lu-J591 is made up of two compounds called J591 and 177Lutetium (177Lu) that are joined together by a connecting molecule called "DOTA". J591 is a monoclonal antibody, or a type of protein. 177Lu is a radioactive molecule that is being tested for the possible treatment of cancer when joined to monoclonal antibodies. J591 attaches to a protein called prostate specific membrane antigen (PSMA) found in the body. PSMA is mostly found in normal and cancerous prostate cells. In addition, however, PSMA has also been found on the vasculature (blood vessels) that supply multiple types of cancer including colorectal, kidney, bladder, head and neck, breast, non-small cell lung, pancreas, ovary, esophagus and gliomas.

  We hope that 177Lu-J591 will seek out blood vessels that supply these tumors and deliver a dose of radiation (from the 177Lu molecule) to the areas of cancer, without affecting target blood vessel that are not associated with the cancer.

  Zirconium-89 (89Zr) is a radioactive tracer that allows special scans to be performed prior to administration of the study drug to determine where the antibody goes in the body and to screen the tumor's blood vessels to see if they attract J591. Again, DOTA is used to join the radioactive material to J591. 89Zr-J591 is not being given to treat cancer.

- **Study Type**

  Interventional

- **Study Phase**

  N/A

Condition

- Kidney Cancer
- Head and Neck Cancer
- Breast Cancer
- Non-small Cell Lung Cancer
- Colorectal Cancer
- Pancreatic Cancer
- Ovarian Cancer
- Esophageal Cancer
- Gliomas

Intervention

Drug: 177Lu-J591

> 70 mCi/m2 of 177Lu-J591 will be administered on Day 1.

Other Names:

> monoclonal antibody J591

Study Arms

Experimental: J591

Recruitment Information

Recruitment Status

Recruiting

Estimated Enrollment

50

Completion Date

December 2019

Primary Completion Date

June 2019

Eligibility Criteria

Inclusion Criteria:

- Histologically, or cytologically documented, advanced stage, malignant adult solid tumors (except prostate cancer) that are refractory to, or recurrent from, standard therapy or for which no curative standard therapy exists. This will include, but is not limited to patients with cancers of the kidney, urothelium, head and neck, breast, non-small cell lung, colorectal, pancreas, ovary, esophagus and gliomas.
- Metastatic or recurrent solid tumor malignancy defined by abnormal CT, MRI, PET scan, CXR and/or bone scan
- Progressive disease manifest by: Development of new lesions or an increase in size of preexisting lesions on imaging study or by physical examination.
- Subjects must have recovered from the acute toxicities of any prior therapy, and not received chemotherapy, radiation therapy or other investigational anticancer therapeutic drug for at least 4 weeks prior to J591 administration in this trial
- All subjects must have archived or current tissue (from a primary or metastatic focus) available for PSMA determination.
- Subjects on bisphosphonate therapy or denosumab must be on a stable dose and must have started therapy > 4 weeks prior to protocol therapy.
- Subjects will be informed as to the potential risk of procreation while participating on this trial and will be advised to use effective contraception during the entire study period. Females of child-bearing potential must have a negative pregnancy test.

Exclusion Criteria:

- Use of red blood cell or platelet transfusions within 4 weeks of treatment.
- Use of hematopoietic growth factors within 4 weeks of treatment.
- Prior cytotoxic chemotherapy and/or radiation therapy within 4 weeks of treatment.
- Prior radiation therapy encompassing >25% of skeleton.
- Prior treatment with 89Strontium or 153Samarium containing compounds (e.g. Metastron®, Quadramet®)
- Platelet count <150,000/mm3 or history of platelet count abnormality or dysfunction.
- Absolute neutrophil count (ANC) <2,000/mm3
- Hematocrit <30 percent or Hemoglobin < 10 g/dL
- Abnormal coagulation profile (PT or INR, PTT) > 1.3x upper limit of normal (ULN)
- Serum creatinine > 2x ULN
- AST (SGOT) >2.5x ULN
- Bilirubin (total) >1.5x ULN
- Active serious infection

- Active angina pectoris or NY Heart Association Class III-IV
- ECOG Performance Status > 2
- Deep vein thrombosis and/or pulmonary embolus within 1 month of enrollment.
- Other serious illness(es) involving the cardiac, respiratory, CNS, renal, hepatic or hematological organ systems which might preclude completion of this study or interfere with determination of causality of any adverse effects experienced in this study.
- Prior investigational therapy (medications or devices) within 6 weeks of treatment.
- Known history of HIV.
- Known leukemia or myelodysplastic syndrome
- Prior allergic reaction to Gadolinium contrast.

▩ Sex/Gender

All

▩ Ages

18 Years to N/A

▩ Accepts Healthy Volunteers

No

▩ Contacts

GUONC Research Team　　guonc@med.cornell.edu

Hydroxychloroquine + Vorinostat in Advanced Solid Tumors

Study ID:

NCT01023737

Sponsor:

Sukeshi Patel

Information provided by (Responsible Party):

The University of Texas Health Science Center at San Antonio (Sukeshi Patel)

Tracking Information

▩ First Submitted Date

July 22, 2009

▩ Start Date

November 2009

▩ Primary Completion Date

July 2018

▩ Last Update Posted Date

August 21, 2017

▩ Current Primary Outcome Measures

Maximum tolerated dose (MTD) of Hydroxychloroquine (HCQ) in combination with Vorinostat in patients with advanced solid tumors[Time Frame: 6+ months, MTD is assessed during the 1st cycle]

▩ Current Secondary Outcome Measures

To evaluate the safety and tolerability of HCQ in combination with Vorinostat in this patient population as determined by toxicity profile, incidence and rating according to NCI/CTC v3.0 criteria.[Time Frame: 1 year]

To evaluate the antitumor activity of HCQ in combination with Vorinostat as determined by response rate and progression free survival (exploratory)[Time Frame: 1 year]

Descriptive Information

▩ Offical Title

Inhibition of Autophagy in Solid Tumors: A Phase I Pharmacokinetic and Pharmacodynamic Study of Hydroxychloroquine in Combination With the HDAC Inhibitor Vorinostat for the Treatment of Patients With Advanced Solid Tumors With an Expansion Study in Advanced Renal and Colorectal Cancer

▩ Brief Summary

This study is an open label non randomized study of hydroxychloroquine (HCQ) with histone deacetylase (HDAC) inhibitor

Vorinostat in patients with advanced solid tumors to determine the maximum tolerated dose (MTD) and to evaluate the safety and antitumor activity of this drug combination.

■ **Study Type**

Interventional

■ **Study Phase**

Phase 1

■ **Condition**

- Malignant Solid Tumour

■ **Intervention**

Drug: Hydroxychloroquine

The HCQ study dose levels are defined as 400mg/day, 600mg/day, 800mg/day and 1000mg/day (oral dosing)during the phase I MTD determination. HCQ will be administered starting on Day 2 of Cycle 1 and will be continued daily thereafter until progression of disease or unacceptable toxicity develops.

Other Names:

HCQ

Drug: Vorinostat

Oral administration of Vorinostat will be begin on Cycle 1 Day 1 at 300mg and will be continued daily thereafter until progression of disease or unacceptable toxicity develops.

Other Names:

Suberoylanilide Hydroxamic Acid

■ **Study Arms**

Experimental: Hydroxychloroquine and Vorinostat

Oral administration of Vorinostat will be begin on Cycle 1 Day 1 at 300mg and will be continued daily and HCQ will be administered starting on Day 2 of Cycle 1 and both will be continued daily thereafter until progression of disease or unacceptable toxicity develops.

Recruitment Information

■ **Recruitment Status**

Recruiting

■ **Estimated Enrollment**

48

■ **Completion Date**

September 2018

■ **Primary Completion Date**

July 2018

■ **Eligibility Criteria**

Inclusion Criteria:

- Patients must be at least 16 years of age
- Patients must have a histologically confirmed non-hematological malignancy. Patients must have received and failed standard treatment for their malignancy; patients for whom no standard treatment is available will also be eligible.
- Patients must have an ECOG PS at 0, 1, or 2
- Patients must have adequate hematologic, renal and liver function (i.e. absolute Neutrophil count > 1000/mm3, platelets > 75,000/mm3); creatinine
- 2 times the upper limits of normal (ULN) total bilirubin ≤ 1.5 mg/dl, ALT and AST £ 3 times above the upper limits of the institutional norm ALT, AST can be < 5 times upper limits of normal if patients have hepatic involvement.
- Patients must be able to provide written informed consent.
- Patients with the potential for pregnancy or impregnating their partner must agree to follow acceptable birth control methods to avoid conception. Women of childbearing potential must have a negative pregnancy test. The anti-proliferative activity of this experimental drug may be harmful to the developing fetus or nursing infant.
- Complete supportive and palliative care will continue to be provided to ameliorate signs and symptoms that were pre-existing or may arise while on study and which do not interfere with the objectives of the study.
- Tumor blocks available from previous surgery/biopsy.

At the tumor specific expansion, only patients with metastatic colorectal and renal cell cancers will be enrolled. Patients with metastatic colorectal and renal cancer must have been treated and progressed or intolerant to standard care therapy.

Patients with colorectal cancer must been treated in the past with Irinotecan and/or Oxaliplatin and/or AvastinIEGFR therapy or intolerant to these agents. No more than 4 lines of therapy permitted in the metastatic setting. Patients with colorectal cancer may enroll irrespective of K-Ras mutational status, although this will be documented.

Patients with renal cell cancer must have been treated with a VEGF targeted therapy and/or mTOR inhibitor. No more than 4 lines of therapy permitted in the metastatic setting.

Prior treatment with Vorinostat and HCQ are not permitted in each tumor type.

Exclusion Criteria:

- Patients with uncontrolled brain metastases.
- Due to risk of disease exacerbation patients with porphyria are not eligible.
- Due to risk of disease exacerbation patients with psoriasis are ineligible unless the disease is well controlled and they are under the care of a specialist for the disorder who agrees to monitor the patient for exacerbations.
- Patients with previously documented macular degeneration or diabetic retinopathy.
- Patients who have had chemotherapy or radiotherapy within 2 weeks (6 weeks for Nitrosoureas or Mitomycin C) prior to entering the study or those who have not recovered from adverse events to ≤ grade 1 due to agents administered more than 4 weeks earlier. For targeted therapies patients will need to clear for 5 half lives.
- Patients may not be receiving any other investigational agents.
- Patients should not have taken valproic acid or another histone deacetylase inhibitor for at least 2 weeks prior to enrollment.
- History of allergic reactions attributed to compounds of similar chemical or biologic composition to vorinostat or HCQ.
- Uncontrolled intercurrent illness including, but not limited to, ongoing or active infection, symptomatic congestive heart failure, unstable angina pectoris, cardiac arrhythmia, or psychiatric illness/social situations that would limit compliance with study requirements.
- Major surgery or significant traumatic injury occurring within 21 days prior to treatment.
- Clinically significant hypercalcemia (including vomiting, dehydration and neurological symptoms).
- QTc > 500 ms at baseline (average of 3 determinations at 10 minutes interval).
- Gastrointestinal tract disease resulting in an inability to take oral medication or a requirement for IV alimentation, prior surgical procedures affecting absorption, or active peptic ulcer disease. Patients with NJ, J or G tube will not be allowed to participate.
- Pregnant women are excluded from this study because SAHA has the potential for teratogenic or abortifacient effects
- Patients with known hepatitis B or C or HIV infection.

Sex/Gender

All

Ages

16 Years to N/A

Accepts Healthy Volunteers

No

Contacts

Epp Goodwin   210-450-5798   CTRCReferral@uthscsa.edu

PHASE II TRIAL OF THE CYCLIN-DEPEDENT KINASE INHIBITOR PD 0332991 IN PATIENTS WITH CANCER

Study ID:

NCT01037790

Sponsor:

Abramson Cancer Center of the University of Pennsylvania

Information provided by (Responsible Party):

Abramson Cancer Center of the University of Pennsylvania (Abramson Cancer Center of the University of Pennsylvania)

Tracking Information

First Submitted Date

December 10, 2009

Start Date

October 2009

Primary Completion Date

October 2016

Last Update Posted Date

August 25, 2016

Current Primary Outcome Measures

Response rates[Time Frame: 5 years]
Safety and tolerability[Time Frame: 5 years]

Current Secondary Outcome Measures

Pharmacodynamic effects on tumor and non-tumor tissue[Time Frame: 5 years]
Relationship between selected biomarkers, pharmacokinetics, and/or efficacy and safety outcomes[Time Frame: 5 years]

Population pharmacokinetic for PD 0332991 and correlation with efficacy outcomes[Time Frame: 5 years]

Descriptive Information

Offical Title

Phase II Trial of the Cyclin-Dependent Kinase Inhibitor PD 0332991 in Patients With Cancer

Brief Summary

RATIONALE: PD 0332991 may stop the growth of tumor cells by blocking some of the enzymes needed for cell growth.

PURPOSE: This phase II trial is studying the side effects and how well PD 0332991 works in treating patients with refractory solid tumors.

Detailed Description

PRIMARY OBJECTIVES:

I. To determine the response rates following treatment with PD 0332991 in the following malignancies: 1) Metastatic breast cancer, 2) Metastatic colorectal cancer, 3) Metastatic melanoma with CDK4 mutation or amplification, or 4) Cisplatin-refractory, unresectable germ cell tumors.

II. To evaluate the safety and tolerability of PD 0332991 administered to subjects with refractory solid tumors.

SECONDARY OBJECTIVES:

I. To assess the pharmacodynamic effects of PD0332991 on tumor and non-tumor tissue.

II. To investigate the relationship between selected biomarkers, PK and/or efficacy and safety outcomes.

III. To estimate the population pharmacokinetic for PD 0332991 and to correlate PK with efficacy outcomes.

IV: To perform a Phase II evaluation of PD 0332991 in a population defined as potential responders on the basis of CCND1 gene amplification.

OUTLINE:

Patients receive oral PD 0332991 once daily on days 1-21. Treatment repeats every 28 days for up to 12 courses in the absence of unacceptable toxicity or disease progression.

Study Type

Interventional

Study Phase

Phase 2

Condition

- Adult Solid Tumor
- Adenocarcinoma of the Colon
- Adenocarcinoma of the Rectum
- Adult Central Nervous System Germ Cell Tumor
- Adult Teratoma
- Benign Teratoma
- Estrogen Receptor-negative Breast Cancer
- Estrogen Receptor-positive Breast Cancer
- Familial Testicular Germ Cell Tumor
- HER2-negative Breast Cancer
- HER2-positive Breast Cancer
- Male Breast Cancer
- Ovarian Immature Teratoma
- Ovarian Mature Teratoma
- Ovarian Monodermal and Highly Specialized Teratoma
- Progesterone Receptor-negative Breast Cancer
- Progesterone Receptor-positive Breast Cancer
- Recurrent Breast Cancer

- Recurrent Colon Cancer
- Recurrent Extragonadal Germ Cell Tumor
- Recurrent Extragonadal Non-seminomatous Germ Cell Tumor
- Recurrent Extragonadal Seminoma
- Recurrent Malignant Testicular Germ Cell Tumor
- Recurrent Melanoma
- Recurrent Ovarian Germ Cell Tumor
- Recurrent Rectal Cancer
- Stage III Extragonadal Non-seminomatous Germ Cell Tumor
- Stage III Extragonadal Seminoma
- Stage III Malignant Testicular Germ Cell Tumor
- Stage III Ovarian Germ Cell Tumor
- Stage IV Breast Cancer
- Stage IV Colon Cancer
- Stage IV Extragonadal Non-seminomatous Germ Cell Tumor
- Stage IV Extragonadal Seminoma
- Stage IV Melanoma
- Stage IV Ovarian Germ Cell Tumor
- Stage IV Rectal Cancer
- Testicular Immature Teratoma
- Testicular Mature Teratoma

Intervention

Drug: PD-0332991

Given orally, 125 mg QD on a 21-day

Other: pharmacological study

Correlative study

Other Names:

pharmacological studies

Study Arms

Experimental: Arm 1

Metastatic breast cancer

Experimental: Arm 2

Metastatic colorectal cancer that harbors the Kras or BRAF mutation

Experimental: Arm 3

Advanced or metastatic esophageal and/or gastric cancer

Experimental: Arm 4

Cisplatin-refractory, unresectable germ cell tumors

Experimental: Arm 5

Any tumor type if tissue tests positive for CCND1 amplification, CDK4/6 mutation , CCND2 amplification OR any other functional alteration at the G1/S checkpoint.

Recruitment Information

Recruitment Status

Recruiting

Estimated Enrollment

205

Eligibility Criteria

Inclusion Criteria:

- Disease Characteristics:

All Subjects: All subjects treated under this protocol will have histologically documented cancer of one of the following

Completion Date

N/A

Primary Completion Date

October 2016

types:

A. Metastatic breast cancer (7 triple negative, 23 ER+ after the first 15 patients are enrolled on the non-CCND1cohort; in addition 10 HER2+ for combination trastuzumab and PD0332991 therapy) up to 55 total enrollment slots B. Metastatic colorectal cancer that harbors the Kras or BRAF mutation (15-30 enrollment slots) C. Advanced or metastatic esophageal and/or gastric cancer (15-30 enrollment slots) D. Cisplatin-refractory, unresectable germ cell tumors (15-30 enrollment slots) E. Any tumor type if tissue tests positive for CCND1 amplification, CDK4/6 mutation, CCND2 amplification OR any other functional alteration at the G1/S checkpoint. (15-30 enrollment slots)

- Biopsy Requirements: For Subjects with accessible disease amenable to biopsy: A biopsy will be obtained pre-treatment and in during cycle 1 (while patient is receiving drug) for molecular markers of the cell cycle, and its inhibition.

- Subjects will be > 18 years old

- The subject has disease that is assessable by tumor marker, physical, or radiologic means.

- The subject has an Eastern Cooperative Oncology Group (ECOG) performance status of 0 or 1.

- The subject has adequate organ function, defined as follows A. Bilirubin ≤ 1.5 x the upper limit of normal (ULN) B. Serum creatinine ≤ 1.5 x UNL or calculated creatinine clearance ≥ 60 mL/min, and C. For subjects without liver metastases: alanine aminotransferase (ALT) and aspartate aminotransferase (AST) ≤ 2.5 x ULN D. For subjects with liver metastases: alanine aminotransferase (ALT) and aspartate aminotransferase ≤ 5 x ULN

- **All tumors must test positive for Rb expression except:**

A. ER positive metastatic breast tumors (data now shows all to be Rb positive.) B. Any tumor type if tissue tests positive for CCND1 amplification, CDK4/6 mutation, CCND2 amplification OR any other functional alteration at the G1/S checkpoint.

- The subject has adequate marrow function, defined as follows: A. Absolute neutrophil count (ANC) >1500/mm3 B. Platelets >100,000/mm3, and C. Hemoglobin > 9 g/dL

- The subject is capable of understanding and complying with the protocol requirements and has signed the informed consent document.

- Sexually active subjects (male and female) must use accepted methods of contraception during the course of the study and for 3 months after the last dose of protocol drug(s).

- Female subjects of childbearing potential must have a negative pregnancy test at screening. Females of childbearing potential are defined as sexually mature women without prior hysterectomy or who have had any evidence of menses in the past 12 months.

- However, women who have been amenorrheic for 12 or more months are still considered to be of childbearing potential if the amenorrhea is possibly due to prior chemotherapy, antiestrogens, or ovarian suppression.

Exclusion Criteria

- The subject has received cytotoxic chemotherapy (including investigational cytotoxic chemotherapy) within 3 weeks (or nitrosoureas or mitomycin C within 6 weeks) before the first dose of PD 0332991. . Patients with HER2-overexpressing tumors may receive trastuzumab up to the date of starting therapy, and may continue to receive trastuzumab while receiving PD0332991.

- The subject has received any other type of investigational agent within 28 days before the first dose of study treatment.

- The subject has not recovered from clinically-meaningful toxicity due to prior therapy (i.e., back to baseline or Grade ≤ 1), with the exception of neurotoxicity and alopecia.

- The subject has untreated or uncontrolled brain metastases or evidence of leptomeningeal involvement of disease unless the subject has a teratoma in which case s/he may be eligible if all other eligibility criteria are met

- **The subject has uncontrolled intercurrent illness including, but not limited to:**

1. ongoing or active infection

2. diabetes mellitus

3. hypertension

4. symptomatic congestive heart failure, unstable angina pectoris, stroke or myocardial infarction within 3 months

- The subject has a baseline corrected QT interval (QTc) > 470 ms.

- The subject is pregnant or breastfeeding.

- **The subject is known to be positive for the human immunodeficiency virus (HIV). Note:**

baseline HIV screening is not required

- The subject is unable or unwilling to abide by the study protocol or cooperate fully with the investigator or designee.

Sex/Gender

All

Ages

18 Years to N/A

Accepts Healthy Volunteers

No

Contacts

Peter O Dwyer, MD   855-216-0098   PennCancerTrials@emergingmed.com

Open-Label Phase 2 Efficacy Trial of Cancer Macrobeads in Patients With Treatment-Resistant Pancreatic or Colorectal Cancer

Study ID:

NCT01053013

Sponsor:

The Rogosin Institute

Information provided by (Responsible Party):

The Rogosin Institute (The Rogosin Institute)

Tracking Information

- **First Submitted Date**

  January 20, 2010

- **Start Date**

  February 2010

- **Current Primary Outcome Measures**

  Tumor volume and number of metastases[Time Frame: 16 months]

- **Current Secondary Outcome Measures**

  Progression-free survival[Time Frame: 16 months]

- **Primary Completion Date**

  December 2018

- **Last Update Posted Date**

  January 29, 2018

Descriptive Information

- **Offical Title**

  An Open-Label Phase 2 Efficacy Trial of the Implantation of Mouse Renal Adenocarcinoma Cell-Containing Agarose-Agarose Macrobeads in the Treatment of Patients With Treatment-Resistant, Metastatic Pancreatic or Colorectal Adenocarcinoma

- **Brief Summary**

  This is a clinical research study of an investigational (FDA IND-BB 10091) treatment for patients with pancreatic cancer (all stages) and advanced colorectal cancer that no longer responds to standard therapies.

  The treatment is being evaluated for its effect on tumor growth. It consists of the placement (implantation) of small beads that contain mouse renal adenocarcinoma cells (RENCA macrobeads). The cells in the macrobeads produce substances that have been shown to slow or stop the growth of tumors in experimental animals and veterinary patients. It has been tested in 31 human subjects with different types of cancers in a Phase I safety trial. Phase II studies in patients with colorectal, pancreatic or prostate cancers are in progress.

- **Study Type**

  Interventional

- **Study Phase**

  Phase 2

- **Condition**

  - Pancreatic Cancer
  - Colorectal Cancer

- **Intervention**

  Biological: Cancer macrobead placement in abdominal cavity
    8 macrobeads per kilogram

  Other Names:
    cancer macrobeads

- **Study Arms**

  Experimental: Cancer macrobeads
    Cancer macrobead placement in abdominal cavity

Recruitment Information

Recruitment Status

Recruiting

Estimated Enrollment

60

Eligibility Criteria

Inclusion Criteria:

- Cancer of pancreas, colon or rectum
- Evidence of metastasis
- Failed available therapies (pancreatic cancer may be treated without previous therapies)
- Resolution of any toxic effects of previous therapies
- Performance status (ECOG PS) 0-2
- Adequate hematologic, coagulation (INR 2-3 max), hepatic and renal function
- Life expectancy of at least 6 weeks
- For females, a negative pregnancy test
- Agrees to contraceptive use while on study if sexually active
- Informed consent

Exclusion Criteria:

- Any condition presenting an unacceptably high anesthetic or surgical risk
- HIV positive
- Cognitive impairment such as to preclude informed consent
- Surgical treatment or chemotherapy within three weeks of scheduled macrobead implantation or within four weeks of bevacizumab (or similar drugs), or radiation therapy within four weeks of scheduled macrobead implantation
- Inadequate hematologic, coagulation (INR >3), hepatic, renal function
- Hepatic blood flow abnormalities and/or large-volume ascites
- Concurrent cancer of any other type except skin cancer (excluding melanoma)
- History of allergic reactions to mouse antigens
- Active infection, congestive heart failure, unstable angina, serious cardiac arrhythmias, psychiatric illness, difficult social situations not permitting reliable participation, active bleeding

Sex/Gender

All

Ages

18 Years to N/A

Accepts Healthy Volunteers

No

Contacts

Barry H Smith, MD, PhD   212-746-1551   bas2005@nyp.org

Nathaniel Berman, MD   212-746-9766   nab2009@nyp.org

Completion Date

December 2018

Primary Completion Date

December 2018

Biweekly Intraperitoneal Oxaliplatin With Systemic Capecitabine and Bevacizumab for Patients With Peritoneal Carcinomatosis From Appendiceal or Colorectal Cancer

Study ID:

NCT01061515

Sponsor:

Washington University School of Medicine

Information provided by (Responsible Party):

Washington University School of Medicine (Washington University School of Medicine)

Tracking Information

First Submitted Date

February 1, 2010

Start Date

May 10, 2011

Primary Completion Date

May 31, 2018

Last Update Posted Date

January 8, 2018

Current Primary Outcome Measures

To determine the maximum tolerated dose of IP oxaliplatin with systemic intravenous bevacizumab and oral capecitabine after surgical debulking and peritoneal scan documenting functional of intraperitoneal ports in patients with peritoneal carcinomatosis[Time Frame: Completion of enrollment (approximately 6 years)]

Assess the safety and tolerability of IP oxaliplatin and intravenous (i.v.) bevacizumab and oral capecitabine after surgical debulking and functional intraperitoneal ports in patients with peritoneal carcinomatosis of appendiceal or colorectal etiology[Time Frame: 30 days after completion of treatment]

To describe the progression rate, progression-free survival and overall survival in patients treated with this regimen.[Time Frame: 1 year post treatment]

Descriptive Information

Offical Title

A Phase I Dose-Escalation Trial of Biweekly Intraperitoneal Oxaliplatin With Systemic Capecitabine and Bevacizumab Following Cytoreduction in Patients With Peritoneal Carcinomatosis From Appendiceal or Colorectal Cancer

Brief Summary

This study is to test escalating doses of intraperitoneal (IP) oxaliplatin in conjunction with systemic bevacizumab and capecitabine in patients with Peritoneal Carcinomatosis (PC) from either appendiceal or colorectal adenocarcinoma that have been adequately cytoreduced and have undergone a peritoneal scan demonstrating patency of at least one of the intraperitoneal ports that were placed at the time of debulking.

Detailed Description

- To determine the maximum tolerated dose of IP oxaliplatin with systemic intravenous bevacizumab and oral capecitabine after adequate surgical debulking and peritoneal scan documenting function of intraperitoneal ports in patients with peritoneal carcinomatosis of appendiceal or colorectal etiology.
- To assess the safety and tolerability of repeated delayed intraperitoneal chemotherapy with oxaliplatin and systemic intravenous bevacizumab and oral capecitabine after adequate surgical debulking and peritoneal scan documenting function of intraperitoneal ports in patients with peritoneal carcinomatosis of appendiceal or colorectal etiology.
- To describe the progression rate, progression-free survival and overall survival in patients treated with this regimen.

Study Type

Interventional

Study Phase

Phase 1

Condition

- Carcinoma

Intervention

Drug: Intraperitoneal Oxaliplatin

  Other Names:

  Eloxatin

  Drug: Bevacizumab

  Other Names:

  Avastin

Drug: Capecitabine

  Other Names:

  Xeloda

Study Arms

Experimental: Dose Level 1

Intraperitoneal oxaliplatin 25 mg/m2 IP on day 1 of each cycle

Bevacizumab 5 mg/kg CIVI on day 1 of each cycle

Capecitabine 850 mg/m2 PO BID on days 1-7 of each cycle.

Each cycle is 14 days long.

Experimental: Dose Level 2

Intraperitoneal oxaliplatin 50 mg/m2 IP on day 1 of each cycle

Bevacizumab 5 mg/kg CIVI on day 1 of each cycle

Capecitabine 850 mg/m2 PO BID on days 1-7 of each cycle.

Each cycle is 14 days long.

Experimental: Dose Level 3

Intraperitoneal oxaliplatin 65 mg/m2 IP on day 1 of each cycle

Bevacizumab 5 mg/kg CIVI on day 1 of each cycle

Capecitabine 850 mg/m2 PO BID on days 1-7 of each cycle.

Each cycle is 14 days long.

Experimental: Dose Level 4

Intraperitoneal oxaliplatin 85 mg/m2 IP on day 1 of each cycle

Bevacizumab 5 mg/kg CIVI on day 1 of each cycle

Capecitabine 850 mg/m2 PO BID on days 1-7 of each cycle.

Each cycle is 14 days long.

Experimental: Dose Level 5

Intraperitoneal oxaliplatin 100 mg/m2 IP on day 1 of each cycle

Bevacizumab 5 mg/kg CIVI on day 1 of each cycle

Capecitabine 850 mg/m2 PO BID on days 1-7 of each cycle.

Each cycle is 14 days long.

Recruitment Information

Recruitment Status

Recruiting

Estimated Enrollment

24

Completion Date

May 31, 2019

Primary Completion Date

May 31, 2018

Eligibility Criteria

Inclusion Criteria:

- Histological Diagnosis: Patients must have a histologically documented peritoneal carcinomatosis from either colorectal or appendiceal adenocarcinoma.
- Prior Surgical Debulking: Patients must have undergone debulking surgery with peritonectomy and have been allowed at least 4 weeks to recover prior to receiving chemotherapy.
- Port Placement: Intraperitoneal ports may be placed during or at any time separate from surgical debulking. Provided the patient has been allowed at least 4 weeks to recover from surgical debulking, no additional recovery time is required for port placement.
- Active port: Patients must undergo a peritoneal scan documenting at least one working intraperitoneal port prior to receiving chemotherapy.
- Patients may have received prior chemotherapy.
- Age: Patients must be ≥18 years of age. Because no dosing or toxicity data are currently available on the use of oxaliplatin in patients <18 years of age.
- Performance Status: (Eastern cooperativeOncology Group) ECOG 0-2.
- Recovery from Intercurrent Illness: Patients must have recovered from uncontrolled intercurrent illness including, but not limited to, ongoing or active infection, symptomatic congestive heart failure, unstable angina pectoris, or cardiac arrhythmias.
- Informed Consent: All patients must be consented prior to chemotherapy. The patient should not have any serious medical of

psychiatric illness that would prevent either the giving of informed consent or the receipt of treatment.
- **Hematological Status:**
- absolute neutrophil count ≥1,500/mm³
- platelet count ≥100,000/mm³
- hemoglobin ≥8 g/dl.
- **Hepatic function:**
- Total bilirubin must be <2X the institutional upper limit of normal (ULN)
- Transaminases (SGOT and/or SGPT) must be ≤3X the institutional upper limit of normal (ULN)
- Alkaline phosphatase must be ≤4X the institutional upper limit of normal (ULN)
- Renal Function: Patients must have adequate renal function prior to chemotherapy defined as serum creatinine ≤ 2.0 mg/dl or creatinine clearance ≥60 ml.min/1.73 m² for patients with creatinine levels above 2.0 mg/dl.

Exclusion Criteria:
- Pregnant or breast feeding: For all sexually active patients, the use of adequate contraception (hormonal or barrier method of birth control) will be required during therapy, prior to study entry, and for the duration of study participation. Non-pregnant status will be determined in all women of childbearing potential.
- Prior history of hypersensitivity reactions to oxaliplatin, bevacizumab, 5-FU or capecitabine.
- Gastrointestinal ailments that may alter the absorption of oral medications (i.e. bowel obstruction, short-gut syndrome).
- Patients receiving antiretroviral therapy Highly Active Anti Retroviral Treatment (HAART) for HIV infection are excluded from the study because of possible pharmacokinetic interactions. Appropriate studies will be undertaken in patients receiving HAART therapy, when indicated.
- Patients with Grade 2 or higher peripheral neuropathy.

Sex/Gender

All

Ages

18 Years to N/A

Accepts Healthy Volunteers

No

Contacts

Benjamin Tan, M.D.   314-362-9115   btan@wustl.edu

Immunotherapy Using Tumor Infiltrating Lymphocytes for Patients With Metastatic Cancer

Study ID:

NCT01174121

Sponsor:

National Cancer Institute (NCI)

Information provided by (Responsible Party):

National Institutes of Health Clinical Center (CC) (National Cancer Institute (NCI))

Tracking Information

First Submitted Date

July 31, 2010

Primary Completion Date

December 29, 2023

Start Date

July 15, 2010

Last Update Posted Date

February 9, 2018

Current Primary Outcome Measures

Rate of tumor regression[Time Frame: 6 and 12 weeks after cell infusion, then every 3 months x 3, then every 6 months x 2 years, then per PI discretion]

Number of patients who have a clinical response to treatment

Current Secondary Outcome Measures

Frequency of treatment related to adverse events[Time Frame: 30 days after end of treatment]

Aggregate of all adverse events and their frequency

Descriptive Information

▨ Offical Title

A Phase II Study Using Short-Term Cultured, Autologous Tumor-Infiltrating Lymphocytes Following a Lymphocyte Depleting Regimen in Metastatic Cancers Plus the Administration of Pembrolizumabat Time of Progression

▨ Brief Summary

Background:

The NCI Surgery Branch has developed an experimental therapy that involves taking white blood cells from patients' tumors, growing them in the laboratory in large numbers, and then giving the cells back to the patient. These cells are called Tumor Infiltrating Lymphocytes, or TIL and we have given this type of treatment to over 200 patients with melanoma. Researchers want to know if TIL shrink s tumors in people with digestive tract, urothelial, breast, or ovarian/endometrial cancers. In this study, we are selecting a specific subset of white blood cells from the tumor that we think are the most effective in fighting tumors and will use only these cells in making the tumor fighting cells.

Objective:

The purpose of this study is to see if these specifically selected tumor fighting cells can cause digestive tract, urothelial, breast, or ovarian/endometrial tumors to shrink and to see if this treatment is safe.

Eligibility:

- Adults age 18-70 with metastatic digestive tract, urothelial, breast, or ovarian/endometrial cancer who have a tumor that can be safely removed.

Design:

Work up stage: Patients will be seen as an outpatient at the NIH clinical Center and undergo a history and physical examination, scans, x-rays, lab tests, and other tests as needed.

Surgery: If the patients meet all of the requirements for the study they will undergo surgery to remove a tumor that can be used to grow the TIL product.

Leukapheresis: Patients may undergo leukapheresis to obtain additional white blood cells. {Leukapheresis is a common procedure, which removes only the white blood cells from the patient.}

Treatment: Once their cells have grown, the patients will be admitted to the hospital for the conditioning chemotherapy, the TIL cells and aldesleukin. They will stay in the hospital for about 4 weeks for the treatment.

Follow up: Patients will return to the clinic for a physical exam, review of side effects, lab tests, and scans about every 1-3 months for the first year, and then every 6 months to 1 year as long as their tumors are shrinking. Follow up visits will take up to 2 days.

▨ Detailed Description

Background:

- Metastatic digestive tract cancers, in particular esophageal, gastric, pancreatic and hepatobiliary carcinomas, are associated with poor survival beyond five years and poor response to existing therapies.
- Data from the Surgery Branch and from the literature support that metastatic cancers are potentially immunogenic and that TIL can be grown and expanded from these tumors.
- In metastatic melanoma, TIL can mediate the regression of bulky disease at any site when administered to an autologous patient with high dose aldesleukin (IL-2) following a nonmyeloablative but lymphodepleting chemotherapy preparative regimen.
- The recent young-TIL approach, in which TIL are minimally cultured in vitro, not selected for tumor recognition, before rapid expansion and infusion to metastatic melanoma patients, has lead to objective response rates comparable to previous trials relying on TIL screened for tumor recognition, with no added toxicities.
- In pre-clinical models, the administration of an anti-PD-1 antibody enhances the anti-tumor activity of transferred T-cells.
- With the approval of amendment Z, we propose to investigate the feasibility, safety, and efficacy of TIL adoptive transfer therapy with the addition of pembrolizumab at the time of progressive disease as treatment in Arm 4, including a 7th cohort (glioblastoma).

Objectives:

-With Amendment Z, to determine the ability of autologous TIL infused after minimal in vitro culture in conjunction with high dose aldesleukin following a non-myeloablative lymphodepleting preparative regimen and then the addition of anti-PD-1 at time of progressive disease per RECIST criteria to mediate tumor regression in patients with metastatic cancers.

Eligibility:

Patients who are 18 years of age or older must have:

- Metastatic digestive tract, urothelial, breast, ovarian/endometrial cancer, or glioblastoma refractory to standard chemotherapy, originating from the a) gastric, gastroesophageal junction, b) pancreas, liver or biliary tree, c) colon or rectum, d) bladder, e) breast, or f) ovarian/endometrial;
- Normal basic laboratory values.

Patients may not have:

- Concurrent major medical illnesses
- Severe hepatic function impairment due to liver metastatic burden
- Unpalliated biliary or bowel occlusion, cholangitis, or digestive tract bleeding
- Any form of immunodeficiency
- Severe hypersensitivity to any of the agents used in this study

Design:

- Patients will undergo resection or biopsy to obtain tumor for generation of autologous TIL cultures and autologous cancer cell lines, and for frozen tissue archive. Lymph nodes, ascites,peritoneal implants, and normal tissue adjacent to metastatic deposit will also be obtained when possible for ongoing and future research as described in 03-C-0277.
- With the approval of amendment X, all patients on Arm 4 will receive a non-myeloablative lymphocyte depleting preparative regimen of cyclophosphamide and fludarabine followed by the infusion of autologous TIL and then begin high-dose aldesleukin (720,000 IU/kg IV every 8 hours for up to 12 doses).
- Once patients meet progressive disease by RECIST criteria, Pembrolizumab will be administered within 4 weeks after PD for up to 8 doses..
- Clinical and immunologic response will be evaluated at the first follow-up evaluation following the last dose of study drug.
- Twenty-one patients will be initially enrolled in each group to assess toxicity and tumor responses. If two or more of the first 21 patients per groups shows a clinical response (PR or CR), accrual will continue to 41 patients, targeting a 20% goal for objective response.
- Up to 332 patients may be enrolled over 3-8 years.

Study Type

Interventional

Study Phase

Phase 2

Condition

- Metastatic Colorectal Cancer
- Metastatic Gastric Cancer
- Metastatic Pancreatic Cancer
- Metastatic Hepatocellular Carcinoma
- Progressive Glioblastoma

Intervention

Biological: Young TIL

On day 0, cells will be infused intravenously over 20 to 30 minutes (one to four days after the last dose of fludarabine).

Drug: Aldesleukin

Aldesleukin 720,000 IU/kg IV (based on total body weight) over 15 minutes approximately every eight hours (+/1hr) beginning within 24 hours of cell infusion and continuing for up to 5 days (maximum of 15 doses.)

Drug: Cyclophosphamide

On day -7 and day -6: Cyclophosphamide 60 mg/kg/day X 2 days IV in 250 ml D5W over 1 hr.

Drug: Fludarabine

On day -5 to day -1: Fludarabine 25 mg/m2/day IVPB daily over 30 minutes for 5 days.

Drug: Pembrolizumab

Day -2, day 21, day 42, and day 63, Pembrolizumab 2mg/kg IV over approximately 30 minutes.

Study Arms

Experimental: Arm 2

Young unselected TIL (CLOSED)

Experimental: Arm 4

Young unselected TIL + pembrolizumab at time of progression for a total of 4 doses.

Experimental: Arm 3

Young unselectedTIL + pembrolizumab prior to cell administration and continuing for a total of 4 doses (CLOSED)

Experimental: Arm 1

Young CD8+ enriched TIL (CLOSED)

Publications

(Includes publications given by the data provider as well as publications identified by ClinicalTrials.gov Identifier (NCT Number) in Medline.)Chiba T, Ohtani H, Mizoi T, Naito Y, Sato E, Nagura H, Ohuchi A, Ohuchi K, Shiiba K, Kurokawa Y, Satomi S. Intraepithelial CD8+ T-cell-count becomes a prognostic factor after a longer follow-up period in human colorectal carcinoma: possible association with suppression of micrometastasis. Br J Cancer. 2004 Nov 1;91(9):1711-7. (https://www.ncbi.nlm.nih.gov/pubmed/15494715)

Fong Y, Fortner J, Sun RL, Brennan MF, Blumgart LH. Clinical score for predicting recurrence after hepatic resection for metastatic colorectal cancer: analysis of 1001 consecutive cases. Ann Surg. 1999 Sep;230(3):309-18; discussion 318-21. (https://www.ncbi.nlm.nih.gov/pubmed/10493478)

Tomlinson JS, Jarnagin WR, DeMatteo RP, Fong Y, Kornprat P, Gonen M, Kemeny N, Brennan MF, Blumgart LH, D'Angelica M. Actual 10-year survival after resection of colorectal liver metastases defines cure. J Clin Oncol. 2007 Oct 10;25(29):4575-80. (https://www.ncbi.nlm.nih.gov/pubmed/17925551)

Recruitment Information

Recruitment Status

Recruiting

Estimated Enrollment

332

Completion Date

December 27, 2024

Primary Completion Date

December 29, 2023

Eligibility Criteria

-INCLUSION CRITERIA:

1. Measurable metastatic (stage IV) gastric, gastroesophageal, pancreatic, hepatocellular carcinoma, cholangiocarcinoma, gallbladder, colorectal, urothelial, breast, ovarian/endometrial carcinoma, or glioblastoma with at least one lesion that is resectable for TIL generation with minimal morbidity preferentially using minimal invasive laparoscopic or thoracoscopic surgery for removal of superficial tumor deposit, plus one other lesion that can be measured.

2. All patients must be refractory to approved standard systemic therapy.

Specifically :

- Metastatic colorectal patients must have received oxaliplatin or irinotecan.
- Hepatocellular carcinoma patients must have received sorafenib (Nexavar), since level 1 data support a survival benefit with this agent.
- Breast and Ovarian cancer patients must be refractory to both 1st line and 2nd line treatments and must have received at least one second line chemotherapy regimen.
- Patients with recurrent glioblastoma that have received standard surgery, radiation therapy, and chemotherapy for their primary tumors and require resection of their tumors for palliative or other clinical indications. These patients will not undergo surgery solely for treatment on this protocol.

3. Patients with 3 or fewer brain metastases that are less than 1 cm in diameter and asymptomatic are eligible. Lesions that have been treated with stereotactic radiosurgery must be clinically stable for 1 month after treatment for the patient to be eligible.

4. Clinical performance status of ECOG 0 or 1.

5. Greater than or equal to 18 years of age and less than or equal to 70 years of age.

6. Willing to practice birth control during treatment and for four months after receiving the treatment.

7. Willing to sign a durable power of attorney.

8. Able to understand and sign the Informed Consent Document.

9. Hematology:

- Absolute neutrophil count greater than 1000/mm(3) without support of filgrastim.
- Normal WBC (> 3000/mm(3)).
- Hemoglobin greater than 8.0 g/dl. Subjects may be transfused to reach this cut-off.
- Platelet count greater than 100,000/mm(3).
- Normal prothrombin time (less than or equal to 15.2 seconds).

10. Serology:

- Seronegative for HIV antibody. (The experimental treatment being evaluated in this protocol depends on an intact immune system. Patients who are HIV seropositive can have decreased immune competence and thus may be less responsive to the experimental treatment and more susceptible to its toxicities.)
- Seronegative for active hepatitis B, and seronegative for hepatitis C antibody. If hepatitis C antibody test is positive, then patient must be tested for the presence of antigen by RT-PCR and be HCV RNA negative.

11. Chemistry:

- Serum ALT/AST less than five times the upper limit of normal.
- Serum creatinine less than or equal to 1.6 mg/dl.
- Total bilirubin less than or equal to 2 mg/dl, except in patients with Gilbert's Syndrome, who must have a total bilirubin less than or equal to 3 mg/dl.

12. More than four weeks must have elapsed since any prior systemic therapy at the time the patient receives the preparative regimen, and patients' toxicities must have recovered to a grade 1 or less. Patients may have undergone minor surgical procedures with the past 3 weeks, as long as all toxicities have recovered to grade 1 or less.

13. Four weeks must have elapsed since any prior antibody therapies to allow antibody levels to decline.

14. Subjects must be co-enrolled in protocol 03-C-0277.

EXCLUSION CRITERIA:

1. Women of child-bearing potential who are pregnant or breastfeeding because of the potentially dangerous effects of the treatment on the fetus or infant.

2. Concurrent systemic steroid therapy. (Note: Patients with recurrent glioblastoma who require steroids for clinical indications are eligible.)

3. Active systemic infections (e.g.: requiring anti-infective treatment), coagulation disorders or any other active major medical illnesses

4. Advanced primary with impeding occlusion, perforation or bleeding, dependant on transfusion.

5. Any form of primary immunodeficiency (such as Severe Combined Immunodeficiency Disease and AIDS).

6. History of major organ autoimmune disease.

7. Grade 3 or 4 major organ Immune-Related Adverse Events (IRAEs) following treatment with anti-PD-1/PD-L1

8. Concurrent opportunistic infections (The experimental treatment being evaluated in this protocol depends on an intact immune system. Patients who have decreased immune competence may be less responsive to the experimental treatment and more susceptible to its toxicities.)

9. History of severe immediate hypersensitivity reaction to any of the agents used in this study.

10. History of coronary revascularization or ischemic symptoms.

11. Any patient known to have an LVEF less than or equal to 45%.

12. Documented LVEF of less than or equal to 45% tested in patients with:

- Clinically significant atrial and/or ventricular arrhythmias including but not limited to: atrial fibrillation, ventricular tachycardia, second or third degree heart block
- Age greater than or equal to 60 years old

13. Documented Child-Pugh score of B or C for hepatocellular carcinoma patients with known underlying liver dysfunction.

14. Documented FEV1 less than or equal to 60% predicted tested in patients with:

- A prolonged history of cigarette smoking (20 pk/year of smoking within the past 2 years).
- Symptoms of respiratory dysfunction

15. Patients who are receiving any other investigational agents.

Sex/Gender

All

Ages

18 Years to 70 Years

Accepts Healthy Volunteers

No

Contacts

Mary E. Link, R.N.   (866) 820-4505   ncisbirc@mail.nih.gov
Steven A Rosenberg, M.D.   (866) 820-4505   sar@mail.nih.gov

Study of Hepatic Arterial Infusion With Intravenous Irinotecan, 5FU and Leucovorin With or Without Panitumumab, in Patients With Wild Type RAS Who Have Resected Hepatic Metastases From Colorectal Cancer

Study ID:
NCT01312857

Sponsor:
Memorial Sloan Kettering Cancer Center

Information provided by (Responsible Party):

Memorial Sloan Kettering Cancer Center (Memorial Sloan Kettering Cancer Center)

Tracking Information

First Submitted Date

March 8, 2011

Start Date

March 2011

Primary Completion Date

March 2018

Last Update Posted Date

April 4, 2017

Current Primary Outcome Measures

to determine if panitumumab with Hepatic Arterial Infusion (HAI) in combination with systemic chemotherapy can increase the recurrence free survival (RFS) for colorectal cancer patients with resected liver metastases[Time Frame: 2 years]

Current Secondary Outcome Measures

to assess toxicity as per the NCI Common Toxicity Criteria[Time Frame: Day 1 of each cycle]

Toxicities will be recorded as adverse events on the Adverse Event case report form and must be graded using The National Cancer Institute's Common Toxicity Criteria (CTC)version 4.0 with the exception of skinor nail-related toxicities, which must be graded using CTC version 3.0 with modifications

to determine survival[Time Frame: 2 years]

to analyze tumor tissue for predictive biomarkers[Time Frame: 2 years]

(such as NRAS, BRAF, PIK3CA, AKT1 and MEK1), and correlate with patient progression and survival following therapy.

Descriptive Information

Offical Title

A Randomized Phase II Study of Hepatic Arterial Infusion With Intravenous Irinotecan, 5FU and Leucovorin With or Without Panitumumab, in Patients With Wild Type RAS Who Have Resected Hepatic Metastases From Colorectal Cancer

Brief Summary

The purpose of this study is to see if Panitumumab plus the other treatments will increase the time of remission. Remission means that there is no sign of the cancer.

Study Type

Interventional

Study Phase

Phase 2

Condition

- Metastatic Colorectal Cancer

Intervention

Drug: panitumumab

All patients receive HAI FUDR (0.12 mg/kg/day X kg X pump volume) / pump flow rate and Dexamethasone flat dose of 25 mg on days 1.

All patients receive CPT-11 (150 mg/m2 IV over 30 min to an hour), Leucovorin (400 mg/m2 IV, over 30 min to an hour) and 5FU (1000 mg/m2/day continuous infusion over two days) on days 15 and 29 Randomization to panitumumab 6 mg/kg day 15 and 29 Each cycle repeats every 36 days for a total of 6 cycles

Drug: Randomization to No Panitumumab

All patients receive HAI FUDR (0.12 mg/kg/day X kg X pump volume) / pump flow rate and Dexamethasone flat dose of 25 mg on days 1.

All patients receive CPT-11 (150 mg/m2 IV over 30 min to an hour), Leucovorin (400 mg/m2 IV, over 30 min to an hour) and 5FU (1000 mg/m2/day continuous infusion over two days) on days 15 and 29 Randomization (to no panitumumab) Each cycle repeats every 36 days for a total of 6 cycles

Study Arms

Experimental: Randomization to panitumumab

Patients whose liver metastases have been completely resected will be randomized Arm A will receive Panitumumab in addition to HAI FUDR/Dexamethasone plus systemic CPT-11/5FU/LV

Experimental: Randomization to No Panitumumab

Patients whose liver metastases have been completely resected will be randomized and patients randomized to Arm B will receive HAI FUDR/Dex plus systemic CPT-11/5FU/LV alone.

Recruitment Information

Recruitment Status

Recruiting

Estimated Enrollment

78

Completion Date

March 2018

Primary Completion Date

March 2018

Eligibility Criteria

Inclusion Criteria:

- History of histologically confirmed colorectal adenocarcinoma metastatic to the liver with no clinical or radiographic evidence of extrahepatic disease. Confirmation of diagnosis must be performed at MSKCC.
- Completely resected hepatic metastases without current evidence of other metastatic disease.
- **Lab values ≤ 14 days prior to registration:**
- WBC ≥ 3.0 K/uL
- ANC > 1.5 K/uL
- Platelets ≥ 100,000/uL
- Creatinine <1.5 mg/dL
- HGB ≥ 9 gm/dL Renal function (≤ 14 days prior to registration).
- Creatinine ≤1.5 mg/dL or creatinine clearance ≥ 50 mL/min calculated by the

Cockcroft-Gault method as follows:

- Male creatinine clearance = (140 -age in years) x (weight in Kg) / (serum Cr in mg/dl x 72)
- Female creatinine clearance = (140 age in years) x (weight in Kg) x 0.85 / (serum Cr in mg/dl x 72) (use of creatinine clearance per protocol based on chemotherapy regimen) Hepatic function, as follows: (≤ 14 days prior to registration)
- Aspartate aminotransferase (AST) (≤ 5 x ULN)
- Alanine aminotransferase (ALT) (≤ 5 x ULN)
- Total Bilirubin ≤ 1.5 mg/dl
- Magnesium ≥ lower limit of normal (≤ 48 hours prior to registration.)
- Calcium ≥ lower limit of normal (≤ 48 hours prior to registration.)
- Prior chemotherapy is acceptable if last dose given ≥ 3 weeks prior to registration to this study. [Note: no chemotherapy to be given after resection of liver lesions prior to treatment on this study.]
- Any investigational agent is acceptable if administered ≤ 30 days before registration
- KPS ≥ 60% (ECOG (or Karnofsky) performance status (preferably 0 or 1/≥ 60% for Karnofsky)
- Histologically confirmed all RAS wild type.
- Paraffin-embedded tumor tissue obtained from the primary tumor or metastasis

Exclusion Criteria:

- Patients < 18 years of age.
- Prior radiation to the liver (Prior radiation therapy to the pelvis is acceptable if completed at least 4 weeks prior to registration.)
- Active infection, ascites, hepatic encephalopathy.
- Prior treatment with HAI FUDR.
- Patients who have had prior anti EGFR antibody therapy inhibitors and who have not responded to this treatment will be excluded. However, patients who have responded to prior anti-EGFR therapy are eligible.)
- Female patients who are pregnant or lactating or planning to become pregnant within 6 months after the end of the treatment (female patients of child-bearing potential must have negative pregnancy test ≤ 72 hours before registration).
- If a patient has any serious medical problems which may preclude receiving this type of treatment.
- Patients with current evidence of hepatitis A, B, C (ie, active hepatitis)
- Patients with history or known presence of primary CNS tumors, seizures not well controlled with standard medical therapy, or history of stroke will also be excluded.
- History of allergic reactions attributed to compounds of similar chemical or biologic composition to Panitumumab.
- Serious or non-healing active wound, ulcer, or bone fracture.
- History of interstitial lung disease e.g. pneumonitis or pulmonary fibrosis or evidence of interstitial lung disease on baseline chest CT scan.
- Patients who have a diagnosis of Gilbert's disease.
- **History of other malignancy, except:**
- Malignancy treated with curative intent and with no known active disease present for ≥ 3 years prior to registration and felt to

be at low risk for recurrence by the treating physician

- Adequately treated non-melanomatous skin cancer or lentigo maligna without evidence of disease
- Adequately treated cervical carcinoma in situ without evidence of disease

▨ **Sex/Gender**

All

▨ **Ages**

18 Years to N/A

▨ **Accepts Healthy Volunteers**

No

▨ **Contacts**

Nancy Kemeny, MD   646-888-4180
Michael D'Angelica, MD   212-639-3226

S0820, Adenoma and Second Primary Prevention Trial

Study ID:

NCT01349881

Sponsor:

Southwest Oncology Group

Information provided by (Responsible Party):

Southwest Oncology Group (Southwest Oncology Group)

Tracking Information

▨ **First Submitted Date**

May 5, 2011

▨ **Start Date**

March 2013

▨ **Primary Completion Date**

June 2024

▨ **Last Update Posted Date**

January 4, 2018

▨ **Current Primary Outcome Measures**

3-year event rate after registration among Stage 0-III colon cancer patients. (An event is defined as high-risk adenoma or second primary colorectal cancer.)[Time Frame: 3 years]

> The primary objective is to assess whether eflornithine 500 mg or sulindac 150 mg are effective in reducing the 3-year event rate, defined as high risk adenoma or 2nd primary colorectal cancer, in Stage 0, I, II, and III colon cancer patients.

▨ **Current Secondary Outcome Measures**

Incidence of colorectal lesions with respect to high-grade dysplasia, adenomas with villous features, adenomas 1 cm or greater, multiple adenomas, polyps >/= 0.3 cm, total advanced colorectal events or total colorectal events at 3 years.[Time Frame: 3 years and 8 years]

> Incidence of colorectal lesions with respect to high grade dysplasia, adenomas with villous features, adenomas 1 cm or greater, multiple adenomas, polyps >/= 0.3 cm, total advanced colorectal events (defined as the number of patients with at least one high risk adenoma, 2nd primary colorectal cancer, colorectal cancer recurrence, or metastasis) or total colorectal cancer events (defined as the number of patients with at least one advanced colorectal event or polyp)at 3 years and 8 years.

Toxicity by CTCAE v.4.0 at 3 years[Time Frame: 3 years]

> Quantitative and qualitative toxicities at 3 years.

Examine interaction of treatment arm and genotype expression with respect to different outcomes.[Time Frame: 3 years and 8 years]

Interaction of intervention arm and baseline statin use with respect to 3-year event rate.[Time Frame: 3 year]

> Interaction of intervention arm and baseline statin use with respect to 3-year event rate will be examined.

Evaluate SNPs associated with decreased adenoma/second primary CRC risk and AEs[Time Frame: 3 years and 8 years]

> Evaluate a minimal set of tagging single nucleotide polymorphisms across multiple genes relevant to eflornithine and sulindac, in order to characterize associations with decreased adenoma/second primary CRC risk and adverse events.

Descriptive Information

Offical Title

- A Double Blind Placebo-Controlled Trial of Eflornithine and Sulindac to Prevent Recurrence of High Risk Adenomas and Second Primary Colorectal Cancers in Patients With Stage 0-III Colon or Rectal Cancer, Phase III Preventing Adenomas of the Colon With Eflornithine and Sulindac (PACES)

Brief Summary

The investigators hypothesize that the combination of eflornithine and sulindac will be effective in reducing a three-year event rate of adenomas and second primary colorectal cancers in patients previously treated for Stages 0 through III colon cancer.

Detailed Description

The purpose of this study is to assess whether eflornithine 500 mg or sulindac 150 mg are effective in reducing the 3-year event rate of high risk adenoma or second primary colorectal cancer in Stage 0, I II and III colon cancer patients. The primary hypothesis will test the main effect of each agent, as well as the comparison of placebo alone to the combination of sulindac and eflornithine.

Study Type

Interventional

Study Phase

Phase 3

Condition

- Colorectal Neoplasms

Intervention

Drug: Eflornithine placebo & sulindac placebo

Eflornithine placebo 2 tablets PO daily for 3 years. Sulindac placebo 1 tablet PO daily for 3 years

Drug: eflornithine & sulindac placebo

Eflornithine two 250 mg tablets PO daily for 3 years. Sulindac placebo 1 tablet PO daily for 3 years.

Drug: Eflornithine placebo & sulindac

Eflornithine placebo 2 tablets PO daily for 3 years. Sulindac one 150 mg tablet PO daily for 3 years.

Drug: Eflornithine plus sulindac

Eflornithine two 250 mg tablets PO daily for 3 years. Sulindac one 150 mg tablet PO daily for 3 years.

Study Arms

Placebo Comparator: eflornithine placebo & sulindac placebo

Eflornithine placebo 2 tablets, PO, daily for 3 years. Sulindac placebo, 1 tablet, PO, daily for 3 years.

Experimental: Eflornithine & sulindac placebo

Eflornithine two 250 mg tablets PO daily for 3 years. Sulindac placebo one tablet PO daily for 3 years.

Experimental: Eflornithine placebo & sulindac

Eflornithine placebo 2 tablets PO daily for 3 years. Sulindac one 150 mg tablet PO daily for 3 years.

Experimental: Eflornithine plus sulindac

Eflornithine two 250 mg tablets PO daily for 3 years. Sulindac one 150 mg tablet PO daily for 3 years.

Recruitment Information

Recruitment Status

Recruiting

Estimated Enrollment

1340

Completion Date

June 2029

Primary Completion Date

June 2024

Eligibility Criteria

Inclusion Criteria:

- History of Stage 0-III colon or rectal cancer with primary resection 1 year previously
- Post-operative colonoscopy and CT scans of chest, abdomen & pelvis showing no evidence of disease
- Must not have cardiovascular risk factors including unstable angina, history of myocardial infarction, or cerebrovascular accident, coronary artery bypass surgery, or NY Heart Assoc Class III or IV heart failure.

- Patients must not have known uncontrolled hyperlipidemia (defined as LDL-C >/= 190 mg/dL or triglycerides >/= 500 mg/dL within the past 3 years or uncontrolled high blood pressure (systolic blood pressure > 150 mm Hg) within 28 days prior to registration
- At least 30 days from completion of adjuvant chemo and RT.
- Presence of gastroesophageal reflux disease acceptable if controlled with medications
- Not receiving or planning to receive concomitant corticosteroids,nonsteroidal anti-inflammatory drugs(NSAIDs), nor anticoagulants. Maximum aspirin dose
- 100 mg per day or ≤ two 325 mg tablets per week.
- Able to swallow oral medications
- Laboratory: WBC ≥ 4.0 x 103/mcL, platelets ≥ 100,000/mcL and hemoglobin > 11.0 g/dL. Serum bilirubin ≤ 2.0 mg/dL and AST (SGOT) or ALT(SGPT) ≤ 2 x IULN. Serum creatinine ≤ 1.5 x IULN
- Zubrod PS 0-1, 18 years of age or older
- Will not participate in any other clinical trial for the treatment or prevention of cancer unless off protocol treatment, on follow-up phase only
- Offered opportunity to participate in blood specimen banking

Exclusion Criteria:
- History of colon resection > 40 cm
- Mid-low rectal cancer
- Recurrent or metastatic disease
- High cardiovascular risk; Uncontrolled hypertension
- Planned radiation therapy or additional chemotherapy
- Documented history of gastric/duodenal ulcer within last 12 months and/or current treatment or active symptoms of gastric/duodenal ulcer
- Known history of familial adenomatous polyposis, hereditary nonpolyposis colorectal cancer, or inflammatory bowel disease
- ≥ 30 dB uncorrectable hearing loss for age of any of the five tested frequencies on prestudy audiogram
- Known hypersensitivity to sulindac or excipient byproducts. Previous asthma, urticaria, or allergic-type reaction to aspirin or other NSAIDs
- Significant medical or psychiatric condition that would preclude study completion (8 years)
- No other prior malignancy except adequately treated basal cell or squamous cell skin cancer, in situ cervical cancer, or other cancer for which the patient has been disease-free for > 5 years
- Pregnant or nursing women. Women/men of reproductive potential must agree to use effective contraception

▨ **Sex/Gender**

All

▨ **Ages**

18 Years to N/A

▨ **Accepts Healthy Volunteers**

No

▨ **Contacts**

Patricia N. O'Kane, B.S.   210-614-8808   pokane@swog.org
Kimberly J Kaberle, B.S.   210-614-8808   kkaberle@swog.org

A Study of LGK974 in Patients With Malignancies Dependent on Wnt Ligands

Study ID:

NCT01351103

Sponsor:

Novartis Pharmaceuticals

Information provided by (Responsible Party):

Novartis (Novartis Pharmaceuticals)

Tracking Information

First Submitted Date

May 4, 2011

Start Date

December 1, 2011

Primary Completion Date

September 25, 2018

Last Update Posted Date

January 4, 2018

Current Primary Outcome Measures

Maximum Tolerated Dose or Recommended Dose for Expansion of LGK974 as a single agent or in combination with PDR001 in patients treated[Time Frame: 34 months]

> Determine the Maximum Tolerated Dose (MTD) or Recommended Dose for Expansion (RDE) of LGK974 as a single agent and in combination with PDR001 when administered orally to adult patients with malignancies dependent on Wnt ligands.

Current Secondary Outcome Measures

Type and category of study drug related adverse events (AE)[Time Frame: 61 months]

> The incidence of treatment-emergent adverse events (new or worsening from baseline) will be summarized by primary system organ class, severity based on the Common Terminology Criteria for Adverse Events (CTCAE) version 4.03, type of AE, relationship to study drug by dose group. Deaths reportable as SAEs and non-fatal serious adverse events will be listed by patient and tabulated by primary system organ clase, type of AE and dose group.

Absorption and plasma concentrations of LGK974[Time Frame: 61 months]

> Evaluate pharmacokinetic (PK) parameters such as AUClast, AUCtau, Cmax, the apparent elimination T1/2 and Racc for LGK974 and its pharmacologically metabolite. This will include but is not limited to the following timepoints: 8 times at C1D1; C1D2, C1D8, C1D16 and C1D22 pre-dose; 8 times at C1D15; and then pre-dose for each subsequent cycles D1.

Biomarkers related to the Wnt pathway[Time Frame: 61 months]

> Assessing percent change from baseline to post-treatment of biomarkers related to the Wnt pathway.

Overall response rate of tumor[Time Frame: 61 months]

> Patients with an Objective Overall Response (OOR) were those whose best response to treatment was a complete response (CR) or a partial response (PR) assessed by RECIST 1.1 or irRC . A patient had a CR if the target tumors disappeared. A patient had a PR if there was a ≥ 30% reduction in the sum of the products of the largest perpendicular diameters of the target tumors compared to the baseline value. Duration of Response (DOR) will also be summarized and is defined as the time from first observation of response to the first time of progression or death.

Absorportion and plasma concentrations of PDR001[Time Frame: 61 months]

> Evaluate pharmacokinetic (PK) parameters such as AUClast, AUCtau, Cmax, the apparent elimination T1/2 and Racc for LGK974, its pharmacologically metabolite and PDR001. Serial timpoints will be obtained on C1D1 and within C1 dosing, pre-dose samples may also be obtained during study treatment..

Biomarkers related to immunomodulation[Time Frame: 61 months]

> Evaluate biomarkers of immunomodulation after treatment with LGK974 and PDR001.

Descriptive Information

Offical Title

A Phase I, Open-label, Dose Escalation Study of Oral LGK974 in Patients With Malignancies Dependent on Wnt Ligands

Brief Summary

This primary purpose of this study is to find the recommended dose of LGK974 as a single agent and in combination with PDR001 that can be safely given to adult patients with selected solid malignancies for whom no effective standard treatment is available.

Study Type

Interventional

Study Phase

Phase 1

Condition

- Pancreatic Cancer
- BRAF Mutant Colorectal Cancer
- Other Tumor Types With Documented Genetic Alterations Upstream in the Wnt Signaling Pathway
- Melanoma
- Triple Negative Breast Cancer

- Head and Neck Cancer

- ## Intervention

  Drug: LGK974
  > Biological: PDR001

- ## Study Arms

  Experimental: LGK974
  Experimental: LGK974 in combination with PDR001

Recruitment Information

- ### Recruitment Status

  Recruiting

- ### Estimated Enrollment

  170

- ### Completion Date

  January 10, 2020

- ### Primary Completion Date

  September 25, 2018

- ### Eligibility Criteria

  Inclusion Criteria:

  Diagnosis of locally advanced or metastatic cancer that has progressed despite standard therapy or for which no effective standard therapy exists and histological confirmation of one of the following diseases indicated below:

  Single Agent Dose escalation part:documented B-RAF mutant colorectal cancer or pancreatic adenocarcinoma. In addition, tumors of any histological origin with documented genetic alterations upstream in the Wnt signaling pathway are eligible with prior agreement with Novartis.

  Single Agent Dose expansion part: documented B-RAF mutant colorectal cancer with documented RNF43 mutation and/or RSPO fusion or pancreatic adenocarcinoma with documented RNF43 mutation. In addition, patients with tumors of any histological origin with documented genetic alterations upstream in the Wnt signaling pathway (e.g. RNF43 or RSPO fusion) are eligible with prior agreement with Novartis

  LGK974 with PDR001: Dose escalation: melanoma patients primary refractory to anti-PD-1 inhibitor. Dose expansion: patients with pancreatic cancer, or TNBC, or melanoma, or head and neck cancer.

  Exclusion Criteria:

  - Impaired cardiac function
  - Impairment of gastrointestinal function or gastrointestinal disease that may significantly alter the absorption of oral LGK974 (e.g., ulcerative diseases, uncontrolled nausea, vomiting, diarrhea, malabsorption syndrome, small bowel resection)
  - Brain metastases that have not been adequately treated
  - Malignant disease other than that being treated in this study
  - Laboratory abnormalities as specified in the protocol
  - Osteoporosis, severe or untreated osteopenia
  - Bone fractures within the past year
  - Pathologic bone fracture
  - Active, known or suspected autoimmune disease or severe hypersensitivity reactions to other monoclonal antibodies

  Other protocol-defined inclusion/exclusion criteria may apply

- ### Sex/Gender

  All

- ### Ages

  18 Years to N/A

- ### Accepts Healthy Volunteers

  No

- ### Contacts

  Novartis Pharmaceuticals   1-888-669-6682   Novartis.email@novartis.com
  Novartis Pharmaceuticals   +41613241111

Vaccine Therapy in Treating Patients With Metastatic Solid Tumors

Study ID:

NCT01376505

Sponsor:

Pravin Kaumaya

Information provided by (Responsible Party):

Ohio State University Comprehensive Cancer Center (Pravin Kaumaya)

Tracking Information

First Submitted Date

June 9, 2011

Start Date

June 2011

Primary Completion Date

December 2017

Last Update Posted Date

June 16, 2017

Current Primary Outcome Measures

Type and duration of immune response measured over time to repeat vaccine administration[Time Frame: up to 6 months]

Immune response will be defined by Enzyme-linked immunosorbent assay (ELISA), Flow cytometry, T-cell proliferation and cytokine. The magnitude of antibody levels will be assessed to the vaccine and HER-2 over-expressing cells (e.g.,BT474). Lymphoproliferative responses will be assessed by a non radioactive cell proliferation assay Bioplex human isotyping kit will be used to assess antibody types and cytokine profiles.

Clinical benefit will be assessed[Time Frame: up to 6 months]

Will re-evaluate disease status with tumor markers and RESIST criteria,or full evaluation upon development of new symptoms

Current Secondary Outcome Measures

Evaluation of safety and toxicity at regular intervals by NCI common toxicity criteria (CTCAE v 4.0)[Time Frame: up to 6 months]

Safety will be defined if patients are able to receive all 3 vaccinations without dose-limiting toxicity (DLT), any incidence of grade 3 hematologic and non-hematologic toxicity or any incidence of Grade 4 toxicity. The development of a positive skin test to the vaccine immediate hypersensitivity

Descriptive Information

Offical Title

Phase I Active Immunotherapy Trial With a Combination of Two Chimeric (Trastuzumab-like and Pertuzumab-like)Human Epidermal Growth Factor Receptor 2 (HER-2) B Cell Peptide Vaccine Emulsified in ISA 720 and Nor-MDP Adjuvant in Patients With Advanced Solid Tumors

Brief Summary

This phase I trial studies the side effects and best dose of vaccine therapy in treating patients with metastatic solid tumors. Vaccines made from antibodies and peptides combined with tumor cells may help the body build an effective immune response to kill tumor cells.

Detailed Description

PRIMARY OBJECTIVES:

I. To perform early phase clinical trial assessing safety and clinical toxicity of immunization, and as well as to establish an optimal biological dose (OBD) of combination vaccines with n-muramyldipeptide derivative (nor-MDP) as adjuvant emulsified in Montanide (ISA 720).

II. To establish whether an OBD of two combination vaccines is achieved. III. To measure both humoral and cellular immune responses including the specificity, class and kinetics of anti-human epidermal growth factor receptor-2 (HER-2) peptide.

IV. To evaluate whether the combination of HER-2 epitopes show therapeutic benefit, provide synergistic and/or additive effects and to enumerate mechanisms of action.

SECONDARY OBJECTIVES:

I. To collect and analyze post-immune sera and peripheral blood cells for additional six months post the last injection.

II. To document any clinical responses that may occur.

OUTLINE: This is a dose-escalation study.

Patients receive a HER2/neu peptide vaccine comprising measles virus epitope MVF-HER-2 (266-296) and MVF-HER-2 (597-

626) emulsified with nor-MDP in ISA 720 intramuscularly (IM) on day 1. Treatment repeats every 21 days for up to 3 courses in the absence of disease progression or unacceptable toxicity.

After completion of study treatment, patients are followed up for 30 days.

OUTLINE: EXTENSION TRIAL AT OBD

The dose-escalation (4 cohorts) has successfully completed with the accrual of 24 patients and the Optimum biological dose (OBD) has been determined as the dose at cohort level 2.

The next phase of the study progresses directly into an extension trial at the OBD. 12 patients will be accrued at that level. The extension cohort will be open to only HER-2 and/or EGFR overexpressing cancers. Patients (all gastrointestinal,ovarian and breast must have received no more than three prior cytotoxic chemotherapy regimens in the last two years after standard therapy. Patients (breast, ovarian and gastrointestinal cancers) must have received no more than three prior cytotoxic chemotherapy regimens in the last two years after standard therapy.

■ **Study Type**

Interventional

■ **Study Phase**

Phase 1

■ **Condition**

- Malignant Solid Tumour
- Breast Cancer
- Malignant Tumor of Colon
- GIST
- Ovarian Cancer

■ **Intervention**

Biological: HER-2 vaccine

Three intramuscular (IM) injections (separated by 21 days) of a mixture of two peptides {MVF-HER-2(597-626) and MVF-HER-2 (266-296)} vaccine emulsified with nor-MDP in ISA 720 vehicle. Increasing doses of the combined vaccine preparation emulsified with nor-MDP (0.025) mg and Montanide ISA 720 will be administered in a final volume of 1.0 ml. Starting at dose level 1, 1.0mg of each peptide will be used for vaccination. In increasing dosing cohorts 1.5mg, 2.0mg and 2.5mg will be used. Patients may also receive 6 months booster shots.

Other Names:

Synthetic peptides of HER-2 comprising B cell epitopes with a Promiscuous T cell epitope of Measles Virus.

Biological: Extension HER-2 vaccine trial at OBD

Three intramuscular (IM) injections (separated by 21 days) of a mixture of two peptides {MVF-HER-2(597-626) and MVF-HER-2 (266-296)} vaccine emulsified with nor-MDP in ISA 720 vehicle. The dose level has been determined to be cohort 2. The combined vaccine preparation consists of 1.5mg of each of the HER-2 vaccine emulsified with nor-MDP (0.025) mg and Montanide ISA 720 will be administered in a final volume of 1.0 ml. Patients may also receive 6 months booster shots.

■ **Study Arms**

Experimental: HER-2 Vaccine

combination of MVF-HER-2 (597-626) and MVF-HER-2 (266-296) emulsified with nor-MDP and ISA 720

This escalation arm has completed. The trial has moved on to the extension arm

Experimental: EXTENSION HER-2 Vaccine at OBD

Combination of MVF-HER-2 (597-626) and MVF-HER-2 (266-296) emulsified with nor-MDP and ISA 720 at dose level cohort 2

This extension arm is ongoing

Recruitment Information

■ **Recruitment Status**

Recruiting

■ **Estimated Enrollment**

36

■ **Completion Date**

December 2017

■ **Primary Completion Date**

December 2017

■ **Eligibility Criteria**

Inclusion Criteria:

- Must have histologically confirmed metastatic solid tumor; the malignancy should be considered incurable using standard treatment

- Patients are not required to have HER-2 over-expression to be on this study
- If the patient has had HER-2 expression measured prior to enrollment, the report alone will be accepted
- If the patient has not had HER-2 expression measured prior to enrollment on this study tumor tissue blocks and/or freshly isolated tissue must be available for determination of HER-2 expression
- Patients are not required to have epidermal growth factor receptor (EGFR) over-expression to be on this study
- If the patient has had EGFR expression measured prior to enrollment, the report alone will be accepted
- If the patient has not had EGFR expression measured prior to enrollment on this study tumor tissue blocks and/or freshly isolated tissue must be available for determination of EGFR expression
- Patients with prior history of treated brain metastases who are off steroids and have stable metastatic brain disease for at least 3 months are eligible
- Patients must be ambulatory with an Eastern Cooperative Oncology Group (ECOG) performance status of 0, 1, or 2
- White blood cells > 3500/mm^3
- Platelet count > 100,000/mm^3
- Serum bilirubin < 1.5 mg %, regardless of whether patients have liver involvement secondary to tumor
- Alanine aminotransferase (ALT) must be < 2 times upper limit of normal
- Creatinine < 1.5 mg/dL or calculated creatinine clearance > 60 mL/min
- Patients will be tested for reactivity to a panel of four common microbial skin test antigens: candida, trichophyton, intermediate strength purified protein derivative (PPD), and tetanus toxoid; determination of patient eligibility for this trial will proceed independently of these skin test results; patients who have previously been tested for these antigens but were excluded from participation in the trial due to non-reactivity may be considered as eligible provided that all other eligibility criteria are met
- Patients must be at least 4 weeks past any prior surgery, cytotoxic, chemotherapy, other immunotherapy, hormonal therapy, or radiation therapy; patients having been treated with monoclonal antibodies may enter the trial after a specified period of time (2 times the mean half life of the agent); patients must have recovered from any toxicity of prior therapy prior to enrolling on study except for neuropathy where patients need to recover to less than grade 2
- Women of child-bearing potential must not be pregnant and must have a negative pregnancy test; men and women must agree to practice effective contraception while on this study
- Patients must obtain a base line Echocardiogram or multi gated acquisition scan (MUGA) and require the left ventricular ejection fraction to be within normal limits (or 50% or higher)
- Ability to understand and the willingness to sign a written informed consent document; the patient must be aware that his/her disease is neoplastic in nature and willingly consent after being informed of the procedure to be followed, the experimental nature of the therapy, alternatives, potential benefits, side-effects, risks, and discomforts

Exclusion Criteria:
- Patients who are {MVF-HER-2(266-296) and MVF-HER-2 (597-626)} immediate hypersensitivity skin test positive
- Patients who have evidence of active infection that requires antibiotic therapy; patients must have been off antibiotic treatment for at least 3 weeks prior to initiating treatment and must be confirmed to be clear of the infection; if patient develops an infection requiring antibiotic treatment while on the treatment portion of the study patients will be treated for the active infection with antibiotics and will resume vaccine treatment when the infection is healed
- Patients with known active human immunodeficiency virus (HIV), hepatitis A, hepatitis B, or hepatitis C infection
- Patients with serious cardiopulmonary disorders, including congestive heart failure, symptomatic coronary artery disease, serious cardiac arrhythmia, and symptomatic chronic obstructive pulmonary disease or patients with other serious uncontrolled medical diseases
- Patients who require or likely to require corticosteroids or other immunosuppressives for intercurrent disease are NOT eligible
- Splenectomized patients
- Autoimmune diseases including rheumatoid arthritis, systemic lupus erythematosus, scleroderma, polymyositis dermatomyositis, or a vasculitic syndrome
- Patients who have developed anaphylactic responses to other vaccines
- History of congestive heart failure, coronary artery disease and myocardial infarction; active or unstable cardiovascular disease or cardiac disease requiring drug or device intervention

ADDITIONAL KEY ELIGIBILITY CRITERIA FOR EXTENSION & EXPANSION COHORT:
- Histologically documented metastatic or unresectable breast, ovarian and gastrointestinal cancers
- Progressive disease after at least one line of standard therapy
- Patients must have received or refused first line standard systemic therapy for their metastases (if applicable)
- Patients (pancreatic and esophageal cancers) must have received no more than two prior cytotoxic chemotherapy regimens in the last two years after standard therapy. Patients (breast and gastrointestinal cancers) must have received no more than three prior cytotoxic chemotherapy regimens in the last two years after standard therapy.
- Measurable disease, defined as ≥ 1 lesions that can be accurately measured in ≥ 1 dimensions as ≥ 20 mm with conventional techniques or as ≥ 10 mm with spiral CT scan
- Disease that is amenable to biopsy and be willing to undergo tumor biopsy

- ▩ **Sex/Gender**

  All
- ▩ **Ages**

  18 Years to N/A
- ▩ **Accepts Healthy Volunteers**

  No
- ▩ **Contacts**

  Pravin Kaumaya, PhD   614-292-7028   pravin.kaumaya@osumc.edu

Efficacy Evaluation of TheraSphere Following Failed First Line Chemotherapy in Metastatic Colorectal Cancer

Study ID:

NCT01483027

Sponsor:

BTG International Inc.

Information provided by (Responsible Party):

BTG International Inc. (BTG International Inc.)

Tracking Information

- ▩ **First Submitted Date**

  November 24, 2011
- ▩ **Start Date**

  January 2012
- ▩ **Current Primary Outcome Measures**

  Progression free survival[Time Frame: From date of randomization until the date of first documented progression or date of death from any cause, whichever comes first, assessed up to 36 months]

- ▩ **Primary Completion Date**

  September 2018
- ▩ **Last Update Posted Date**

  September 1, 2017

Descriptive Information

- ▩ **Offical Title**

  A Phase III Clinical Trial Evaluating TheraSphere® in Patients With Metastatic Colorectal Carcinoma of the Liver Who Have Failed First Line Chemotherapy
- ▩ **Brief Summary**

  The effectiveness and safety of TheraSphere will be evaluated in patients with colorectal cancer with metastases in the liver, who are scheduled to receive second line chemotherapy. All patients receive the standard of care chemotherapy with or without the addition of TheraSphere.
- ▩ **Study Type**

  Interventional
- ▩ **Study Phase**

  Phase 3
- ▩ **Condition**

  - Colorectal Cancer Metastatic
- ▩ **Intervention**

  Device: TheraSphere
     yttrium 90 microspheres
- ▩ **Study Arms**

  Experimental: Treatment group

Standard of care second-line chemotherapy plus TheraSphere

No Intervention: Control group
Standard of care second-line chemotherapy with no added therapy

Recruitment Information

▨ **Recruitment Status**

Recruiting

▨ **Estimated Enrollment**

340

▨ **Completion Date**

February 2019

▨ **Primary Completion Date**

September 2018

▨ **Eligibility Criteria**

Inclusion Criteria

- Must be male or female, 18 years of age or older, and of any ethnic or racial group
- Not resected primary tumor; must be clinically stable
- Colorectal cancer with unresectable metastatic disease to the liver (unresectable unilobar or bilobar disease) who have disease progression in the liver with oxaliplatin or irinotecan based first line chemotherapy
- Eligible to receive second-line standard-of-care chemotherapy with either 1) an oxaliplatin-based chemotherapy regimen, or 2) an irinotecan-based chemotherapy regimen
- Baseline efficacy images with measurable target tumors in the liver according to RECIST 1.1 using standard imaging techniques taken within 28 days prior to randomization. Images must be taken after, or at the time of completion of first line chemotherapy
- Tumor replacement <50% of total liver volume
- Eastern Cooperative Oncology Group (ECOG) of 0-1 through screening to first treatment
- First line chemotherapy regimen completed at least 14 days prior to initiation of 2nd line chemotherapy under the protocol
- Patient is willing to participate in the study and has signed the study informed consent
- Serum creatinine ≤ 2.0 mg/dL
- Serum bilirubin up to 1.2 x upper limit of normal
- Albumin ≥ 3.0 g/dL
- Neutrophil count >1200/cubic mm

Exclusion Criteria

- History of hepatic encephalopathy
- Contraindications to angiography and selective visceral catheterization such as bleeding diathesis or coagulopathy that is not correctable by usual therapy of hemostatic agents
- History of severe peripheral allergy or intolerance to contrast agents, narcotics, sedatives or atropine that cannot be managed medically
- Presentation of pulmonary insufficiency or clinically evident chronic obstructive pulmonary disease
- Cirrhosis or portal hypertension
- Prior external beam radiation treatment to the liver
- Prior intra-arterial liver directed therapy, including transcatheter arterial chemoembolization (TACE) or Y-90 microsphere therapy
- Planned treatment with biological agents within 28 days prior to receiving TheraSphere (may resume after Y-90 treatment or immediately if in control arm)
- Planned liver directed therapy or radiation therapy
- Intervention for, or compromise of, the Ampulla of Vater
- Clinically evident ascites (trace ascites on imaging is acceptable)
- Toxicities due to prior cancer therapy that have not resolved before the initiation of study treatment, if the Investigator determines that the continuing complication will compromise the safe treatment of the patient
- Significant life-threatening extra-hepatic disease, including patients who are on dialysis, have unresolved diarrhea, have serious unresolved infections including patients who are known to be human immunodeficiency virus (HIV) positive or have acute hepatitis B virus (HBV) or hepatitis C virus (HCV)
- confirmed extra-hepatic metastases. Limited indeterminate extra-hepatic lesions in the lung and/or lymph nodes are permitted (up to 5 lesions in the lung, with each individual lesion <1 cm; any number of lymph nodes with each individual nodes <1.5 cm)
- Contraindications to the planned second line standard-of-care chemotherapy regimen
- Women of childbearing potential must have a negative serum pregnancy test within 14 days prior to randomization, and must not be breastfeeding and must agree to use contraceptive for duration of study.
- Participation in a clinical trial with an investigational therapy within 30 days prior to randomization
- Co-morbid disease or condition that would place the patient at undue risk and preclude safe use of TheraSphere treatment, in

the Investigator's judgment

■ **Sex/Gender**

All

■ **Ages**

18 Years to N/A

■ **Accepts Healthy Volunteers**

No

■ **Contacts**

John Saliba   +79 81 881 6336   John.Saliba@chiltern.com
Judith Koehnen   +49 (0)221-80068367   judith.Koehnen@Chiltern.com

PROSPECT: Chemotherapy Alone or Chemotherapy Plus Radiation Therapy in Treating Patients With Locally Advanced Rectal Cancer Undergoing Surgery

Study ID:

NCT01515787

Sponsor:

Alliance for Clinical Trials in Oncology

Information provided by (Responsible Party):

Alliance for Clinical Trials in Oncology (Alliance for Clinical Trials in Oncology)

Tracking Information

■ **First Submitted Date**

January 18, 2012

■ **Start Date**

January 2012

■ **Current Primary Outcome Measures**

Pelvic R0 resection rate (Phase II)[Time Frame: Up to 8 years]
DFS (Phase III)[Time Frame: Up to 8 years]

Time to local recurrence (TLR)[Time Frame: Up to 8 years]

■ **Primary Completion Date**

January 2021

■ **Last Update Posted Date**

February 6, 2018

■ **Current Secondary Outcome Measures**

Pathologic complete response[Time Frame: Up to 8 years]
Overall survival[Time Frame: Up to 8 years]

Adverse event (AE) profiles[Time Frame: Up to 8 years]

- Rates of receiving preor post-operative 5FUCMT[Time Frame: Up to 8 years]

Descriptive Information

■ **Offical Title**

A Phase II/III Trial of Neoadjuvant FOLFOX With Selective Use of Combined Modality Chemoradiation Versus Preoperative Combined Modality Chemoradiation for Locally Advanced Rectal Cancer Patients Undergoing Low Anterior Resection With Total Mesorectal Excision (PROSPECT)

■ **Brief Summary**

The standard treatment for locally advanced rectal cancer involves chemotherapy and radiation, known as 5FUCMT, (the chemotherapy drugs 5-fluorouracil/capecitabine and radiation therapy) prior to surgery. Although radiation therapy to the pelvis has been a standard and important part of treatment for rectal cancer and has been shown to decrease the risk of the cancer coming back in the same area in the pelvis, some patients experience undesirable side effects from the radiation and there have been important advances in chemotherapy, surgery, and radiation which may be of benefit. The purpose of this study is to compare the effects, both good and bad, of the standard treatment of chemotherapy and radiation to chemotherapy using a combination regimen known as FOLFOX, (the drugs 5-fluorouracil (5-FU), oxaliplatin and leucovorin) and selective use of the standard treatment, depending on response to the FOLFOX. The drugs in the FOLFOX regimen are all FDA (Food and Drug Administration) approved and have been used routinely to treat patients with advanced colorectal cancer.

Detailed Description

OUTLINE: This is a multicenter, phase II/III study. Patients are stratified according to ECOG performance status (0 or 1 vs 2) and randomized to 1 of 2 treatment regimens. Patients will receive full supportive care while on this study.

OBJECTIVES:

Primary

1. Phase II component: To assure that neoadjuvant FOLFOX followed by selective use of 5FUCMT group (Group 1) maintains the current high rate of pelvic R0 resection and is consistent with non-inferiority for time to local recurrence (TLR).

2. Phase III component: To compare neoadjuvant FOLFOX followed by selective use of 5FUCMT (Group 1) to standard 5FUCMT (Group 2) with respect to the co-primary endpoints of the Time to Local Recurrence (TLR) and Disease-Free Survival (DFS).

Secondary

1. To determine if the neoadjuvant FOLFOX followed by selective use of 5FUCMT (Group 1) is non-inferior to the standard group 5FUCMT (Group 2) with respect to the proportion of patients who achieve a pathologic complete response (pCR) at the time of surgical resection.

2. To determine if the neoadjuvant FOLFOX followed by selective use of 5FUCMT (Group 1) is non-inferior to the standard 5FUCMT (Group 2) with respect to overall survival.

3. To evaluate and compare the adverse event profile and surgery complications between two groups.

- 4. To estimate the proportion of patients in the selective group (Group 1) who receive: 1) pre-operative 5FUCMT; 2) post-operative 5FUCMT; 3) either preor post-operative 5FUCMT.

Event monitoring of patients will continue up to 8 years post randomization.

Study Type

Interventional

Study Phase

Phase 2/Phase 3

Condition

- Colorectal Cancer

Intervention

Drug: FOLFOX (chemotherapy)

Oxaliplatin 85 mg/m^2 IV over 2 hours on day 1, leucovorin 400 mg/m^2 bolus IV over 2 hours on day 1 and 5-fluorouracil 400 mg/m^2 bolus over 5-15 minutes then 2400 mg/m^2 continual over 46-48 hours total dose IV on days 1-2. The treatment schedule repeats based on the group. Dose modifications are allowed based on adverse events.

Other: 5 FUCMT (chemoradiation)

5-fluorouracil 225 mg/m^2 per day continuous IV infusion administered concurrently with radiation therapy for 5 or 7 days per week OR capecitabine 825 mg/m^2 twice daily administered orally and concurrently with radiation therapy for 5 days per week. Dose modifications are allowed based on adverse events.

Procedure: surgery

low anterior resection with total mesorectal excision

Procedure: magnetic resonance imaging or endorectal ultrasound

Study Arms

Experimental: Group 1

Patients will receive FOLFOX chemotherapy once every two weeks for 6 cycles total over a period of 12 weeks. After completing FOLFOX chemotherapy, the patient will have an MRI scan or endorectal ultrasound (ERUS) to examine the tumor. If the tumor has not decreased in size by at least 20%, the patient will receive 5FUCMT (radiation with chemotherapy). If the tumor has decreased in size by 20%, then the patient will proceed directly to surgery.

If all borders of the tumor are normal post surgery, then the patient receives six additional cycles of FOLFOX chemotherapy. If all borders of the tumor are not normal then the patient receives chemoradiation therapy for 5.5 weeks after surgery. After chemoradiation, additional cycles of FOLFOX or similar chemotherapy will be recommended for 4 cycles or 8 weeks. Patient observation with follow up evaluations and event monitoring will occur up to 8 years post randomization.

Active Comparator: Group 2

Patients receive 5FUCMT including chemotherapy and radiation therapy for 5.5 weeks. Patients will be given either 5-fluorouracil or capecitabine and radiation therapy. After the chemoradiation therapy is completed, patients will proceed directly to surgery. Post-surgery, patients will receive FOLFOX chemotherapy once every two weeks for 8 cycles total over a period of 16 weeks. Patient observation with follow up evaluations and event monitoring will occur up to 8 years post randomization.

Recruitment Information

Recruitment Status

Recruiting

Estimated Enrollment

1120

Completion Date

N/A

Primary Completion Date

January 2021

Eligibility Criteria

Registration Inclusion Criteria:

1. Age ≥ 18 years at diagnosis

2. Diagnosis of rectal adenocarcinoma

3. Radiologically measurable or clinically evaluable disease as defined in the protocol

4. ECOG Performance Status (PS): 0, 1 or 2

5. For this patient, the standard treatment recommendation in the absence of a clinical trial would be combined modality neoadjuvant chemoradiation followed by curative intent surgical resection

6. Candidate for sphincter-sparing surgical resection prior to neoadjuvant therapy according to the primary surgeon

7. Primary surgeon is credentialed or is willing to be credentialed in Total Mesorectal Excision (TME), which entails submission of photos of a single TME specimen either before enrolling the first patient or by using the surgeon's 1st accrued case.

8. Clinical Stage: T2N1, T3N0, T3N1.

- N2 disease is to be estimated as four or more lymph nodes that are ≥ 10 mm.

- Clinical staging should be estimated based on the combination of the following assessments: physical exam by the primary surgeon, CT or PET/CT scan of the chest/abdomen/pelvis and either a pelvic MRI or an ultrasound (ERUS). If a pelvic MRI is peformed, it is acceptable to perform CT of the chest/abdomen, ommitting CT imaging of the pelvis.

9. The following laboratory values obtained ≤ 28 days prior to registration:

- Absolute neutrophil count (ANC) ≥ 1500/mm^3

- Platelet count ≥ 100,000/mm^3

- Hemoglobin > 8.0 g/dL

- Total bilirubin ≤ 1.5 x upper limit of normal (ULN)

- SGOT (AST) ≤ 3 x ULN

- SGPT (ALT) ≤ 3 x ULN

- Creatinine ≤1.5 x ULN

10. Negative pregnancy test done ≤ 7 days prior to registration, for women of childbearing potential only

11. Patient of child-bearing potential is willing to employ adequate contraception

12. Provide informed written consent

13. Willing to return to enrolling medical site for all study assessments

Registration Exclusion Criteria:

1. Clinical T4 tumors

2. Primary surgeon indicates need for abdominoperineal (APR) at baseline

3. Evidence that the tumor is adherent to or invading the mesorectal fascia on imaging studies such that the surgeon would not be able to perform an R0 resection (one with negative margins)

4. Tumor is causing symptomatic bowel obstruction (patients who have had a temporary diverting ostomy are eligible).

5. Chemotherapy within 5 years prior to registration. Hormonal therapy is allowable if the disease free interval is ≥ 5 years.

6. Any prior pelvic radiation

7. Other invasive malignancy ≤ 5 years prior to registration. Exceptions are colonic polyps, non-melanoma skin cancer, ductal carcinoma in situ, bladder carcinoma in situ, or carcinoma-in-situ of the cervix.

8. Any of the following because this study involves an agent that has known genotoxic, mutagenic and teratogenic effects.

- Pregnant women

- Nursing women

- Men or women of childbearing potential who are unwilling to employ adequate contraception

9. Co-morbid illnesses or other concurrent disease which, in the judgment of the clinician obtaining informed consent, would make the patient inappropriate for entry into this study or interfere significantly with the proper assessment of safety and toxicity of the prescribed regimens.

Sex/Gender

All

Ages

18 Years to N/A

Dose Finding Study of Once or Twice Weekly IMMU-130 in Metastatic Colorectal Cancer

Study ID:

NCT01605318

Sponsor:

Immunomedics, Inc.

Information provided by (Responsible Party):

Immunomedics, Inc. (Immunomedics, Inc.)

Tracking Information

- First Submitted Date

  May 22, 2012

- Start Date

  September 2012

- Primary Completion Date

  December 2016

- Last Update Posted Date

  March 21, 2016

- Current Primary Outcome Measures

  Safety[Time Frame: Safety during treatment and every 3 months after treatment]

  Safety and tolerability will be evaluated from adverse events, standard safety laboratories (CBC with differential and platelet count, serum chemistries, urinalysis), physical examination, vital signs, and EKG. Adverse events will be classified according to the MedDRA system of preferred terms and system organ class, and all adverse events and abnormal laboratories will be classified for severity using NCI CTCAE v4.0 toxicity grades. Descriptive statistics will be used to characterize adverse events, cytopenias, and other abnormal laboratories.

- Current Secondary Outcome Measures

  Efficacy[Time Frame: measured every 8 weeks during treatement & every 3 months after treatment]

  CT (chest, abdomen, pelvis; other if needed) and serum CEA are done every 8 weeks after first dose until the end of treatment or progression of disease and then every 3 months during follow up. CT may be obtained more frequently at the physician discretion to assess disease status.for up to 2 years or until progression of disease.

Descriptive Information

- Offical Title

  A Phase I/II Study of Once or Twice Weekly IMMU-130 (hMN-14-SN38, Antibody-Drug Conjugate) in Patients With Colorectal Cancer.

- Brief Summary

  This is a Phase I/II, open-label study of IMMU-130 administered in 21-day treatment cycles, once or twice weekly for 2 consecutive weeks followed by one week of rest to patients with metastatic colorectal cancer who have been previously treated with at least one prior irinotecan-containing regimen. The study is being done to evaluate whether the study drug is safe and tolerable at different dose levels with these dosing schedules and to obtain preliminary information on its efficacy.

- Study Type

  Interventional

- Study Phase

  Phase 1/Phase 2

- Condition

  - Metastatic Colorectal Cancer
  - Colon Cancer
  - Rectal Cancer

Intervention

Drug: IMMU-130

This is a Phase I/II, open-label study of IMMU-130 administered in 21-day treatment cycles, once or twice weekly for 2 consecutive weeks followed by one week of rest to patients with metastatic colorectal cancer who have been previously treated with at least one prior irinotecan-containing regimen.

Other Names:

hMN14-SN38

Labetuzumab-SN38

Antibody-Drug Conjugate

Study Arms

Experimental: IMMU-130

All patients receive IMMU-130 administered in 21-day treatment cycles consisting of once or twice weekly for 2 consecutive weeks followed by a 1-week rest period. Treatment can be continued in the absence of unacceptable toxicity for a period of up to 8 cycles until the first documentation of Progressive Disease by CT (physician discretion), but must terminate study treatment upon the second documentation of Progressive Disease.

Publications

(Includes publications given by the data provider as well as publications identified by ClinicalTrials.gov Identifier (NCT Number) in Medline.)Govindan SV, Goldenberg DM. New antibody conjugates in cancer therapy. ScientificWorldJournal. 2010 Oct 12;10:2070-89. doi: 10.1100/tsw.2010.191. Review. (https://www.ncbi.nlm.nih.gov/pubmed/20953556)

Govindan SV, Cardillo TM, Moon SJ, Hansen HJ, Goldenberg DM. CEACAM5-targeted therapy of human colonic and pancreatic cancer xenografts with potent labetuzumab-SN-38 immunoconjugates. Clin Cancer Res. 2009 Oct 1;15(19):6052-61. doi: 10.1158/1078-0432.CCR-09-0586. Epub 2009 Sep 29. (https://www.ncbi.nlm.nih.gov/pubmed/19789330)

Moon SJ, Govindan SV, Cardillo TM, D'Souza CA, Hansen HJ, Goldenberg DM. Antibody conjugates of 7-ethyl-10-hydroxycamptothecin (SN-38) for targeted cancer chemotherapy. J Med Chem. 2008 Nov 13;51(21):6916-26. doi: 10.1021/jm800719t. Epub 2008 Oct 22. (https://www.ncbi.nlm.nih.gov/pubmed/18939816)

Govindan SV, Griffiths GL, Hansen HJ, Horak ID, Goldenberg DM. Cancer therapy with radiolabeled and drug/toxin-conjugated antibodies. Technol Cancer Res Treat. 2005 Aug;4(4):375-91. Review. (https://www.ncbi.nlm.nih.gov/pubmed/16029057)

Recruitment Information

Recruitment Status

Recruiting

Estimated Enrollment

104

Completion Date

December 2016

Primary Completion Date

December 2016

Eligibility Criteria

Inclusion Criteria:

- Male or female patients, ≥ 18 years of age, able to understand and give written informed consent.
- Histologically or cytologically confirmed colorectal adenocarcinoma.
- Stage IV (metastatic) disease.
- Previously treated with at least one prior irinotecan-containing regimen for colorectal cancer.
- Adequate performance status (ECOG 0 or 1). (Appendix 1)
- Expected survival > 6 months.
- CEA plasma levels > 5 ng/mL.
- Measurable disease by CT or MRI.
- At least 4 weeks beyond treatment (chemotherapy, immunotherapy and/or radiation therapy) or major surgery and recovered from all acute toxicities.
- At least 2 weeks beyond corticosteroids.
- Adequate hematology without ongoing transfusional support (hemoglobin > 9 g/dL, ANC > 1,500 per mm3, platelets > 100,000 per mm3).
- Adequate renal and hepatic function (creatinine ≤ 1.5 x IULN, bilirubin ≤ IULN, AST and ALT ≤ 3.0 x IULN or 5 x IULN if know liver metastases).
- Otherwise, all toxicity at study entry ≤ Grade 1 by NCI CTC v4.0.

Exclusion Criteria:

- Women who are pregnant or lactating.
- Women of childbearing potential and fertile men unwilling to use effective contraception during study until conclusion of 12-

week post-treatment evaluation period.
- Patients with Gilbert's disease or known CNS metastatic disease.
- Patients with CEA plasma levels > 1000 ng/mL are excluded during dose escalation, but may be included after the MTD is determined.
- Presence of bulky disease (defined as any single mass > 10 cm in its greatest dimension).
- Patients with active ≥ grade 2 anorexia, nausea or vomiting, and/or signs of intestinal obstruction.
- Patients with non-melanoma skin cancer or carcinoma in situ of the cervix are eligible, while patients with other prior malignancies must have had at least a 3-year disease-free interval.
- Patients known to be HIV positive, hepatitis B positive, or hepatitis C positive.
- Known history of unstable angina, MI, or CHF present within 6 months or clinically significant cardiac arrhythmia (other than stable atrial fibrillation) requiring anti-arrhythmia therapy.
- Known history of clinically significant active COPD, or other moderate-to-severe chronic respiratory illness present within 6 months.
- Infection requiring intravenous antibiotic use within 1 week.
- Other concurrent medical or psychiatric conditions that, in the Investigator's opinion, may be likely to confound study interpretation or prevent completion of study procedures and follow-up examinations.

Sex/Gender

All

Ages

18 Years to N/A

Accepts Healthy Volunteers

No

Contacts

Pius Maliakal, PhD   973-605-8200   pmaliakal@immunomedics.com
Roman Gomez, CCRP   973-605-8200   rgomez@immunomedics.com

Pilot 3D Contrast-Enhanced Ultrasound Imaging to Predict Treatment Response in Liver Metastases

Study ID:

NCT01631318

Sponsor:

Stanford University

Information provided by (Responsible Party):

Stanford University (Stanford University)

Tracking Information

First Submitted Date

June 26, 2012

Start Date

November 2012

Primary Completion Date

April 2019

Last Update Posted Date

January 12, 2017

Current Primary Outcome Measures

Measurements of blood flow, in terms of comparison of the perfusion parameters of the lesion as a predictor of tumor response to treatment and use as a biomarker for response to treatment[Time Frame: Baseline]

Descriptive statistics will be presented for lesion size, by lesion type, and across lesion types. Lesion shape, depth, vascularization, and border definition will also be categorized by dose and lesion type. Based on the unenhanced ultrasound, the target lesion to liver echogenicity will be categorized by lesion type. Based on the Definity®-enhanced ultrasound, the pattern of enhancement of the target lesion will be summarized by lesion type.

Measurements of blood flow, in terms of comparison of the perfusion parameters of the lesion as a predictor of tumor response to treatment and use as a biomarker for response to treatment[Time Frame: 2 weeks after chemotherapy initiation]

Descriptive statistics will be presented for lesion size, by lesion type, and across lesion types. Lesion shape, depth, vascularization, and border definition will also be categorized by dose and lesion type. Based on the unenhanced ultrasound, the target lesion to liver echogenicity will be categorized by lesion type. Based on the Definity®-enhanced ultrasound, the pattern of enhancement of the target lesion will be summarized by lesion type.

Measurements of blood flow, in terms of comparison of the perfusion parameters of the lesion as a predictor of tumor response to treatment and use as a biomarker for response to treatment[Time Frame: 2 months post-treatment]

Descriptive statistics will be presented for lesion size, by lesion type, and across lesion types. Lesion shape, depth, vascularization, and border definition will also be categorized by dose and lesion type. Based on the unenhanced ultrasound, the target lesion to liver echogenicity will be categorized by lesion type. Based on the Definity®-enhanced ultrasound, the pattern of enhancement of the target lesion will be summarized by lesion type.

Descriptive Information

▦ Offical Title

Pilot Technical Feasibility Study on 3D Contrast-enhanced Ultrasound Imaging and to Assess Whether Change in Ultrasound 3D Perfusion Pattern Can Predict Treatment Response

▦ Brief Summary

Patients are invited to participate in a research study of liver perfusion (how blood flows to the liver over time). Researchers hope to learn whether perfusion characteristics of liver metastases may be predictive of response to treatment and whether liver perfusion characteristics can be used to follow response to treatment. Patients were selected as a possible participant in this study because they are identified as having liver metastases

▦ Detailed Description

PRIMARY OBJECTIVES:

I. The purpose of this study is to perform a pilot feasibility study on 3-dimensional (3D) ultrasound imaging of liver metastases and to evaluate whether perfusion characteristics (measurements of blood-flow) of hepatic metastases can predict tumor response to treatment in patients with liver metastases. The investigators long term goal is to assess whether early perfusion changes at 2 weeks after chemotherapy initiation can be used as a non-invasive early biomarker for treatment response assessment.

OUTLINE:

Patients undergo 3D dynamic contrast-enhanced ultrasound imaging before initiation of chemotherapy, at 2 weeks, and at 2 months.

▦ Study Type

Interventional

▦ Study Phase

N/A

▦ Condition

- Liver Metastases
- Colon Cancer

▦ Intervention

Procedure: dynamic contrast-enhanced ultrasound imaging
Undergo 3D contrast enhanced ultrasound imaging

Other Names:
DCE-USI

▦ Study Arms

Experimental: Diagnostic (3D contrast-enhanced ultrasound imaging)
Patients undergo 3D dynamic contrast-enhanced ultrasound imaging before initiation of chemotherapy and at 2 weeks.

Recruitment Information

▦ Recruitment Status

Recruiting

▦ Estimated Enrollment

10

▦ Eligibility Criteria

Inclusion Criteria
- Provides written Informed Consent and is willing to comply with protocol requirements.

▦ Completion Date

N/A

▦ Primary Completion Date

April 2019

- Has at least 1 focal lesion in liver or kidney
- Patient may be (i) in the process of receiving treatment (1 scan session), (ii) never treated (3 scan sessions) or (iii) changing treatment regimen/ type and/or receiving a new form of treatment and/or has been on a treatment break ('holiday')(3 scan session)
- Is at least18 years of age.

Exclusion Criteria
- Is determined by the Investigator that the subject is clinically unsuitable for the study.
- Known right to left cardiac shunt, bidirectional or transient.
- Hypersensitivity to perflutren.
- Hypersenstivity to the contrast agent Definity.
- Pregnant and lactating women

Sex/Gender

All

Ages

18 Years to N/A

Accepts Healthy Volunteers

No

Phase I/II Study of IMMU-132 in Patients With Epithelial Cancers

Study ID:

NCT01631552

Sponsor:

Immunomedics, Inc.

Information provided by (Responsible Party):

Immunomedics, Inc. (Immunomedics, Inc.)

Tracking Information

First Submitted Date

June 26, 2012

Start Date

February 2013

Primary Completion Date

June 2018

Last Update Posted Date

June 14, 2017

Current Primary Outcome Measures

Safety[Time Frame: During treatment, at the final evaluation and at follow up after treatment]

Safety will be assessed by monitoring the patient for adverse events, monitoring the change in lab values during and after treatment compared to baseline over an average of 6 months.

Current Secondary Outcome Measures

Efficacy[Time Frame: Efficacy will be assessed every 8 weeks during treatment and then every 12 weeks after treatment]

Efficacy will be evaluated from CT scans (or MRI studies), using RECIST 1.1 to classify tumor response, time to onset of objective response, duration of objective response, and time to progression. Efficacy will be assessed every 8 weeks until the end of treatment or progression of disease and every 12 weeks at the follow up, over an average of 6 months.

Descriptive Information

Offical Title

A Phase I/II Study of IMMU-132 (hRS7-SN38 Antibody Drug Conjugate) in Patients With Epithelial Cancers

Brief Summary

The primary objective is to evaluate the safety and tolerability of IMMU-132 as a single agent administered in 3-week treatment cycles for up to 8 cycles, in previously treated patients with advanced epithelial cancer.The secondary objectives are to obtain initial data concerning pharmacokinetics, immunogenicity, and efficacy with this dosing regimen. IMMU-132 targets the TROP-

2 antigen which is expressed on a variety of cancers. The antibody, RS7, is attached to SN38, which is the active metabolite of irinotecan. This is planned as a multi-center study. In Phase II, up to 130 patients (assessable) in triple-negative breast cancer, up to 100 patients (assessable) in non-small cell and small-cell lung cancer and up to 50 patients (assessable) per other cancer types included in the protocol will be studied at the 10 mg/kg dose.

Detailed Description

This is a Phase I/II, open-label study of IMMU-132 in previously treated patients with advanced epithelial cancers, including ovarian, breast, prostate (hormone refractory), lung (non-small cell and small cell), head & neck (squamous cell), esophageal, gastric, colorectal, pancreatic, hepatocellular, renal (clear cell), endometrial, cervical, urothelial, thyroid cancers and glioblastoma multiforme. Patients receive IMMU-132 administered once-weekly for the first 2 weeks of 3-week treatment cycles. Patients may receive up to a maximum total of 8 cycles (16 doses), but patients with a partial response or stable disease at that time, or patients who had achieved an objective response but relapsed after discontinuing treatment, may continue to be treated based on physician discretion. Treatment will continue until unacceptable toxicity or progression of disease. Both safety and efficacy will be assessed.

Study Type

Interventional

Study Phase

Phase 1/Phase 2

Condition

- Colorectal Cancer
- Gastric Adenocarcinoma
- Esophageal Cancer
- Hepatocellular Carcinoma
- Non-small Cell Lung Cancer
- Small Cell Lung Cancer
- Ovarian Epithelial Cancer
- Carcinoma Breast Stage IV
- Hormone-refractory Prostate Cancer
- Pancreatic Ductal Adenocarcinoma
- Head and Neck CancersSquamous Cell
- Renal Cell Cancer
- Urinary Bladder Neoplasms
- Cervical Cancer
- Endometrial Cancer
- Follicular Thyroid Cancer
- Glioblastoma Multiforme
- Triple Negative Breast Cancer

Intervention

Drug: IMMU-132

  IMMU-132 is administered on days 1 & 8 of 3 week treatment cycles. Up to 8 cycles will be given.

Other Names:

  hRS7-SN38

  Sacituzumab Govitecan

Study Arms

Experimental: IMMU-132

  IMMU-132 (hRS7-SN38) is an Antibody Drug Conjugate where the antibody, hRS7 is attached to SN38. SN38 is the active metabolite of irinotecan (CPT-11).

Recruitment Information

Recruitment Status

Recruiting

Estimated Enrollment

250

Completion Date

June 2018

Primary Completion Date

June 2018

Eligibility Criteria

Inclusion Criteria:

- Male or female patients, >18 years of age, able to understand and give written informed consent.
- Histologically or cytologically confirmed epithelial cancer of one of the following types:
- Colorectal
- Gastric adenocarcinoma
- Esophageal cancer
- Hepatocellular carcinoma
- Non-small cell lung cancer
- Small cell lung cancer
- Ovarian epithelial cancer
- Cervical Cancer
- Endometrial Cancer
- Breast cancer
- Hormone-refractory prostate cancer
- Pancreatic ductal adenocarcinoma
- Head and neck cancerssquamous cell
- Renal cell cancer (clear cell)
- Urothelial cancers
- Glioblastoma multiforme
- Follicular thyroid cancer

(Note: Confirmation of Trop-2 expression by immunohistology or other means is not required, but the Sponsor will request tissue specimens from archived materials for determination of Trop-2 expression.)

- Stage IV (metastatic) disease.
- Refractory to or relapsed after at least one prior standard therapeutic regimen (Appendix 1 lists approved or standard chemotherapeutic agents for each cancer type. Patients who have not received all approved or standard treatments for their cancer must be informed that these alternatives to receiving IMMU-132 are available prior to consenting to participate in this trial.)
- Adequate performance status (ECOG 0 or 1)
- Expected survival > 6 months.
- Measurable disease by CT or MRI.
- At least 2 weeks beyond treatment (chemotherapy, investigational drugs including small molecular inhibitors, immunotherapy and/or radiation therapy) or major surgery and recovered from all acute toxicities to Grade 1 or less (except alopecia).
- At least 2 weeks beyond high dose systemic corticosteroids (however, low dose corticosteroids < 20 mg prednisone or equivalent daily are permitted).
- Adequate hematology without ongoing transfusional support (hemoglobin > 9 g/dL, ANC > 1,500 per mm3, platelets > 100,000 per mm3).
- Adequate renal and hepatic function (creatinine ≤ 2.0 x IULN, bilirubin ≤ 1.5 IULN, AST and ALT ≤ 3.0 x IULN or 5 x IULN if know liver metastases).
- Otherwise, all toxicity at study entry < Grade 1.

Exclusion Criteria:

- •Women who are pregnant or lactating.
- Women of childbearing potential and fertile men unwilling to use effective contraception during study until conclusion of 12-week post-treatment evaluation period.
- Patients with Gilbert's disease.
- Patients with brain metastases can be enrolled only if treated, non-progressive brain metastases and off high-dose steroids (>20 mg prednisone or equivalent) for at least 4 weeks.
- Presence of bulky disease (defined as any single mass > 7 cm in its greatest dimension). Patients with a mass over 7 cm, but otherwise eligible, may be considered for enrollment after discussion and approval with the medical monitor.
- Patients with active ≥ grade 2 anorexia, nausea or vomiting, and/or signs of intestinal obstruction.
- Patients with non-melanoma skin cancer or carcinoma in situ of the cervix are eligible, while patients with other prior malignancies must have had at least a 3-year disease-free interval.
- Patients known to be HIV positive, hepatitis B positive, or hepatitis C positive.
- Known history of unstable angina, MI, or CHF present within 6 months or clinically significant cardiac arrhythmia (other than stable atrial fibrillation) requiring anti-arrhythmia therapy.
- Known history of clinically significant active COPD, or other moderate-to-severe chronic respiratory illness present within 6 months.

- Prior history of clinically significant bleeding, intestinal obstruction, or GI perforation within 6 months of initiation of study treatment.
- Infection requiring intravenous antibiotic use within 1 week.
- history of an anaphylactic reaction to irinotecan or ≥ Grade 3 GI toxicity to prior irinotecan,
- Other concurrent medical or psychiatric conditions that, in the Investigator's opinion, may be likely to confound study interpretation or prevent completion of study procedures and follow-up examinations.

▦ **Sex/Gender**

All

▦ **Ages**

18 Years to N/A

▦ **Accepts Healthy Volunteers**

No

▦ **Contacts**

Heather Horne   973-605-8200   hhorne@immunomedics.com
Finn Augensen   973-605-8200   faugensen@Immunomedics.com

Romidepsin in Treating Patients With Lymphoma, Chronic Lymphocytic Leukemia, or Solid Tumors With Liver Dysfunction

Study ID:

NCT01638533

Sponsor:

National Cancer Institute (NCI)

Information provided by (Responsible Party):

National Cancer Institute (NCI) (National Cancer Institute (NCI))

Tracking Information

▦ **First Submitted Date**

July 9, 2012

▦ **Primary Completion Date**

June 30, 2018

▦ **Start Date**

June 12, 2012

▦ **Last Update Posted Date**

December 19, 2017

▦ **Current Primary Outcome Measures**

Dose-limiting toxicity of romidepsin in groups of patients with varying degree of hepatic dysfunction according to the National Cancer Institute Common Toxicity Criteria for Adverse Events version 4.0[Time Frame: 28 days]

In order to define levels of hepatic impairment at which dose modifications of romidepsin are required, data will be combined across hepatic dysfunction groups to evaluate the association between toxicity, dose, and liver assay level(s). The outcome variable, drug tolerance and dose-limiting toxicities will be modeled as function of dose and liver assay using multivariate linear regression. Higher order terms of the predictor variables and interactions will be included if there is evidence of non-linear and/or non-additive associations.

Maximum tolerated dose of romidepsin in groups of patients with varying degree of hepatic dysfunction according to the National Cancer Institute Common Toxicity Criteria for Adverse Events version 4.0[Time Frame: 28 days]

Analyses will be descriptive in nature. The observed toxicities will be characterized by dose level within each category of liver dysfunction (mild, moderate, severe, and liver transplant). These results will be summarized in relation to what is known about romidepsin in a population without liver dysfunction (as defined in this protocol).

Pharmacokinetic (PK) profile of romidepsin in patients with varying degrees of hepatic dysfunction using liquid chromatography-electrospray ionization tandem mass spectrometric method[Time Frame: 0, 1, 2, 3, 4, 4.25, 4.5, 5, 6, 8, 10, 24, and 48 hours after initiation of the infusion on day 1]

Pharmacokinetic variables will be tabulated and descriptive statistics calculated for each function group. Geometric means and coefficients of variation will be presented for maximum concentration and area under the curve for each group.

Antitumor activity assessed using Response Evaluation Criteria in Solid Tumors and the International Workshop Lymphoma Response Criteria[Time Frame: Up to 30 days]

Association of antitumor activity and romidepsin treatment will be documented.

Child-Pugh classification of hepatic dysfunction[Time Frame: Baseline]

Correlations of the Child-Pugh classification of hepatic dysfunction with the observed toxicities and plasma PK of romidepsin administration will be explored.

Descriptive Information

■ Offical Title

A Phase 1 and Pharmacokinetic Single Agent Study of Romidepsin in Patients With, Lymphomas, Chronic Lymphocytic Leukemia and Select Solid Tumors and Varying Degrees of Liver Dysfunction

■ Brief Summary

This phase I trial studies the side effects and best dose of romidepsin in treating patients with lymphoma, chronic lymphocytic leukemia, or solid tumors with liver dysfunction. Romidepsin may stop the growth of cancer cells by entering the cancer cells and by blocking the activity of proteins that are important for the cancer's growth and survival.

■ Detailed Description

PRIMARY OBJECTIVES:

I. To establish the safety and tolerability of romidepsin given on days 1, 8, and 15 of a 28 day cycle to patients with varying degrees of liver dysfunction (mild, moderate and severe).

II. To establish the maximum tolerated dose (MTD) and appropriate dosing recommendations for romidepsin in such patients.

III. To characterize the pharmacokinetics (PK) of romidepsin in patients with varying degrees of liver dysfunction.

SECONDARY OBJECTIVES:

I. To explore correlations of the Child-Pugh classification of liver dysfunction with the observed toxicities and plasma PK of romidepsin administration.

II. To document any preliminary evidence of antitumor activity at tolerable doses of romidepsin in patients with varying degrees of liver dysfunction.

OUTLINE: This is a dose-escalation study.

Patients receive romidepsin intravenously (IV) over 4 hours on days 1, 8, and 15. Courses repeat every 28 days in the absence of disease progression or unacceptable toxicity.

After completion of study treatment, patients are followed up for 30 days.

■ Study Type

Interventional

■ Study Phase

Phase 1

■ Condition

- Glioma
- Lymphoma
- Metastatic Malignant Solid Neoplasm
- Neuroendocrine Neoplasm
- Recurrent Adult Soft Tissue Sarcoma
- Recurrent Bladder Carcinoma
- Recurrent Breast Carcinoma
- Recurrent Chronic Lymphocytic Leukemia
- Recurrent Colorectal Carcinoma
- Recurrent Head and Neck Carcinoma
- Recurrent Lung Carcinoma
- Recurrent Malignant Solid Neoplasm
- Recurrent Melanoma
- Recurrent Pancreatic Carcinoma
- Recurrent Primary Cutaneous T-Cell Non-Hodgkin Lymphoma
- Recurrent Prostate Carcinoma
- Recurrent Renal Cell Carcinoma

- Recurrent Thyroid Gland Carcinoma
- Refractory Chronic Lymphocytic Leukemia
- Refractory Mature T-Cell and NK-Cell Non-Hodgkin Lymphoma
- Refractory Primary Cutaneous T-Cell Non-Hodgkin Lymphoma
- Stage III Breast Cancer AJCC v7
- Stage III Colorectal Cancer AJCC v7
- Stage III Cutaneous Melanoma AJCC v7
- Stage III Lung Cancer AJCC v7
- Stage III Pancreatic Cancer AJCC v6 and v7
- Stage III Prostate Cancer AJCC v7
- Stage III Renal Cell Cancer AJCC v7
- Stage III Soft Tissue Sarcoma AJCC v7
- Stage IIIA Breast Cancer AJCC v7
- Stage IIIA Colorectal Cancer AJCC v7
- Stage IIIA Cutaneous Melanoma AJCC v7
- Stage IIIB Breast Cancer AJCC v7
- Stage IIIB Colorectal Cancer AJCC v7
- Stage IIIB Cutaneous Melanoma AJCC v7
- Stage IIIC Breast Cancer AJCC v7
- Stage IIIC Colorectal Cancer AJCC v7
- Stage IIIC Cutaneous Melanoma AJCC v7
- Stage IV Breast Cancer AJCC v6 and v7
- Stage IV Colorectal Cancer AJCC v7
- Stage IV Cutaneous Melanoma AJCC v6 and v7
- Stage IV Lung Cancer AJCC v7
- Stage IV Pancreatic Cancer AJCC v6 and v7
- Stage IV Prostate Cancer AJCC v7
- Stage IV Renal Cell Cancer AJCC v7
- Stage IV Soft Tissue Sarcoma AJCC v7
- Stage IVA Colorectal Cancer AJCC v7
- Stage IVB Colorectal Cancer AJCC v7
- Unresectable Solid Neoplasm

Intervention

Other: Pharmacological Study

Correlative studies

Drug: Romidepsin

Given IV

Other Names:

Antibiotic FR 901228

Depsipeptide

FK228

FR901228

Istodax

N-[(3S,4E)-3-Hydroxy-7-mercapto-1-oxo-4-heptenyl]-D-valyl-D-cysteinyl-(2Z)-2-amino-2-butenoyl-L-valine, (4->1) Lactone, Cyclic

Study Arms

Experimental: Treatment (romidepsin)

Patients receive romidepsin IV over 4 hours on days 1, 8, and 15. Courses repeat every 28 days in the absence of disease progression or unacceptable toxicity.

Recruitment Information

Recruitment Status

Recruiting

Estimated Enrollment

132

Completion Date

N/A

Primary Completion Date

June 30, 2018

Eligibility Criteria

Inclusion Criteria:

- Patients must have histologically or cytologically confirmed (at original diagnosis or subsequent recurrence or progression) lymphoma, chronic lymphocytic lymphoma (CLL) or solid tumor; patients with lymphoma or CLL must have radiologically or clinically evaluable disease, and be refractory to standard therapy as defined by relapse within 6 months of last treatment (see note below); patients with solid tumors must have radiologically or clinically evaluable disease that is metastatic, unresectable, progressive, or recurrent, and for which standard curative measures do not exist or are no longer effective
- Patients with a liver mass, raised alpha-fetoprotein level (>= 500 ng/mL) and positive serology for hepatitis, consistent with a diagnosis of hepatocellular carcinoma will be eligible without the need for pathologic confirmation of the diagnosis
- Patients with prostate cancer, renal cell cancer, neuroendocrine tumors, lung cancer, colorectal cancers, soft tissue sarcomas, glioma and thyroid cancer are excluded in the normal and mild cohorts due to a lack of efficacy in these tumor types in phase 2 studies; patients with breast, pancreatic, bladder, head and neck cancers, as well as melanoma and other malignancies are eligible
- Note: patients with prostate cancer, renal cell cancer, lung cancer, colorectal cancers, soft tissue sarcomas, glioma and thyroid cancer are allowed to enroll in the moderate and severe cohorts provided the patients:
- Sign a separate consent form which outlines the lack of efficacy observed in prior studies
- Are consented to the study by a protocol-specified designee who is not their longitudinal oncologist; patients with neuroendocrine tumors are still excluded from the moderate and severe cohorts
- Note: as romidepsin is approved for patients with relapsed or refractory peripheral T-cell lymphoma (PTCL) or cutaneous T cell lymphoma (CTCL), these patients would be eligible WITHOUT the requirement of having 'relapsed within 6 months of last treatment'
- Life expectancy of > 3 months
- Eastern Cooperative Oncology Group (ECOG) performance status =< 2 (Karnofsky >= 60%)
- Hemoglobin >= 9 g/dL (transfusions and/or erythropoietin are permitted)
- Absolute neutrophil count (ANC) >= 1.5 x 10^9/L
- Platelets >= 100 x 10^9/L (or platelet count >= 30 × 10^9 cells/L in patients with lymphoma or CLL if bone marrow disease involvement is documented)
- Creatinine =< twice upper limit institutional normal
- Patients with abnormal liver function will be eligible and will be grouped according to the criteria below
- Group A (normal hepatic function)
- Bilirubin =< upper limit of normal (ULN) and aspartate aminotransferase (AST) =< ULN
- Group B (mild hepatic dysfunction)
- B1: bilirubin =< ULN and AST > ULN
- B2: bilirubin > ULN but =< 1.5 x ULN and any AST
- Group C (moderate hepatic dysfunction)
- Bilirubin > 1.5 x ULN to =< 3 x ULN and any AST
- Group D (severe hepatic dysfunction)
- Bilirubin > 3 x ULN and up to investigators discretion and any AST
- Patients with active hemolysis should be excluded; no distinction will be made between liver dysfunction due to metastases and liver dysfunction due to other causes; registration laboratory investigations will be used to assign a patient to a hepatic function group; liver function tests should be repeated within 24 hours prior to starting initial therapy and may result in the patients' group assignment being altered if different to registration test results
- Patients with brain metastases who require corticosteroids or non-enzyme inducing anticonvulsants must be on a stable dose of corticosteroids and seizure free for 1 month prior to enrollment; patients with known brain metastases should have completed brain irradiation (whole brain or gamma knife) more than 4 weeks before starting the protocol; patients on enzyme inducing anticonvulsants are not eligible; note that patients should have had their steroids tapered to low dose (i.e. < 1.5 mg of dexamethasone/day) due to the potential for higher dexamethasone doses to induce cytochrome P450, family 3, subfamily A, polypeptide 4 (CYP3A4)
- Patients with biliary obstruction for which a stent has been placed are eligible, provided the shunt has been in place for at least 10 days prior to the first dose of romidepsin and the liver function has stabilized; two measurements at least 2 days apart that put the patient in the same hepatic dysfunction stratum will be accepted as evidence of stable hepatic function; there should be no evidence of biliary sepsis
- Eligibility of patients receiving any medications or substances known to affect or with the potential to affect the activity or PK of romidepsin will be determined following review of their case by the site principal investigator

- Patients treated with any of the medications prohibited must discontinue their use at least 7 days prior to the first dose of romidepsin; certain other agents that interact with the CYP3A4 system may be used with caution
- Women of childbearing potential and men must agree to use adequate contraception (hormonal or barrier method of birth control; abstinence) prior to study entry and for the duration of study participation; should a woman become pregnant or suspect she is pregnant while participating in this study, she should inform her treating physician immediately; note: since romidepsin binds to the estrogen receptor, the effectiveness of estrogen containing contraceptives may be reduced
- Human immunodeficiency virus (HIV)-positive patients who are not receiving: agents with the potential for PK interactions with romidepsin or hepatotoxic antiretrovirals (nucleoside reverse-transcriptase inhibitors [NRTIs]: abacavir, didanosine, emtricitabine, lamivudine, stavudine, and zidovudine), dual protease inhibitor (PI)-based regimens except low-dose boosting with ritonavir, atazanavir, indinavir, maraviroc, and nevirapine may be eligible; additionally, the HIV-positive patients should have a cluster of differentiation (CD)4 count > 250/mm^3; if the specific cause of hepatic dysfunction is unknown, the patient should be worked up for other viral causes of hepatitis and their eligibility determined after consultation with the principal investigator
- Patients who have received prior romidepsin use are eligible
- Ability to understand and the willingness to sign a written informed consent document

Exclusion Criteria:

- Patients who have had (prior to entering the study): major surgery is not permitted within 4 weeks of romidepsin administration; anti-cancer therapy including chemotherapy, radiotherapy, hormonal (with the exception of hormones for thyroid conditions), and other investigational agents will not be allowed within 14 days or five (5) half-lives (whichever is longer) prior to the first dose of romidepsin (6 weeks for nitrosoureas or mitomycin C); additionally, participants must have recovered to less than grade 2 clinically significant adverse effect(s)/toxicity(ies) of the previous therapy, with the exception of alopecia, unless approved by the principal investigator; biologics or immunotherapy will not be allowed within 28 days prior to, or during, romidepsin administration
- Patients with prostate cancer, renal cell cancer, neuroendocrine tumors, lung cancer, colorectal cancers, soft tissue sarcomas, glioma, and thyroid cancer are excluded in the normal and mild cohorts due to a lack of efficacy in these tumor types in phase 2 studies; patients with prostate cancer, renal cell cancer, lung cancer, colorectal cancers, soft tissue sarcomas, glioma and thyroid cancer are allowed to enroll in the moderate and severe cohorts only; patients with neuroendocrine tumors are still excluded from the moderate and severe cohorts
- Patients may not be receiving any other investigational agents
- History of allergic reactions attributed to compounds of similar chemical or biologic composition to romidepsin, including cyclic tetrapeptide compounds
- Concurrent medications associated with a known risk of corrected QT interval (QTc) prolongation and/or Torsades de Pointes are not allowed within 2 weeks of initiation of study treatment; those medications listed as a possible risk for causing QTc prolongation and Torsades de Pointes will be allowed, although if an alternative medication can be substituted, that would be preferable; granisetron is an acceptable antiemetic on this study, but if a patient must take ondansetron, they may NOT take any other concomitant agents which might impact their QTc
- Thiazolidinedione agents such as rosiglitazone and pioglitazone are not permitted
- Uncontrolled intercurrent illness including, but not limited to ongoing or active infection, or psychiatric illness/social situations that would limit compliance with study requirements
- Patients with current evidence of significant cardiovascular disease (New York Heart Association class III or IV cardiac disease), symptomatic congestive heart failure, dilated/hypertrophic or restrictive cardiomyopathy, myocardial infarction (within the past 6 months), unstable angina, unstable arrhythmia or a need for anti-arrhythmic therapy (use of medications for rate control for atrial fibrillation is allowed such as calcium channel blockers and beta-blockers, if stable medication for at least last month prior to initiation of romidepsin treatment and medication not listed as causing Torsades de Pointes), or evidence of acute ischemia on electrocardiogram (ECG); marked baseline prolongation of QT/QTc interval, e.g., repeated demonstration of a QTc interval > 450 msec

; long QT syndrome; the required use of concomitant medication that may cause Torsades de Pointes or may cause a significant prolongation of the QTc

- Note: due to difficulties assessing QTc in patients with heart block, they may be eligible if deemed safe by a cardiologist; if a patient must take ondansetron as their antiemetic, their QTc may NOT be over 450 (no exception for patients with heart block)
- Pregnant women are excluded from this study; breastfeeding should be discontinued if the mother is treated with this drug
- Warfarin is not permitted

■ Sex/Gender

All

■ Ages

18 Years to N/A

■ Accepts Healthy Volunteers

No

18F FPPRGD2 PET/CT or PET/MRI in Predicting Early Response in Patients With Cancer Receiving Anti-Angiogenesis Therapy

Study ID:

NCT01806675

Sponsor:

Sanjiv Sam Gambhir

Information provided by (Responsible Party):

Stanford University (Sanjiv Sam Gambhir)

Tracking Information

▣ **First Submitted Date**

March 5, 2013

▣ **Start Date**

March 2013

▣ **Current Primary Outcome Measures**

▣ **Primary Completion Date**

March 2018

▣ **Last Update Posted Date**

March 14, 2017

Change in maximum standard uptake values (SUVmax) on 18F FPPRGD2 and 18F FDG PET[Time Frame: From baseline up to 6 weeks]

Response to treatment is based on the change in PET uptake, change in CT tumor size, PET European Organization for Research and Treatment of Cancer (EORTC) response criteria, and CT Response Evaluation Criteria In Solid Tumors (RECIST) response criteria. Each of the four response criteria will be dichotomized into responding or non-responding to treatment. The Mann-Whitney test and logistic regression of response/non-response will be performed.

▣ **Current Secondary Outcome Measures**

Progression-free survival[Time Frame: Up to 1 year]

For each SUV measure patients will be divided into two groups based on whether their SUV uptake is above or below the median. Kaplan-Meir curves for the two groups will be plotted and a log-rank test for difference in PFS will be performed. A Cox proportional-hazards regression of PFS on group will be performed.

Descriptive Information

▣ **Offical Title**

Phase I/II 18F FPPRGD2 PET/CT or PET/MRI Imaging of $\alpha v \beta 3$ Integrins Expression as a Biomarker of Angiogenesis

▣ **Brief Summary**

The purpose of the study is to conduct research of a new PET radiopharmaceutical in cancer patients. We will assess the uptake of this novel radiopharmaceutical in subjects with breast cancer, lung cancer, glioblastoma multiforme (GBM) and other cancers requiring antiangiogenesis treatment.

▣ **Detailed Description**

PRIMARY OBJECTIVES:

I. Evaluate 18F FPPRGD2 PET/CT or PET/MRI for prediction and early assessment of response to anti-angiogenesis therapy in patients with non-small cell lung cancer (NSCLC), breast cancer, glioblastoma multiforme (GBM) and other cancers.

OUTLINE:

Patients undergo 18F FPPRGD2 PET/CT or PET/MRI at baseline, 1 week, and 6 weeks (or standard of care follow-up) and 18F FDG PET/CT at baseline and 6 weeks (or standard of care follow-up) .

After completion of study imaging, patients are followed up at 12 months.

▣ **Study Type**

Interventional

▣ **Study Phase**

Phase 1/Phase 2

▣ **Condition**

- Adult Giant Cell Glioblastoma
- Adult Glioblastoma

- Adult Gliosarcoma
- Male Breast Cancer
- Metastatic Squamous Neck Cancer With Occult Primary Squamous Cell Carcinoma
- Recurrent Adenoid Cystic Carcinoma of the Oral Cavity
- Recurrent Adult Brain Tumor
- Recurrent Basal Cell Carcinoma of the Lip
- Recurrent Breast Cancer
- Recurrent Colon Cancer
- Recurrent Esthesioneuroblastoma of the Paranasal Sinus and Nasal Cavity
- Recurrent Hypopharyngeal Cancer
- Recurrent Inverted Papilloma of the Paranasal Sinus and Nasal Cavity
- Recurrent Laryngeal Cancer
- Recurrent Lip and Oral Cavity Cancer
- Recurrent Lymphoepithelioma of the Nasopharynx
- Recurrent Lymphoepithelioma of the Oropharynx
- Recurrent Metastatic Squamous Neck Cancer With Occult Primary
- Recurrent Midline Lethal Granuloma of the Paranasal Sinus and Nasal Cavity
- Recurrent Mucoepidermoid Carcinoma of the Oral Cavity
- Recurrent Nasopharyngeal Cancer
- Recurrent Non-small Cell Lung Cancer
- Recurrent Oropharyngeal Cancer
- Recurrent Pancreatic Cancer
- Recurrent Paranasal Sinus and Nasal Cavity Cancer
- Recurrent Rectal Cancer
- Recurrent Renal Cell Cancer
- Recurrent Salivary Gland Cancer
- Stage IIIA Breast Cancer
- Stage IIIA Non-small Cell Lung Cancer
- Stage IIIB Breast Cancer
- Stage IIIB Non-small Cell Lung Cancer
- Stage IIIC Breast Cancer
- Stage IV Breast Cancer
- Stage IV Non-small Cell Lung Cancer
- Stage IV Pancreatic Cancer
- Stage IV Renal Cell Cancer
- Stage IVA Colon Cancer
- Stage IVA Rectal Cancer
- Stage IVA Salivary Gland Cancer
- Stage IVB Colon Cancer
- Stage IVB Salivary Gland Cancer
- Stage IVC Salivary Gland Cancer
- Tongue Cancer
- Unspecified Adult Solid Tumor, Protocol Specific

■ Intervention

Drug: fludeoxyglucose F 18
    Undergo 18F FDG PET/CT

Other Names:
    18FDG

    FDG

    Drug: 2-fluoropropionyl-labeled pegylated dimeric RGD peptide

    Undergo 18F FPPRGD2 PET/CT or PET/MRI

Other Names:
    104150

18F-FPPRGD2

[18F] FPPRGD2

fluorine 18 ((18)F) FPPRGD2

PEG3-E[c(RGDyk)]2

Diagnostic Test: positron emission tomography

Undergo 18F FPPRGD2 PET/CT or PET/MRI

Other Names:

FDG-PET

PET

PET scan

tomography, emission computed

magnetic resonance imaging

Diagnostic Test: computed tomography

Undergo 18F FPPRGD2 PET/CT or PET/MRI

Other Names:

tomography, computed

magnetic resonance imaging

Diagnostic Test: positron emission tomography

Undergo 18F FDG PET/CT

Other Names:

FDG-PET

PET

PET scan

tomography, emission computed

Diagnostic Test: computed tomography

Undergo 18F FDG PET/CT

Other Names:

tomography, computed

Other: laboratory biomarker analysis

Correlative studies

Study Arms

Experimental: Diagnostic (18F FPPRGD2 PET/CT or PET/MRI)

Patients undergo 18F FPPRGD2 PET/CT or PET/MRI imaging at baseline, 1 week, and 6 weeks (or standard of care follow-up) and 18F FDG PET/CT at baseline and 6 weeks (or standard of care follow-up) .

Recruitment Information

Recruitment Status

Recruiting

Estimated Enrollment

150

Completion Date

March 2019

Primary Completion Date

March 2018

Eligibility Criteria

Inclusion Criteria:

- Provides written informed consent
- Diagnosed with advanced NSCLC, breast cancer, GBM or other cancers (such as head and neck, colorectal, pancreatic, renal cancers); patients will undergo anti-angiogenesis treatment
- Able to remain still for duration of each imaging procedure (about one hour)

Exclusion Criteria:

- Pregnant or nursing

- **Sex/Gender**

  All
- **Ages**

  18 Years to N/A
- **Accepts Healthy Volunteers**

  No
- **Contacts**

  Krithika Rupnarayan   650-736-0959   krupnara@stanford.edu

Panitumumab and Chemotherapy in Patients With Advanced Colorectal Cancer After Prior Therapy With Bevacizumab

Study ID:

NCT01814501

Sponsor:

John Hays

Information provided by (Responsible Party):

Ohio State University Comprehensive Cancer Center (John Hays)

Tracking Information

- **First Submitted Date**

  February 25, 2013
- **Start Date**

  February 2013
- **Primary Completion Date**

  December 31, 2018
- **Last Update Posted Date**

  February 5, 2018
- **Current Primary Outcome Measures**

  Progression free survival(PFS)[Time Frame: Time from study day 1 to the time the patient is first recorded as having disease progression or death, assessed up to 2 years]

  > Continuous variables will be expressed by means, standard deviations and 95% confidence intervals. Estimated using the Kaplan-Meier estimator with confidence interval calculated based on the Brookmeyer-Crowley method.

- **Current Secondary Outcome Measures**

  Frequency and severity of toxicities of the regimens, graded according to the NCI CTCAE v4.0[Time Frame: Up to 2 years]

  > Frequencies will be computed for discrete data.

  Overall response rate, as described in RECIST v1.1 criteria[Time Frame: Up to 2 years]

  Overall survival[Time Frame: Time from study day 1 to the date of death or the last date the patient was known to be alive, assessed up to 1 year]

  > Continuous variables will be expressed by means, standard deviations and 95% confidence intervals. Kaplan-Meier estimator will be used.

Descriptive Information

- **Offical Title**

  A Phase II Study of Panitumumab in Combination With FOLFIRI After Progression on FOLFIRI Plus Bevacizumab in KRAS(Kirsten Rat Sarcoma) and NRAS Wild-Type Metastatic Colorectal Cancer.

- **Brief Summary**

  This phase II trial studies how well panitumumab and combination chemotherapy works in treating patients with metastatic colorectal cancer previously treated with combination chemotherapy and bevacizumab. Monoclonal antibodies, such as panitumumab, can block tumor growth in different ways. Some block the ability of tumor cells to grow and spread. Others find tumor cells and help kill them or carry tumor-killing substances to them. Drugs used in chemotherapy, such as leucovorin calcium, fluorouracil, and irinotecan hydrochloride, work in different ways to stop the growth of tumor cells, either by killing the cells or by stopping them from dividing. Giving panitumumab and combination chemotherapy together may kill more tumor cells

Detailed Description

PRIMARY OBJECTIVES:

I. To determine the median progression-free survival in patients treated with leucovorin calcium, fluorouracil, and irinotecan hydrochloride (FOLFIRI) and panitumumab for K-ras and NRAS wild-type, metastatic colorectal carcinoma who have already progressed on FOLFIRI + Bevacizumab.

SECONDARY OBJECTIVES:

I. To determine the frequency and severity of toxicities of the regimens. II. To determine overall response rate. III. To determine the median overall survival and the overall survival rate at 1 year.

OUTLINE:

Patients receive panitumumab intravenously (IV) over 60-90 minutes, leucovorin calcium IV over 90 minutes, fluorouracil IV continuously over 46 hours, and irinotecan hydrochloride IV over 90 minutes on days 1 and 15. Courses repeat every 28 days in the absence of disease progression or unacceptable toxicity.

After completion of study treatment, patients are followed up periodically.

Study Type

Interventional

Study Phase

Phase 2

Condition

- Mucinous Adenocarcinoma of the Colon
- Mucinous Adenocarcinoma of the Rectum
- Recurrent Colon Cancer
- Recurrent Rectal Cancer
- Signet Ring Adenocarcinoma of the Colon
- Signet Ring Adenocarcinoma of the Rectum
- Stage IV Colon Cancer
- Stage IV Rectal Cancer

Intervention

Biological: panitumumab

Given IV

Other Names:

ABX-EGF

MOAB ABX-EGF

monoclonal antibody ABX-EGF

Vectibix

Drug: irinotecan hydrochloride

Given IV

Other Names:

Campto

Camptosar

CPT-11

irinotecan

U-101440E

Drug: fluorouracil

Given IV

Other Names:

5-fluorouracil

5-Fluracil

5-FU

Drug: leucovorin calcium

Given IV

Other Names:
  CF

  CFR

  LV

■ **Study Arms**

Experimental: Treatment (panitumumab, combination chemotherapy)
  5-Fluorouracil, irinotecan, and panitumumab

Recruitment Information

■ **Recruitment Status**

Recruiting

■ **Estimated Enrollment**

35

■ **Completion Date**

December 31, 2018

■ **Primary Completion Date**

December 31, 2018

■ **Eligibility Criteria**

Inclusion Criteria:

- Patients with advanced adenocarcinoma of the colon or rectum not curable with surgery or radiotherapy and have been previously treated for their disease with FOLFIRI plus bevacizumab in the first line metastatic setting; patients will only be eligible if their last line of therapy prior to enrolling onto the study was FOLFIRI and bevacizumab received no more than 6 months prior to enrolling in this study; they should have been treated with FOLFIRI plus bevacizumab until disease progression is radiographically documented
- Patients' tumors will need to tested for the K-RAS and N-RAS mutation status; only those patients with wild-type or unmutated K-RAS and N-RAS oncogene are eligible to participate in this study
- Provide written informed consent prior to study-specific screening procedures, with the understanding that the patient has the right to withdraw from the study at any time, without prejudice
- Prior cetuximab is allowed in the adjuvant but not in the metastatic setting, but must have been completed at least 6 months before starting this trial
- Eastern Cooperative Oncology Group (ECOG) performance status =< 1
- Life expectancy greater than 12 weeks
- No active brain metastasis; previously surgically treated or irradiated lesions are allowed if not clinically active
- Has a negative serum pregnancy test within 7 days prior to registration (female patients of childbearing potential)
- Ability to understand and willingness to sign a written informed consent
- No history of severe reactions to fluorouracil (5-FU), irinotecan (irinotecan hydrochloride), or a monoclonal antibody
- Leukocytes >= 3000/uL
- Absolute neutrophil count >= 1500/uL
- Platelets >= 100,000/uL
- Hemoglobin >= 9 mg/dL
- Total bilirubin =< 1.5 X upper limit of normal (ULN)
- Aspartate aminotransferase (AST)/alanine aminotransferase (ALT) =< 3 X ULN (or < 5 x ULN with liver metastases)
- Creatinine clearance (CrCl) >= 30 ml/min (Cockroft-Gault equation)
- Magnesium >= lower limit of normal
- Measurable disease is required according to Response Evaluation Criteria in Solid Tumors (RECIST) 1.1 criteria
- The effects of Panitumumab on the developing human fetus are unknown; for this reason and because monoclonal antibodies as well as other therapeutic agents used in this trial are known to be teratogenic, women of child-bearing potential and men must agree to use adequate contraception (hormonal or barrier method of birth control; abstinence) prior to study entry and for the duration of study participation and up to 6 months after completing therapy; should a woman become pregnant or suspect she is pregnant while participating in this study, she should inform her treating physician immediately

Exclusion Criteria:

- Pregnant or lactating women; women of childbearing potential with either a positive or no pregnancy test at baseline; woman or men of childbearing potential not using a reliable and appropriate contraceptive method; (postmenopausal woman must have been amenorrheic for at least 12 months to be considered of non-childbearing potential)
- Sexually active males unwilling to practice contraception during the study and 6 months beyond
- Uncontrolled intercurrent illness including but not limited to clinically significant cardiac disease not well controlled with medication (e.g. congestive heart failure, symptomatic coronary artery disease and cardiac arrhythmias) or myocardial

infarction within the last 12 months, and serious concurrent infections

- History of interstitial lung disease (eg, pneumonitis or pulmonary fibrosis) or evidence of interstitial lung disease on baseline chest computed tomography (CT) scan
- KRAS or NRAS mutant tumors
- Active inflammatory bowel disease or other bowel disease causing chronic diarrhea (defined as >= Common Toxicity Criteria [CTC] grade 2 [Common Terminology Criteria for Adverse Events (CTCAE) version 4.0])
- Clinically significant cardiovascular disease (including myocardial infarction, unstable angina, symptomatic congestive heart failure, serious uncontrolled cardiac arrhythmia) =< 1 year
- Bevacizumab within the last 4 weeks before starting treatment on trial
- Patient is more than 6 months since the last dose of FOLFIRI
- Patients who have required toxicity related dose reductions of no less than 50% of the original dose of infusional 5-FU and/or irinotecan during the administration of FOLFIRI + bevacizumab
- Prior exposure to panitumumab in any setting
- Prior exposure to cetuximab in the metastatic (stage IV) setting
- Radiotherapy =< 14 days prior to enrollment; patients must have recovered from all radiotherapy-related toxicities
- Prior unanticipated severe reaction to fluoropyrimidine therapy, or known sensitivity to 5-fluorouracil, leucovorin (leucovorin calcium), irinotecan, or panitumumab
- Treatment for other carcinomas within the last three years, except cured non-melanoma skin and treated in-situ cervical cancer
- Participation in any investigational drug study within 4 weeks preceding the start of study treatment
- Other serious uncontrolled medical conditions that the investigator feels might compromise study participation
- Major surgery within 4 weeks of the start of study treatment, without complete recovery
- Unwillingness to give written informed consent
- Unwillingness to participate or inability to comply with the protocol for the duration of the study
- Patients with human immunodeficiency virus (HIV)/acquired immune deficiency syndrome (AIDS) and those severely immunocompromised will be excluded; however, no patients will be tested for HIV

Sex/Gender

All

Ages

18 Years to N/A

Accepts Healthy Volunteers

No

Contacts

Ohio State University Comprehensive Cancer Center   1-800-293-5066   OSUCCCClinicaltrials@osumc.edu

Hamida Umar   614-685-6406   Hamida.Umar@osumc.edu

ICARuS Post-operative Intraperitoneal Chemotherapy (EPIC) and Hyperthermic Intraperitoneal Chemotherapy (HIPEC) After Optimal Cytoreductive Surgery (CRS) for Neoplasms of the Appendix, Colon or Rectum With Isolated Peritoneal Metastasis

Study ID:

NCT01815359

Sponsor:

Memorial Sloan Kettering Cancer Center

Information provided by (Responsible Party):

Memorial Sloan Kettering Cancer Center (Memorial Sloan Kettering Cancer Center)

Tracking Information

First Submitted Date

March 13, 2013

Start Date

March 2013

Primary Completion Date

March 2019

Last Update Posted Date

January 19, 2018

Current Primary Outcome Measures

disease-free survival[Time Frame: 3 years]

> Documentation of tumor recurrence will be made based on surveillance CT scans at time points as determined by attending radiologist, with clinical correlation from the treating physician.

Current Secondary Outcome Measures

surgical toxicity grade 3 to 5[Time Frame: up to 60 days]

> We will evaluate toxicity up to 30 days postoperatively for any surgical Grade 3-5 complications/toxicites or chemotherapy related Grade 4 or 5 toxicities. Surgical morbidity will be graded using the Common Terminology Criteria for Adverse Events (CTCAE) Version 4.0

chemotherapy toxicity grade 3 to 5[Time Frame: up to 60 days]

> We will evaluate toxicity up to 30 days postoperatively for any surgical Grade 3-5 complications/toxicities or chemotherapy related Grade 4 or 5 toxicities.

Descriptive Information

Offical Title

ICARuS (Intraperitoneal Chemotherapy After cytoReductive Surgery): A Multi-center, Randomized Phase II Trial of Early Post-operative Intraperitoneal Chemotherapy (EPIC) and Hyperthermic Intraperitoneal Chemotherapy (HIPEC) After Optimal Cytoreductive Surgery (CRS) for Neoplasms of the Appendix, Colon or Rectum With Isolated Peritoneal Metastasis

Brief Summary

This is the first randomized trial comparing Early post-operative intraperitoneal chemotherapy (EPIC) and hyperthermic intraperitoneal chemotherapy (HIPEC) for appendiceal and colorectal cancer. The purpose of this study is to find out what effects, good and/or bad, EPIC and HIPEC after cytoreductive surgery have on the patient and the appendiceal, rectal or colon cancer.

Study Type

Interventional

Study Phase

Phase 2

Condition

- Appendix Cancer
- Colorectal Cancer

Intervention

Procedure: Cytoreductive Surgery

> Optimal Surgical Debulking

> Drug: HIPEC with Mitomycin-C

> Drug: EPIC with FUDR and Leucovorin

Study Arms

Experimental: Appendiceal, no chemotherapy within 6 months prior to surgery

> First, patients will be stratified by previous systemic chemotherapy and by the organ of origin as determined by the Colorectal Disease Management Team.

> Exposure to chemotherapy in the prior 6 months vs. no such exposure

> Appendix vs. Colon or Rectum Then, patients will be randomly assigned in the operating room, by envelope, to either HIPEC (Group A) or EPIC (Group B) after the operating surgeon determines that the patient is optimally cytoreduced to nodules no greater than 2.5mm.

Experimental: Appendiceal, chemotherapy within 6 months prior to surgery

> First, patients will be stratified by previous systemic chemotherapy and by the organ of origin as determined by the Colorectal

Disease Management Team.

Exposure to chemotherapy in the prior 6 months vs. no such exposure

Appendix vs. Colon or Rectum • Then, patients will be randomly assigned in the operating room, by envelope, to either HIPEC (Group A) or EPIC (Group B) after the operating surgeon determines that the patient is optimally cytoreduced to nodules no greater than 2.5mm.

Experimental: Colorectal, no chemotherapy within 6 months prior to surgery

First, patients will be stratified by previous systemic chemotherapy and by the organ of origin as determined by the Colorectal Disease Management Team.

Exposure to chemotherapy in the prior 6 months vs. no such exposure

Appendix vs. Colon or Rectum • Then, patients will be randomly assigned in the operating room, by envelope, to either HIPEC (Group A) or EPIC (Group B) after the operating surgeon determines that the patient is optimally cytoreduced to nodules no greater than 2.5mm.

Experimental: Colorectal, chemotherapy within 6 months prior to surgery

First, patients will be stratified by previous systemic chemotherapy and by the organ of origin as determined by the Colorectal Disease Management Team.

Exposure to chemotherapy in the prior 6 months vs. no such exposure

Appendix vs. Colon or Rectum • Then, patients will be randomly assigned in the operating room, by envelope, to either HIPEC (Group A) or EPIC (Group B) after the operating surgeon determines that the patient is optimally cytoreduced to nodules no greater than 2.5mm.

Recruitment Information

Recruitment Status

Recruiting

Completion Date

March 2019

Estimated Enrollment

220

Primary Completion Date

March 2019

Eligibility Criteria

Inclusion Criteria:

- Patient's age 18 years or older, both genders.
- Clinical diagnosis of appendiceal or colorectal neoplasm with peritoneal mucinosis or metastasis.
- Patient must be planning to undergo complete cytoreduction of all peritoneal disease.
- ECOG performance status ≤ 1.
- Hematology: ANC ≥ 1,500/ µL; Platelets > 75,000/ µL.
- Adequate Renal function Creatinine <1.5 x the upper limit of normal (ULN) or calculated creatinine clearance of ≥ 50ml/min.
- Adequate Hepatic function: Bilirubin less than 1.5mg/dL; (except in patients with Gilbert's Syndrome, who must have a total bilirubin less than 3.0mg/dL).
- Women with childbearing potential who are negative for pregnancy test (urine or blood) and who agree to use effective contraceptive method. Reliable contraception should be used from trial screening and must be continued throughout the study. A woman of childbearing potential is defined as one who is biologically capable of becoming pregnant.
- A man participating in this study must agree to utilize reliable barrier form of contraception for the duration of the study.
- Signed and dated written informed consent to participate in this clinical trial must be obtained prior to any study procedure.
- Subjects with a history of endometrial cancer are eligible only if they presented with a stage lower than 1A and if the histology was a subtype other than poorly differentiated.

Exclusion Criteria:

- Subjects who have previously undergone intraperitoneal chemotherapy.
- Subjects with classical carcinoid
- Tumors of low malignant potential
- Other prior malignancies, except for cured non-melanoma skin cancer, curatively treated in situ carcinoma of the cervix, adequately treated malignancies for which there has been no evidence of activity for more than 3 years or indolent tumors for which observation over three years is a reasonable option.
- Presence of clinically apparent or suspected metastasis to sites other than lymph nodes or peritoneal surfaces.
- Women who are pregnant or lactating.
- Subjects with a condition which may interfere with the subjects' ability to understand the requirements of the study.
- Known HIV
- Active coronary artery disease (defined as unstable angina or a positive cardiac stress test).

- Subjects with a history of coronary artery disease may be included if they have had a normal stress test within 60 days of enrollment.

Uncontrolled hypertension defined as >140/90 and not cleared for surgery at the time of consent.

- New York Heart Association (NYHA) Class II or higher Congestive heart failure.
- Restrictive or obstructive pulmonary disease that would limit study compliance or place the patient at unacceptable risk for participation in the study.
- History of cerebrovascular disease. that would limit study compliance or place the patient at unacceptable risk for participation in the study.
- Subjects with other concurrent severe medical problems unrelated to the malignancy that would significantly limit full compliance with the study, or places them at an unacceptable risk for participation in the study.
- Patients with known floxuridine, leucovorin ,or mitomycin allergy.
- Evidence of extensive intraperitoneal adhesions at the time of surgery which prohibits intraperitoneal therapy, as determined by the operating surgeon.
- Any condition that would preclude the ability to deliver appropriate IP therapy.
- Use of an oral medication, lacking a suitable non-oral substitute, that if held for up to ten days, would be felt an unacceptable risk by the investigator.
- Life expectancy < 12 weeks.

■ **Sex/Gender**

All

■ **Ages**

18 Years to N/A

■ **Accepts Healthy Volunteers**

No

■ **Contacts**

Garrett Nash, MD, MPH   212-639-8668

Andrea Cercek, MD   646-888-4189

Evaluation of Low-dose Irinotecan and Cyberknife® SBRT to Treat Colorectal Cancer With Limited Liver Metastasis

Study ID:

NCT01847495

Sponsor:

Advocate Health Care

Information provided by (Responsible Party):

Advocate Health Care (Advocate Health Care)

Tracking Information

■ **First Submitted Date**

April 12, 2013

■ **Start Date**

October 2013

■ **Primary Completion Date**

October 2020

■ **Last Update Posted Date**

January 27, 2017

■ **Current Primary Outcome Measures**

Number of participants with adverse events related to toxicities from concurrent SBRT and irinotecan[Time Frame: 3 years]

■ **Current Secondary Outcome Measures**

Tumor response rate[Time Frame: 3 years]

Progression free survival[Time Frame: 3 years]

Overall survival[Time Frame: 3 years]

Descriptive Information

Offical Title

Prospective Evaluation of Low-dose Irinotecan and Cyberknife® Stereotactic Body Radiotherapy in the Treatment of Patients With Colorectal Cancer and Limited Liver Metastasis

Brief Summary

The purpose of this study is to determine the effects of CyberKnife stereotactic body radiotherapy in combination with irinotecan chemotherapy in patients with colon or rectal cancer that has spread to the liver.

Conventional radiation therapy has a limited role in the treatment of patients with liver metastases because the radiation doses are limited by liver toxicity. The CyberKnife system is a type of radiation machine that precisely focuses large doses of x-rays on the tumor, so that injury from radiation to the nearby normal tissue will be minimal. It is approved by the U.S. Food and Drug Administration to treat tumors, lesions and conditions anywhere in the body when radiation therapy is required. While the device is no longer classified as "investigational", the best treatment dose and times are still being evaluated.

Chemotherapy delivered with radiation therapy can increase the effectiveness of treatment, and may allow for a lower dose of radiation therapy to be utilized, thereby limiting negative side effects.

In this study, patients will receive Cyberknife radiosurgery directed to liver metastasis for 3-5 treatments, given every other day. Irinotecan 40mg/m2 will be administered intravenously daily for 3-5 days (5 treatments within 10 elapsed days), and prior to radiation therapy. Patients will have follow-up visits at months 1,2,4,6,9,12,15,18, 24, 30, 36, and every 6 months thereafter for 3 years.

Study Type

Interventional

Study Phase

N/A

Condition

- Colorectal Cancer

Intervention

Drug: Irinotecan
   40mg/m2 x 3-5 days

Other Names:

   Camptosar

   Irinotecan Hydrochloride

   Irinotecan HCl

   CPT-11

   Radiation: CyberKnife

45-60 Gy for 3-5 days CyberKnife SBRT to liver metastasis within 10 elapsed days. Irinotecan will be administered on the same day, prior to SBRT.

Other Names:
   Stereotactic Radiosurgery

Study Arms

Experimental: Low-Dose Irinotecan & CyberKnife SBRT
   Irinotecan 40mg/m2 x 3-5 days + CyberKnife SBRT 45-60Gy x 3-5 fractions

Recruitment Information

Recruitment Status

Recruiting

Estimated Enrollment

41

Eligibility Criteria

- Age>18 years
- Histologically confirmed primary colorectal cancer
- Stage IV colorectal cancer with </= 3 metastases, up to 5cm in size.

Completion Date

October 2025

Primary Completion Date

October 2020

- CT scan or MRI of the abdomen with contrast, 60days prior to enrollment
- If patient is allergic to contrast, imaging without contrast is acceptable
- Positron-Emission Tomography 60 days prior to enrollment
- No additional sites of metastasis at the time of protocol enrollment. History of other sites of metastasis that are currently controlled are acceptable.
- No malignant ascites
- At least 4 weeks from any chemotherapy
- No prior liver radiation therapy
- ECOG performance status 0-1
- Life expectancy>3months
- Laboratory evaluations completed 60 days prior to treatment including CMP, CBC with differential, liver function test, and prothrombin time.

Sex/Gender

All

Ages

18 Years to N/A

Accepts Healthy Volunteers

No

Contacts

Arica Hirsch, MD   847 723-8030

TRC102 and Temozolomide for Relapsed Solid Tumors and Lymphomas

Study ID:

NCT01851369

Sponsor:

National Cancer Institute (NCI)

Information provided by (Responsible Party):

National Institutes of Health Clinical Center (CC) (National Cancer Institute (NCI))

Tracking Information

First Submitted Date

May 8, 2013

Start Date

May 8, 2013

Primary Completion Date

December 24, 2019

Last Update Posted Date

December 14, 2017

Current Primary Outcome Measures

Establish safety, tolerability, and maximum tolerated dose of oral TRC102 in combination with oral TMZ in patients with refractory solid tumors.[Time Frame: DLT determined first cycle (28) daysdays)]

To explore the response rate of this combination in patients with colon cancer, NSCLC, and granulosa cell ovarian cancer[Time Frame: Response rate one year]

Current Secondary Outcome Measures

Evaluate the pharmacokinetic (PK) profile of oral TRC102 when administered in combination with TMZ[Time Frame: First 5 days]

To explore the progression free survival rate of this combination in patients with colon cancer, NSCLC, and granulosa cell ovarian cancer[Time Frame: Duration on study]

Descriptive Information

Offical Title

A Phase I/II Trial of TRC102 (Methoxyamine HCl) in Combination With Temozolomide in Patients With Relapsed Solid Tumors and Lymphomas

Brief Summary

Background:

- TRC102 is a new cancer treatment drug that may help improve the results of chemotherapy. It blocks tumor cells' attempts to repair damaged DNA, which may allow chemotherapy to kill the cells more easily. Researchers want to see how well it works with temozolomide, a chemotherapy drug that is designed to damage tumor cell DNA. These drugs will be given to people who have advanced solid tumors or lymphomas that have not responded to earlier treatments.

Objectives:

- To test the safety and effectiveness of TRC102 and temozolomide for advanced solid tumors and lymphomas.

Eligibility:

- Individuals at least 18 years of age who have advanced solid tumors or lymphomas that have not responded to earlier treatments.

Design:

- Participants will be screened with a physical exam and medical history. Blood and urine samples will be collected. Tumor samples may also be collected. The size and location of the tumors will be determined with imaging studies.
- Participants will take TRC102 and temozolomide for 28-day cycles of treatment. They will take temozolomide and TRC 102 by mouth once a day on days 1-5. Participants will keep a diary to record doses and any side effects.
- Treatment will be monitored with frequent blood tests and imaging studies. Tumor samples will also be collected.
- Participants will continue their treatment as long as the cancer does not grow and there are no severe side effects.

Detailed Description

Background:

-Base excision repair (BER) of DNA repair pathway has been implicated in resistance to both alkylating and antimetabolite chemotherapy.

-TRC102 (methoxyamine HCl) acts through a novel mechanism to inhibit BER and has demonstrated the ability to potentiate the activity of the alkylating agent temozolomide (TMZ), in vitro and in vivo. We hypothesize that TRC102 can be safely co-administered with TMZ and would potentiate DNA damage caused by TMZ, resulting in antitumor responses.

- Based on responses measured during the Phase I portion of the trial, we will further explore the efficacy of this combination in patients with metastatic colon carcinoma, nonsmall cell lung cancer (NSCLC), and granulosa cell ovarian cancer

Primary Objective:

-To establish the safety, tolerability, and maximum tolerated dose (MTD) of oral TRC102 in combination with oral TMZ in patients with refractory solid tumors

-Evaluate the pharmacokinetic (PK) profile of oral TRC102 when administered in combination with TMZ.

-To explore the response rate of this combination in patients with colon cancer, NSCLC, and granulosa cell ovarian cancer

Secondary Objectives:

- Determine the effects of the study treatment on the level of histone gammaH2AX in circulating tumor cells (CTCs) and tumor and correlate the gammaH2AX response in tumor and CTCs
- Determine the effects of the study treatment on the levels of cleaved caspase 3, epithelialmesenchymal transition, and APE in tumor and CTCs
- To explore resistance mechanisms to the study drug combination
- Determine and characterize the effects of study treatment on erythrocytes
- Characterize the clinical presentation of hemolysis observed in earlier study subjects and explore the possible mechanisms

-To explore the progression free survival rate of this combination in patients with colon cancer, NSCLC, and granulosa cell ovarian cancer

Eligibility:

-Phase I: histologically confirmed solid tumors that have progressed on standard therapy known to prolong survival or for which no standard treatment options exist

-Phase II: histologically confirmed adenocarcinoma of the colon post at least two lines of therapy, NSCLC post at least two lines of therapy, or granulosa cell ovarian cancer post at least one line of therapy

- No major surgery, radiation, or chemotherapy within 4 weeks prior to entering the study
- Adequate organ function
- Healthy adult volunteers greater than or equal to 18 years of age will be consented to donate research blood

Study Design: Phase I

- This is an open-label Phase I trial; traditional 3+3 design.
- Oral TRC102 and oral TMZ will be administered daily, days 1-5 in 28-day cycles
- Once the MTD is established, up to 15 additional patients will be enrolled at the MTD to further evaluate that dose for PK and PD endpoints for evidence of DNA damage and apoptosis.

-During the escalation phase, tumor biopsies will be optional. During the expansion phase, (once MTD is reached), mandatory paired tumor biopsies will be pursued in the 15 additional patients enrolled to further evaluate PD endpoints.

Phase II

-This is a 3-arm Simon 2-stage design trial evaluating independently the response rate of patients with colon, NSCLC, and granulosa cell ovarian cancer.

- Patients with a body surface area (BSA) of greater than or equal to 1.6 m(2) will receive 125 mg of TRC 102 and 150 mg/m2 of TMZ PO qday x 5 every 28 days (DL6). Patients with a BSA of <1.6 m(2) will receive 100 mg of TRC 102 and 150 mg/m2 of TMZ PO qday x 5 every 28 days (DL5).. Each cycle will be 28 days.
- The accrual ceiling for the Phase II portion is 75 patients.
- Mandatory paired tumor biopsies will be pursued to further evaluate PD endpoints.

Study Type

Interventional

Study Phase

Phase 1/Phase 2

Condition

- Lymphomas
- Solid Tumors
- NSCLC
- Metastatic Colon Carcinoma
- Granulosa Cell Ovarian Cancer

Intervention

Drug: TRC 102

TRC102 has been shown to potentiate the activity of temozolomide by preventing BER and allowing cleavage of TRC102 bound DNA, which will cause DNA strand breaks in cancer cells. We hypothesize that oral TRC102 can be safely co administered with TMZ and would potentiate DNA damage caused by TMZ resulting in antitumor responses.

Publications

(Includes publications given by the data provider as well as publications identified by ClinicalTrials.gov Identifier (NCT Number) in Medline.)Liu L, Nakatsuru Y, Gerson SL. Base excision repair as a therapeutic target in colon cancer. Clin Cancer Res. 2002 Sep;8(9):2985-91. (https://www.ncbi.nlm.nih.gov/pubmed/12231545)

Yan L, Bulgar A, Miao Y, Mahajan V, Donze JR, Gerson SL, Liu L. Combined treatment with temozolomide and methoxyamine: blocking apurininc/pyrimidinic site repair coupled with targeting topoisomerase IIalpha. Clin Cancer Res. 2007 Mar 1;13(5):1532-9. (https://www.ncbi.nlm.nih.gov/pubmed/17332299)

Kinders RJ, Hollingshead M, Lawrence S, Ji J, Tabb B, Bonner WM, Pommier Y, Rubinstein L, Evrard YA, Parchment RE, Tomaszewski J, Doroshow JH; National Cancer Institute Phase 0 Clinical Trials Team. Development of a validated immunofluorescence assay for γH2AX as a pharmacodynamic marker of topoisomerase I inhibitor activity. Clin Cancer Res. 2010 Nov 15;16(22):5447-57. doi: 10.1158/1078-0432.CCR-09-3076. Epub 2010 Oct 5. (https://www.ncbi.nlm.nih.gov/pubmed/20924131)

Recruitment Information

Recruitment Status

Recruiting

Estimated Enrollment

65

Completion Date

December 24, 2019

Primary Completion Date

December 24, 2019

Eligibility Criteria

- Eligibility Criteria (Patients)
- Phase I: histologically confirmed solid tumors that have progressed on standard therapy known to prolong survival or for which no standard treatment options exist.
- Phase II: histologically confirmed colorectal adenocarcinoma post at least two lines of therapy, NSCLC post at least two lines of therapy, or granulosa cell ovarian cancer post at least one line of therapy. Patients must have measurable disease.
- Age greater than18 years. Because no dosing or adverse event data are currently available on the use of TRC102 in combination with TMZ in patients less than 18 years of age, children are

excluded from this study.

- Patients enrolling in the expansion cohorts must have disease amenable to biopsy and be willing to undergo pre-and post-treatment biopsies.
- ECOG performance status less than 2 (Phase I), less than or equal to 1(Phase II).
- Life expectancy of greater than 3 months
- Patients must have normal organ and marrow function as defined below:
- Absolute neutrophil count greater than 1,500/mcL
- Hemoglobin greater than or equal to 10 g/dL without transfusion within 1 week prior to enrollment

Platelets greater than 100,000/mcL

Total bilirubin less than or equal to1.5 X institutional ULN

AST(SGOT)/ALT(SGPT) less than 3 X institutional upper limit of normal; 5.0 x ULN in cases of liver metastases

creatinine less than or equal to 1.5 X institutional ULN

OR

creatinine clearance greater than 60 mL/min/1.73 m2 for patients with creatinine levels greater than 1.5 mg/dL

-The effects of study drug on the developing human fetus are unknown. For this reason, women of child-bearing potential and men must agree to use adequate contraception (hormonal or barrier method of birth control; abstinence) prior to study entry and for the

duration of study participation and for at least 3 months after dosing with study drugs ceases. Should a woman become pregnant or suspect she is pregnant while she or her partner is participating in this study, she should inform her treating physician

immediately. Men treated or enrolled on this protocol must also agree to use adequate contraception prior to the study, for the duration of study participation, and 3 months after completion of study drug administration.

- Patients must have completed any chemotherapy, radiation therapy, or biologic therapy greater than or equal to 4 weeks (or 5 half-lives, whichever is shorter) prior to entering the study (6 weeks for nitrosoureas or mitomycin C). Patients must be greater than or equal to 2 weeks since any prior administration of a study drug in a Phase 0 or equivalent study and greater than or equal to 1 week from palliative radiation therapy. Patients must have recovered to eligibility levels from prior toxicity or adverse events. Treatment with bisphosphonates is permitted.
- Patients must be able to swallow whole tablets or capsules; nasogastric or G-tube administration is not allowed.
- Ability to understand and the willingness to sign a written informed consent document and to undergo tumor biopsies in the expansion phase.

Exclusion Criteria (Patients)

- Patients who are actively receiving any other investigational agents.
- Patients with active brain metastases or carcinomatous meningitis are excluded from this clinical trial. Patients with treated brain metastases, whose brain metastatic disease has remained stable for greater than or equal to 4 weeks without requiring steroid and anti-seizure medications are eligible to participate.
- Phase II only: patient must not have been diagnosed with another cancer within the last 3 years.
- Phase II only: patients with colorectal cancer with known MSI-high disease who have previously been treated with immunotherapy.
- History of allergic reactions attributed to compounds of similar chemical or biologic composition to TRC102 or TMZ.
- Uncontrolled intercurrent illness including, but not limited to, serious untreated infection, symptomatic congestive heart failure, unstable angina pectoris, cardiac arrhythmia, or psychiatric illness/social situations that would limit compliance with study requirements.
- Pregnant women are excluded from this study because the effects of the study drugs on the developing fetus are unknown. Because there is an unknown but potential risk for adverse events in nursing infants secondary to treatment of the mother with the study drugs, breastfeeding should be discontinued prior to the first dose of study drug and women should refrain from nursing throughout the treatment period and for 3 months following the last dose of study drug.
- HIV-positive patients on combination antiretroviral therapy are ineligible because of possible PK interactions with TRC102.

Eligibility Criteria (Healthy volunteer blood donors)

- Age greater than 18 years; hemoglobin greater than or equal to 12 g/dL; no history of bleeding problems; not taking aspirin or any medication that may affect erythrocyte biochemistry
- Willingness to sign the healthy volunteer informed consent form.

- **Sex/Gender**

  All

- **Ages**

  18 Years to 120 Years

- **Accepts Healthy Volunteers**

  Accepts Healthy Volunteers

- **Contacts**

  Jennifer H Zlott   (301) 435-5664   zlottjh@mail.nih.gov

  Alice P Chen, M.D.   (240) 781-3320   chenali@mail.nih.gov

A Phase I Study of Nilontinib and Cetuximab in Patients With Solid Tumors

Study ID:

NCT01871311

Sponsor:

Georgetown University

Information provided by (Responsible Party):

Georgetown University (Georgetown University)

Tracking Information

- **First Submitted Date**

  June 4, 2013

- **Start Date**

  May 2014

- **Current Primary Outcome Measures**

  Maximum tolerated dose[Time Frame: 18 months]

  The dose at which </= 1 out of 6 subjects experiences a dose limiting toxicity

- **Primary Completion Date**

  December 2017

- **Last Update Posted Date**

  February 2, 2017

Descriptive Information

- **Offical Title**

  A Phase I Study of the BCR-ABL Tyrosine Kinase Inhibitor Nilontinib and Cetuximab in Patients With Solid Tumors That Can be Treated With Cetuximab

- **Brief Summary**

  The purpose of this study is to determine the recommended Phase II dose of nilotinib when used in combination with cetuximab in the treatment of patients with recurrent and/or metastatic Kras wildtype colorectal cancer or squamous cell carcinoma of the head and neck.

- **Detailed Description**

  ABL1 has been suggested to play a key role in the resistance mechanism to anti EGFR therapy in cancer. Therefore, this study aims to evaluate the safety and possible effect of targeting both EGFR using cetuximab along with ABL1 using nilotinib. Correlative studies assess the changes in tumor proteome in response to therapy and magnitude of ADCC as a marker of antibody activity.

- **Study Type**

  Interventional

- **Study Phase**

  Phase 1

- **Condition**

  - Colorectal Cancer

- Head and Neck Cancer

Intervention

Drug: Nilotinib + Cetuximab

Nilotinib BID for a 28-day cycle + Cetuximab 400 mg/m2 on day 1 dose then 250 mg/m2 weekly

Three dose levels for nilotinib:

Dose level -1 200-mg daily Dose level 1 200-mg BID Dose level 2 300-mg BID

Cycle duration will be 4 weeks, with weekly evaluation of toxicity. Assessment of tumor progression will occur every 2 cycles. Subjects will be treated until disease progression or cessation due to intolerable toxicity.

Study Arms

Experimental: Nilotinib + Cetuximab

All patients with receive Nilotinib BID for a 28-day cycle + Cetuximab 400 mg/m2 on day 1 dose then 250 mg/m2 weekly

Recruitment Information

Recruitment Status

Recruiting

Estimated Enrollment

22

Completion Date

December 2017

Primary Completion Date

December 2017

Eligibility Criteria

Inclusion Criteria:

1. Recurrent and/or metastatic Kras wildtype colorectal cancer or squamous cell carcinoma of the head and neck

2. Previous therapy:

1. Patients must have progressed after standard therapy for metastatic/recurrent disease, including irinotecan and oxaliplatin-containing regimens for patients with CRC and platinum-containing regimens for patients with H&NSCC.

2. Patients may have received cetuximab or panitumumab previously

3. Ability to swallow medication tablets by mouth (which may include taking nilotinib mixed in apple sauce)

4. At least one measurable lesion by RECIST criteria

5. A tumor lesion that can be readily biopsied using a core needle via clinical exam or image-guidance.

6. Over the age of 18 years and able to provide informed consent

7. Adequate kidney, liver, and bone marrow function as follows:

1. Hemoglobin >/= 8.0 gm/dL

2. Absolute neutrophil count >/= 1500

3. Platelet count >/= 100,000

4. Creatinine within institutional normal limits or glomerular filtration rate > 60

5. Total bilirubin f. AST and ALT

8. Life expectancy of greater than 3 months

9. ECOG performance status

10. Normal left ventricular ejection fraction, defined as EF > 50%

Exclusion Criteria:

1. Chemotherapy or surgery within 4 weeks prior to treatment start

2. Radiation treatment within 3 weeks prior to treatment start

3. Prior therapy with nilotinib, ponatinib, dasatinib, or imatinib

4. Untreated brain metastases or neurologically unstable central nervous system metastases; CNS metastases will be considered stable if there is no new nor enlarging lesions for one month, and the patient remains off steroids and anti-epileptics for the same time period

5. Any severe or uncontrolled medical condition or other condition that could affect participation in this study, including: unstable angina, uncontrolled hypertension, serious uncontrolled cardiac arrhythmia, uncontrolled infection, or myocardial infarction

6. Diarrhea > Grade 1 at baseline

7. Concomitant medication or herbal therapy known to inhibit CYP3A4

8. Gastrointestinal tract disease resulting in the inability to take oral medication or a requirement for IV alimentation, prior surgical procedures affecting absorption, or active peptic ulcer disease

9. Ongoing ventricular cardiac dysrhythmias of NCI CTCAE grade >/= 2

10. Subjects with a history of serious ventricular arrhythmia (ventricular tachycardia or ventricular fibrillation >/= 3 beats in a row)

11. Serious cardiac arrhythmia requiring medication

12. QTc interval > 500 msec

13. Female patients who are pregnant or breast feeding, or adults who are of reproductive potential and are unwilling to refrain from conceiving a child during study treatment

14. Patients unwilling or unable to comply with the protocol, or provide informed consent

▦ Sex/Gender

All

▦ Ages

18 Years to N/A

▦ Accepts Healthy Volunteers

No

▦ Contacts

Lisa Ley, RN   202-687-6653   leyl@georgetown.edu
Ann W Gramza, MD   ann.w.gramza@gunet.georgetown.edu

Phase 2 Study of MK-3475 in Patients With Microsatellite Unstable (MSI) Tumors

Study ID:

NCT01876511

Sponsor:

Sidney Kimmel Comprehensive Cancer Center

Information provided by (Responsible Party):

Sidney Kimmel Comprehensive Cancer Center (Sidney Kimmel Comprehensive Cancer Center)

Tracking Information

▦ First Submitted Date

June 10, 2013

▦ Primary Completion Date

June 2021

▦ Start Date

September 2013

▦ Last Update Posted Date

December 15, 2017

▦ Current Primary Outcome Measures

Immune-related progression free survival (irPFS) rate at 20 weeks in patients with MSI positive and negative colorectal adenocarcinoma using immune related response criteria (irRC)[Time Frame: 4 years]

Objective response rate (irORR) at 20 weeks in patients with MSI positive and negative colorectal adenocarcinoma using immune related response criteria (irRC)[Time Frame: 4 years]

Immune-related progression free survival (irPFS) rate in patients with MSI positive non-colorectal adenocarcinoma using immune related response criteria (irRC) at 20 weeks[Time Frame: 4 years]

objective response rate in patients with MSI-negative cancer with a mutator phenotype using RECIST 1.1 criteria[Time Frame: 4 years]

▦ Current Secondary Outcome Measures

Overall survival[Time Frame: 4 years]

irPFS and PFS in patients with MSI positive and negative tumors at 28 weeks using irRC and RECIST 1.1[Time Frame: 4 years]

Best overall response rate and disease control rate in patients with MSI positive and negative tumors[Time Frame: 4 years]

Number of participants experiencing immune-related toxicities (IRAEs)[Time Frame: 4 years]

Does MSI as a marker predict treatment response[Time Frame: 4 years]

Identify alternative markers of MSI status. This includes but is not limited to MLH 1, MSH 2, MSH 6, PMS2, BRAF pV600E, and TGFBR2.[Time Frame: 4 years]

Descriptive Information

Offical Title

Phase 2 Study of MK-3475 in Patients With Microsatellite Unstable (MSI) Tumors

Brief Summary

This study will be looking at whether MK-3475 (an antibody that blocks negative signals to T cells) is effective (anti-tumor activity) and safe in three different patient populations. These include: 1. patients with MSI positive colon cancer, 2. patients with MSI negative colon cancer 3. patients with other MSI positive cancers, and 4. patients with MSI negative cancer with a mutator phenotype.

Study Type

Interventional

Study Phase

Phase 2

Condition

- MSI Positive Colorectal Cancer
- MSI Negative Colorectal Cancer
- MSI Positive Non-Colorectal Cancers

Intervention

Drug: MK-3475

    MK-3475 10 mg/kg every 14 days

    Drug: MK-3475

    MK-3475 200mg flat dose every 21 days

Study Arms

Experimental: MSI Positive Colorectal Cancer
Experimental: MSI Negative Colorectal Cancer
Experimental: MSI Positive Non-Colorectal Cancer
Experimental: MSI Negative with Mutator Phenotype

Recruitment Information

Recruitment Status

Recruiting

Estimated Enrollment

171

Completion Date

June 2021

Primary Completion Date

June 2021

Eligibility Criteria

Inclusion Criteria:

1. Arm 1 only: Patients with MSI positive colorectal cancer 2. Arm 2 only: Patients with MSI negative colorectal cancer 3. Arm 3 only: Patients with MSI positive non-colorectal cancer 4. Arm 4 only: patients with hypermutated MSI negative cancer 4. Have measurable disease 5. ECOG Performance Status of 0 to 1 6. Adequate organ function as defined by study-specified laboratory tests 7. Must use acceptable form of birth control through the study and for 28 days after final dose of study drug 8. Signed informed consent form 9. Willing and able to comply with study procedures 10. Agree to have a biopsy of their cancer 11. Patients with colon cancer must have received at least two prior cancer therapy regimens.

12. Patients with other cancer types must have received at least one prior cancer therapy

Exclusion Criteria:

1. Patients with uncontrolled intercurrent illness, including but not limited to ongoing or active infection, systematic congestive heart failure, unstable angina pectoris, cardiac arrhythmia or psychiatric condition that would limit compliance with study requirements. .

2. Patients who have had chemotherapy or biological cancer therapy within 2 weeks prior to the first dose of study drug

3. Patients who have had radiation within 2 weeks prior to the first dose of study drug

4. Patients who have undergone major surgery within 4 weeks of dosing of investigational agent

5. Patients who have received another investigational product or investigational device within 4 weeks prior to receiving study drug

6. Patients who have received any of the following concomitant therapy: IL-2, interferon, or other non-study immunotherapy regimens, immunosuppressive agents, other investigational therapies or chronic use of systemic corticosteroids within one week

prior to first dose of study drug

7. Patients who have received a live vaccine within 4 weeks prior to or after any dose of MK-3475

8. Patients who have received growth factors, including but not limited to granulocyte-colony stimulating factor (G-CSF), granulocyte macrophage-colony stimulating factor (GM-CSF), erythropoietin, etc. within 2 weeks of study drug administration

9. Patient who have had prior treatment with anti-PD-1, anti-PD-L1, anti-PD-L2, anti-CD137, anti-OX-40, anti-CD40, or anti-CTLA-4 antibodies

10. Patients with history of any autoimmune disease:inflammatory bowel disease, (including ulcerative colitis and Crohn's Disease), rheumatoid arthritis, systemic progressive sclerosis (scleroderma), systemic lupus erythematosus (SLE) autoimmune vasculitis, CNS or motor neuropathy considered to be of autoimmune origin.

11. Patients who have known history of infection with HIV, hepatitis B, or hepatitis C

12. Patients with evidence of interstitial lung disease

13. Systemically active steroid use

14. Patients on home oxygen

15. Patients with oxygen saturation of <92% on room air by pulse oximetry

16. Pregnant or lactating

17. Conditions, including alcohol or drug dependence, or intercurrent illness that would affect the patient's ability to comply with study visits and procedures

18. Patient with known active central nervous system metastases and/or carcinomatous meningitis.

19. Patients with primary brain tumors.

Sex/Gender

All

Ages

18 Years to N/A

Accepts Healthy Volunteers

No

Body Warming in Improving Blood Flow and Oxygen Delivery to Tumors in Patients With Cancer

Study ID:

NCT01896778

Sponsor:

Roswell Park Cancer Institute

Information provided by (Responsible Party):

Roswell Park Cancer Institute (Roswell Park Cancer Institute)

Tracking Information

First Submitted Date

July 8, 2013

Start Date

October 4, 2013

Primary Completion Date

April 11, 2018

Last Update Posted Date

September 28, 2017

Current Primary Outcome Measures

Changes in tumor vascular (blood flow, blood volume)[Time Frame: Baseline to 24-88 hours]

The primary analysis will be implemented using an analysis-of-covariance model for both blood flow and blood volume.

Current Secondary Outcome Measures

Changes in tumor vascular measures[Time Frame: Baseline to 88-264 hours]

Incidence of adverse events graded according to the National Cancer Institute Common Terminology Criteria for Adverse Events version 4.0[Time Frame: Up to 30 days post-treatment]

The frequency of toxicities will be tabulated by grade across all dose levels and cycles. The frequency of toxicities will also be tabulated for the dose estimated to be the maximum tolerated dose.

Descriptive Information

▨ Offical Title

Body Warming to Alter [Thermo] Regulation and the Microenvironment [B-WARM] Therapy: A Pilot Study

▨ Brief Summary

This randomized pilot clinical trial studies body warming in improving blood flow and oxygen delivery to tumors in patients with cancer. Heating tumor cells to several degrees above normal body temperature may kill tumor cells.

▨ Detailed Description

PRIMARY OBJECTIVES:

I. To determine the feasibility and efficacy of 2 different Body Warming to Alter (Thermo) Regulation and the Microenvironment (B-WARM) regimens on altering tumor blood flow in patients with a variety of malignancies.

SECONDARY OBJECTIVES:

I. To determine if duration and thermal dose of B-WARM changes duration and extent of tumor blood flow changes in patients with a variety of malignancies.

OUTLINE: Patients are randomized to 1of 2 arms.

ARM I: Patients undergo B-WARM at 39 degrees Celsius (C) for 30 minutes.

ARM II: Patients undergo B-WARM at 39 degrees C for 2 hours.

After completion of study, patients are followed up at 30 days.

▨ Study Type

Interventional

▨ Study Phase

N/A

▨ Condition

- Adult Liver Carcinoma
- Breast Carcinoma
- Colon Carcinoma
- Kidney Neoplasm
- Lung Carcinoma
- Malignant Head and Neck Neoplasm
- Malignant Neoplasm
- Melanoma
- Ovarian Neoplasm
- Soft Tissue Sarcoma

▨ Intervention

Procedure: Hyperthermia Treatment
  Undergo B-WARM

Other Names:

  Clinical Hyperthermia

  Diathermy

  Hyperthermia

  Hyperthermia Therapy

  Other: Laboratory Biomarker Analysis

  Correlative studies

▨ Study Arms

Experimental: Arm I (B-WARM for 30 minutes)
  Patients undergo B-WARM at 39 degrees C for 30 minutes.

Experimental: Arm II (B-WARM for 2 hours)
  Patients undergo B-WARM at 39 degrees C for 2 hours.

Recruitment Information

Recruitment Status

Recruiting

Estimated Enrollment

20

Eligibility Criteria

Inclusion Criteria:

- Patients with a variety of malignancies (i.e., melanoma, sarcoma, colon, head and neck, renal, breast, lung, ovary, liver)
- Patients must have measurable disease (1.0 cm or greater) by computed tomography (CT) scan
- Have an estimated glomerular filtration rate (eGFR) (using the Cockcroft-Gault equation) of more than 60 mL/min
- Have an Eastern Cooperative Oncology Group (ECOG) performance status of 0-2
- Patients of child-bearing potential must agree to use acceptable contraceptive methods (e.g., double barrier) during treatment
- Patient or legal representative must understand the investigational nature of this study and sign an Independent Ethics Committee/Institutional Review Board approved written informed consent form prior to receiving any study related procedure

Exclusion Criteria:

- History of prior myocardial infarction or arrhythmia
- History of any condition deemed by the principal investigator to be a contraindication to B-WARM therapy (e.g., skin reaction, dysregulation of thermoregulation, etc)
- All patients with transdermal patches (e.g.; fentanyl, Lidoderm, scopolamine, etc)
- Pregnant or nursing female patients
- Unwilling or unable to follow protocol requirements
- Any condition which in the investigator's opinion deems the patient an unsuitable candidate to receive B-WARM
- Received an investigational agent within 30 days prior to enrollment
- Received any systemic therapy within 21 days prior to planned B-WARM therapy
- Patients may be enrolled on study but at least 21 days should elapse prior to date of B-WARM therapy
- Patients should not have either CT scanning or B-WARM if they have a fever at the time
- Fever should be worked up and treated as appropriate
- Patients should be afebrile for 24 hours prior to scanning or B-WARM therapy

Sex/Gender

All

Ages

18 Years to N/A

Accepts Healthy Volunteers

No

Completion Date

April 11, 2019

Primary Completion Date

April 11, 2018

Phase I Study of SGI-110 With Irinotecan Followed by Randomized Phase II Study of SGI-110 With Irinotecan Versus Regorafenib or TAS-102 in Previously Treated Metastatic Colorectal Cancer

Study ID:

NCT01896856

Sponsor:

Sidney Kimmel Comprehensive Cancer Center

Information provided by (Responsible Party):

Sidney Kimmel Comprehensive Cancer Center (Sidney Kimmel Comprehensive Cancer Center)

Tracking Information

■ **First Submitted Date**

July 8, 2013

■ **Start Date**

September 2013

■ **Current Primary Outcome Measures**

Phase 1/2: SGI-110 + irinotecan versus regorafenib or TAS-102 adverse events[Time Frame: 4 years]

In Phase 1, subjects will be assessed for adverse events attributable to SGI-110 and/or irinotecan. In Phase 2, subjects will be assessed for adverse events attributable to SGI-110 and/or irinotecan versus regorafenib or TAS-102.

Phase 1/2: Response[Time Frame: 4]

Subjects will be monitored for response via RECIST 1.1 criteria.

■ **Current Secondary Outcome Measures**

Phase 1/2: survival[Time Frame: 4 years]

Subjects will be monitored for survival (overall survival versus progression free survival).

■ **Primary Completion Date**

September 2018

■ **Last Update Posted Date**

January 23, 2018

Descriptive Information

■ **Offical Title**

A Phase I Study of SGI-110 Combined With Irinotecan Followed by a Randomized Phase II Study of SGI-110 Combined With Irinotecan Versus Regorafenib or TAS-102 in Previously Treated Metastatic Colorectal Cancer Patients

■ **Brief Summary**

This is a phase I/randomized phase II study of the combination of SGI-110 and previously treated metastatic colorectal cancer patients. This study will be conducted in two components. First, patients will be enrolled in a phase I study of SGI-110 combined with irinotecan in a standard 3+3 design. After the maximum tolerated dose (MTD) is determined, patients will subsequently be enrolled in a 2:1 randomized phase II study of SGI-110 and irinotecan versus the standard of care regorafenib or TAS-102.

■ **Study Type**

Interventional

■ **Study Phase**

Phase 2

■ **Condition**

• Previously Treated Metastatic Colorectal Cancer

■ **Intervention**

Drug: SGI-110

Drug: Irinotecan

Drug: regorafenib

Drug: TAS-102

Other Names:

lonsurf

■ **Study Arms**

Active Comparator: Phase 2: Arm B regorafenib or TAS-102

In phase 2, we will compare SGI-110 + irinotecan to regorafenib or TAS-102.

Active Comparator: Phase 2: Arm A SGI-110 + irinotecan

In phase 2, we will compare SGI-110 + irinotecan to regorafenib or TAS-102

Recruitment Information

■ **Recruitment Status**

Recruiting

■ **Estimated Enrollment**

108

■ **Completion Date**

September 2019

■ **Primary Completion Date**

September 2018

Eligibility Criteria

Inclusion Criteria:

- Participants must have histologically or cytologically confirmed adenocarcinoma of the colon or rectum
- Patients in the phase II cohort must be amenable to having two research biopsies. This applies to the first 36 patients enrolled to Arm A, who have both biopsiable disease and are randomized to SGI-110 + Irinotecan.
- Archival tissue must be procured if available
- Participants must have measurable disease, defined as at least one lesion that can be accurately measured in at least one dimension (longest diameter to be recorded) as > 20 mm with conventional techniques or as > 10 mm with spiral CT scan. See section 10 for the evaluation of measureable disease.
- Patients in the phase II cohort must have progressed while receiving irinotecan therapy in the metastatic setting. There are no limitations on number of prior therapies in the metastatic setting.
- Age minimum of 18 years.
- Life expectancy of greater than 12 weeks.
- ECOG performance status <1
- Participants must have normal organ and marrow function
- The effects of SGI-110 on the developing human fetus are unknown. For this reason and because oncological agents are known to be teratogenic, women of child-bearing potential and men must agree to use adequate contraception (hormonal or barrier method of birth control; abstinence) prior to study entry, for the duration of study participation, and for 3 months after completion of the study.

Should a woman become pregnant or suspect she is pregnant while participating in this study or within 30 days of last dose, she should inform her treating physician immediately.

- Ability to understand and the willingness to sign a written informed consent document.

Exclusion Criteria:

- Participants who have had chemotherapy or radiotherapy within 4 weeks (6 weeks for nitrosoureas or mitomycin C) prior to enrolling in the study or those who have not recovered from adverse events due to agents administered more than 4 weeks earlier.
- Participants may not be receiving any other study agents.
- Participants with known brain metastases should be excluded from this clinical trial because of their poor prognosis and because they often develop progressive neurologic dysfunction that would confound the evaluation of neurologic and other adverse events.
- History of allergic reactions attributed to compounds of similar chemical or biologic composition to irinotecan, decitabine or SGI-110.
- Subjects who have received prior therapy with any hypomethylating agents.
- Uncontrolled intercurrent illness including, but not limited to ongoing or active infection, symptomatic congestive heart failure, unstable angina pectoris, cardiac arrhythmia, or psychiatric illness/social situations that would limit compliance with study requirements.
- Pregnant women are excluded from this study because SGI-110 is a/an hypomethylating agent with the potential for teratogenic or abortifacient effects. Because there is an unknown but potential risk of adverse events in nursing infants secondary to treatment of the mother with SGI-110, breastfeeding should be discontinued. These potential risks may also apply to other agents used in this study.
- Individuals with a history of a different malignancy are ineligible except for the following circumstances: Individuals with a history of other malignancies who have been disease-free for at least 5 years and are deemed by the investigator to be at low risk for recurrence of that malignancy. Individuals with the following cancers are eligible if diagnosed and treated within the past 5 years: cervical cancer in situ, definitively treated early stage prostate cancer (confined to prostate with Gleason 6 or below), definitely treated breast ductal or lobular carcinoma in situ, and basal cell or squamous cell carcinoma of the skin.
- HIV-positive individuals on combination antiretroviral therapy are ineligible because of the potential for pharmacokinetic interactions with SGI-110. In addition, as these individuals are at increased risk of lethal infections when treated with marrow-suppressive therapy. Appropriate studies will be undertaken in participants receiving combination antiretroviral therapy when indicated.
- Previous treatment with regorafenib and TAS-102 (This applies to phase II only.) If patients have previously received either regorafenib OR TAS-102, they must be able to receive the alternate regimen if randomized to the standard of care arm).
- Hospitalization for an acute medical issue within 4 weeks prior to screening visit that would not otherwise be managed in an infusion center or outpatient clinic setting (e.g., a patient admitted to complete a transfusion would not be ineligible.).
- Symptomatic bowel obstruction within 6 months prior to enrollment, Patients who undergo surgical correction of obstructing lesion will be eligible within 6 months.

Sex/Gender

All

Ages

18 Years to N/A

Safety of Endoscopic Resection of Large Colorectal Polyps: A Randomized Trial.

Study ID:

NCT01936948

Sponsor:

White River Junction Veterans Affairs Medical Center

Information provided by (Responsible Party):

White River Junction Veterans Affairs Medical Center (White River Junction Veterans Affairs Medical Center)

Tracking Information

■ **First Submitted Date**

September 3, 2013

■ **Start Date**

April 2013

■ **Current Primary Outcome Measures**

Delayed bleeding complications[Time Frame: 30 days following a study polyp resection]

A bleeding event that occurred within 30 days after completion of the colonoscopy with a study polyp resection and is associated with a decrease in hemoglobin by at least 2gm, hemodynamic instability, presentation to the ED, need for hospitalization, repeat colonoscopy, or other interventions.

■ **Primary Completion Date**

December 2020

■ **Last Update Posted Date**

March 3, 2017

■ **Current Secondary Outcome Measures**

Overall complications[Time Frame: 30 days]

Overall complications are defined as an aggregate of all complications that occur at the time of the procedure (immediate complications) or during 30 days of follow-up. They include delayed bleeding complications, perforation, postpolypectomy syndrome, and clinical events that require an ED visit, admission to the hospital, additional testing or an intervention.

Complete polyp resection[Time Frame: 6 months]

Rate of complete study polyp resection at the initial colonoscopy and at first follow-up endoscopy

Polyp recurrence[Time Frame: 3 months to 5 years]

Rate of recurrent polyp at the resection site after complete polyp resection.

Clip complications[Time Frame: 30 days]

Incidence if complications associated with application of clips.

Descriptive Information

■ **Offical Title**

Safety of Endoscopic Resection of Large Colorectal Polyps: A Randomized Trial.

■ **Brief Summary**

The effectiveness of colonoscopy in reducing colorectal cancer mortality relies on the detection and removal of neoplastic polyps. Because the risk of prevalent cancer and of transition to cancer increases with polyp size, effective and safe resection of large polyps is particularly important. Large polyps ≥20mm are removed by so-called endoscopic mucosal resection (EMR) using electrocautery snares. Resection of these large polyps is associated with a risk of severe complications that may require hospitalization and additional interventions. The most common risk is delayed bleeding which is observed in approximately 2-9% of patients. A recent retrospective study suggests that closure of the large mucosal defect after resection may decrease the risk of delayed bleeding. However, significant uncertainty remains about the polypectomy techniques to optimizing resection and minimizing risk. Important aspects that may affect risk include clipping of the mucosal defect and electrocautery setting.

■ Detailed Description

Aim 1. The primary aim of the study is to compare the rate of delayed bleeding complications in patients undergoing endoscopic resection of large polyps between:

- A) Closing the mucosal defect after resection (Clip group) and
- B) Not closing the mucosal defect after resection (No clip group).

Aim 2. The secondary aim of the study is to compare the rate of overall complications in patients undergoing endoscopic resection of large polyps between two cautery settings:

- A) Low power coagulation and
- B) Endocut.

■ Study Type

Interventional

■ Study Phase

N/A

■ Condition

- Colon Polyps

■ Intervention

Procedure: Clip closure

Patients will be randomized to either closing the mucosal defect after polyp removal or not closing the mucosal defect using clips (main intervention and comparison). The resection margins will be approximated using clips. Complete closure is defined as approximated margins with less than 1cm gap between clips. All patients will further be randomized to two different settings of electrocautery (EndoCut or Coagulation) to standardize otherwise variable electrocautery practice, and for explorative analysis.

■ Study Arms

Active Comparator: Clip closure + EndoCut

Clipping of the mucosal defect after resection of a ≥20mm non-pedunculated study polyp using clips. Resection is done using the EndoCut electrocautery mode.

Active Comparator: Clip closure + Coagulation

Clipping of the mucosal defect after resection of a ≥20mm non-pedunculated study polyp using clips. Resection is done using the Coagulation electrocautery mode.

No Intervention: No clip closure + EndoCut

No clipping of the mucosal defect after resection of a ≥20mm non-pedunculated study polyp. Resection is done using the EndoCut electrocautery mode.

No Intervention: No clip closure + Coagulation

No clipping of the mucosal defect after resection of a ≥20mm non-pedunculated study polyp. Resection is done using the Coagulation electrocautery mode.

Recruitment Information

■ Recruitment Status

Recruiting

■ Estimated Enrollment

1020

■ Completion Date

December 2021

■ Primary Completion Date

December 2020

■ Eligibility Criteria

Inclusion Criteria:

- Any patient ≥18 and ≤89 who presents for a colonoscopy and who does not have criteria for exclusion
- Patients with a ≥20mm non-pedunculated colon polyp

Exclusion Criteria:

- Patients with known (biopsy proven) invasive carcinoma in a potential study polyp
- Pedunculated polyps (as defined by Paris Classification type Ip or Isp)
- Patients with ulcerated depressed lesions (as defined by Paris Classification type III)
- Patients with inflammatory bowel disease
- Patients who are receiving an emergency colonoscopy
- Poor general health (ASA class>3)

- Patients with coagulopathy with an elevated INR ≥1.5, or platelets <50
- Poor bowel preparation
- Pregnancy

Sex/Gender

All

Ages

18 Years to 89 Years

Accepts Healthy Volunteers

No

Contacts

Heiko Pohl, MD   802-295-9363   heiko.pohl@dartmouth.edu
Cathy Lombardo   802-295-9363   cathy.lombardo@va.gov

GVAX for Colorectal Cancer

Study ID:

NCT01952730

Sponsor:

Massachusetts General Hospital

Information provided by (Responsible Party):

Massachusetts General Hospital (Massachusetts General Hospital)

Tracking Information

First Submitted Date

April 26, 2013

Start Date

July 2013

Primary Completion Date

July 2018

Last Update Posted Date

January 8, 2018

Current Primary Outcome Measures

number of patients who fail to receive the first six scheduled vaccinations because of toxicity[Time Frame: 2 years]

> To determine the safety of 6 vaccinations with lethally irradiated, autologous colorectal cancer cells engineered by adenoviral mediated gene transfer to secrete GM-CSF in stage IV colorectal cancer patients who are completely resected. Patient safety will be assured by monitoring the number of patients who fail to receive the first six scheduled vaccinations because of toxicity. If three or more patients experience grade 4 or worse toxicity due to the vaccine before completing six immunizations, the study will be terminated.

Current Secondary Outcome Measures

Progression Free Survival[Time Frame: 10 years]

> To determine the progression free survival of stage IV colorectal cancer patients vaccinated with lethally irradiated, autologous colorectal cancer cells engineered by adenoviral mediated gene transfer to secrete GM-CSF.

Immune Response[Time Frame: 2 years]

> To evaluate the immune response elicited by the vaccine. We will evaluate the immune cell composition(CD4+ and CD8+ T cells, T regulatory cells, macrophage, etc) in the resected specimens and in the circulating blood.

Two year survival[Time Frame: 5 years]

> To assess overall survival at 2 years

Descriptive Information

Offical Title

A Pilot Safety Study of Vaccination With Autologous, Lethally Irradiated Colorectal Cancer Cells Engineered by Adenoviral Mediated Gene Transfer to Secrete Human Granulocyte-Macrophage Stimulating Factor

Brief Summary

This study is a Pilot clinical trial. Pilot clinical trials test the safety of an investigational combination of drugs. Pilot studies provide information on what effects, both good and bad, the Investigational agent might have on your disease. "Investigational" means that the intervention is still being studied and that research doctors are trying to find out more about it. It also means that the FDA has not approved the treatment for your type of cancer.

The main purposes of this study are to determine:

- The amount of vaccine that can be made for your colorectal tumor cells
- If the vaccine can be given safely
- What the effects of the vaccine are, both good and bad
- How the vaccine affects your immune system
- Whether this vaccine might have any effect on the return of your cancer in the liver after surgical removal

This study is being done because there are currently no treatments which have demonstrated to cure diseae which has progressed, or moved beyond the site of the primary site of disease (colon or rectum). These vaccinations will be given after you have completed the standard of care treatment as determined by your doctor.

Laboratory research has made vaccines from cancer cells by inserting genetic material from a protein called granulocyte-macrophage colony stimulating factor (GM-CSF) into the cancer cell. Once complete, the cancer cells are able to produce large amounts of GM-CSF. The vaccine made form these cells has a greater anti-tumor effect than cancer cells without GM-CSF. The purpose of this research study is to determine the safety of an investigational vaccine that will be made using your own colorectal cancer cells in the manner described above.

This vaccine has been used in several other research studies for treatment for other cancers (skin, lung, ovarian, sarcoma and leukemia.) Information from these other research studies suggests that this vaccine may help to reduce the risk of your colorectal cancer returning after you have your colorectal cancer surgery.

Due to these results in melanoma and several other tumors we are encouraged to use this vaccine approach in patients with liver metastases from colorectal cancer, after the cancer in the liver has been removed by surgery.

Detailed Description

After you have given your consent to participate in this study, your study doctor will perform some tests to confirm that you are eligible to participate. These tests may take place up to 21 days before the surgery to remove a liver tumor, which will be used to create the vaccines. Many of the following examinations are commonly done to determine diagnosis and/or stage of disease and you may have already had some or all of these evaluations. They may or may not have to be repeated. These tests include a medical history, performance status, blod samples, routine blood tests, tumor assessment and blood pregnancy test (if applicable). If these tests indicate you are eligible for this study and you agree to participate, you will be referred to a surgeon for the surgical removal of tumor tissue from which the vaccine will be made.

The surgery will be performed at Massachusetts General Hospital. You will be asked to sign a separate consent form to give permission to the surgeon to perform this operation. That consent will describe the risks of the operation which involves removing the tumor cells from your liver.

After your surgery, there is a possibility that your physician will recommend other treatment before starting the vaccines if he or she feels it would be beneficial to your care and medically appropriate. This part of the treatment would not be experimental (for example, chemotherapy or radiation therapy).

Then, in this case, the vaccines made from your cancer will not be administered to you until at least 4 weeks after your last chemotherapy or radiation treatment. If the time between your operation and the first scheduled vaccine injection is 8 weeks or longer, we will ask you to undergo another chest, abdomen and pelvic CT scan and clinical blood work to confirm that it is still safe for you to proceed with the vaccines. After this 4 week rest period, vaccine administration will occur as previously outlined.

If these tests indicate you are eligible for this study and you agree to participate, you will be referred to a surgeon for the surgical removal of tumor tissue from which the vaccine will be made.

It is important to know that sometimes we are unable to collect enough cells from the tumor collection. In those cases we can try to grow the tumor cells for a short period of time to get enough cells to make a vaccine, but we can not guarantee that we will always be able to produce vaccine for every participant who undergoes tumor cell collection.

The vaccines created from your colorectal cancer cells are scheduled to be given to you on days 1, 8, 15 and then every two weeks after that until 6 total vaccines have been administered. The amount of vaccines is dependent on the total amount of cells collected when your colorectal cancer liver metastasis is processed and prepared into vaccine in our lab. It is hoped that you will receive at least six vaccines. All scheduled treatment will occur in the outpatient clinic.

The vaccines will be administered in two injections that will be placed underneath your skin. The two injections will be given at the same place on your body. The recommended sites are your arms, thighs or trunk area and the sites will rotate per vaccine.

Day 1 is the first day of treatment on study. The following procedures are planned on this day: update of medical history, physical exam, blood samples for routine labs, required blood sample for immune studies, vaccine administration, and, if enough cells can be grown, you will receive an injection of cancer cells that have been killed but not able to secrete GM-CSF. This is done to measure the amount of reaction of your immune system caused by the vaccine alone.

Punch biopsies will be obtained 2 days after the first and fifth vaccinations. A DTH injection will also be administered at the first and fifth vaccine. Two days after the vaccine and DTH administration punch biopsy will be taken. DTH injections are Delayed-type Hyper-sensitivity Tests. This injection inserts a small amount of the vaccine under your skin to determine if you have any allergic reactions to the vaccine. This will consist of a small piece of skin tissue removed under local anesthesia. A small stitch will be placed after the biopsy. You will sign a separate consent form for this procedure.

The following procedures are planned for Days 8 and 15: update of medical history, weight and vital signs, blood samples for routine labs and immune studies, and vaccine administration.

On day 29 and every two weeks (until no more vaccines are available) you wil undergo an update of medical history, physical exam, weight and vital signs, blood samples for routine labs and immune studies, punch biopsy and vaccine administration. With vaccine #5, you may receive a second DTH injection. Two days after the vaccine and DTH injection, punch biopsies will be taken off both sites to further evaluate your body's response to the treatment.

After the final dose of study drug, your treating physician will determine if you are eligible to receive a second series of vaccinations. In addition, there must be sufficient numbers of cells for vaccine remaining from the original harvest or a new liver metastasis has occurred and been removed to make more vaccine.

If you give consent to participate in the repeat dose phase, you will be required to repeat the screening tests to see if you are still eligible to participate in the study.

It is possible that additional rounds of vaccine therapy may be offered after the second round, as long as it is appropriate in the opinion of your treating physician and additional tumor is available to make vaccine and you continue to meet the eligibility criteria.

Participants will be monitored every 3 months with a blood test for the first 3 years and then every 6-12 months for a total of 5 years. Staging CT scans will be performed 3 months after the last vaccination, then every 6 months for the first three years and then yearly to year 5. After 5 years imaging will be at the discretion of the treating physician. Blood draws for immune research studies will occur every 3 months for 2 years after completing all vaccinations.

Study Type

Interventional

Study Phase

Phase 1

Condition

- Colorectal Cancer

Intervention

Biological: GVAX

Study Arms

Experimental: Experimental Treatment Arm
   GVAX, up to 6 vaccinations, administered via injection

Recruitment Information

Recruitment Status

Recruiting

Estimated Enrollment

15

Completion Date

July 2030

Primary Completion Date

July 2018

Eligibility Criteria

Inclusion Criteria:

- Histologically documented hepatic colorectal cancer metastasis with resectable hepatic lesions
- At least 4 weeks since last dose of chemotherapy, radiotherapy, immunotherapy, systemic glucocorticoid therapy or operation in order to receive vaccine
- Fully recovered from hepatic resection

Exclusion Criteria:

- Pregnant or breastfeeding
- Uncontrolled active infection
- Infection with HIV, Hepatitis B or C
- Other current malignancies except in situ cancer or basal/squamous cell carcinoma
- Active autoimmune disease
- Hepatic metastases involving both branches of the portal vein or all three hepatic veins
- Peritoneal metastases identified at the time of attempted resection
- Greater than 1 month since resection of liver metastasis for vaccine production

Sex/Gender

All

Ages

18 Years to N/A

SGI-110 in Combination With an Allogeneic Colon Cancer Cell Vaccine (GVAX) and Cyclophosphamide (CY) in Metastatic Colorectal Cancer (mCRC)

Study ID:

NCT01966289

Sponsor:

Sidney Kimmel Comprehensive Cancer Center

Information provided by (Responsible Party):

Sidney Kimmel Comprehensive Cancer Center (Sidney Kimmel Comprehensive Cancer Center)

Tracking Information

■ **First Submitted Date**

October 10, 2013

■ **Primary Completion Date**

December 2018

■ **Start Date**

December 2013

■ **Last Update Posted Date**

July 11, 2017

■ **Current Primary Outcome Measures**

Difference in CD45RO+ tumor infiltrating lymphocytes (TILs) measured by immunohistochemistry in pre and post-treatment tumor biopsies from patients with metastatic colorectal cancer[Time Frame: 4 years]

Number of Participants with Adverse Events as a Measure of Safety and Tolerability[Time Frame: 4 years]

■ **Current Secondary Outcome Measures**

Overall Survival (OS)[Time Frame: 4 years]

Time To Progression (TTP)[Time Frame: 4 years]

Progression Free Survival (PFS)[Time Frame: 4 years]

Descriptive Information

■ **Offical Title**

A Pilot Study of SGI-110 in Combination With an Allogeneic Colon Cancer Cell Vaccine (GVAX) and Cyclophosphamide (CY) in Metastatic Colorectal Cancer (mCRC) as Maintenance Therapy

■ **Brief Summary**

This study will be looking at whether CY/GVAX in combination with SGI-110 is effective (recruits CD45RO+ T cells to the tumor which may be a marker of anti-tumor activity) and safe in patients with metastatic colon or rectum cancers.

■ **Study Type**

Interventional

■ **Study Phase**

Phase 1

■ **Condition**

• Metastatic Colorectal Cancer

■ **Intervention**

Drug: CY

CY is administered intravenously at 200 mg/m2

Other Names:

Cyclophosphamide, Cytoxan

Biological: GVAX

GVAX is administered intradermally at 5E8 colon cancer cells + 5E7 GM-CSF secreting cells

Other Names:

Colon cancer tumor vaccine

Drug: SGI-110

SGI-110 is administered subcutaneously at 60 mg/m2

Study Arms

Experimental: Cohort 1:CY/GVAX concurrently with SGI-110

During each of the four cycles, Cyclophosphamide (CY) is administered on Day 1 at 200 mg/m2, the colon cancer tumor vaccine (GVAX) is administered on Day 2 at 5E8 colon cancer cells + 5E7 GM-CSF secreting cells, and SGI-110 is administered on Days 1-5 at 60 mg/m2. Each cycle is 28 days. Enrollment will begin first in Cohort 1 and 2. If a response to the treatment is seen in Cohorts 1 and 2, enrollment in Cohort 3 and 4 will begin.

Experimental: Cohort 2: CY/GVAX after SGI-110

During each of the four cycles, SGI-110 is administered on Days 1-5 at 60 mg/m2, Cyclophosphamide (CY) is administered on Day 8 at 200 mg/m2, and the colon cancer tumor vaccine (GVAX) is administered on Day 9 at 5E8 colon cancer cells + 5E7 GM-CSF secreting cells. Each cycle is 28 days. Enrollment will begin first in Cohort 1 and 2. If a response to the treatment is seen in Cohorts 1 and 2, enrollment in Cohort 3 and 4 will begin.

Experimental: Cohort 3: CY/GVAX

During each of the four cycles, Cyclophosphamide (CY) is administered on Day 1 at 200 mg/m2 and the colon cancer tumor vaccine (GVAX) is administered on Day 2 at 5E8 colon cancer cells + 5E7 GM-CSF secreting cells. Each cycle is 28 days. Enrollment will begin first in Cohort 1 and 2. If a response to the treatment is seen in Cohorts 1 and 2, enrollment in Cohort 3 and 4 will begin.

Experimental: Cohort 4: SGI-110

During each of the four cycles, SGI-110 is administered on Days 1-5 at 60 mg/m2. Each cycle is 28 days. Enrollment will begin first in Cohort 1 and 2. If a response to the treatment is seen in Cohorts 1 and 2, enrollment in Cohort 3 and 4 will begin.

Recruitment Information

Recruitment Status

Recruiting

Estimated Enrollment

32

Completion Date

December 2019

Primary Completion Date

December 2018

Eligibility Criteria

Inclusion Criteria:

1. Documented cancer of the colon or rectum who have received and are stable on first or second-line therapy regimens for metastatic colorectal cancer

2. ECOG Performance Status of 0 to 1

3. Adequate organ function as defined by study-specified laboratory tests

4. Must use acceptable form of birth control through the study and for 28 days after final dose of study drug

5. Signed informed consent form

6. Willing and able to comply with study procedures

Exclusion Criteria:

1. Currently have or have history of certain study-specified heart, liver, kidney, lung, neurological, immune or other medical conditions

2. Systemically active steroid use

3. Another investigational product within 28 days prior to receiving study drug

4. Major surgery or significant traumatic injury (or unhealed surgical wounds) occurring within 28 days prior to receiving study drug

5. Chemotherapy, radiation, hormonal, or biological cancer therapy within 28 days prior to receiving study drug

6. Pregnant or lactating

7. Unwilling or unable to comply with study procedures

- ▨ **Sex/Gender**

  All

- ▨ **Ages**

  18 Years to 100 Years

- ▨ **Accepts Healthy Volunteers**

  No

- ▨ **Contacts**

  Carol Judkins, RN   410-614-5241   judkica@jhmi.edu

  Nilofer Azad, MD   nazad2@jhmi.edu

Cabozantinib and Panitumumab to Treat KRAS Wild-Type Metastatic Colorectal Cancer

Study ID:

NCT02008383

Sponsor:

John Strickler, M.D.

Information provided by (Responsible Party):

Duke University (John Strickler, M.D.)

Tracking Information

- ▨ **First Submitted Date**

  December 3, 2013

- ▨ **Start Date**

  January 2014

- ▨ **Primary Completion Date**

  January 2018

- ▨ **Last Update Posted Date**

  May 2, 2017

- ▨ **Current Primary Outcome Measures**

  Recommended phase II dose (RPTD) for the combination of cabozantinib and panitumumab[Time Frame: RPTD for the study will be determined at the completion of Phase I dose escalation cohort; estimated as 1 year]

  Objective response rate (ORR) of cabozantinib monotherapy in patients with prospectively identified MET amplified metastatic colorectal cancer[Time Frame: Approximately every 8 weeks and/or restaging]

- ▨ **Current Secondary Outcome Measures**

  Non-dose limiting toxicities of cabozantinib and panitumumab.[Time Frame: Continuous, every 4 weeks minimum until end of study estimated at 4 years]

  Adverse events will be recorded

  Response rate of cabozantinib and panitumumab[Time Frame: approximately every 8 weeks and/or restaging]

  Response is assessed at restaging, approximately every 8 weeks.

  Progression free survival associated with the cabozantinib and panitumumab regimen[Time Frame: From date of randomization until the date of first documented progression or date of death from any cause, whichever came first, assessed up to 60 months]

  Overall survival associated with the cabozantinib and panitumumab regimen[Time Frame: From date of randomization until the date of death from any cause assessed up to 60 months]

  Progression free survival associated with cabozantinib monotherapy in patients with MET amplified colorectal cancer[Time Frame: From date of randomization until the date of first documented progression or date of death from any cause, whichever came first, assessed up to 60 months]

  Overall survival associated with cabozantinib monotherapy in patients with MET amplified colorectal cancer[Time Frame: From date of randomization until the date of death from any cause assessed up to 60 months]

  To describe the safety and tolerability of cabozantinib monotherapy in patients with MET amplified colorectal cancer[Time Frame: Continuous, every 4 weeks minimum until end of study estimated at 4 years]

  Adverse events will be recorded

Descriptive Information

Offical Title

Cabozantinib (XL184) With Panitumumab in Subjects With KRAS Wild-Type Metastatic Colorectal Cancer and Cabozantinib Monotherapy in Subjects With MET Amplified Treatment-Refractory Colorectal Cancer

Brief Summary

There will be three parts to this phase I study: 1) the Combination Dose Finding cohort; 2) the Combination Expansion cohort; and 3) the Monotherapy MET Amplified cohort. In the Combination Dose Finding cohort and the Combination Expansion cohort, we will combine cabozantinib and panitumumab in patients with KRAS wild-type metastatic colorectal cancer (CRC). In the Monotherapy MET Amplified cohort, we will screen at least 50 patients for MET gene amplification ("MET amplification"). Patients with MET amplification will receive cabozantinib only (monotherapy).

The primary objective of this open-label phase Ib trial are:

1. To determine the maximum tolerated dose and the recommended phase II dose for the combination of cabozantinib and panitumumab in patients with KRAS wild-type metastatic colorectal cancer and

2. To identify the objective response rate (ORR) of cabozantinib monotherapy in patients with prospectively identified MET amplified metastatic colorectal cancer.

The secondary objectives are:

1. To describe the non-dose limiting toxicities of cabozantinib and panitumumab.

2. To describe the clinical activity (ORR, PFS, OS) of cabozantinib and panitumumab.

3. To describe the safety and tolerability of cabozantinib monotherapy in patients with MET amplified colorectal cancer.

4. To describe the clinical activity (PFS, OS) of cabozantinib monotherapy in patients with MET amplified colorectal cancer.

Study Type

Interventional

Study Phase

Phase 1

Condition

- Colorectal Cancer

Intervention

Biological: Panitumumab

The FDA approved dose for panitumumab is 6mg/kg IV, every two weeks. This is the dose and schedule that will be used in this study.

Other Names:

Vectibix

Drug: Cabozantinib

There will be three parts to this phase I study: 1) the Combination Dose Finding cohort; 2) the Combination Expansion cohort; and 3) the Monotherapy MET Amplified cohort.

Cabozantinib will start at a dose of 60 mg daily with reductions to 40 and 20 mg daily possible in the dose finding cohort. The combination expansion cohort dose will determined by the dose finding cohort. The Monotherapy MET Amplified cohort will recieve 60 mg Cabozantinib daily.

Other Names:

Cometriq

Study Arms

Experimental: Cabozantinib and Panitumumab
60 mg Cabozantinib PO daily and 6 mg/kg Panitumumab IV every 2 weeks.

Experimental: Cabozantinib
60 mg Cabozantinib PO daily.

Recruitment Information

Recruitment Status

Recruiting

Estimated Enrollment

50

Completion Date

January 2019

Primary Completion Date

January 2018

Eligibility Criteria

MET Amplification Screening Test Inclusion Criteria:

1. Histologically and/or cytologically confirmed and radiographically measurable KRAS wild-type adenocarcinoma of the colon or rectum that is metastatic and/ or unresectable. Subjects must have been treated with a fluoropyrimidine (e.g., 5-fluorouracil or capecitabine), oxaliplatin, irinotecan and bevacizumab or have contraindication to such treatment.

2. Prior treatment with anti-EGFR therapy (either panitumumab or cetuximab).

3. At least one site of disease that is measurable by RECIST (version 1.1) criteria that has not been previously irradiated; if the patient has had previous radiation to the target lesion(s), there must be evidence of progression since the radiation.

4. Age ≥ 18 years.

5. Eastern Cooperative Oncology Group (ECOG) performance status of 0, 1, or 2.

6. Life expectancy greater than 3 months.

7. Capable of understanding and complying with the protocol requirements and has signed the informed consent document.

8. Adequate organ and marrow function as defined below:

Absolute neutrophil count ≥ 1,000/μl without colony stimulating factor support

Platelets ≥ 75,000/μl

Hemoglobin ≥ 8 g/dL

AST/ALT ≤ 3 X upper limit of normal (ULN)

Total bilirubin ≤ 1.5 X upper limit of normal (ULN)

Serum albumin ≥ 2.5 g/dL

MET Amplification Screening Test Exclusion Criteria:

1. Presence of or known history of brain/ CNS tumor or metastases.

2. KRAS exon 2 (codons 12 or 13) mutation detected in tumor tissue specimen.

3. Concurrent severe and/or uncontrolled medical conditions which may compromise participation in the study, including impaired heart function or clinically significant heart disease.

4. Concomitant treatment, in therapeutic doses, with anticoagulants such as warfarin or warfarin-related agents, heparin, thrombin or Factor Xa inhibitors, or antiplatelet agents (e.g., clopidogrel). Low dose aspirin (≤ 81 mg/day), low-dose warfarin (≤ 1 mg/day), and prophylactic LMWH are permitted.

5. Previously experienced any of the following:

1. clinically significant gastrointestinal bleeding within the last 6 months

2. hemoptysis of ≥ 0.5 teaspoon (2.5ml) of red blood within the last 3 months

3. any other signs indicative of pulmonary hemorrhage within the last 3 months

6. Radiographic evidence of cavitating pulmonary lesion(s).

7. Tumor in contact with, invading or encasing any major blood vessels.

8. Evidence of endotracheal or endobronchial tumor.

9. Uncontrolled, significant intercurrent or recent illness including, but not limited to, the following conditions:

1. Cardiovascular disorders including:

i. Congestive heart failure (CHF): New York Heart Association (NYHA) Class III (moderate) or Class IV (severe) at the time of screening

ii. Any history of congenital long QT syndrome

iii. Any of the following within the last 6 months:

1. unstable angina pectoris

2. clinically-significant cardiac arrhythmias

3. stroke (including TIA, or other ischemic event)

4. myocardial infarction

5. thromboembolic event requiring therapeutic anticoagulation Note: Subjects with a venous filter (e.g., vena cava filter) are not eligible for this study.

b. Gastrointestinal disorders particularly those associated with a high risk of perforation or fistula formation including: i. Any of the following within the last 28 days:

1. active peptic ulcer disease

2. active inflammatory bowel disease (including ulcerative colitis and Crohn's disease), diverticulitis, cholecystitis, symptomatic cholangitis or appendicitis

3. malabsorption syndrome

ii. Any of the following within the last 6 months:

1. abdominal fistula

2. gastrointestinal perforation

3. bowel obstruction or gastric outlet obstruction

4. intra-abdominal abscess

Note: Complete resolution of an intra-abdominal abscess must be confirmed prior even if the abscess occurred more that 6 months ago.

c. Other disorders associated with a high risk of fistula formation or wound healing complications, including percutaneous endoscopic gastrostomy (PEG) tube placement within the last 3 months.

d. History of chronic pancreatitis.

10. Unable to swallow tablets.

11. Evidence within the last 2 years of another malignancy which required systemic treatment.

12. Known history of HIV seropositivity, hepatitis C virus, acute or chronic active hepatitis B infection, or other serious chronic infection requiring ongoing treatment.

Main Study Inclusion Criteria:

1. For the Monotherapy MET Amplified cohort only: MET gene amplification by prospective screening assay from peripheral blood.

2. Histologically and/or cytologically confirmed and radiographically measurable KRAS wild-type adenocarcinoma of the colon or rectum that is metastatic and/ or unresectable. Subjects must have been treated with a fluoropyrimidine (e.g., 5-fluorouracil or capecitabine), oxaliplatin, irinotecan and bevacizumab or have contraindication to such treatment. In addition, for the monotherapy MET Amplified cohort, must have received prior treatment with anti-EGFR therapy (either panitumumab or cetuximab).

3. At least one site of disease that is measurable by RECIST (version 1.1) criteria that has not been previously irradiated; if the patient has had previous radiation to the target lesion(s), there must be evidence of progression since the radiation.

4. Age ≥ 18 years.

5. Eastern Cooperative Oncology Group (ECOG) performance status of 0 or 1.

6. Life expectancy greater than 3 months.

7. Sexually active subjects (men and women) must agree to use medically accepted barrier methods of contraception (e.g., male or female condom) during the course of the study and for 4 months after the last dose of study drug(s), even if oral contraceptives are also used. All subjects of reproductive potential must agree to use both a barrier method and a second method of birth control during the course of the study and for 4 months after the last dose of study drug(s).

8. Women of childbearing potential must have a negative pregnancy test within 7 days before the first dose of study treatment.

9. Capable of understanding and complying with the protocol requirements and has signed the informed consent document.

10. Adequate organ and marrow function as defined by protocol.

Main Study Exclusion Criteria:

1. Cytotoxic chemotherapy (including investigational cytotoxic chemotherapy) or biologic agents (e.g., cytokines or antibodies) within 3 weeks, or nitrosoureas/ mitomycin C within 6 weeks before the first dose of study treatment.

2. Prior treatment with a small molecule kinase inhibitor or a hormonal therapy (including investigational kinase inhibitors or hormones) within 14 days or five half-lives of the compound or active metabolites, whichever is longer, before the first dose of study treatment.

3. For Combination Dose Finding and Combination Expansion cohorts only: History of hypersensitivity reactions/anaphylaxis attributed to humanized and/or chimeric monoclonal antibodies or other such proteins. Hypersensitivity reactions that are clearly related to cetuximab may be permitted at the discretion of the Lead PI.

4. Radionuclide treatment, including yttrium-90 treatment, within 6 weeks of the first dose of study treatment.

5. Radiation therapy:

a. to the thoracic cavity, abdomen or pelvis within 3 months of the first dose of study treatment or has ongoing complications or is without complete recovery and healing from prior radiation therapy b. to bone metastases within 14 days of the first dose of study treatment c. to any other site(s) within 28 days of the first dose of study treatment

6. Any other type of investigational agent within 28 days before the first dose of study treatment.

7. Not recovered to baseline or CTCAE ≤ Grade 1 from toxicity due to all prior therapies except alopecia, oxaliplatin-related neuropathy, and other non-clinically significant adverse events.

8. Presence of or known history of brain/ CNS tumor or metastases.

9. KRAS exon 2 (codons 12 or 13) mutation detected in tumor tissue specimen.

10. Concurrent severe and/or uncontrolled medical conditions which may compromise participation in the study, including impaired heart function or clinically significant heart disease.

11. Prothrombin time (PT) or partial thromboplastin time (PTT) test ≥ 1.3 x laboratory upper limit of normal (ULN) within 7 days before the first dose of study treatment.

12. Concomitant treatment, in therapeutic doses, with anticoagulants such as warfarin or warfarin-related agents, heparin, thrombin or Factor Xa inhibitors, or antiplatelet agents (e.g., clopidogrel). Low dose aspirin (≤ 81 mg/day), low-dose warfarin (≤ 1 mg/day), and prophylactic LMWH are permitted.

13. Chronic concomitant treatment of strong CYP3A4 inducers or CYP3A4 inhibitors.

14. Previously experienced any of the following:

1. clinically significant gastrointestinal bleeding within 6 months before the first dose of study treatment

2. hemoptysis of ≥ 0.5 teaspoon (2.5ml) of red blood within 3 months before the first dose of study treatment

3. any other signs indicative of pulmonary hemorrhage within 3 months before the first dose of study treatment

15. Radiographic evidence of cavitating pulmonary lesion(s).

16. Tumor in contact with, invading or encasing any major blood vessels.

17. Evidence of endotracheal or endobronchial tumor.

18. Uncontrolled, significant intercurrent or recent illness including, but not limited to, the following conditions:

1. Cardiovascular disorders including:

i. Congestive heart failure (CHF): New York Heart Association (NYHA) Class III (moderate) or Class IV (severe) at the time of screening

ii. Concurrent uncontrolled hypertension defined as sustained BP > 140 mm Hg systolic, or > 90 mm Hg diastolic despite optimal antihypertensive treatment within 7 days of the first dose of study treatment

iii. Any history of congenital long QT syndrome

iv. Any of the following within 6 months before the first dose of study treatment:

1. unstable angina pectoris

2. clinically-significant cardiac arrhythmias

3. stroke (including TIA, or other ischemic event)

4. myocardial infarction

5. thromboembolic event requiring therapeutic anticoagulation

Note: Subjects with a venous filter (e.g., vena cava filter) are not eligible for this study.

b. Gastrointestinal disorders particularly those associated with a high risk of perforation or fistula formation including:

i. Any of the following within 28 days before the first dose of study treatment

1. active peptic ulcer disease

2. active inflammatory bowel disease (including ulcerative colitis and Crohn's disease), diverticulitis, cholecystitis, symptomatic cholangitis or appendicitis

3. malabsorption syndrome

ii. Any of the following within 6 months before the first dose of study treatment:

1. abdominal fistula

2. gastrointestinal perforation

3. bowel obstruction or gastric outlet obstruction

4. intra-abdominal abscess

Note: Complete resolution of an intra-abdominal abscess must be confirmed prior to initiating treatment with cabozantinib even if the abscess occurred more that 6 months before the first dose of study treatment.

c. Other disorders associated with a high risk of fistula formation or wound healing complications, including percutaneous endoscopic gastrostomy (PEG) tube placement within 3 months before the first dose of study therapy.

d. History of chronic pancreatitis.

e. Other clinically significant disorders such as:

i. active infection requiring IV antibiotic within 28 days before the first dose of study treatment

ii. serious non-healing wound/ulcer/bone fracture within 28 days before the first dose of study treatment

iii. history of organ transplant

iv. concurrent uncompensated hypothyroidism or thyroid dysfunction

Note: Patients with newly diagnosed thyroid conditions may participate if stable on a new regimen for at least 7 days before the first dose of study treatment.

v. history of surgery as follows:

1. major surgery within 3 months of the first dose of cabozantinib if there were no wound healing complications or within 6 months of the first dose of cabozantinib if there were wound complications

2. minor surgery, including dental procedures, within 1 month of the first dose of cabozantinib if there were no wound healing complications or within 3 months of the first dose of cabozantinib if there were wound complications

In addition, complete wound healing from prior surgery must be confirmed at least 28 days before the first dose of cabozantinib irrespective of the time from surgery.

19. History of interstitial lung disease (e.g., pneumonitis or pulmonary fibrosis) or evidence of interstitial lung disease on baseline chest CT scan.

20. Unable to swallow tablets.

21. Corrected QT interval calculated by the Fridericia formula (QTcF) > 500 ms within 28 days before start of treatment. Note: At baseline (i.e. screening), three ECGs to be obtained within 30 minutes but approximately 2 minutes apart (i.e. triplicate). If the average of the three consecutive results for QTcF is ≤ 500 ms, the subject meets eligibility in this regard.

22. Pregnant or breastfeeding.

23. For the Combination Dose Finding and Combination Expansion cohorts only: Previously identified allergy or hypersensitivity to components of the study treatment formulation or panitumumab.

24. Unable or unwilling to abide by the study protocol or cooperate fully with the investigator or designee.

25. Evidence within 2 years of the start of study treatment of another malignancy which required systemic treatment.

26. Known history of HIV seropositivity, hepatitis C virus, acute or chronic active hepatitis B infection, or other serious chronic infection requiring ongoing treatment.

▨ Sex/Gender

All

▨ Ages

18 Years to N/A

▨ Accepts Healthy Volunteers

No

▨ Contacts

Christy Arrowood   919-668-1861   christy.arrowood@duke.edu
Anthony Amara, MSW   919-668-1861   anthony.amara@duke.edu

Nonrandomized, Open-Label Phase IIb Efficacy Trial of Cancer Macrobeads Compared With Best Supportive Care in Patients With Treatment-Resistant Colorectal Cancer

Study ID:
NCT02046174

Sponsor:
The Rogosin Institute

Information provided by (Responsible Party):
The Rogosin Institute (The Rogosin Institute)

Tracking Information

▨ First Submitted Date
January 21, 2014

▨ Start Date
January 2014

▨ Primary Completion Date
December 2018

▨ Last Update Posted Date
May 4, 2017

▨ Current Primary Outcome Measures

Overall Survival[Time Frame: 12 months]

This study is to evaluate the efficacy of renal adenocarcinoma (RENCA) macrobead implantation compared with best supportive care, as assessed by overall survival

▨ Current Secondary Outcome Measures

Change in levels of tumor markers (CEA and CA19-9)[Time Frame: 12 months]

Change from baseline over the period after the first RENCA macrobead implantation in levels of tumor markers (including carcinoembryonic antigen [CEA] and carbohydrate antigen 19-9 [CA19-9]

Change in clinical status, as measured by ECOG performance status score and Global clinical assessment[Time Frame: 12 months]

Change from baseline over the period after the first RENCA macrobead implantation in clinical status, as measured by Eastern Cooperative Oncology Group (ECOG) performance status score and Global Clinical Assessment

Change in quality of life, as measured by the EORTC QLQ C30 Questionnaire[Time Frame: 12 months]

Change from baseline over the period after the first RENCA macrobead implantation in quality of life, as measured by the European Organization for Research and Treatment of Cancer Quality of Life Questionnaire (EORTC QLQ C30)

Tumor marker response rate[Time Frame: 12 months]

Tumor marker response rate, defined as the proportion of patients who have a decrease from baseline of 20% or more in CEA or CA 19-9 values

Change in quality of life, as measured by the KPS[Time Frame: 12 months]

Change from baseline over the period after the first RENCA macrobead implantation in quality of life, as measured by the Karnofsky Performance Status Scale (KPS)

Descriptive Information

▦ Offical Title

A Phase IIb, Nonrandomized, Open-Label Trial With Mouse Renal Adenocarcinoma (RENCA) Cell Containing Agarose-Agarose Macrobeads Compared With Best Supportive Care in Patients With Treatment-Resistant, Metastatic Colorectal Carcinoma

▦ Brief Summary

This is a clinical research study of an investigational (FDA IND-BB 10091) treatment for patients with advanced colorectal cancer that no longer responds to standard therapies.

The treatment is being evaluated for its effect on tumor growth. It consists of the placement (implantation) of small beads that contain mouse renal adenocarcinoma cells (RENCA macrobeads). The cells in the macrobeads produce substances that have been shown to slow or stop the growth of tumors in experimental animals and veterinary patients. It has been tested in 31 human subjects with different types of cancers in a Phase I safety trial. Phase II studies in patients with colorectal, pancreatic or prostate cancers are in progress

▦ Detailed Description

This is a Phase IIb, multicenter, nonrandomized, open-label study with RENCA macrobeads in patients with treatment-resistant, metastatic colorectal carcinoma to determine the effect of RENCA macrobead implantation on overall survival compared with best supportive care.

Two treatment groups will be enrolled in this study, as follows:

- Group A (n=40) patients who will undergo up to 4 implantations of RENCA macrobeads, at an amount of 8 RENCA macrobeads /kg body weight
- Group B (n=80) patients who will receive or are receiving best supportive care, defined as management of symptoms aimed at maintaining or improving quality of life, but not including approved therapies targeting the patient's malignancy

▦ Study Type

Interventional

▦ Study Phase

Phase 2

▦ Condition

- Colorectal Cancers

▦ Intervention

Biological: RENCA macrobeads

Other Names:

mouse renal adenocarcinoma (RENCA) macrobeads

macrobead

▦ Study Arms

Experimental: Macrobead Implantation Arm

patients who will undergo up to 4 implantations of RENCA macrobeads, at an amount of 8 RENCA macrobeads /kg body weight

No Intervention: Best Supportive Care Arm

patients who will receive, or are receiving, best supportive care, defined as management of symptoms aimed at maintaining or improving quality of life, but not including approved therapies targeting the patient's malignancy

Recruitment Information

▦ Recruitment Status

Recruiting

▦ Estimated Enrollment

120

▦ Eligibility Criteria

Inclusion Criteria:

▦ Completion Date

December 2019

▦ Primary Completion Date

December 2018

Patients in both treatment groups must meet all of the following criteria to be considered eligible to participate in the study:

- Adult men or women, aged 18 years or older, with histologically-confirmed, metastatic adenocarcinoma of the colon or rectum that is resistant to available treatment options
- Radiographically documented evidence of disease progression.
- Life expectancy of at least 6 weeks, in the investigator's opinion, at the time disease progression is documented.
- Considered surgical candidates on the basis of co-morbidity risks, number and sites of metastases, and ability to withstand general anesthesia.
- Able to provide written informed consent.

Patients in Group A must also meet all of the following additional criteria:

- ECOG performance status score of 0, 1, or 2.
- Adequate hematologic function, defined as follows:

1. absolute neutrophil count (ANC) ≥1500 /mL
2. hemoglobin ≥9 g/dL
3. platelets ≥75,000 /mL

- Adequate hepatic function, defined as follows:

1. bilirubin ≤1.5 times the upper limit of normal (x ULN)
2. aspartate transaminase (AST) ≤3 x ULN, or ≤5 x ULN if liver metastases are present
3. alanine transaminase (ALT) ≤3, x ULN, or ≤5 x ULN if liver metastases are present

- Adequate renal function, defined as creatinine ≤2.0 mg/dL.
- Adequate coagulation function, defined as follows:

1. International Normalized Ratio (INR) ≤1.5 or between 2 and 3 if the patient is receiving anticoagulation
2. partial thromboplastin time (PTT) ≤5 seconds above the ULN Note: Patients receiving full-dose anticoagulation therapy must be receiving a stable dose of oral anticoagulant therapy or low-molecular-weight heparin.

- Clinically significant toxic effects of chemotherapy (excluding alopecia), radiotherapy, hormonal therapy, or prior surgery must have resolved to Grade 1 or better, with the exception of peripheral neuropathy, which must have resolved to Grade 2 or better.
- Agrees to contraceptive use while on study if sexually active

Exclusion Criteria:

Patients in either treatment group who meet any of the following criteria will be excluded from participating in the study:

- Hepatic blood flow abnormalities, i.e., portal vein hypertension and thrombosis, and/or a large volume of ascites.
- Concurrent cancer of any other type, except skin cancers other than melanoma.
- A positive test result for HIV or any hepatitis other than A at screening.
- Considered by the investigator to be unsuitable for participation in the study

Patients in Group A who meet any of the following criteria will be excluded from participating in the study:

- Received FDA-approved chemotherapy within 3 weeks of Day 0, or bevacizumab (or similar drugs) within 4 weeks of Day 0, or radiation therapy at any site within 4 weeks of Day 0
- Investigational anticancer therapy within 4 weeks of Day 0
- Positive reaction to the skin test for allergy to mouse antigen
- History of hypersensitivity reaction that, in the opinion of the investigator, poses an increased risk of an allergic reaction to the RENCA macrobeads, particularly any known allergy to murine antigens or body tissues.
- Ongoing or active infection, symptomatic congestive heart failure, unstable angina pectoris, serious cardiac arrhythmias (with the exception of well controlled atrial fibrillation), active bleeding, or psychiatric illness, or social situations that could interfere with the patient's ability to participate in the study.

Sex/Gender

All

Ages

18 Years to N/A

Accepts Healthy Volunteers

No

Contacts

Barry H. Smith, M.D., Ph.D   212-746-1551   bas2005@nyp.org

Nathaniel Berman, M.D.   212-746-9766   nab2009@nyp.org

An Investigational Immuno-therapy Study of Nivolumab, and Nivolumab in Combination With Other Anti-cancer Drugs, in Colon Cancer That Has Come Back or Has Spread

Study ID:

NCT02060188

Sponsor:

Bristol-Myers Squibb

Information provided by (Responsible Party):

Bristol-Myers Squibb (Bristol-Myers Squibb)

Tracking Information

▓ **First Submitted Date**

December 18, 2013

▓ **Start Date**

March 7, 2014

▓ **Primary Completion Date**

January 29, 2019

▓ **Last Update Posted Date**

January 30, 2018

▓ **Current Primary Outcome Measures**

Objective response rate (ORR) in all MSI-High and non-MSI-High subjects as determined by Investigators[Time Frame: The final analysis of the primary endpoint will occur at least 6 months after the last enrolled subject's first dose of study therapy (Approximately up to 34 months)]

(Tumor imaging assessments will occur every 6 weeks from the date of first dose (+/-1 wk) for the first 24 weeks, then every 12 wks (+/1 wk) thereafter until disease progression or treatment is discontinued (whichever occurs later)) (Tumor imaging assessments will occur every 6 weeks from the date of first dose (+/-1 wk) for the first 24 weeks, then every 12 wks (+/1 wk) thereafter until disease progression or treatment is discontinued (whichever occurs later))

▓ **Current Secondary Outcome Measures**

ORR in all MSI-H and non-MSI-H subjects based on IRRC determination[Time Frame: The final analysis of the secondary endpoint will occur the time of the primary endpoint analysis (Approximately up to 34 months)]

Tumor imaging assessments will occur every 6 weeks from the date of first dose (+/wk) for the first 24 weeks, then every 12 wks (+/1 wk) thereafter until disease progression or treatment is discontinued(whichever occurs later)

Descriptive Information

▓ **Offical Title**

A Phase 2 Clinical Trial of Nivolumab, or Nivolumab Combinations in Recurrent and Metastatic Microsatellite High (MSI-H) and Non-MSI-H Colon Cancer

▓ **Brief Summary**

The purpose of this study is to examine if Nivolumab by itself, or Nivolumab in combination with other anti-cancer drugs, will result in meaningful tumor size reduction, in patients with colon cancer that has come back or has spread, and who have a specific biomarker in their tumors.

▓ **Detailed Description**

Allocation: The Microsatellite Instability High (MSI-High) and C4 and C6 Cohort Parts of the trial are Non-randomized, The Non-MSI high Dose Escalation Phase part of the trial contained a randomized portion

▓ **Study Type**

Interventional

▓ **Study Phase**

Phase 2

▓ **Condition**

- Microsatellite Unstable Colorectal Cancer
- Microsatellite Stable Colorectal Cancer
- Mismatch Repair Proficient Colorectal Cancer
- Mismatch Repair Deficient Colorectal Cancer

▓ **Intervention**

Drug: Ipilimumab

Other Names:

Yervoy

Drug: Nivolumab

Other Names:

BMS-936558

Opdivo

Drug: Cobimetinib

Other Names:

Cotellic

Drug: Daratumumab

Other Names:

Darzalex

Drug: anti-LAG-3 antibody

Other Names:

BMS-986016

Study Arms

Experimental: Nivolumab Monotherapy

Nivolumab administered as IV infusion at a dose of 3mg/kg every 2 weeks until disease progression

Experimental: Nivolumab (Nivo) + Ipilimumab (Ipi)

Nivo 3mg/Kg IV with Ipi 1 mg/Kg IV every 3 week (wk) for 4 doses followed by Nivo 3mg/Kg IV every 2wk until progression

Dose Escalation Phase: (Complete)

Dose Level (DL) 1: Nivo 0.3mg/Kg with Ipi 1 mg/Kg IV every 3wk for 4 doses followed by Nivo 3mg/Kg IV every 2wk until progression

DL 1: Nivo 1mg/Kg IV with Ipi 1 mg/Kg IV every 3 wk for 4 doses followed by Nivo 3mg/Kg IV every 2wk until progression

DL 2a: Nivo 1mg/Kg IV with Ipi 3 mg/Kg IV every 3wk for 4 doses followed by Nivo 3mg/Kg IV every 2 wk until progression

DL 2b: Nivo 3mg/Kg IV with Ipi 1 mg/Kg IV every 3wk for 4 doses followed by Nivo 3mg/Kg IV every 2 wk until progression

Experimental: Nivolumab (Nivo) + Ipilimumab (Ipi) Cohort C3

Nivo IV dosed every 2wk with Ipi IV dosed every 6wk.

Experimental: Nivolumab (Nivo) + Ipilimumab (Ipi) + Cobimetinib Cohort C4

Nivo IV dosed every 2wk, with Ipi IV dosed every 6wk, combined with Cobimetinib dosed orally once daily 21 days on/7 days off.

Experimental: Nivolumab (Nivo) + BMS-986016 Cohort C5

Nivo IV dosed every 2wk with BMS-986016 dosed every 2 wk

Experimental: Nivolumab (Nivo) + Daratumumab Cohort C6

Daratumumab IV dosed weekly for week 1-8; then every 2 wks from Week 9-24; then every 4 wks on week 25; with Nivo dosed every 2 wks starting at week 3 and every 4 wks starting at week 25

Recruitment Information

Recruitment Status

Recruiting

Estimated Enrollment

340

Completion Date

December 31, 2019

Primary Completion Date

January 29, 2019

Eligibility Criteria

For more information regarding BMS clinical trial participation, please visit www.BMSStudyConnect.com

Inclusion Criteria:

- Men and women ≥ 18 years of age

- Eastern Cooperative Oncology Group (ECOG) performance status 0 to 1
- Histologically confirmed recurrent or metastatic colorectal cancer
- Measurable disease by CT or MRI
- Testing for MSI Status (by an accredited lab)

1. Subjects with microsatellite instability high (MSI-H) tumors will enroll in the MSI-H Cohort (mStage and cStage groups), the C3 Cohort, and the C5 Cohort.

- 2. Subjects with phenotypes that are non-microsatellite instability high (non-MSI-H) will enroll in the nonMSI-H Safety Cohort and the C6, C4 Cohorts.
- Adequate organ function as defined by study-specific laboratory tests
- Must use acceptable form of birth control throughout the study. After the final dose of study drug, an acceptable form of birth control must be used for 23 weeks for women of childbearing potential (WOCBP) and 31 weeks for men who are sexually active with WOCBP
- Signed informed consent
- Willing and able to comply with study procedures
- Subjects enrolled into the C3 Cohort must have not had treatment for their metastatic disease

Exclusion Criteria:

- Active brain metastases or leptomeningeal metastases are not allowed.
- Prior treatment with an anti-Programmed Death Receptor (PD)-1, anti-PD-L1, anti-PD-L2, anti-Cytotoxic T-Cell Lymphoma-4 Antigen (CTLA-4) antibody, or any other antibody or drug specifically targeting T-cell co-stimulation or immune checkpoint pathways
- Prior malignancy active within the previous 3 years except for locally curable cancers
- Subjects with active, known or suspected autoimmune disease
- Subjects with a condition requiring systemic treatment with either corticosteroids or other immunosuppressive medications within 14 days of study drug administration

Other protocol defined inclusion/exclusion criteria could apply

Sex/Gender

All

Ages

18 Years to N/A

Accepts Healthy Volunteers

No

Contacts

Recruiting sites have contact information. Please contact the sites directly. If there is no contact information, please email: Clinical.Trials@bms.com

First line of the email MUST contain NCT# and Site #.

Trametinib and Navitoclax in Treating Patients With Advanced or Metastatic Solid Tumors

Study ID:

NCT02079740

Sponsor:

National Cancer Institute (NCI)

Information provided by (Responsible Party):

National Cancer Institute (NCI) (National Cancer Institute (NCI))

Tracking Information

First Submitted Date

March 4, 2014

Start Date

March 7, 2014

Primary Completion Date

March 1, 2019

Last Update Posted Date

December 15, 2017

Current Primary Outcome Measures

Incidence of adverse events graded (Phase Ib and II)[Time Frame: Up to 42 days]

According to National Cancer Institute Common Terminology Criteria for Adverse Events version 4.0.

Progression-free survival (Phase II)[Time Frame: Time from start of treatment to time of progression or death, whichever occurs first, assessed up to 30 days]

Progression-free survival will be assessed.

Response rate (partial response [PR] + complete response [CR]) assessed according to Response Evaluation Criteria in Solid Tumors version 1.1 (Phase II)[Time Frame: Up to 30 days]

The 95% confidence intervals should be provided.

Current Secondary Outcome Measures

Percent change in levels of apoptosis markers (cleaved caspase-3) (Phase Ib and II)[Time Frame: Baseline to up to 30 days]

Results will be reported as a % increase or decrease in level of a given marker after treatment initiation (post treatment biopsy) relative to before treatment (pre-treatment biopsy).

Percent change in levels of proliferation markers (Ki67) (Phase Ib and II)[Time Frame: Baseline to up to 30 days]

Results will be reported as a % increase or decrease in level of a given marker after treatment initiation (post treatment biopsy) relative to before treatment (pre-treatment biopsy).

Percent change in levels of proteins/messenger ribonucleic acid (mRNA)s implicated in B-cell lymphoma 2 family signaling (Phase Ib and II)[Time Frame: Baseline to up to 30 days]

Results will be reported as a % increase or decrease in level of a given marker after treatment initiation (post treatment biopsy) relative to before treatment (pre-treatment biopsy).

Percent change in levels of proteins/messenger ribonucleic acids implicated in mitogen-activated protein kinase signaling (Phase Ib and II)[Time Frame: Baseline to up to 30 days]

Results will be reported as a percent (%) increase or decrease in level of a given marker after treatment initiation (post treatment biopsy) relative to before treatment (pre-treatment biopsy).

Pharmacokinetic parameters (observed plasma drug concentration, area under the curve, half-life) for trametinib and navitoclax when administered in combination (Phase Ib)[Time Frame: Pre-dose trametinib (-1 hours [h]), pre-dose navitoclax (0 h), 2h, 4h, 6h, 8h, day 1 of courses 4, 8, and 12]

Pharmacokinetic parameters will be assessed.

Response rate (partial response + complete response) (Phase Ib)[Time Frame: Up to 30 days]

The 95% confidence intervals should be provided.

Descriptive Information

Offical Title

An Open Label, Two-Part, Phase Ib/II Study to Investigate the Safety, Pharmacokinetics, Pharmacodynamics, and Clinical Activity of the MEK Inhibitor Trametinib and the BCL2-Family Inhibitor Navitoclax (ABT-263) in Combination in Subjects With KRAS or NRAS Mutation-Positive Advanced Solid Tumors

Brief Summary

This phase Ib/II trial studies the side effects and best dose of trametinib and navitoclax and how well they work in treating patients with solid tumors that have spread to other places in the body. Trametinib and navitoclax may stop the growth of tumor cells by blocking some of the enzymes needed for cell growth.

Detailed Description

PRIMARY OBJECTIVES:

I. To determine the dose-limiting toxicities of trametinib in combination with navitoclax, and the maximal doses at which both drugs can be safely administered together. (Phase Ib) II. To determine the response rate of the combination of trametinib and navitoclax in subjects with KRAS or NRAS mutation-positive advanced or metastatic solid tumors in disease-specific expansion cohorts. (Phase II) III. To confirm the safety and tolerability of trametinib and navitoclax in combination at the recommended phase 2 dose (RP2D) determined in the Phase 1b portion. (Phase II)

SECONDARY OBJECTIVES:

I. To determine the pharmacokinetics of both drugs administered together. (Phase Ib) II. To assess for evidence of response to therapy. (Phase Ib) III. To evaluate the pharmacodynamic response to therapy in tumor biopsies. (Phase Ib) IV. To evaluate the pharmacodynamic response to therapy in tumor biopsies (first 15 patients enrolled overall). (Phase II)

OUTLINE: This is a phase Ib, dose-escalation study followed by a phase II study.

Patients receive trametinib orally (PO) once daily (QD) and navitoclax PO QD on days 1-28. Courses repeat every 28 days in the absence of disease progression or unacceptable toxicity. If unacceptable toxicity is observed, patients may receive trametinib PO QD on days 1-14.

After completion of study treatment, patients are followed up for 30 days.

■ **Study Type**

Interventional

■ **Study Phase**

Phase 1/Phase 2

■ **Condition**

- Advanced Malignant Solid Neoplasm
- KRAS Gene Mutation
- Metastatic Malignant Solid Neoplasm
- NRAS Gene Mutation
- Recurrent Colorectal Carcinoma
- Recurrent Lung Carcinoma
- Recurrent Malignant Solid Neoplasm
- Recurrent Pancreatic Carcinoma
- Stage III Colorectal Cancer AJCC v7
- Stage III Lung Cancer AJCC v7
- Stage III Pancreatic Cancer AJCC v6 and v7
- Stage IIIA Colorectal Cancer AJCC v7
- Stage IIIB Colorectal Cancer AJCC v7
- Stage IIIC Colorectal Cancer AJCC v7
- Stage IV Colorectal Cancer AJCC v7
- Stage IV Lung Cancer AJCC v7
- Stage IV Pancreatic Cancer AJCC v6 and v7
- Stage IVA Colorectal Cancer AJCC v7
- Stage IVB Colorectal Cancer AJCC v7
- Unresectable Malignant Neoplasm

■ **Intervention**

Other: Laboratory Biomarker Analysis
  Correlative studies

  Biological: Navitoclax

  Given PO

Other Names:
  A-855071.0

  ABT-263

  Bcl-2 Family Protein Inhibitor ABT-263

  Other: Pharmacological Study

  Correlative studies

  Drug: Trametinib

  Given PO

Other Names:
  GSK1120212

  JTP-74057

  MEK Inhibitor GSK1120212

  Mekinist

■ **Study Arms**

Experimental: Treatment (trametinib, navitoclax)

Patients receive trametinib PO QD and navitoclax PO QD on days 1-28. Courses repeat every 28 days in the absence of disease progression or unacceptable toxicity. If unacceptable toxicity is observed, patients may receive trametinib PO QD on days 1-14.

Recruitment Information

Recruitment Status

Recruiting

Estimated Enrollment

130

Completion Date

N/A

Primary Completion Date

March 1, 2019

Eligibility Criteria

Inclusion Criteria:

- Patients must have histologically or cytologically-confirmed diagnosis of KRAS or NRAS mutation-positive malignancy that is metastatic or unresectable and for which standard curative measures do not exist or are no longer effective; patients must have activating mutations affecting codons 12, 13, 61, or 146 as determined in a Clinical Laboratory Improvement Amendments (CLIA)-certified lab to be eligible for this study
- Patients must have measurable disease by Response Evaluation Criteria in Solid Tumors (RECIST), defined as at least one lesion that can be accurately measured in at least one dimension (longest diameter to be recorded for non-nodal lesions and short axis for nodal lesions) as >= 20 mm by chest x-ray or as >= 10 mm with computed tomography (CT) scan, magnetic resonance imaging (MRI), or calipers by clinical exam
- Participants must have received at least one line of prior systemic chemotherapy and must have experienced documented radiographic progression or intolerance on this therapy
- Paired pre-treatment and post-treatment biopsies are required for all patients on Part 1 and first 15 patients in Part 2; participants must have available archival tumor tissue (at least 20 unstained slides); if archival tissue is not available or is found not to contain tumor tissue, a fresh biopsy is required; if a patient is having a tumor biopsy, less than 20 unstained slides are acceptable with approval of the principal investigator (PI); biopsies will only be performed in a given patient if they are not deemed to involve unacceptable risk based on the sites of disease and other concurrent medical conditions
- Eastern Cooperative Oncology Group (ECOG) performance status =< 1
- Life expectancy of greater than 3 months
- Able to swallow and retain orally-administered medication and does not have any clinically significant gastrointestinal abnormalities that may alter absorption such as malabsorption syndrome or major resection of the stomach or bowels
- All prior treatment-related toxicities must be Common Terminology Criteria for Adverse Events version 4 (CTCAE v 4) grade =< 1 (except alopecia) at the time of enrollment; this requirement to return to =< grade 1 does not apply to immune checkpoint inhibitor related endocrinopathies (e.g. thyroiditis, hypophysitis, etc.) that necessitate hormone replacement therapy including, but not limited to levothyroxine, cortisol, and testosterone
- Leukocytes >= 3,000/mcL
- Absolute neutrophil count (ANC) >= 1,200/mcL (subjects may be treated with hematopoietic growth factors to achieve or maintain this level)
- Hemoglobin >= 9 g/dL
- Platelets >= 100 x 10^9/L
- Albumin >= 2.5 g/dL
- Total bilirubin =< 1.5 x institutional upper limit of normal (ULN) (patients with Gilbert's syndrome may have serum bilirubin > 1.5 × ULN)
- Aspartate aminotransferase (AST) and alanine aminotransferase (ALT) =< 2.5 x institutional ULN
- Serum creatinine =< 1.5 mg/dL OR calculated creatinine clearance (Cockroft-Gault formula) >= 50 mL/min OR 24-hour urine creatinine clearance >= 50 mL/min
- Prothrombin time (PT)/international normalized ratio (INR) and partial thromboplastin time (PTT) =< 1.2 x institutional ULN
- Left ventricular ejection fraction >= institutional lower limit of normal (LLN) by echocardiogram (ECHO) or multi gated acquisition scan (MUGA)
- **Women of child-bearing potential and men with a female partner of child bearing potential must agree to use adequate contraception using one of the methods listed below prior to study entry, for the duration of study participation, and up to 4 months following completion of therapy:**
- Total abstinence from sexual intercourse (minimum one complete menstrual cycle prior to study drug administration)
- Vasectomized male subject or vasectomized partner of female subjects
- Hormonal contraceptives (oral, parenteral, transdermal or vaginal ring) for at least 3 months prior to study drug administration; if the subject is currently using a hormonal contraceptive, she should also use a barrier method during this study and for 1 month after study completion
- Intrauterine device (IUD)
- Double-barrier method: male condom plus diaphragm or vaginal cap with spermicide (contraceptive sponge, jellies or creams)
- Men with a female partner of childbearing potential must have either had a prior vasectomy or agree to use effective contraception; additionally, male subjects (including those who are vasectomized) whose partners are pregnant or might be pregnant must agree to use condoms for the duration of the study and for 4 months following completion of therapy
- Women of childbearing potential must have a negative serum pregnancy test within 7 days prior to initiation of treatment;

women will be considered not of childbearing potential if they are surgically sterile (bilateral oophorectomy or hysterectomy) and/or post-menopausal (amenorrheic for at least 12 months); should a woman become pregnant or suspect she is pregnant while she or her partner is participating in this study, she should inform her treating physician immediately; the potential hazard to the fetus should be explained to the patient and partner (as applicable)

- Ability to understand and the willingness to sign a written informed consent document

Exclusion Criteria:

- History of another malignancy; exception: patients who have been disease-free for 3 years, or patients with a history of completely resected non-melanoma skin cancer or any carcinoma in situ and/or patients with indolent second malignancies, are eligible; consult the Cancer Therapy Evaluation Program (CTEP) medical monitor if unsure whether second malignancies meet the requirements

- History of interstitial lung disease or pneumonitis

- Any major surgery, extensive radiotherapy (> 15 days of treatment), chemotherapy with delayed toxicity, biologic therapy, or immunotherapy within 21 days prior to first dose of study treatment and/or daily or weekly chemotherapy without the potential for delayed toxicity within 14 days prior to first dose of study treatment

- Use of other investigational drugs within 28 days (or five half-lives, whichever is shorter; with a minimum of 14 days from the last dose) preceding the first dose of study drug(s) and during the study

- Patients with known brain metastases should be excluded from this clinical trial; exception: patients with brain metastases will be allowed on study if they have clinically controlled neurologic symptoms, defined as surgical excision and/or radiation therapy followed by 21 days of stable neurologic function and no evidence of central nervous system (CNS) disease progression as determined by computed tomography (CT) or magnetic resonance imaging (MRI) within 21 days prior to the first dose of study drug

- Have a known immediate or delayed hypersensitivity reaction or idiosyncrasy to drugs chemically related to trametinib, or excipients or to dimethyl sulfoxide (DMSO), or to compounds of similar chemical or biologic composition to navitoclax

- Current use of a prohibited medication; the following medications or non-drug therapies are prohibited:

- Other anti-cancer therapy while on study treatment; (note: megestrol [Megace] if used as an appetite stimulant is allowed)

- Concurrent treatment with bisphosphonates is permitted; however, treatment must be initiated prior to the first dose of study therapy; prophylactic use of bisphosphonates in patients without bone disease is not permitted, except for the treatment of osteoporosis

- The concurrent use of all herbal supplements is prohibited during the study (including, but not limited to, St. John's wort, kava, ephedra [ma huang], ginkgo biloba, dehydroepiandrosterone [DHEA], yohimbe, saw palmetto, or ginseng)

- The following concomitant medications are not allowed during navitoclax administration: warfarin, clopidogrel (Plavix), ibuprofen, tirofiban (Aggrastat), and other anticoagulants, drugs, or herbal supplements that affect platelet function are excluded, with the exception of low-dose anticoagulation medications (such as heparin) that are used to maintain the patency of a central intravenous catheter; aspirin will not be allowed within 7 days prior to the first dose of navitoclax or during navitoclax administration; however, subjects who have previously received aspirin therapy for thrombosis prevention may resume a low dose (i.e., maximum 100 mg QD) of aspirin if platelet counts are stable (>= 50,000/mm^3) through 6 weeks of navitoclax administration; all decisions regarding treatment with aspirin therapy will be determined by the investigator in conjunction with the medical monitor

- Caution should be exercised when dosing navitoclax concurrently with cytochrome P450, family 2, subfamily C, polypeptide 8 (CYP2C8) and cytochrome P450, family 2, subfamily C, polypeptide 9 (CYP2C9) substrates; common CYP2C8 substrates include paclitaxel, statins, and glitazones, whereas CYP2C9 substrates include phenytoin and warfarin; when possible, investigators should switch to alternative medications or monitor the patients closely (particularly in the case of medications that have a narrow therapeutic window such as warfarin; use of warfarin is specifically prohibited while on study); cytochrome P450, family 3, subfamily A (CYP3A) inhibitors such as ketoconazole and clarithromycin are not allowed 7 days prior to the first dose of navitoclax or during navitoclax administration; as part of the enrollment/informed consent procedures, the patient will be counseled on the risk of interactions with other agents, and what to do if new medications need to be prescribed or if the patient is considering a new over-the-counter medicine or herbal product; patient instructions and information of possible drug interactions will be given to all patients upon enrollment in this study

- History or current evidence/risk of retinal vein occlusion (RVO)

- History or evidence of cardiovascular risk including any of the following:

- Left ventricle ejection fraction (LVEF) < LLN

- A QT interval corrected for heart rate using the Bazett's formula QTcB >= 480 msec

- History or evidence of current clinically significant uncontrolled arrhythmias (exception: patients with controlled atrial fibrillation for > 30 days prior to enrollment are eligible)

- History of acute coronary syndromes (including myocardial infarction and unstable angina), coronary angioplasty, or stenting within 6 months prior to randomization

- History or evidence of current >= class II congestive heart failure as defined by the New York Heart Association (NYHA) functional classification system

- Treatment-refractory hypertension defined as a blood pressure of systolic > 140 mmHg and/or diastolic > 90 mmHg which cannot be controlled by anti-hypertensive therapy

- Known cardiac metastases

- Patients with intra-cardiac defibrillators

- Known hepatitis B virus (HBV), or hepatitis C virus (HCV) infection (patients with chronic or cleared HBV and HCV infection are eligible); patients with human immunodeficiency virus (HIV) are not eligible if on anti-retroviral medications

- Uncontrolled intercurrent illness including, but not limited to, ongoing or active infection, symptomatic congestive heart failure, unstable angina pectoris, cardiac arrhythmia, or psychiatric illness/social situations that would limit compliance with study requirements
- Subject has an underlying condition predisposing them to bleeding or currently exhibits signs of clinically significant bleeding
- Subject has a recent history of non-chemotherapy-induced thrombocytopenic-associated bleeding within 1 year prior to the first dose of study drug
- Subject has a significant history of cardiovascular disease (e.g., myocardial infarction [MI], thrombotic or thromboembolic event in the last 6 months)
- Pregnant women or nursing mothers

Sex/Gender

All

Ages

18 Years to N/A

Accepts Healthy Volunteers

No

Ph 1 Study ADI-PEG 20 Plus FOLFOX in Subjects With Advanced Gastrointestinal Malignancies

Study ID:

NCT02102022

Sponsor:

Polaris Group

Information provided by (Responsible Party):

Polaris Group (Polaris Group)

Tracking Information

First Submitted Date

March 28, 2014

Start Date

November 2014

Primary Completion Date

August 2019

Last Update Posted Date

September 19, 2017

Current Primary Outcome Measures

- Number of Participants with Adverse Events as a Measure of Safety and Tolerability of ADI-PEG 20 in combination with folinic acid (leucovorin), fluorouracil and oxaliplatin (FOLFOX) in advanced GI malignancies.[Time Frame: course of study 1 year expected]

Descriptive Information

Offical Title

Phase 1 Study of ADI PEG 20 Plus FOLFOX in Subjects With Advanced Gastrointestinal Malignancies

Brief Summary

Assessment of safety and tolerability of ADI-PEG 20 in combination with folinic acid (leucovorin), fluorouracil and oxaliplatin (FOLFOX) in advanced GI malignancies.

Study Type

Interventional

Study Phase

Phase 1

Condition

- Advanced Gastrointestinal (GI) Malignancies

- Hepatocellular Carcinoma
- Gastric Cancer
- Colorectal Cancer

Intervention

Drug: ADI-PEG 20

Other Names:

arginine deiminase formulated with polyethylene glycol

Study Arms

Experimental: ADI-PEG 20

Recruitment Information

Recruitment Status

Recruiting

Estimated Enrollment

148

Completion Date

October 2019

Primary Completion Date

August 2019

Eligibility Criteria

Inclusion Criteria:

For Advanced GI Malignancies (Dose Escalation and MTD Cohorts):

1. Advanced histologically proven GI cancer.

2. First line or progressive disease if already treated with any form of therapy, including but not limited to chemotherapy, radiotherapy, local therapy, surgery or immuno-therapy. Patients with HCC who failed sorafenib, with documented PD or AEs that resulted in discontinuance of that agent. Patients with pancreatic cancer (dose escalation only) who have progressed following a gemcitabine based regimen. Subjects failing prior platinum containing regimens are eligible. Gastric cancer subjects that express tumor HER-2 amplification must be treated with trastuzumab prior to enrollment, unless trastuzumab is not available for those indications in a particular country.

3. Measurable disease using RECIST 1.1 criteria (Appendix A). At least 1 measurable lesion must be present. Subjects who have received local-regional therapy such as (but not limited to) chemoembolization, embolization, cryoablation, hepatic artery therapy, percutaneous ethanol injection, radiation therapy, radiofrequency ablation or surgery are eligible, provided that they have either a target lesion which has not been treated with local therapy and/or the target lesion(s) within the field of the local regional therapy has shown an increase of ≥ 20% in size. Local-regional therapy must be completed at least 4 weeks prior to the baseline CT scan.

- 4. ECOG performance status of 0 1.

5. Expected survival of at least 3 months.

For HCC (Dose Escalation and MTD Expansion):

19. Prior treatment with sorafenib, with documented PD or AEs that resulted in discontinuance of that agent. Patient may have been treated with other lines off therapy as well excluding ADI-PEG 20.

20. Cirrhotic status of Child-Pugh grade A. Child-Pugh status should be determined based on clinical findings and laboratory data during the screening period (Appendix C). Subjects on Coumadin anti-coagulants are to receive only 1 point for their INR status.

21. Serum albumin level ≥ 2.8 g/dl. 22. Prothrombin time (PT)-international normalized ratio (INR): PT <6 seconds above control or INR <1.7. Subjects on Coumadin anti-coagulants are to receive only 1 point for their INR status.

23. Subjects with active hepatitis B or C on anti-viremic compounds may remain on such treatment, except for interferon.

Exclusion Criteria:

1. Serious infection requiring treatment with systemically administered antibiotics at the time of study entrance, or an infection requiring systemic antibiotic therapy within 7 days prior to the first dose of study treatment.

2. Pregnancy or lactation.

3. Expected non-compliance.

4. Uncontrolled intercurrent illness including, but not limited to, ongoing or active infection, symptomatic congestive heart failure (New York Heart Association Class III or IV), cardiac arrhythmia, or psychiatric illness, social situations that would limit compliance with study requirements.

5. Subjects who have had any anticancer treatment prior to entering the study and have not recovered to baseline (except alopecia) or ≤ Grade 1 AEs, or deemed irreversible from the effects of prior cancer therapy. AEs > Grade 1 that are not considered a safety risk by the Sponsor and investigator may be allowed upon agreement with both.

Sex/Gender

All

Ages

18 Years to N/A

■ **Accepts Healthy Volunteers**

No

■ **Contacts**

John Bomalaski, M.D.   858-452-6688   jbomalaski@polarispharma.com

Jessica Frick   858-452-6688   jfrick@polarispharma.com

Irinotecan-Eluting Beads in Treating Patients With Refractory Metastatic Colon or Rectal Cancer That Has Spread to the Liver

Study ID:

NCT02110953

Sponsor:

Fox Chase Cancer Center

Information provided by (Responsible Party):

Fox Chase Cancer Center (Fox Chase Cancer Center)

Tracking Information

■ **First Submitted Date**

April 8, 2014

■ **Start Date**

January 2016

■ **Current Primary Outcome Measures**

Maximum tolerated dose of irinotecan-eluting beads, determined by dose limiting toxicities, graded according to National Cancer Institute Common Terminology Criteria for Adverse Events version 4.0[Time Frame: 3 weeks]

■ **Primary Completion Date**

April 2018

■ **Last Update Posted Date**

April 14, 2017

■ **Current Secondary Outcome Measures**

Response rate, classified using Response Evaluation Criteria in Solid Tumors (RECIST) criteria version 1.1[Time Frame: 8 weeks following administration of irinotecan-eluting beads]

Duration of overall response[Time Frame: From the time measurement criteria are met for complete response or partial response until the first date that recurrent or progressive disease is objectively documented, assessed up to 2 years]

Time to progression[Time Frame: From start of treatment to progression in the treated lobe, assessed up to 2 years]

Descriptive Information

■ **Offical Title**

Phase I Study of Drug-Eluting Irinotecan Beads (DEBIRI) in Refractory Metastatic Colorectal Cancer With Liver-Only or Liver-Predominant Disease

■ **Brief Summary**

This phase I trial studies the side effects and best dose of irinotecan-eluting beads in treating patients with colon or rectal cancer that has spread to the liver and does not respond to treatment with standard therapy. Irinotecan-eluting beads are tiny beads that have been loaded with irinotecan hydrochloride, a chemotherapy drug. Drugs used in chemotherapy, such as irinotecan hydrochloride, work in different ways to stop the growth of tumor cells, either by killing the cells or stopping them from dividing. This treatment delivers the chemotherapy directly to the tumor area inside the liver instead of to the whole body as with systemic delivery of the drug. Irinotecan-eluting beads may work better that standard chemotherapy in treating patients with colon or rectal cancer that has spread to the liver.

■ **Detailed Description**

PRIMARY OBJECTIVES:

I. To determine the maximum tolerated dose of drug eluting irinotecan (irinotecan hydrochloride) beads (irinotecan-eluting beads), delivered intrahepatically for the treatment of liver only or liver-predominantly colorectal metastatic disease.

SECONDARY OBJECTIVES:

123

I. To determine the response rate of colorectal liver metastases treated with drug-eluting irinotecan beads in refractory metastatic colorectal patients with liver only or liver predominant disease.

II. To determine the time to progression of colorectal liver metastases treated with drug-eluting irinotecan beads in refractory metastatic colorectal patients with liver only or liver predominant disease.

III. To determine the overall survival of patients treated with drug-eluting irinotecan beads for liver only or liver predominant metastatic disease from colorectal cancer.

OUTLINE: This is a dose-escalation study.

Patients receive irinotecan-eluting beads via hepatic artery embolization every 3 weeks for a total of 2 treatments in the absence of disease progression or unacceptable toxicity. Patients with bi-lobular disease and no evidence of progression in the treated lobe may repeat treatment at the discretion of the treating physician.

After completion of study treatment, patients are followed up at 30 days and then every 3 months for 2 years.

■ **Study Type**

Interventional

■ **Study Phase**

Phase 1

■ **Condition**

- Liver Metastases
- Mucinous Adenocarcinoma of the Colon
- Mucinous Adenocarcinoma of the Rectum
- Recurrent Colon Cancer
- Recurrent Rectal Cancer
- Signet Ring Adenocarcinoma of the Colon
- Signet Ring Adenocarcinoma of the Rectum
- Stage IVA Colon Cancer
- Stage IVA Rectal Cancer
- Stage IVB Colon Cancer
- Stage IVB Rectal Cancer

■ **Intervention**

Combination Product: irinotecan-eluting beads

Receive irinotecan hydrochloride-eluting beads via hepatic artery embolization

Procedure: hepatic artery embolization

Receive irinotecan hydrochloride-eluting beads via hepatic artery embolization

■ **Study Arms**

Experimental: Treatment (irinotecan-eluting beads)

Patients receive irinotecan-eluting beads via hepatic artery embolization every 3 weeks for a total of 2 treatments in the absence of disease progression or unacceptable toxicity. Patients with bi-lobular disease and no evidence of progression in the treated lobe may repeat treatment at the discretion of the treating physician.

Recruitment Information

■ **Recruitment Status**

Recruiting

■ **Estimated Enrollment**

30

■ **Completion Date**

April 2019

■ **Primary Completion Date**

April 2018

■ **Eligibility Criteria**

Inclusion Criteria:

- Patients must have a histologically or cytologically confirmed adenocarcinoma of the colon or rectum that is metastatic to the liver and unresectable and for which standard curative measures do not exist or are no longer effective
- Patients must have received prior fluoropyrimidine, oxaliplatin and irinotecan-based therapy for their disease and had progression or intolerance to these agents that resulted in treatment discontinuation
- Liver disease must not be amenable to potentially curative surgical resection
- Patients must have liver-only or liver-predominant disease to be eligible for this study; liver predominant disease is defined dominant metastatic burden in the liver, with extra-hepatic disease that is judged by the investigator as unlikely to be life threatening within 3 months

- Patients must have a patent portal vein as documented by computed tomography (CT), magnetic resonance imaging (MRI), or ultrasound
- Prior radiation therapy is allowed but must have been completed >= 4 weeks prior to study entry; patients with history of prior radiation to the liver including radio-labeled microspheres cannot take part in this study
- Eastern Cooperative Oncology Group performance status 0 or 1
- Previous surgery or radiofrequency ablation (RFA) to the liver is allowed; patients with history of chemoembolization or radio-labeled microspheres are excluded
- Life expectancy of >= 12 weeks
- Leukocytes >= 3,000/µL
- Absolute neutrophil count >= 1,500/µL
- Platelets >= 100,000/µL
- Total bilirubin =< 1.5 X upper limit of normal (ULN)
- Aspartate aminotransferase (AST) (serum glutamic oxaloacetic transaminase [SGOT])/alanine aminotransferase (ALT) (serum glutamate pyruvate transaminase [SGPT]) =< 2 X ULN
- Alkaline phosphatase =< 2 X ULN
- Creatinine =< 2.0 X mg/dL
- Prothrombin time (PT)/partial thromboplastin time (PTT) =< 1.5 X ULN
- Women of childbearing potential (WOCBP) and sexually active males must agree to use an accepted and effective method of contraception prior to study entry and for the duration of the study; WOCBP include any female who has experienced menarche and who has not undergone successful surgical sterilization (hysterectomy, bilateral tubal ligation or bilateral oophorectomy) or is not postmenopausal; women who use oral, implanted or injectable contraceptive hormones, or mechanical products such as an intrauterine device or barrier methods (diaphragm, condoms, spermicides) to prevent pregnancy or practicing abstinence or where partner is sterile (e.g., vasectomy) should be considered to be of child bearing potential
- Patients must demonstrate ability to understand and the willingness to sign a written informed consent document
- Patients must discontinue any medication that causes strong cytochrome P450, family 3, subfamily A, polypeptide 4 (CYP3A4) induction 2 weeks prior to treatment initiation; patients who are not able to discontinue these drugs are considered ineligible
- Patients must discontinue any medication that causes a strong CYP3A4 inhibition 1 week prior to treatment initiation; patients who are not able to discontinue these drugs are considered ineligible

Exclusion Criteria:

- Patients who have had chemotherapy (including targeted therapy i.e. cetuximab, panitumumab) or radiotherapy =< 4 weeks or treatment with bevacizumab =< 6 weeks prior to entering the study or those who have not recovered from acute adverse events due to agents administered more than 4 weeks earlier, with the exclusion of alopecia or neuropathy; patients with history of radiation to the liver including radio-labeled microspheres at any point in their past will be excluded
- Patients may not be receiving nor have received any other investigational agent =< 4 weeks prior to study registration
- Pregnant or nursing women may not participate in this trial
- Patients with known brain metastases are excluded from this study
- Known human immunodeficiency virus (HIV)-positive patients and those with known hepatitis B or C are excluded from the study
- Patients with uncontrolled intercurrent illness including, but not limited to, ongoing or active bacterial infection, symptomatic congestive heart failure, unstable angina pectoris, cardiac arrhythmia, or psychiatric illness/social situations that would limit compliance with study requirements
- Patients with clinically evident ascites requiring medical management or paracentesis, or Childs-Pugh score B/C are not eligible
- Patients with evidence of other cancer within 5 years, excluding adequately treated basal cell carcinoma of the skin
- Patient with significant cardiac, renal or hematologic or pulmonary dysfunction
- Patients with previous chemoembolization to liver metastases

Sex/Gender

All

Ages

18 Years to N/A

Accepts Healthy Volunteers

No

Low Glycemic Load Diet in Patients With Stage I-III Colon Cancer

Study ID:

NCT02129218

Sponsor:

Case Comprehensive Cancer Center

Information provided by (Responsible Party):

Case Comprehensive Cancer Center (Case Comprehensive Cancer Center)

Tracking Information

First Submitted Date

April 17, 2014

Start Date

February 16, 2015

Primary Completion Date

September 22, 2017

Last Update Posted Date

March 20, 2017

Current Primary Outcome Measures

Individual patient compliance, defined by following assigned target glycemic load index >= 75% of the time between weeks 4 and 12[Time Frame: Up to week 12]

> This compliance rate will be determined through conducting a 24 hour telephone recall, every 2 weeks at random and calculating the glycemic load. For each dose cohort, the number and percentage of patients who are compliant will be summarized, with 90% confidence interval that accounts for the two-stage design.

Current Secondary Outcome Measures

Food acceptability score[Time Frame: Up to 12 weeks]

> Results of the acceptability survey will be tabulated and described (the questions use a 7 point likert scale), separately for each cohort.

Hours of nutritionist time per week[Time Frame: Up to 12 weeks]

> The median number of hours will be calculated based on time spent with each patient, separately for each cohort.

Descriptive Information

Offical Title

A Pilot Study to Determine the Feasibility of a Low Glycemic Load Diet in Patients With Stage I-III Colon Cancer

Brief Summary

This pilot clinical trial studies the feasibility of a low glycemic load diet in patients with stage I-III colon cancer. A low glycemic load diet includes foods that have low scores on the glycemic index. The glycemic index is a scale that measures how much a certain carbohydrate causes a person's blood sugar to rise. A low glycemic load diet may help decrease the chance of cancer coming back and improve the survival in patients with colon cancer.

Detailed Description

PRIMARY OBJECTIVES:

I. To determine the feasibility of following a low or medium glycemic load diet in patients with stage I-III (local-regional) colon cancer.

SECONDARY OBJECTIVES:

I. To determine patient-reported acceptability of diet. II. To determine nutritionist resources utilized. III. To evaluate the effect of lowering dietary glycemic load on body mass index (BMI), lipid metabolism and pro-oncogenic intermediaries of cellular metabolism.

OUTLINE: Patients are sequentially enrolled in 1 of 4 possible cohorts as needed based on the feasibility of the prior cohort.

COHORT 1: Patients follow a low glycemic load diet with standard dietary intervention (contact with nutritionist in person every 2 weeks with phone contact on the alternating weeks) for 12 weeks.

COHORT 2: Patients follow a low glycemic load diet with intensified dietary intervention (contact with nutritionist in person every week) for 12 weeks.

COHORT 3: Patients follow a medium glycemic load diet with standard dietary intervention for 12 weeks.

COHORT 4: Patients follow a medium glycemic load diet with intensified dietary intervention for 12 weeks.

Study Type

Interventional

- **Study Phase**

  N/A

- **Condition**

  - Stage I Colon Cancer
  - Stage II Colon Cancer
  - Stage III Colon Cancer
  - Stage I Rectal Cancer
  - Stage II Rectal Cancer
  - Stage III Rectal Cancer

- **Intervention**

  Other: questionnaire administration

  > Ancillary studies including three day food record, twenty-four hour dietary recall, and a food acceptability questionnaire.

  Other: laboratory biomarker analysis

  Correlative studies

  Behavioral: Standard Dietary Intervention

  > Participants will be contacted by a nutritionist, in person every 2 weeks with phone contact on the alternating weeks. At the initial visit, each participant will be given verbal and written patient education materials, including low glycemic load diet recipes, meal plans, food preparation, and grocery shopping information. Individual instruction will be tailored to their baseline dietary preferences (e.g. vegan, allergies, etc).

  Behavioral: Intensified Dietary Intervention

  > Patients will be contacted weekly, in person, by a nutritionist . Participants will take part in a cooking demonstration at the time of their initial visit. The demonstration will be hands-on and participants will be able to sample foods and recipes. In addition to grocery shopping information, participants will be accompanied by a nutritionist to their local grocery store to practice new shopping habits for their target dietary glycemic load. Each participant will also receive weekly random phone calls to assess his or her progress.

  Behavioral: Low glycemic load

  Behavioral: Medium Glycemic Load

- **Study Arms**

  Experimental: Cohort 1: Low glycemic load with standard diet

  > Patients follow a low glycemic load diet with a standard dietary intervention for 12 weeks.

  Experimental: Cohort 2: Low glycemic load with intensified diet

  > Patients follow a low glycemic load diet with intensified dietary intervention for 12 weeks.

  Active Comparator: Cohort 3: Medium glycemic load with standard diet

  > Patients follow a medium glycemic load diet with standard dietary intervention for 12 weeks.

  Active Comparator: Cohort 4: Medium glycemic load with intensified diet

  > Patients follow a medium glycemic load diet with intensified dietary intervention for 12 weeks.

Recruitment Information

- **Recruitment Status**

  Recruiting

- **Completion Date**

  September 22, 2017

- **Estimated Enrollment**

  72

- **Primary Completion Date**

  September 22, 2017

- **Eligibility Criteria**

  Inclusion Criteria:

  - Patients must have stage I-III colon or rectal cancer and have undergone definitive therapy; definitive therapy may have included surgery alone, or surgery plus neoadjuvant and/or adjuvant therapy
  - Patients must regularly consume a diet with a glycemic load > 150 as estimated through the 3 day food recall
  - Patients must readily be available for a 3 month period and agree to participate in regular dietary adherence assessments (surveys and phone interviews)

  Exclusion Criteria:

  - Current participation in an intervention targeting diet or exercise

- ▣ **Sex/Gender**

  All

- ▣ **Ages**

  18 Years to N/A

- ▣ **Accepts Healthy Volunteers**

  No

A Pilot Study Treatment of Malignant Tumors Using [18F] Fluorodeoxyglucose (FDG)

Study ID:

NCT02130492

Sponsor:

Northwell Health

Information provided by (Responsible Party):

Northwell Health (Northwell Health)

Tracking Information

- ▣ **First Submitted Date**

  May 1, 2014

- ▣ **Start Date**

  May 2014

- ▣ **Primary Completion Date**

  July 2019

- ▣ **Last Update Posted Date**

  September 11, 2017

- ▣ **Current Primary Outcome Measures**

  Number of Participants with Serious and Non-Serious Adverse Events and Type of Serious and Non-Serious Adverse Events[Time Frame: Up to 1 year post administration of FDG]

- ▣ **Current Secondary Outcome Measures**

  Efficacy Outcome Measure[Time Frame: Up to one year post FDG treatment]

  Tumor responses in terms of size (CT scans) or FDG uptake (FDG-PET scans) will be carefully recorded and monitored using RECIST Criteria.

Descriptive Information

- ▣ **Offical Title**

  A Pilot Study Treatment of Malignant Tumors Using [18F] Fluorodeoxyglucose (FDG)

- ▣ **Brief Summary**

  The objectives of this Pilot study are to investigate the toxicity and safety of high doses of [18F]-Fluorodeoxyglucose (FDG) used as a therapeutic agent in patients with advanced stage IV malignant tumors that failed standard of care treatment, have a good performance status and bear radiosensitive tumors with a high [18F]-FDG uptake.

  The investigators hypothesize that [18F]FDG may have a significant tumoricidal effect on cancer cells and radionuclide therapy of cancers with high doses of [18F]FDG administered as a single dose or in multiple doses (dose fractionation regimen) can be safe and well tolerated with minimal toxicities. Advantages of FDG are its uptake in many different human tumors, its short half-life (110 minutes) and the possibility to monitor its effect closely with the FDG-PET scan. The rationale for using high doses of this radiopharmaceutical agent for treatment is that most malignant lesions have accentuated glucose metabolism, which is mirrored by increased uptake of FDG. Since FDG cannot be metabolized within the cell like glucose, it is effectively confined within the cancer cells; thus, FDG treatment is potentially a novel form of targeted therapy for tumors with increased FDG uptake.

- ▣ **Study Type**

  Interventional

- ▣ **Study Phase**

  Phase 1

- ▣ **Condition**

128

- Radiosensitive Stage IV Solid and Hematological Tumors With High FDG Uptake Not Responding to Standard of Care
- Lung Cancer, Head and Neck Cancer, Breast Cancer, Gastric Cancer, Pancreatic Cancer, Colon Cancer, Lymphomas, Sarcomas, Etc

▨ Intervention

Radiation: FDG

> The intervention arm consists of treatment with increasing doses of [18F]-Fluorodeoxyglucose.

Other Names:

> [18F]-Fluorodeoxyglucose

▨ Study Arms

Experimental: FDG arm

> Patients will receive increasing doses of FDG.

Recruitment Information

▨ Recruitment Status

Recruiting

▨ Estimated Enrollment

6

▨ Completion Date

July 2019

▨ Primary Completion Date

July 2019

▨ Eligibility Criteria

Inclusion Criteria:

- Provision of informed consent.
- Adults 21 years and older.
- Stage IV solid cancers and stage IV lymphomas that failed to respond to two or more regimens of standard chemotherapy.
- Life expectancy more than 3 months.
- ECOG performance status equal to or less than 2.
- Pathologically documented solid tumors and lymphoma.
- SUV in the primary tumor and/or at least one of the metastatic lesions will need to have an SUV ratio tumor to liver at least greater than 5 and the SUV in the bladder should not be above 100.
- Adequate bone marrow, hepatic and renal function as evidenced by:
- Liver function: bilirubin < 1.5x upper limit of normal (ULN) and SGOT (AST) < 2.5x ULN.
- Renal function: Serum creatinine <1.5 times the ULN or creatinine clearance above 50.
- Bone marrow function: WBC above 4,000/μl; platelet count above 100,000/mm3, absolute neutrophil count above 1,500/mm3, Hemoglobin above 10 g/dl.
- Absence of brain metastases.
- No patients under the age of 21 and no pregnant or nursing women will be enrolled. Women who are not of child bearing potential, and women of child bearing potential who agree to use, while on study, an effective form of contraception and who have a negative serum pregnancy test within 72 hours prior to initial study treatment. Two forms of approved contraception measures should be used simultaneously while on trial in premenopausal women.
- Men willing to use, while on study, an effective form of contraception.
- Ability to comply with all the aspects of the protocol and to come to the follow up visits as per protocol.

Exclusion Criteria:

- Unacceptable uptakes to normal organs as determined after pre-enrollment PET imaging and serum and urinary dosimetry.
- Patients with uncontrolled diabetes.
- Patients with Stage IV lymphoma that involves the bone marrow or patients with solid tumors/ metastatic disease that involves more than 25 % of the bones.
- Patients with radioresistant tumors (i.e. melanoma).
- Patients with primary or metastatic disease to the marrow, heart or brain will be enrolled in order to prevent potential toxicity to these organs.
- Patients with neurological disorders including strokes, seizure disorder, dizziness, vertigo, preexisting grade 2 or higher neuropathy, tremors.
- Mini Mental Test score less than 24.
- Unexplained temperature > 101F or <95F for any 7 consecutive days or chronic diarrhea defined as > 3 stools/day persisting for 15 consecutive days, within the 30 days prior to treatment.
- Prior chemotherapy or surgery within one month, or prior radiotherapy within 2 months.
- Immunotherapy or biologic therapy within 1 month.

- Radiation to more than 50% of the bone marrow.
- Concurrent radiotherapy, chemotherapy. Post-menopausal women who are already using estrogens/progestins as hormone replacement therapy are permitted to enter and to continue using the hormones Tamoxifen and/or Aromatase Inhibitors will be accepted.
- Significant cardiac disease (i.e. uncontrolled high blood pressure, unstable angina, congestive heart failure, myocardial infarction within the previous year) or serious cardiac arrhythmia requiring medication.
- Active acute infection or inflammation, as determined by increased wbc and fever or abnormal CXR. Inflammation in general can cause FDG uptake that may be severe enough to be confused with malignant lesions, especially when there is granulomatous inflammation such as tuberculosis, sarcoidosis, histoplasmosis, and aspergillosis among others and patients with inflammatory disorders are excluded.
- Recent fractures within 2 months.
- Psychiatric illness/social situations that may affect the patient's compliance with the treatment.
- Current use of illicit drugs that may affect the patient's compliance with the treatment.

▨ Sex/Gender

All

▨ Ages

21 Years to N/A

▨ Accepts Healthy Volunteers

No

▨ Contacts

Doru Paul, MD   516-734-8775   dpaul4@northwell.edu

Genotype-Directed Study Of Irinotecan Dosing In FOLFIRI + BevacizumabTreated Metastatic Colorectal Cancer

Study ID:

NCT02138617

Sponsor:

UNC Lineberger Comprehensive Cancer Center

Information provided by (Responsible Party):

UNC Lineberger Comprehensive Cancer Center (UNC Lineberger Comprehensive Cancer Center)

Tracking Information

▨ First Submitted Date

May 1, 2014

▨ Start Date

May 2014

▨ Primary Completion Date

May 2021

▨ Last Update Posted Date

January 30, 2018

▨ Current Primary Outcome Measures

Progression Free Survival[Time Frame: From date of registration until date of first documented progression up to 8 years.]

Tumor measurements within 5 days prior to D1 every 2 cycles starting with cycle 3 to include CT/MRI scans of chest, abdomen and pelvis---any additional suspected sites of disease should be evaluated per treating physician discretion. Progression Free Survival is defined as time from day 1 (D1) of treatment to progression or death from any cause.

▨ Current Secondary Outcome Measures

Toxicity[Time Frame: From date of registration up to 8 years.]

Evaluate toxicity profile when irinotecan is dosed according to UGT1A1 genotype. Toxicity will be classified and graded according to the National Cancer Institute's Common Terminology Criteria for Adverse Events (CTCAE, version 4.03)

Overall Response[Time Frame: 5 years]

Estimate Overall Response (OR =Complete Response +Partial Response) in previously untreated mCRC patients receiving FOLFIRI + bevacizumab when irinotecan dose is based on UGT1A1 genotype. OR will be defined per Response Evaluation Criteria in Solid Tumors version 1.1 (RECIST 1.1).

Overall Survival[Time Frame: 8 years]

Estimate Overall Survival (OS) in previously untreated mCRC patients receiving FOLFIRI + bevacizumab when irinotecan dose is based on UGT1A1 genotype. OS is defined as the time from D1 of treatment to death from any cause

Descriptive Information

Offical Title

Genotype-Directed Phase II Study Of Higher Dose Of Irinotecan In First-Line Metastatic Colorectal Cancer Patients Treated With Folfiri Plus Bevacizumab

Brief Summary

This study involves standard combination chemotherapy treatment for colon cancer, 5-Fluorouracil (5FU), leucovorin and irinotecan (known as FOLFIRI), plus bevacizumab (Avastin). The study is designed to test the FOLFIRI regimen based on certain characteristics of a person's genetic makeup or "genes". Genes are made of DNA and determine not only inherited traits or appearance (hair and eye color, height, body type, etc.) but also play an important role in health and how the body responds to illness and treatments for those illnesses.

In this study, the investigators will examine the relationship between a patient's genes (DNA), or "genotype", and how the patient's body breaks down and removes or "metabolizes" the anti-cancer drug irinotecan. Circulating blood level of irinotecan plays an important role in how well this drug works against a patient's cancer as well as the adverse side effects the patient may experience. The current standard dose of irinotecan was determined in clinical trials without knowing individual genotypes and thus does not take into account a patient's ability to metabolize irinotecan. This means that based on one genotype the current standard dose of irinotecan may be correct or based on other genotypes the standard dose could result in lower and possibly less effective blood levels and result in significant under-dosing of irinotecan.

Based on genotype the patient will be assigned to one of the following doses of irinotecan:

- 180 mg/m2 (standard dose)
- 260 mg/m2
- 310 mg/m2

The purpose of this research study is to determine if dosing irinotecan based on genotype is effective and safe for patients with colon cancer. Patient genotype will be determined from a small sample of blood and a laboratory test or "assay" performed at UNC Laboratories. For the purpose of this study, this assay is new and considered to be "investigational". This means that the genotype assay used in this study has not yet been approved by the FDA for determining irinotecan dose levels in patients with colon cancer.

Detailed Description

This phase II multicenter clinical trial will use a genotype-guided dosing strategy for irinotecan to prospectively analyze efficacy in 100 metastatic colorectal cancer patients (mCRC) receiving FOLFIRI (5-fluorouracil (5-FU), leucovorin, irinotecan) plus bevacizumab. Irinotecan is detoxified and excreted primarily by glucuronidation in the liver via the isoenzyme uridine diphosphate glucuronosyl transferase (UGT1A1). Common variants in UGT1A1 alter the rate of glucuronidation and thus alter exposure to irinotecan.

The UGT1A1

28 allele results in slower irinotecan glucuronidation, and thus greater exposure to its active metabolite SN-38. At the standard irinotecan dose used in FOLFIRI (180 mg/m2; established prior to our understanding of the importance of genotype in the rate of this drug's metabolism), there is a small increased risk of neutropenia in

28 homozygotes. However, the risk of clinically important consequences of neutropenia, such as febrile neutropenia and infection, are not significantly increased. Patients with other genotypes have a quite low risk of adverse effects suggesting patients with these low risk genotypes may tolerate higher doses of irinotecan in FOLFIRI. This finding was demonstrated in a phase I study in which

1/

28 and

1/

1 genotypes were able to tolerate escalating doses of irinotecan up to 260 mg/m2 and 310 mg/m2, respectively.

The central hypothesis of this trial is that increasing the irinotecan dose in

1/

28 and

1/

1 genotypes will increase the overall benefit of FOLFIRI for patients with mCRC as these two groups are likely under-dosed with the current dosing regimen. Eligible patients will be genotyped for UGT1A1 and assigned into 1 of 3 different dosing groups, based on their relative rate of metabolism. The primary objective of this trial is to estimate progression-free survival (PFS), and secondary objectives include characterization of toxicity and objective response rate (OR; complete response (CR) + partial response (PR)).

Study Type

Interventional

- ■ **Study Phase**

  Phase 2

- ■ **Condition**

  - Colon Cancer

- ■ **Intervention**

  Drug: 5-Fluorouracil

  400 mg/m2 IV bolus followed by 2400 mg/m2 IV over 46 hours, Day 1 and Day 15 .

  Other Names:

  5-FU

  Adrucil

  Drug: Leucovorin

  200-400 mg/m2 IV over 2 hours, Day 1 and Day 15

  Other Names:

  LV

  leucovorin calcium

  folinic acid

  citrovorum factor

  Drug: Irinotecan

  IV infusion over 90 minutes, dosed at 180, 260 or 310 mg/m2 based on genotype.

  Other Names:

  Camptosar

  Novaplus Irinotecan Hydrochloride

  Drug: Bevacizumab

  Bevacizumab (5 mg/kg IV infused as per institutional policy, IV, Day 1, 15)

  Other Names:

  Avastin

- ■ **Study Arms**

  Experimental:

  1/

  1 Genotype

  FOLFIRI (5-fluorouracil (5-FU), leucovorin, irinotecan) Irinotecan dose 310 mg/m2,(IV, Day 1, 15); Bevacizumab (IV, Day 1, 15), repeat treatment cycle every 28 days.

  Experimental:

  1/

  28 Genotype

  FOLFIRI (5-fluorouracil (5-FU), leucovorin, irinotecan) Irinotecan dose 260 mg/m2, FOLFIRI (IV, Day 1, 15); Bevacizumab (IV, Day 1, 15), repeat treatment cycle every 28 days.

  Experimental:

  28/

  28

  FOLFIRI (5-fluorouracil (5-FU), leucovorin, irinotecan) Irinotecan dose 180 mg/m2, FOLFIRI (IV, Day 1, 15); Bevacizumab (IV, Day 1, 15), repeat treatment cycle every 28 days.

Recruitment Information

- ■ **Recruitment Status**

  Recruiting

- ■ **Estimated Enrollment**

  100

- ■ **Completion Date**

  May 2022

- ■ **Primary Completion Date**

  May 2021

Eligibility Criteria

Inclusion Criteria:

Subjects must meet all of the inclusion criteria to participate in this study:

1. IRB-approved informed consent obtained and signed

2. Age ≥ 18 years

3. Histological or cytological documentation of adenocarcinoma of the colon or rectum

4. Measurable or non-measurable (but evaluable) disease as defined via RECIST 1.1

5. Metastatic disease not amenable to surgical resection with curative intent

6. No prior chemotherapy for metastatic disease

7. Eastern Cooperative Oncology Group (ECOG) performance status ≤ 2 (see section 11.1, Appendix A)

8. **Adequate bone marrow, renal and hepatic function, as evidenced by the following:**

- absolute neutrophil count (ANC) ≥1,500/mm3
- platelets ≥100,000/mm3
- hemoglobin ≥9.0 g/dL
- serum creatinine ≤1.5 x upper limit of normal (ULN)
- AST and ALT ≤3x ULN (≤5.0 × ULN for patients with liver involvement of their cancer
- Bilirubin ≤1.5 X ULN
- Alkaline phosphatase ≤3 x ULN (≤5 x ULN with liver involvement of their cancer)

9. Willing to undergo UGT1A1 genotyping

10. Negative pregnancy test (urine or serum), within 7 day prior to Day 1 of FOLFIRI in women of childbearing potential

11. Women of childbearing potential and male subjects must agree to use adequate contraception for the duration of study participation. Adequate contraception is defined as any medically recommended method (or combination of methods) as per standard of care.

Exclusion Criteria

1. UGT1A1 genotype other than

1/

1,

1/

28, or

28/

28

2. Known dihydropyrimidine dehydrogenase (DPD) deficiency

3. Prior treatment with irinotecan and/or bevacizumab

4. Unable or unwilling to discontinue (and substitute if necessary) use of prohibited drugs for at least 14 days (fruits and juices for at least 7 days) prior to Day 1 of FOLFIRI + bevacizumab initiation (see section 11.2, Appendix B, for list of prohibited drugs)

5. Inadequately controlled hypertension (defined as systolic blood pressure > 140 mmHg and/or diastolic blood pressure > 90 mmHg)

6. Prior history of hypertensive encephalopathy

7. **Active cardiac disease including any of the following:**

- New York Heart Association (NYHA) Grade II or greater congestive heart failure (see section 11.3, Appendix C)
- History of myocardial infarction or unstable angina within 6 months prior to Day 1
- History of stroke or transient ischemic attack within 6 months prior to Day 1 of FOLFIRI + bevacizumab initiation

8. Significant vascular disease (e.g., aortic aneurysm, requiring surgical repair or recent peripheral arterial thrombosis) within 6 months prior to Day 1 of FOLFIRI + bevacizumab initiation

9. History of hemoptysis (≥ 1/2 teaspoon of bright red blood per episode) within 1 month prior to Day 1 of FOLFIRI + bevacizumab initiation

10. Evidence of bleeding diathesis or significant coagulopathy (in the absence of therapeutic anticoagulation)

11. Major surgical procedure, open biopsy, or significant traumatic injury within 28 days prior to Day 1 of FOLFIRI + bevacizumab initiation or anticipation of need for major surgical procedure during the course of the study

12. Core biopsy or other minor surgical procedure, excluding placement of a vascular access device, within 7 days prior to Day 1 of FOLFIRI + bevacizumab initiation

13. History of abdominal fistula or gastrointestinal perforation within 6 months prior to Day 1 of FOLFIRI + bevacizumab initiation

14. Serious, non-healing wound, active ulcer, or untreated bone fracture

15. **Proteinuria as demonstrated by:**

Urine protein: creatinine (UPC) ratio ≥ 1.0 at screening OR Urine dipstick for proteinuria ≥ 2+ (patients discovered to have ≥2+

proteinuria on dipstick urinalysis at baseline should undergo a 24 hour urine collection and must demonstrate ≤ 1g of protein in 24 hours to be eligible)

16. Any serious uncontrolled medical disorder that would impair the ability of the subject to receive protocol-driven therapy

17. Other anti-cancer or investigational therapy while patients are on study therapy

◼ **Sex/Gender**

All

◼ **Ages**

18 Years to N/A

◼ **Accepts Healthy Volunteers**

No

◼ **Contacts**

Bob Broomer   919-966-9257   bob   broomer@med.unc.edu

Study to Identify Transcriptional Targets of Vitamin D in Patients With Stage I-III Colon Cancer or Resectable Colon Cancer Liver Metastases Receiving Preoperative Vitamin D Supplementation.

Study ID:

NCT02172651

Sponsor:

Dana-Farber Cancer Institute

Information provided by (Responsible Party):

Dana-Farber Cancer Institute (Dana-Farber Cancer Institute)

Tracking Information

◼ **First Submitted Date**

June 17, 2014

◼ **Start Date**

July 2014

◼ **Current Primary Outcome Measures**

◼ **Primary Completion Date**

April 2018

◼ **Last Update Posted Date**

February 9, 2018

VDR Binding Sites[Time Frame: 14 to 28 days]

Compare VDR binding sites between supplementation arms (high-dose versus standard-dose), between malignant versus adjacent benign colon or liver tissue in those receiving high-dose vitamin D, and between primary colon tumors versus liver metastases in patients exposed to high-dose vitamin D. Laboratory procedures for enriching epithelial cells from the surgical specimen, sonicating cross-linked chromatin, immunoprecipitating VDR-chromatin complexes, and preparing DNA libraries for massively parallel sequencing will be refined.

◼ **Current Secondary Outcome Measures**

RNA transcriptome[Time Frame: 28 days]

The goal is to infer direct transcriptional targets of VDR by determining which loci bind VDR and also alter gene expression in response to high-dose vitamin D supplementation. RNA-Seq libraries, prepared from poly(A)+ mRNA and sequenced by Illumina Hi-seq, will be analyzed using Tophat, Cufflinks60 and other new statistical packages to identify consistent differences in transcript levels between tissues exposed to high-dose versus standard-dose vitamin D3 at pre-determined FDRs on the order of 0.01. Stringent tests for statistically significant differences in RNA levels between samples are built into the algorithms for RNA-seq analysis.

Number of Participants with Serious and Non-Serious Adverse Events[Time Frame: Baseline, 14 days to 28 days]

Grade of severity in accordance with the NCI-CTCAE version 4.0 guideline

Descriptive Information

Offical Title

Study to Identify Transcriptional Targets of Vitamin D in Patients With Stage I-III Colon Cancer or Resectable Colon Cancer Liver Metastases Receiving Preoperative Vitamin D Supplementation.

Brief Summary

This study seeks to learn more about the vitamin D receptor and its relationship to colon cancer. The Vitamin D receptor is found in colon cancer cells. When Vitamin D binds to the receptor in the cancer cells, it may stop cancer cells from growing abnormally and may cause cancer cell death. Vitamin D has been used in other research studies and information from those other research studies suggests that Vitamin D may help in the treatment of colon cancer.

Participants will receive either high-dose vitamin D or standard-dose vitamin D. The study drug will be given 14-28 days prior to your surgery. The number of days will depend on when the surgery is scheduled.

Detailed Description

- The participant will be given a study drug-dosing diary to keep track of when they take the study drug. The participant will be taking the study drug once every day, for 14 28 days, prior to their surgery.
- Run-In Phase: The first 6-12 participants will receive high-dose vitamin D prior to surgery. The number of participants in this phase will be based on the results of the analyzed research samples.
- Randomized Phase: Because no one knows which of the study options is best, the participant will be "randomized" into one of the study groups: high dose vitamin D or standard dose vitamin D.
- 48 Participants will be randomized to receive high-dose vitamin D or standard-dose vitamin D. Randomization means that the participants are put into a group by chance. Neither the participant nor the research doctor will choose what group the participant will be in. The participant will have an equal chance of getting assigned to each arm (like flipping a coin). The randomized phase will enroll to two groups at the same time:
- Group A: 24 participants with a recent diagnosis of stage I, II or III colon cancer will be randomized to receive high-dose vitamin D or standard-dose vitamin D.
- Group B: 24 participants with resectable liver metastases from colon cancer will be randomized to receive high-dose vitamin D or standard-dose vitamin D.

Additional research procedures to be performed on study:

- Blood samples will be collected for research purposes (a little more than 2 teaspoons of blood). The samples will be collected immediately prior to the participant's surgery and used to study the vitamin D receptor and pathway, as well as its relationship to colon cancer. Some of this blood will be stored to be used for future cancer research.
- Tumor tissue will be collected for research purposes at the time of the participant surgery. This tissue will also be used to study the vitamin D receptor and pathway, as well as its relationship to colon cancer. Some of the tumor tissue collected will be sent for use in a separate, but related study. In this study, the participant's tumor will be used to grow cell lines. This means the participant's tumor cells will be multiplied in the lab. These cell lines will be used to study the binding sites in the genes of participants and learn more about vitamin D's role in preventing colon cancer.

Study Type

Interventional

Study Phase

Early Phase 1

Condition

- Stage, Colon Cancer
- Stage I-III Colon Cancer
- Stage IV Colon Cancer With Resectable Liver Metastases

Intervention

Drug: Vitamin D3

Other Names:

cholecalciferol (vitamin D3)

Study Arms

Experimental: Vitamin D-Run in phase

One capsule of vitamin D3 10,000 IU orally once daily for 14 days until the date of surgery. To allow for some flexibility in the scheduling of surgery, patients can be treated with preoperative vitamin D3 for up to 28 days. On the morning of surgery, prior to operating, a second blood sample will be collected for follow-up 25(OH)D, calcium, and albumin determination. Colon and liver resection will occur per institutional standards of care, and malignant and adjacent benign tissue will be collected for the laboratory endpoints described in this protocol.

Recruitment Information

Recruitment Status

Recruiting

Estimated Enrollment

12

Completion Date

May 2020

Primary Completion Date

April 2018

Eligibility Criteria

Inclusion Criteria:

Participants must meet the following criteria on screening examination to be eligible to participate in the study:

- Participants must have histologically confirmed adenocarcinoma of the colon that is localized, with no evidence of distant metastasis (stage I, II, or III), and for which surgical resection of the primary tumor is being planned;

  --OR

- Participants must have histologically or cytologically confirmed adenocarcinoma of the colon with resectable liver metastases for which liver resection is being planned.

- No prior radiation therapy or systemic treatment is allowed for patients undergoing resection of stage I, II, or III colon cancer.

- Prior systemic treatment or radiation therapy is allowed for patients with resectable liver metastases.

- The last dose of chemotherapy or radiation must have been administered at least 4 weeks prior to liver surgery.

- The last dose of bevacizumab must have been administered at least 6 weeks prior to liver resection.

- Age ≥18 years.

- ECOG performance status ≤ 1 (see Appendix A)

- Participants must have normal organ and marrow function as defined below:

- Total bilirubin ≤1.5× institutional upper limit of normal (ULN)

- AST(SGOT)/ALT(SGPT) ≤ 2.5 × institutional ULN, or <5x ULN if clearly attributable to liver metastases

- Serum calcium (corrected for albumin level) ≤ 1x institutional ULN

- Serum creatinine within normal institutional limits or creatinine clearance ≥60 mL/min/1.73 m2 for subjects with creatinine levels above institutional normal.

- Participants on full-dose anticoagulation are eligible if the following criteria are met:

- Participant has an in-range INR (usually 2-3) on a stable dose of warfarin or is on a stable dose of low molecular weight heparin

- Participant has no active bleeding or pathological condition that carries a high risk of bleeding (i.e., tumor involving major vessels or known varices)

- Participants receiving anti-platelet agents are eligible. In addition, patients who are on daily prophylactic aspirin or anticoagulation for atrial fibrillation are eligible.

- Discontinuation of anticoagulation, aspirin, and/or anti-platelet agents prior to surgery will occur according to institutional standards of care.

- Non-pregnant and not nursing

- Women of child-bearing potential must have a negative serum or urine pregnancy test (minimum sensitivity 25 IU/L or equivalent units of HCG) within 14 days prior to study entry. Women of child-bearing potential include any female who has experienced menarche and who has not undergone surgical sterilization (hysterectomy, bilateral tubal ligation, or bilateral oophorectomy) or is not postmenopausal (defined as amenorrhea ≥12 consecutive months; or women on hormone replacement therapy with documented serum follicle stimulating hormone level >35 mIU/mL). Women who are using oral, implanted, or injectable contraceptive hormones or mechanical products such as intrauterine device or barrier methods (diaphragm, condoms, spermicides) to prevent pregnancy, or who are practicing abstinence or where partner is sterile (e.g., vasectomy), should be considered to be of child-bearing potential.

- The effects of higher-dose vitamin D3 and colon or liver surgery (and associated perioperative medications and anesthesia) on the developing human fetus are unknown and may pose unacceptable risk. For this reason, women of child-bearing potential and men must agree to use adequate contraception (hormonal or barrier method of birth control; abstinence) prior to study entry and for the duration of study participation. Should a woman become pregnant or suspect she is pregnant while participating in this study, she should inform her treating physician immediately.

- Ability to understand and the willingness to sign a written informed consent document.

Exclusion Criteria:

Participants who exhibit any of the following conditions at screening will not be eligible for admission into the study.

- Prior systemic therapy, radiotherapy, or investigational agent in participants undergoing surgery for stage I, II, or III colon cancer.

- Participants who have had chemotherapy or radiotherapy within 4 weeks (6 weeks for bevacizumab) of liver resection.

- Concurrent use of other anti-cancer therapy, including chemotherapy agents, targeted agents, biological agents, immunotherapy, or investigational agents not otherwise specified in this protocol.

- Inability to swallow pills.

- History of malabsorption or uncontrolled vomiting or diarrhea, or any other disease significantly affecting gastrointestinal function that could interfere with absorption of oral medications.

- History of allergic reactions attributed to compounds of similar chemical or biologic composition to vitamin D.
- Regular use of supplemental vitamin D totaling ≥ 2,000 IU/day in the past year.
- Use of supplemental vitamin D or supplements containing vitamin D beyond the protocol-prescribed study treatment is not allowed during the treatment period of this clinical trial.
- In order to maintain blinding, vitamin D levels should not be routinely checked at screening or during the study by the treating investigator. Vitamin D levels will be assayed only as part of the research blood samples collected during the study. If there are concerns related to a participant's vitamin D status, the lead Principal Investigator should be contacted for further discussion.
- Use of chronic oral corticosteroid therapy, lithium, phenytoin, quinidine, isoniazid, and/or rifampin (all of which can cause vitamin D depletion). Short-term use of corticosteroids as anti-emetic therapy for chemotherapy is permitted.
- Regular use of thiazide diuretics (i.e., hydrochlorothiazide), which can lead to hypercalcemia, and unwillingness or inability to discontinue or switch to an alternative anti-hypertensive agent.
- Pre-existing hypercalcemia (defined as baseline serum calcium above the institutional ULN, corrected for albumin level if albumin is not within institutional limits of normal).
- -The use of supplemental calcium or supplements containing calcium is prohibited during the treatment period of this clinical trial.
- Known active hyperparathyroid disease or other serious disturbance of calcium metabolism in the past 5 years.
- History of symptomatic genitourinary stones within the past year.
- Any uncontrolled intercurrent illness including, but not limited to, ongoing or active infection, symptomatic congestive heart failure, unstable angina pectoris, cardiac arrhythmia, or psychiatric illness/social situations that, in the opinion of the investigator, may increase the risks associated with study participation or study treatment, limit compliance with study requirements, or interfere with the interpretation of study results.
- Pregnant or nursing women or men/women of child-bearing potential who are unwilling to employ adequate contraception.
- -Pregnant and nursing women are excluded from this study because there is an unknown but potential risk of adverse events related to higher-dose vitamin D3 and colon or liver surgery (and associated perioperative medications and anesthesia) on the human fetus. Consequently, breastfeeding should be discontinued if the mother is enrolled on the study.
- **History of prior or synchronous malignancy except:**
- A malignancy that was treated with curative intent, for which there has been no known active disease for >3 years prior to randomization, and for which the risk of recurrence is low as determined by the investigator.
- Curatively treated non-melanoma skin malignancy, cervical cancer in situ, or prostatic intraepithelial neoplasia without evidence of prostate cancer.
- Known positive test for human immunodeficiency virus (HIV), hepatitis C virus, or acute or chronic hepatitis B infection.
- Participants with these infections are ineligible because they are at increased risk of significant complications in the perioperative period, particularly for active hepatitis B or C patients undergoing liver resection. Appropriate studies will be undertaken in participants receiving combination antiretroviral therapy when indicated.

Sex/Gender

All

Ages

18 Years to N/A

Accepts Healthy Volunteers

No

Contacts

Kimmie Ng, MD   617-632-5960

A Phase 1/2 Study Exploring the Safety, Tolerability, and Efficacy of Pembrolizumab (MK-3475) in Combination With Epacadostat (INCB024360) in Subjects With Selected Cancers (INCB 24360-202 / MK-3475-037 / KEYNOTE-037/ ECHO-202)

Study ID:

NCT02178722

Sponsor:

Incyte Corporation

Information provided by (Responsible Party):

Incyte Corporation (Incyte Corporation)

Tracking Information

▒ **First Submitted Date**

June 26, 2014

▒ **Start Date**

June 2014

▒ **Primary Completion Date**

November 2019

▒ **Last Update Posted Date**

December 11, 2017

▒ **Current Primary Outcome Measures**

Phase 1: Number of subjects with dose limiting toxicities (DLTs) of INCB024360 in combination with MK-3475[Time Frame: 56 days]

   Phase 2: Objective response rate[Time Frame: Assessed every 9 weeks for duration of study participation which is estimated to be 18 months]

▒ **Current Secondary Outcome Measures**

Progression free survival[Time Frame: Response is measured every 9 weeks for duration of study participation which is estimated to be 18 months]

   Number of subjects with Adverse Events as a Measure of Safety and Tolerability of INCB024360 in combination with MK-3475[Time Frame: Adverse events are assessed every 3 weeks for duration of study participation which is estimated to be 18 months]

   Overall survival (OS)[Time Frame: Patients are checked for survival every 12 weeks for duration of study participation which is estimated to be 18 months]

Descriptive Information

▒ **Offical Title**

A Phase 1/2 Study Exploring the Safety, Tolerability, and Efficacy of Pembrolizumab (MK-3475) in Combination With Epacadostat (INCB024360) in Subjects With Selected Cancers (KEYNOTE-037/ ECHO-202)

▒ **Brief Summary**

The purpose of this study is to assess the safety, tolerability, and efficacy when combining MK-3475 and INCB024360 in subjects with certain cancers. This study will be conducted in 2 phases, Phase 1 and Phase 2.

▒ **Study Type**

Interventional

▒ **Study Phase**

Phase 1/Phase 2

▒ **Condition**

- Solid Tumors and Hematologic Malignancy
- Endometrial Cancer
- NSCLC (Non-small Cell Lung Carcinoma)
- HNSCC (Head and Neck Squamous Cell Cancer)
- Gastric Cancer

- HCC (Hepatocellular Carcinoma)
- Lymphoma, Large B-Cell, Diffuse (DLBCL)
- CRC (Colorectal Cancer)
- Ovarian Cancer
- RCC (Renal Cell Carcinoma)
- UC (Urothelial Cancer)
- Breast Cancer
- Melanoma

Intervention

Drug: MK-3475

  IV infusion

  Drug: INCB024360

  Oral daily dosing

Study Arms

Experimental: Phase 1: MK-3475 + INCB024360

  Phase 1: MK-3475 + INCB024360 25 mg twice a day (BID) as starting dose, followed by dose escalations (Phase 1) until recommended phase 2 dose of INCB024360 is determined

Experimental: Phase 2: MK-3475 + INCB024360

  (recommended phase 2 dose)

Recruitment Information

Recruitment Status

Recruiting

Estimated Enrollment

508

Completion Date

February 2020

Primary Completion Date

November 2019

Eligibility Criteria

Inclusion Criteria:

- Subjects with histologically or cytologically NSCLC, melanoma, transitional cell carcinoma of the genitourinary (GU) tract, renal cell cancer, triple negative breast cancer, adenocarcinoma of the endometrium or squamous cell carcinoma of the head and neck (Phase 1).
- Subjects with histologically confirmed melanoma, NSCLC, transitional cell carcinoma of the GU tract, TNBC, SCCHN, ovarian cancer, MSI high colorectal cancer (CRC), RCC, gastric cancer, HCC and DLBCL (Phase 2).
- Life expectancy > 12 weeks.
- Eastern Cooperative Oncology Group (ECOG) performance status 0 1.
- Presence of measurable disease per Response Evaluation Criteria in Solid Tumors (RECIST) 1.1 or Lugano Classification for subjects with DLBCL.
- Laboratory and medical history parameters within protocol-defined range.
- For Phase 1: Subjects who have advanced or metastatic disease as noted above that have received at least one prior therapy or have advanced or metastatic disease for which no curative treatment is available may be enrolled.
- For Phase 2 expansion cohorts: Subjects with NSCLC, melanoma (checkpoint inhibitor naïve, primary refractory melanoma, relapsed melanoma), transitional cell carcinoma of the GU tract, SCCHN, ovarian cancer, MSI high CRC, RCC, DLBCL, and TNBC.
- Phase 2 expansion: NSCLC
- Subjects who have received at least 1 prior platinum-based therapy. Subjects who have a non-platinum-based regimen may be enrolled with medical monitor approval.
- Tumors with epidermal growth factor receptor mutation positive or anaplastic lymphoma kinase fusion oncogene positive treated with a tyrosine kinase inhibitor are permitted; however, subjects should have progressed on or be intolerant to the targeted therapy.
- Subjects must not have received immunotherapy with programmed death receptor-1 (PD-1) or cytotoxic T-lymphocyte antigen (CTLA-4) targeted therapy.
- Phase 2 expansion: Melanoma
- Documentation of V600E-activating BRAF mutation status.
- Prior systemic therapy requirements.
- Melanoma immune checkpoint-naïve: Subjects must not have received immunotherapy with anti-PD-1, anti-PD-L1, or anti-

CTLA-4 therapy. Exception: Prior anti–CTLA-4 in the adjuvant setting would be permitted.

- Primary refractory melanoma: Subjects must have received prior treatment with anti-PD-1 or anti-PD-L1 therapy (alone or as part of a combination) in the advanced or metastatic setting and have progressive disease as their best response to treatment that is confirmed 4 weeks later.
- Relapsed melanoma: Subjects must have received prior anti–PD-1 or anti–PD-L1 therapy (alone or as part of a combination) in the advanced or metastatic setting and achieved partial response ore complete response but later have confirmed progressive disease.
- Subjects enrolling in the primary refractory or relapsed melanoma must be willing to undergo mandatory pretreatment and on-treatment biopsies.
- Ocular melanoma is excluded.
- Phase 2 expansion: Transitional cell carcinoma of the GU tract
- Metastatic or locally advanced and not amenable to curative therapy with disease progression on or after platinum-based chemotherapy or alternative therapy if platinum-based therapy is not appropriate.
- Prior PD-1 or CTLA-4 targeted therapies are excluded
- Phase 2 expansion: SCCHN
- Histologically confirmed metastatic or recurrent squamous cell carcinoma not amenable to local therapy with curative intent (surgery or radiation with or without chemotherapy). Carcinoma of the nasopharynx, salivary gland, or

Subjects must have received at least 1 prior systemic chemotherapy regimen that must have included a platinum-based therapy.

- Prior PD-1 or CTLA-4 targeted therapies are excluded.
- Phase 2 expansion: Ovarian cancer
- Subjects with FIGO Stage Ic, Stage II, Stage III, Stage IV, recurrent, or persistent (unresectable) histologically confirmed epithelial ovarian cancer, primary peritoneal cancer, or fallopian tube carcinoma.
- Subjects must have received a platinum-taxane-based regimen as first-line therapy.
- Prior PD-1 or CTLA-4 targeted therapies are excluded.
- Borderline, low-malignant-potential epithelial carcinoma per histopathology is excluded.
- Phase 2 expansion: Relapsed or refractory DLBCL
- Prior allogeneic stem-cell transplantation is excluded.
- Must have received > or = 1 prior treatment regimen.
- Not a candidate for curative therapy or hematopoietic stem-cell transplantation (either due to disease burden, fitness, or preference).
- Prior PD-1 or CTLA-4 targeted therapies are excluded.
- Phase 2 expansion: TNBC
- Histologically confirmed breast adenocarcinoma that is unresectable loco regional, or metastatic
- **Pathologically confirmed as triple negative, source documented, defined as both of the following:**
- Estrogen receptor (ER) and progesterone receptor (PgR) negative.
- Human epidermal growth factor receptor 2 (HER2) negative as per American Society of Clinical Oncology/College of American Pathologists guidelines.
- Subject must have received at least 1 prior systemic regimen for advanced or metastatic disease
- Prior PD-1 or CTLA-4 targeted therapies are excluded.
- Phase 2 expansion: RCC
- Subjects with histological or cytological confirmation of clear cell RCC.
- Not curable by surgery.
- Subjects must have received prior antiangiogenic therapy.
- Subjects must not have received prior immunotherapy with anti-PD-1, anti-PD-L1, or anti-CTLA-4 therapy.
- Phase 2 expansion: MSI high CRC
- Subjects with histological confirmation of locally advanced unresectable or metastatic MSI high CRC.
- MSI status is, respectively, determined by examining CRC tumor.
- Subjects may have received no more than 2 lines of prior therapy for advanced disease.
- Phase 2 expansion: Gastric Cancer
- Must have histologically or cytologically confirmed diagnosis of gastric or gastroesophageal junction adenocarcinoma.
- Must have progression on or after therapy containing platinum/fluoropyrimidine or refused standard therapy.
- Subjects may have received no more than 2 lines of prior therapy for advanced disease.
- Prior PD-1 or CTLA-4 targeted therapies are excluded.
- Phase 2 expansion: HCC
- Must have histologically or cytologically confirmed diagnosis of HCC (fibrolamellar and mixed hepatocellular/cholangiocarcinoma subtypes are not eligible).
- Barcelona Clinic Liver Cancer (BCLC) Stage C disease (Llovet et al 1999), or BCLC Stage B disease.

- Subjects may have received no more than 2 lines of prior therapy for the advanced disease
- Must have progressed on, refused, or were intolerant of sorafenib.
- The following are excluded: Subjects with liver transplants, clear invasion of the bile duct or main portal branch(es), or hepatorenal syndrome, or subjects who have required esophageal variceal ablation within 28 days of starting study treatment.
- Prior PD-1 or CTLA-4 targeted therapies are excluded.
- Tumor biopsies are required. If a subject has inaccessible lesions, such as in ovarian cancer, HCC, or gastric cancer, or highly vascular lesions, such as RCC, enrollment may be considered with medical monitor approval, and archived tissue may be acceptable.
- Females of child-bearing potential and males who use adequate birth control through 120 days post dose.

Exclusion Criteria:

- Subjects who participated in any other study in which receipt of an investigational study drug or device occurred within 2 weeks or 5 half-lives (whichever is longer) prior to first dose.
- Has received prior therapy with an anti-PD-1, anti-PD-L1, anti-PD-L2, anti-CD137, or anti-Cytotoxic T-lymphocyte-associated antigen-4 (CTLA-4) antibody (including ipilimumab or any other antibody or drug specifically targeting T-cell co-stimulation or checkpoint pathways). Exception: Prior anti–CTLA-4 in the adjuvant setting for subjects with melanoma would be permitted.
- Has known active central nervous system (CNS) metastases and/or carcinomatous meningitis. Subjects with previously treated brain metastases may participate provided they are stable.
- Has an active autoimmune disease.
- Has evidence of noninfectious pneumonitis that required steroids or current pneumonitis.
- Live vaccine use within 30 days of first dose of study medication.
- Monoamine oxidase inhibitors.

Sex/Gender

All

Ages

18 Years to N/A

Accepts Healthy Volunteers

No

Contacts

Incyte Call Center   1-855-463-3463

Cancer Associated Thrombosis and Isoquercetin (CAT IQ)

Study ID:

NCT02195232

Sponsor:

Dana-Farber Cancer Institute

Information provided by (Responsible Party):

Dana-Farber Cancer Institute (Dana-Farber Cancer Institute)

Tracking Information

First Submitted Date

May 13, 2014

Start Date

January 2015

Primary Completion Date

August 2018

Last Update Posted Date

February 6, 2018

Current Primary Outcome Measures

Percentage of Participants with Reduced D-dimer values[Time Frame: Baseline, 56 Day]

D-dimer concentrations will be compared for each patient at day 0 and day 56 by a paired-t test analysis. Analysis will be performed on an intention to treat basis for patients who undergo randomization and completed the baseline and day 56 D-dimer assessments.

Safety[Time Frame: study visits until day 56]

Will evaluate toxicity of isoquercetin

Descriptive Information

■ Offical Title

Randomized, Placebo-controlled, Double-blind Phase II/III Trial of Oral Isoquercetin to Prevent Venous Thromboembolic Events in Cancer Patients.

■ Brief Summary

This research study is evaluating a drug called isoquercetin to prevent venous thrombosis (blood clots), in participants who have pancreas, non small cell lung cancer or colorectal cancer.

■ Detailed Description

- This research study is a Phase II/III clinical trial.

--The goal of this trial is to evaluate if isoquercetin can prevent blood clots in patients with pancreas, non small cell lung cancer or colorectal cancer. In the Phase II part of this study, the investigators are looking for the dose of isoquercetin to reduce D-dimer and demonstrate safety.

- Phase III Endpoint and Treatment Plan
- Primary Endpoint for Phase III portion of protocol: Cumulative incidence of VTE.
- Following the completion of the phase II portion, enrolled patients will be randomized 1:1 to Arm C (isoquercetin) or Arm D (placebo). The dose for Arm C will be determined after evaluation of the Phase II portion of the trial. The protocol will be amended when the decision is made whether to proceed to Phase III and what dose to use for Arm C. The study will be double-blinded to treatment arm. Lower extremity ultrasound will be performed at 56 days. Baseline D-dimer and correlative labs will be drawn at Day 1 and at 56 days. Patients will be followed for survival after completion of 56 days.
- At BIDMC, optional blood draw will be performed at time 0 and 4 hours following the first dose of study drug.

■ Study Type

Interventional

■ Study Phase

Phase 2/Phase 3

■ Condition

- Thromboembolism of Vein VTE in Colorectal Cancer
- Thromboembolism of Vein in Pancreatic Cancer
- Thromboembolism of Vein in Non-small Cell Lung Cancer

■ Intervention

Drug: Isoquercetin

Other Names:

quercetin-3-O-glucoside

482-35-9

■ Study Arms

Experimental: Isoquercetin

Isoquercetin:

Cohort A: 500 mg, Once daily, 28 days or

Cohort B: 1000 mg, Once daily, 28 days

For both cohorts A and B, lower extremity ultrasound will be performed at 56 days. Baseline D-dimer and correlative labs will be drawn at Day 1 and at 56 days. Patients will be followed for survival after completion of 56 days.

Recruitment Information

■ Recruitment Status

Recruiting

■ Estimated Enrollment

618

■ Eligibility Criteria

■ Completion Date

April 2023

■ Primary Completion Date

August 2018

Inclusion Criteria:

- Participants must meet the following criteria on screening examination to be eligible to participate in phase 2 and 3 of the study:
- Participants must have histologically confirmed malignancy that is metastatic or currently unresectable.
- Eligible malignancies include:
- Adenocarcinoma of the pancreas (currently unresectable or metastatic)
- Colorectal (stage IV)
- Non-small cell lung cancer (currently unresectable stage III or stage IV)
- Receiving or scheduled to receive first or second line chemotherapy (within 30 days of registration)
- Minimum age 18 years. Because limited dosing or adverse event data are currently available on the use of isoquercetin in participants <18 years of age, children are excluded from this study but will be eligible for future pediatric isoquercetin trials.
- Life expectancy of greater than 4 months.
- ECOG performance status ≤2 (see Appendix B).
- Patient must be able to swallow capsules (phase III only)
- Participants must have preserved organ and marrow function as defined below:
- Absolute neutrophil count ≥1,000/mcL
- Platelets ≥ 90,000/mcL
- PT and PTT ≤ 1.5 x upper limit of normal
- Total bilirubin < 2.0 mg/dl
- AST (SGOT)/ALT (SGPT) ≤ 2.5 X institutional upper limit of normal Creatinine < 2.0 mg/dl
- The effects of isoquercetin on the developing human fetus are unknown. For this reason, women of child-bearing potential and men must agree to use adequate contraception (hormonal or barrier method of birth control; abstinence) prior to study entry and for the duration of study participation. Should a woman become pregnant or suspect she is pregnant while participating in this study, she should inform her treating physician immediately.
- Ability to understand and the willingness to sign a written informed consent document.

Exclusion Criteria:

- Participants may not be receiving any other study agents.
- Participants with known brain metastases should be excluded from this clinical trial because of their poor prognosis and because they often develop progressive neurologic dysfunction that would confound the evaluation of neurologic and other adverse events.
- Prior history of documented venous thromboembolic event within the last 2 years (excluding central line associated events whereby patients completed anticoagulation).
- Active bleeding or high risk for bleeding (e.g. known acute gastrointestinal ulcer)
- History of significant hemorrhage (requiring hospitalization or transfusion) outside of a surgical setting within the last 24 months
- Familial bleeding diathesis
- Known diagnosis of disseminated intravascular coagulation (DIC)
- Currently receiving anticoagulant therapy
- Current daily use of aspirin (>81mg daily), Clopidogrel (Plavix), cilostazol (Pletal), aspirin-dipyridamole (Aggrenox) (within 10 days) or considered to use regular use of higher doses of non-steroidal anti-inflammatory agents as determined by the treating physician (e.g ibuprofen > 800 mg daily or equivalent).
- Uncontrolled intercurrent illness including, but not limited to ongoing or active infection, symptomatic congestive heart failure, unstable angina pectoris, cardiac arrhythmia, or psychiatric illness/social situations that would limit compliance with study requirements.
- Known intolerance of niacin or ascorbic acid (including known G6PD deficiency)
- Pregnant women are excluded from this study because isoquercetin is a PDI inhibitor with the potential for teratogenic or abortifacient effects. Because there is an unknown but potential risk of adverse events in nursing infants secondary to treatment of the mother with isoquercetin, breastfeeding should be discontinued if the mother is treated with isoquercetin. These potential risks may also apply to other agents used in this study.

- Sex/Gender

  All

- Ages

  18 Years to N/A

- Accepts Healthy Volunteers

  No

Evaluate the Efficacy of MEDI4736 in Immunological Subsets of Advanced Colorectal Cancer

Study ID:
NCT02227667

Sponsor:
Memorial Sloan Kettering Cancer Center

Information provided by (Responsible Party):
Memorial Sloan Kettering Cancer Center (Memorial Sloan Kettering Cancer Center)

Tracking Information

■ **First Submitted Date**

July 17, 2014

■ **Start Date**

December 2, 2014

■ **Primary Completion Date**

July 2019

■ **Last Update Posted Date**

February 12, 2018

■ **Current Primary Outcome Measures**

best response rate[Time Frame: 2 years]
  according to RECIST 1.1.

■ **Current Secondary Outcome Measures**

Safety[Time Frame: 2 years]

  Subjects will be evaluated for occurrence of AEs at each visit. Events will be characterized and reported. Safety will also be monitored by performing physical exams and routine laboratory procedures. Terminology Criteria for Adverse Events" V4.0 (CTCAE).

Progression-free survival[Time Frame: 2 years]

  Progression-free survival will be measured from the start of treatment with MEDI4736 until the documentation of disease progression or death due to any cause, whichever occurs first.

Overall survival[Time Frame: 2 years]

  Overall survival will be determined as the time from the start of treatment with MEDI4736 until death

Descriptive Information

■ **Offical Title**

Phase II Study to Evaluate the Efficacy of MEDI4736 in Immunological Subsets of Advanced Colorectal Cancer

■ **Brief Summary**

The purpose of this study is to find out what effects, good and/or bad, MEDI4736 has on the patient and cancer.

MEDI4736 is a type of medication called an antibody. Antibodies are normal proteins in the body that help fight infections and possibly cancer. MEDI4736 is a special type of an antibody produced in a laboratory. MEDI4736 works by blocking a specific protein called the Programmed Death Ligand-1 (PDL-1), located on tumor cells.

■ **Study Type**

Interventional

■ **Study Phase**

Phase 2

■ **Condition**

• Advanced Colorectal Cancer

■ **Intervention**

Drug: MEDI4736

Patients will be seen the day of administration of MEDI4736. A medical history, with particular reference to toxicities, including medication review, and physical examination will be conducted at each treatment visit.

Study Arms

Experimental: Patients with Advanced Colorectal Cancer

This will be a Simon two-stage design, single arm, phase II study. All subjects will receive MEDI4736 via IV infusion. Subjects will continue treatment for 12 months, or until progression of disease, initiation of alternative cancer therapy, unacceptable toxicity, or other reasons to discontinue treatment occur. Following the 12-month treatment period, subjects without evidence for progressive disease or other reason to discontinue treatment will be monitored without further treatment. Upon evidence of PD (with or without confirmation according to RECIST 1.1) during the monitoring period, administration of MEDI4736 may resume at the Q2W schedule, for up to another 12 months. The same treatment guidelines followed during the initial 12-month treatment period will be followed during the retreatment period, including the same dose and frequency of treatments and the same schedule of assessments.

Recruitment Information

Recruitment Status

Recruiting

Estimated Enrollment

48

Completion Date

July 2019

Primary Completion Date

July 2019

Eligibility Criteria

Inclusion Criteria:

- Written informed consent obtained.
- Histologicallyor cytologicallyconfirmed CRC.
- Microsatelite-high colorectal cancer (also known as MSI-H, DNA mismatch repair deficient, or sometimes Lynch syndrome); or increased Tumor-Infiltrating Lymphocytes in an archived tumor specimen or fresh biopsy.
- Locally advanced or metastatic CRC
- Subjects have received two or more standard available therapies known to prolong survival and for which they would be considered eligible. At a minimum, such therapies should include regimens containing oxaliplatin and irinotecan in combination with a fluoropyrimidine (e.g., FOLFOX and FOLFIRI or their variants).
- Age ≥ 18 years at time of study entry.
- Eastern Cooperative Oncology Group (ECOG) status of 0 or 1
- Adequate organ and marrow function as defined below:
- Absolute neutrophil count ≥ 1,500/mm3.
- Platelet count ≥ 90,000/mm3.
- AST and ALT ≤ 3 × institutional upper limit of normal (ULN) or ≤ 5 × ULN for subjects with liver metastases.
- Bilirubin ≤ 1.5 × ULN or ≤ 3 × ULN for subjects with documented/suspected Gilbert's disease.
- Serum creatinine ≤ 1.5 x ULN;
- Radiographically measurable disease per RECIST 1.1.
- Life expectancy ≥ 16 weeks.
- Willingness to provide consent for use of archived tissue for research purposes.
- Subjects will be required to agree to a biopsy performed at baseline and again at week 8 of the study in order to be eligible for enrollment in stage 1 of the study
- Females of childbearing potential who are sexually active with a nonsterilized male partner must use 2 methods of effective contraception from screening, and must agree to continue using such precautions for 90 days after the final dose of investigational product; cessation of birth control after this point should be discussed with a responsible physician. Periodic abstinence, the rhythm method, and the withdrawal method are not acceptable methods of birth control.
- Females of childbearing potential are defined as those who are not surgically sterile (ie, bilateral tubal ligation, bilateral oophorectomy, or complete hysterectomy) or postmenopausal (defined as 12 months with no menses without an alternative medical cause).
- Subjects must use 2 acceptable methods of effective contraception as described in below.
- Nonsterilized males who are sexually active with a female partner of childbearing potential must use 2 acceptable methods of effective contraception from Day 1 and for 90 days after receipt of the final dose of investigational product.

Exclusion Criteria:

- Anticancer therapy, monoclonal antibody or major surgery within 4 weeks prior to the first dose of MEDI4736.
- Concurrent use of hormones for non-cancer-related conditions (e.g., insulin for diabetes and hormone replacement therapy) is acceptable.
- Any prior Grade ≥ 3 irAE while receiving immunotherapy (including anti-CTLA-4 or anti-CD137 MAb) or any unresolved irAE of any grade (controlled irAE endocrinopathies are allowed).

- Prior exposure to any anti-PD-1 or anti-PD-L1 antibody.
- Current or prior use of immunosuppressive medication within 28 days before the first dose of MEDI4736, with the exceptions of intranasal and inhaled corticosteroids or systemic corticosteroids at physiological doses, which are not to exceed 10 mg/day of prednisone, or an equivalent corticosteroid.
- Any unresolved toxicity CTCAE >Grade 2 from previous anti-cancer therapy.
- Active autoimmune disease within the past 2 years, except for mild conditions not requiring systemic treatment, such as vitiligo.
- Any concurrent chemotherapy, immunotherapy, biologic or hormonal therapy for cancer treatment. NOTE: Local treatment of isolated lesions, excluding target lesions, for palliative intent is acceptable (e.g., by local ablation, surgery or radiotherapy).
- Active or prior documented inflammatory bowel disease (e.g., Crohn's disease, irritable bowel syndrome, ulcerative colitis).
- Receipt of radiation therapy within 4 weeks prior to starting investigational product, or limited field of radiation for palliation within 2 weeks of the first dose of investigational product.
- Known allergy or reaction to any component of the MEDI4736 formulation or its excipients.
- Known central nervous system (CNS) metastases requiring treatment, such as surgery, radiation or steroids.
- Known history of confirmed primary immunodeficiency.
- History of organ transplant requiring therapeutic immunosuppression.
- Other malignancy within 3 years, except for noninvasive malignancies such as cervical carcinoma in situ (CIS), non-melanomatous carcinoma of the skin or ductal carcinoma in situ (DCIS) of the breast that has/have been surgically cured, or prior malignancy considered by the investigator to be of low likelihood for recurrence.
- Uncontrolled intercurrent illness including, but not limited to, ongoing or active infection, symptomatic congestive heart failure, uncontrolled hypertension, unstable angina pectoris, cardiac arrhythmia, active peptic ulcer disease or gastritis, active bleeding diatheses including any patient known to have active hepatitis B, hepatitis C or human immunodeficiency virus (HIV), or psychiatric illness/social situations that would limit compliance with study requirements or compromise the ability of the patient to give written informed consent.
- Women who are pregnant, breast-feeding or male or female patients of reproductive potential who are not employing an effective method of birth control.
- Any other condition(s) that, in the opinion of the investigator, would interfere with evaluation of the investigational product or interpretation of subject safety or study results.
- Subjects who are known to be HIV positive.
- Receipt of live attenuated vaccination within 30 days prior to receiving MEDI4736

Sex/Gender

All

Ages

18 Years to N/A

Accepts Healthy Volunteers

No

Contacts

Neil Segal, MD PhD   646 888-4187
Leonard Saltz, MD   646-888-4286

CPI-613 and Fluorouracil in Treating Patients With Metastatic Colorectal Cancer That Cannot Be Removed by Surgery

Study ID:

NCT02232152

Sponsor:

Wake Forest University Health Sciences

Information provided by (Responsible Party):

Wake Forest University Health Sciences (Wake Forest University Health Sciences)

Tracking Information

First Submitted Date

September 2, 2014

Start Date

December 2014

Primary Completion Date

December 2018

Last Update Posted Date

January 23, 2018

Current Primary Outcome Measures

MTD of 6,8-bis(benzylthio)octanoic acid in combination with fluorouracil based on the incidence of dose-limiting toxicities graded according to the National Cancer Institute (NCI) Common Terminology Criteria for Adverse Events (CTCAE) version 4.0[Time Frame: Up to 2 weeks]

Current Secondary Outcome Measures

Incidence of toxicity of 6,8-bis(benzylthio)octanoic acid and fluorouracil combination graded according to NCI CTCAE version 4.0[Time Frame: Up to 3 years]

> Examine toxicities by assessing each toxicity by grade.

PK parameters (maximum observed concentration, area under the curve, half-life, elimination rate constant, drug clearance, and volume of distribution) of 6,8-bis(benzylthio)octanoic acid in plasma samples[Time Frame: Week 1: days 1 and 4 before infusion of 6,8-bis(benzylthio)octanoic acid and at 30 minutes, 1, 1.5, 2, 4, 6 and 8 (optional) hours after the completion of infusion]

Progression-free survival (PFS)[Time Frame: Time from the first dose of 6,8-bis(benzylthio)octanoic acid to disease progression, assessed up to 3 years]

> Plot a PFS curve using Kaplan-Meier methods, examine median PFS.

Overall response rate (ORR) (i.e., sum of complete response [CR] and partial response [PR])[Time Frame: Up to 3 years]

> Assess ORR and its 95% confidence interval.

Disease control rate (DCR) (i.e., sum of CR, PR, and stable disease)[Time Frame: Up to 3 years]

> Assess DCR and its 95% confidence interval.

Descriptive Information

Offical Title

A Phase I Clinical Trial of Fluorouracil (5-FU) + CPI-613 Combination in Previously Treated Metastatic Colorectal Cancer Patients

Brief Summary

This pilot phase I trial studies the side effects and best dose of CPI-613 when given together with fluorouracil in treating patients with colorectal cancer that has spread to other parts of the body and cannot be removed by surgery. CPI-613 may kill tumor cells by turning off their mitochondria. Mitochondria are used by tumor cells to produce energy and are the building blocks needed to make more tumor cells. By shutting off these mitochondria, CPI-613 deprives the tumor cells of energy and other supplies that they need to survive and grow in the body. Drugs used in chemotherapy, such as fluorouracil, work in different ways to stop the growth of tumor cells, either by killing the cells, by stopping them from dividing, or by stopping them from spreading. Giving CPI-613 with fluorouracil may kill more tumor cells.

Detailed Description

PRIMARY OBJECTIVES:

I. To determine the maximum tolerated dose (MTD) of CPI-613 (6,8-bis[benzylthio]octanoic acid), when used in combination with 5-FU (fluorouracil), in patients with non-resectable metastatic colorectal cancer who have failed FOLFOX (leucovorin calcium, fluorouracil and oxaliplatin), FOLFIRI (leucovorin calcium, fluorouracil, and irinotecan hydrochloride) and, if Kirsten rat sarcoma viral oncogene homolog (KRAS) wild type, then a epidermal growth factor receptor (EGFR) inhibitor-based regimen.

SECONDARY OBJECTIVES:

I. To assess the pharmacokinetic (PK), safety and efficacy of various doses of CPI-613, when used in combination with 5-FU, in patients with non-resectable metastatic colorectal cancer.

OUTLINE: This is a dose-escalation study of 6,8-bis(benzylthio)octanoic acid.

Patients receive 6,8-bis(benzylthio)octanoic acid intravenously (IV) over 2 hours on days 1-4 and fluorouracil IV over 46 hours on days 2-4. Courses repeat every 2 weeks for 6 months in the absence of disease progression or unacceptable toxicity.

After completion of study treatment, patients are followed up every 2 months for 3 years.

Study Type

Interventional

Study Phase

Phase 1

- Condition
  - Mucinous Adenocarcinoma of the Colon
  - Mucinous Adenocarcinoma of the Rectum
  - Recurrent Colon Cancer
  - Recurrent Rectal Cancer
  - Signet Ring Adenocarcinoma of the Colon
  - Signet Ring Adenocarcinoma of the Rectum
  - Stage IIIA Colon Cancer
  - Stage IIIA Rectal Cancer
  - Stage IIIB Colon Cancer
  - Stage IIIB Rectal Cancer
  - Stage IIIC Colon Cancer
  - Stage IIIC Rectal Cancer
  - Stage IVA Colon Cancer
  - Stage IVA Rectal Cancer
  - Stage IVB Colon Cancer
  - Stage IVB Rectal Cancer
- Intervention

  Drug: 6,8-bis(benzylthio)octanoic acid
  - Given IV

  Other Names:
  - alpha-lipoic acid analogue CPI-613

  - CPI-613

  - Drug: fluorouracil

  - Given IV

  Other Names:
  - 5-fluorouracil

  - 5-Fluracil

  - 5-FU

  - Other: pharmacological study

  - Correlative studies

  Other Names:
  - pharmacological studies

  - Other: laboratory biomarker analysis

  - Correlative studies

- Study Arms

  Experimental: Treatment (6,8-bis(benzylthio)octanoic acid, fluorouracil)

  Patients receive 6,8-bis(benzylthio)octanoic acid IV over 2 hours on days 1-4 and fluorouracil IV over 46 hours on days 2-4. Courses repeat every 2 weeks for 6 months in the absence of disease progression or unacceptable toxicity.

Recruitment Information

- **Recruitment Status**

  Recruiting

- **Estimated Enrollment**

  40

- **Eligibility Criteria**

  Inclusion Criteria:
  - Histologically and cytologically confirmed metastatic colorectal adenocarcinoma (colon, rectal or colorectal cancer) that is not resectable

- **Completion Date**

  December 2018

- **Primary Completion Date**

  December 2018

- Have failed or have not tolerated FOLFOX, FOLFIRI and, if KRAS wild type, then a EGFR inhibitor-based regimen
- Eastern Cooperative Oncology Group (ECOG) performance status being 0-2
- Women of child-bearing potential (i.e., women who are pre-menopausal or not surgically sterile) must use accepted contraceptive methods (abstinence, intrauterine device [IUD], oral contraceptive or double barrier device) during the study, and must have a negative serum or urine pregnancy test within 1 week prior to treatment initiation
- Fertile men must practice effective contraceptive methods during the study, unless documentation of infertility exists
- At least 2 weeks must have elapsed from any prior surgery
- Granulocyte count >= 1500/mm^3
- White blood cell (WBC) >= 3500 cells/mm^3 or >= 3.5 bil/L
- Platelet count >= 100,000 cells/mm^3 or >= 100 bil/L
- Absolute neutrophil count (ANC) >= 1500 cells/mm^3 or >= 1.5 bil/L
- Hemoglobin >= 9 g/dL or >= 90 g/L
- Aspartate aminotransferase (AST/serum glutamic oxaloacetic transaminase [SGOT]) =< 3 x upper normal limit (UNL), alanine aminotransferase (ALT/serum glutamate pyruvate transaminase [SGPT]) =< 3 x UNL (=< 5 x UNL if liver metastases present)
- Bilirubin =< 1.5 x UNL
- Serum creatinine =< 1.5 mg/dL or 13 umol/L
- International normalized ratio or INR must be =< 1.5 unless on therapeutic blood thinners
- No evidence of active infection and no serious infection within the past month
- Mentally competent, ability to understand and willingness to sign the informed consent form
- At least one measurable lesion as assessed by computed tomography (CT) scan using Response Evaluation Criteria in Solid Tumors (RECIST) criteria

Exclusion Criteria:

- Therapy with CPI-613 prior to participating in this trial
- Known hypersensitivity to 5-FU injection, poor nutritional state, known dipyrimidine dehydrogenase deficiency, or taking sorivudine (such as Usevir, brovavir, etc.)
- History of hypersensitivity to active or inactive excipients of any component of treatment
- Previous radiotherapy for central nervous system metastases
- Patients receiving any other standard or investigational treatment for their cancer, or any other investigational agent for any indication, within the past 2 weeks prior to initiation of treatment with study drugs
- Serious medical illness that would potentially increase patients' risk for toxicity
- Any active uncontrolled bleeding, and any patients with a bleeding diathesis (e.g., active peptic ulcer disease)
- History of abdominal fistula or gastrointestinal perforation =< 6 months prior to treatment with study drugs
- Pregnant women, or women of child-bearing potential not using reliable means of contraception
- Lactating females
- Fertile men unwilling to practice contraceptive methods during the study period
- Any condition or abnormality which may, in the opinion of the investigator, compromise the safety of patients
- Unwilling or unable to follow protocol requirements
- Symptomatic heart disease including but not limited to symptomatic congestive heart failure, symptomatic coronary artery disease, symptomatic angina pectoris, symptomatic myocardial infarction or symptomatic congestive heart failure
- Patients with a history of myocardial infarction that is < 3 months prior to registration
- Evidence of active infection, or serious infection within the past month
- Patients with known human immunodeficiency virus (HIV) infection, hepatitis B, or hepatitis C
- Patients who have received cancer immunotherapy of any type within the past 2 weeks prior to initiation of CPI-613 treatment; steroid use for management of refractory pain or for contrast induced allergy is allowed
- Requirement for immediate palliative treatment of any kind including surgery
- Any condition or abnormality which may, in the opinion of the investigator, compromise the safety of the patient

■ Sex/Gender

All

■ Ages

18 Years to N/A

■ Accepts Healthy Volunteers

No

Phase 1 Study of MGD007 in Relapsed/Refractory Metastatic Colorectal Carcinoma

Study ID:

NCT02248805

Sponsor:

MacroGenics

Information provided by (Responsible Party):

MacroGenics (MacroGenics)

Tracking Information

▥ **First Submitted Date**

September 18, 2014

▥ **Start Date**

September 2014

▥ **Primary Completion Date**

June 2018

▥ **Last Update Posted Date**

January 17, 2018

▥ **Current Primary Outcome Measures**

Characterize dose limiting toxicity and establish a maximum tolerated dose and schedule[Time Frame: Cycle 1 of a 6 week cycle]

Safety is based on evaluation of adverse events (AEs) and serious adverse events (SAEs) from the time of study drug administration through the End of Study visit. The MTD will be defined separately for both the weekly and every three week schedules of MGD007 administration, and will be determined as the highest dose level at which the incidence of DLT is < 33% during the first cycle of MGD007 treatment.

▥ **Current Secondary Outcome Measures**

Characterize the PK and Immunogenicity of MGD007[Time Frame: Beginning of treatment through end of treatment, an expected duration of less than 12 months]

Serum concentrations of MGD007 will be monitored. PK modeling will be performed and an appropriate model will be selected to describe the data.

Describe any evidence of anti-tumor activity[Time Frame: Every 6 weeks until End of Study, an expected duration of less than 12 months]

Obtain regular radiographic and clinical evaluations to assess treatment response.

Descriptive Information

▥ **Offical Title**

A Phase 1, First-in-Human, Open Label, Dose Escalation Study of MGD007, A Humanized gpA33 x CD3 Dual-Affinity Re-Targeting (DART®) Protein in Patients With Relapsed/Refractory Metastatic Colorectal Carcinoma

▥ **Brief Summary**

The primary goal of this Phase 1 study is to characterize the safety and tolerability of MGD007 and establish the maximum tolerated dose (MTD) and schedule of MGD007 administered to patients with metastatic colorectal carcinoma. Pharmacokinetics, pharmacodynamics, and the anti-tumor activity of MGD007 will also be assessed.

▥ **Detailed Description**

This is an open-label, multi-center, Phase 1 dose-escalation study to define a MTD, describe preliminarily safety, and to assess PK, immunogenicity, and potential anti-tumor activity of MGD007 in patients with relapsed or refractory metastatic colorectal cancer.

In the initial phase of the study, two dose schedules will be assessed in dose escalation, once weekly and once every three weeks administration of single agent MGD007. Following the establishment of an MTD, additional patients will enroll in four separate dose expansion cohorts to further optimize the dose and schedule of MGD007 administration.

In all segments of the study, patients who benefit from MGD007 treatment and continue to meet eligibility may continue treatment in Cycles 2 and beyond.

▥ **Study Type**

Interventional

▥ **Study Phase**

Phase 1

▥ **Condition**

- Colorectal Carcinoma

Intervention

Drug: MGD007

MGD007 is a gpA33 x CD3 bi-specific antibody-based molecular construct referred to as a DART molecule. MGD007 will be administered as a single agent.

Study Arms

Experimental: Does Escalation Arm A
MGD007 treatment once weekly

Experimental: Dose Escalation Arm B
MGD007 treatment once every 3 weeks

Experimental: Dose Expansion Arm C
MGD007 once every 3 weeks for K-ras wild-type and mutant metastatic CRC

Experimental: Dose Expansion Arms
MGD007 2, 3, 6, or 12 doses/cycle

Recruitment Information

Recruitment Status

Recruiting

Estimated Enrollment

103

Completion Date

March 2019

Primary Completion Date

June 2018

Eligibility Criteria

Inclusion Criteria:

- For the dose escalation cohorts, histologically-proven metastatic colorectal adenocarcinoma that is refractory to 2 prior standard treatment regimens or standard treatment was declined.
- For the dose expansion cohorts, histologically-proven metastatic colorectal adenocarcinoma that is refractory to 1 prior standard treatment regimen or standard therapy was declined.
- Eastern Cooperative Oncology Group (ECOG) performance status of 0 or 1
- Life expectancy of at least 12 weeks
- Measurable disease
- Intolerance to at least 2 prior standard therapy regimens
- Acceptable laboratory parameters
- Adult (≥18 years old)

Exclusion Criteria:

- Known brain metastasis
- Any prior history of or suspected current autoimmune disorders (with the exception of vitiligo, resolved childhood atopic dermatitis, prior Grave's disease)
- Prior history of allogeneic bone marrow, stem-cell, or solid organ transplantation
- Prior treatment with checkpoint inhibitors and other immunotherapy treatments, including anti-LAG-3, anti-PD-1, anti-PD-L1 or anti-CTLA-4 antibodies, if less than 5 half lives before study drug administration
- Prior history of Grade 3 or greater drug-related diarrhea/colitis during treatment with checkpoint inhibitors or other immunotherapy treatments.
- Treatment with any local or systemic anti-neoplastic therapy or any other investigational agent in the 4 weeks prior to study drug administration
- Require, at the time of study entry, treatment with steroids > 10 mg/day of oral prednisone (or equivalent), except topical use, steroid inhaler, nasal spray or ophthalmic solution
- History of clinically significant cardiovascular disease, gastrointestinal disorder, or significant pulmonary compromise.
- Second primary malignancy that has not been in remission for greater than 3 years, with the exception of non-melanoma skin cancer, cervical carcinoma in situ,or squamous intraepithelial lesion on PAP smear, localized prostate cancer (Gleason score <6), or resected melanoma in situ.

Sex/Gender

All

Ages

18 Years to N/A

■ **Accepts Healthy Volunteers**

No

■ **Contacts**

Joanna Lohr   240-552-8030   lohrj@macrogenics.com
Susan Brann   240-552-8023   branns@macrogenics.com

Role of Omalizumab in Reducing the Incidence of Oxaliplatin-induced Hypersensitivity Reaction

Study ID:

NCT02266355

Sponsor:

Yale University

Information provided by (Responsible Party):

Yale University (Yale University)

Tracking Information

■ **First Submitted Date**

October 10, 2014

■ **Start Date**

November 2014

■ **Current Primary Outcome Measures**

Incidence of Recurrent HSR[Time Frame: up to 12 months]
   Recurrent Oxaliplatin HSR in subjects treated with omalizumab

■ **Current Secondary Outcome Measures**

Safety of Omalizumab[Time Frame: up to 12 months]

   Evaluate the safety of omalizumab by assessment of frequency of adverse events and serious adverse events as categorized by CTCAE version 4

■ **Primary Completion Date**

December 2017

■ **Last Update Posted Date**

November 8, 2017

Descriptive Information

■ **Offical Title**

A Pilot Study of the Role of Omalizumab (Xolair) in Reducing the Incidence of Oxaliplatin-induced Hypersensitivity Reaction (HSR)

■ **Brief Summary**

Pilot study to evaluate the activity of omalizumab in the prevention of recurrent oxaliplatin hypersensitivity reaction (HSR) in oxaliplatin-sensitive patients. The study will also evaluate the safety of omalizumab (Xolair) when administered in this setting.

■ **Detailed Description**

This is an open label single arm pilot study studying the effects of omalizumab in the treatment of oxaliplatin hypersensitivity reaction (HSR) for patients with stage IV GI cancer.

■ **Study Type**

Interventional

■ **Study Phase**

Phase 1

■ **Condition**

• Colon Cancer

■ **Intervention**

Drug: Omalizumab

Omalizumab 300 mg SQ every 2 weeks

Other Names:
  Xolair

- ## Study Arms

  Experimental: OmalizumabTreatment Group
    Omalizumab (Xolair) 300 mg SQ every 2 weeks

Recruitment Information

- ## Recruitment Status

  Recruiting

- ## Estimated Enrollment

  12

- ## Completion Date

  March 2018

- ## Primary Completion Date

  December 2017

- ## Eligibility Criteria

  Inclusion Criteria:

  - Clinically evident HSR to oxaliplatin, with symptoms of flushing, urticaria, pruritus, rash, and/or dyspnea without bronchospasm that emerge during or shortly after of oxaliplatin infusion
  - Responding (complete or partial) or stable disease according to RECIST criteria while undergoing treatment with oxaliplatin containing regimen or need to resume an oxaliplatin based regimen in the setting of well-documented recent oxaliplatin hypersensitivity reaction
  - Histologically confirmed stage IV GI cancer (AJCC 7th edition) currently sensitive to oxaliplatin containing chemotherapy regimen
  - Age 18 years or older
  - ECOG performance status 0-2
  - Adequate bone marrow, liver, and kidney function. (WBC > 1500 cells/uL, platelets > 50,000/uL, ALT/AST < 5xULN (unless due to liver metastasis), Creatinine < 2.0 mg/ld)
  - Willing to give written informed consent, adhere to the visit schedules and meet study requirements

  Exclusion Criteria:

  - Prior history of severe reactions to oxaliplatin as characterized by the presence of hemodynamic instability, significant respiratory symptoms or potential airway compromise
  - History of hypersensitivity reaction to Xolair or any ingredient of Xolair
  - Concurrent therapy with investigational agents
  - Use of any other investigational agent in the last 15 days and all toxicity of prior therapy resolved
  - Psychological, familial, or sociological condition potentially hampering compliance with the study protocol and follow-up schedule
  - Women of childbearing potential not using the contraception method(s), as well as women who are breastfeeding
  - Patients with severe medical conditions that in the view of the investigator prohibits participation in the study

- ## Sex/Gender

  All

- ## Ages

  18 Years to N/A

- ## Accepts Healthy Volunteers

  No

- ## Contacts

  Howard Hochster, MD   203-785-5756   howard.hochster@yale.edu
  Howard S Hochster, MD   203-785-5756   howard.hochster@yale.edu

Irinotecan and Cetuximab With or Without Bevacizumab in Treating Patients With RAS Wild-Type Locally Advanced or Metastatic Colorectal Cancer That Cannot Be Removed by Surgery

Study ID:

NCT02292758

Sponsor:

Academic and Community Cancer Research United

Information provided by (Responsible Party):

Academic and Community Cancer Research United (Academic and Community Cancer Research United)

Tracking Information

▨ **First Submitted Date**

November 13, 2014

▨ **Start Date**

December 12, 2014

▨ **Primary Completion Date**

June 1, 2019

▨ **Last Update Posted Date**

November 17, 2017

▨ **Current Primary Outcome Measures**

Progression-free survival (PFS)[Time Frame: From the date of randomization to the date of 1st documented disease progression or death due to any cause, whichever occurs first, assessed up to 12 months]

The distribution of PFS by group will be estimated using the method of Kaplan-Meier. Six and 12 month PFS rates by treatment group with confidence intervals will be estimated based on Kaplan-Meier curves. The hazard ratio (HR) with confidence interval will be estimated based on stratified Cox models (stratified by levels of stratification factors), without and with adjusting for baseline clinical/pathological factors.

▨ **Current Secondary Outcome Measures**

Disease control rate (DCR) maintaining complete response (CR) or partial response (PR) or stable disease[Time Frame: Up to 3 years]

Will be compared between two treatment groups using Chi-square test (or Fisher?s exact test if the data in the contingency table is sparse). Logistic regression models will be used to estimate the odds ratio (OR) and confidence interval without and with adjusting for baseline clinical/pathological factors.

Duration of response (DOR)[Time Frame: From the date of first tumor assessment with the response status being CR or PR to the date of 1st documented progressive disease, assessed up to 12 months]

The distribution of DOR by treatment group will be estimated using the method of Kaplan-Meier. Six and 12 month durable response (i.e. maintaining CR or PR without progressive disease [PD]) rates by treatment group with confidence intervals will be estimated based on Kaplan-Meier curves. The HR with confidence interval will be estimated based on stratified Cox models (stratified by levels of stratification factors), without and with adjusting for baseline clinical/pathological factors.

Incidence of adverse events assessed by National Cancer Institute Common Terminology Criteria for Adverse Events version 4.0[Time Frame: Up to 30 days from last dose of study treatment]

The maximum grade of each adverse event and its attribution will be recorded for each patient. The frequency tables will be reviewed to evaluate for patterns of toxicity. The overall adverse event rates for grade 3 or higher adverse events will be compared between the two treatment groups using Chi-square test (or Fisher?s exact test if the data in the contingency table is sparse).

Overall response rate (ORR) defined as achieving complete response (CR) or partial response (PR)[Time Frame: Up to 3 years]

Will be compared between the two treatment groups using Chi-square test (or Fisher?s exact test if the data in the contingency table is sparse). Logistic regression models will be used to estimate the odds ratio (OR) and confidence interval without and with adjusting for baseline clinical/pathological factors.

Overall survival (OS)[Time Frame: From randomization to the date of death due to any cause, assessed up to 24 months]

The distribution of OS by group will be estimated using the method of Kaplan-Meier. Twelve, 18and 24-month survival rates by treatment group with confidence intervals will be estimated based on Kaplan-Meier curves. The HR with confidence interval will be estimated based on stratified Cox models (stratified by levels of stratification factors), without and with adjusting for baseline clinical/pathological factors.

Relative dose intensity (RDI)[Time Frame: Up to 3 years]

Separate RDIs will be calculated for irinotecan and cetuximab. Agent-specific RDI will be summarized by means, 25th percentiles, medians, 75th percentiles, and min and max values, all of which will be compared between the two treatment groups by the Wilcoxon Rank sum test.

Time to treatment failure (TTF)[Time Frame: Time from the date of randomization to the date of treatment discontinuation due to PD, death, or severe AE, assessed at 6 months]

The distribution of TTF by treatment group will be estimated using the method of Kaplan-Meier. Six month event-free rates by treatment group with confidence intervals will be estimated based on Kaplan-Meier curves. The HR with confidence interval will be estimated based on stratified Cox models (stratified by levels of stratification factors), without and with adjusting for baseline clinical/pathological factors.

Descriptive Information

▨ Offical Title

BOND-3: A Randomized, Double-Blind, Placebo-Controlled Phase II Trial of Irinotecan, Cetuximab, and Bevacizumab Compared With Irinotecan, Cetuximab, and Placebo in RAS-Wildtype, Irinotecan-Refractory, Metastatic Colorectal Cancer

▨ Brief Summary

This randomized phase II trial studies how well irinotecan and cetuximab with or without bevacizumab work in treating patients with RAS wild-type colorectal cancer that has spread to other places in the body and cannot be removed by surgery. Irinotecan may stop the growth of tumor cells by blocking some of the enzymes needed for cell growth. Monoclonal antibodies, such as cetuximab and bevacizumab, may interfere with the ability of tumor cells to grow and spread. Giving irinotecan and cetuximab with or without bevacizumab may work betting in treating patients with colorectal cancer.

▨ Detailed Description

PRIMARY OBJECTIVES:

I. To assess and compare the progression-free survival (PFS) of patients receiving irinotecan, cetuximab, and bevacizumab with patients receiving irinotecan, cetuximab and placebo, in the population of patients with RAS wild-type, irinotecan-refractory metastatic colorectal cancer (mCRC) who also previously received bevacizumab in at least one prior line therapy.

SECONDARY OBJECTIVES:

I. To assess the adverse event (AE) profile and safety of the proposed treatment in this population.

II. To assess and compare the overall survival (OS) between treatment arms in this population.

III. To assess and compare the disease control rate (DCR) between treatment arms in this population.

IV. To assess and compare the overall response rate (ORR) between treatment arms in this population.

V. To assess and compare the duration of response between treatment arms in this population.

VI. To assess and compare time to treatment failure between treatment arms in this population.

VII. To assess relative dose intensity of treatment agents between treatment arms in this population.

TERTIARY OBJECTIVES:

I. Determine the change in genotype concentrations of prespecified gene mutations in circulating cell-free deoxyribonucleic acid (DNA) (cfDNA) collected serially during protocol treatment.

II. Explore the predictive value of pretreatment mutation status, germline single nucleotide polymorphisms (SNPs), and gene expression signatures for cetuximab sensitivity and resistance.

III. Explore the predictive value of dynamic changes in mutation status and gene expression signatures for cetuximab sensitivity and resistance.

OUTLINE: Patients are randomized to 1 of 2 arms.

ARM I: Patients receive cetuximab intravenously (IV) over 90-120 minutes, bevacizumab IV over 30-90 minutes, and irinotecan IV over 90 minutes on day 1. Courses repeat every 14 days in the absence of disease progression or unacceptable toxicity.

ARM II: Patients receive cetuximab IV over 90-120 minutes, placebo IV over 30-90 minutes, and irinotecan IV over 90 minutes on day 1. Courses repeat every 14 days in the absence of disease progression or unacceptable toxicity.

After completion of study treatment, patients are followed up for up to 3 years.

▨ Study Type

Interventional

▨ Study Phase

Phase 2

▨ Condition

- Colorectal Adenocarcinoma
- RAS Wild Type
- Stage IV Colorectal Cancer AJCC v7
- Stage IVA Colorectal Cancer AJCC v7
- Stage IVB Colorectal Cancer AJCC v7

▨ Intervention

Biological: Bevacizumab
  Given IV
Other Names:
  Anti-VEGF

  Anti-VEGF Humanized Monoclonal Antibody

  Anti-VEGF rhuMAb

  Avastin

  Bevacizumab Biosimilar BEVZ92

  Bevacizumab Biosimilar BI 695502

  Bevacizumab Biosimilar CBT 124

  Bevacizumab Biosimilar FKB238

  Immunoglobulin G1 (Human-Mouse Monoclonal rhuMab-VEGF Gamma-Chain Anti-Human Vascular Endothelial Growth Factor), Disulfide With Human-Mouse Monoclonal rhuMab-VEGF Light Chain, Dimer

  Recombinant Humanized Anti-VEGF Monoclonal Antibody

  rhuMab-VEGF
Biological: Cetuximab
  Given IV
Other Names:
  Chimeric Anti-EGFR Monoclonal Antibody

  Chimeric MoAb C225

  Chimeric Monoclonal Antibody C225

  Erbitux

  IMC-C225
Drug: Irinotecan
  Given IV
Other: Laboratory Biomarker Analysis
  Correlative studies
Other: Placebo
  Given IV
Other Names:
  placebo therapy

  PLCB

  sham therapy

- Study Arms

Experimental: Arm I (cetuximab, bevacizumab, irinotecan)
  Patients receive cetuximab IV over 90-120 minutes, bevacizumab IV over 30-90 minutes, and irinotecan IV over 90 minutes on day 1. Courses repeat every 14 days in the absence of disease progression or unacceptable toxicity.

Active Comparator: Arm II (cetuximab, placebo, irinotecan)
  Patients receive cetuximab IV over 90-120 minutes, placebo IV over 30-90 minutes, and irinotecan IV over 90 minutes on day 1. Courses repeat every 14 days in the absence of disease progression or unacceptable toxicity.

Recruitment Information

- Recruitment Status
  Recruiting
- Estimated Enrollment
  60
- Eligibility Criteria

- Completion Date
  December 1, 2021
- Primary Completion Date
  June 1, 2019

Inclusion Criteria:

- Metastatic or locally advanced (unresectable) colorectal cancer with histological confirmation of adenocarcinoma
- Measurable disease
- RAS wild-type tumor; Note: evidence of EGFR expression in the tumor is not required
- Previous failure of at least one fluoropyrimidineand irinotecan-containing chemotherapy regimen for metastatic disease; Note: previous failure is defined as disease progression while receiving treatment or within 6 weeks after the last dose of irinotecan; failure for this assessment is defined as any enlargement of measurable or assessable lesion(s) or the development of any new lesion; a rising tumor marker alone is not sufficient to define failure; patients can have received irinotecan in any previous line of therapy
- Treatment with bevacizumab in at least one prior line of therapy for metastatic disease
- Negative serum or urine pregnancy test done =< 7 days prior to registration, for women of childbearing potential only
- Eastern Cooperative Oncology Group (ECOG) performance status (PS): 0 or 1
- Total serum bilirubin =< institutional upper limit of normal (ULN) obtained =<14 days prior to randomization
- Absolute neutrophil count (ANC) >= 1500/mm^3 obtained =<14 days prior to randomization
- Platelet count >= 100,000/mm^3 obtained =<14 days prior to randomization
- Hemoglobin >= 9.0 g/dL (hemoglobin may be supported by transfusion) obtained =<14 days prior to randomization
- Alanine aminotransferase (ALT) and aspartate aminotransferase (AST) =< 2.5 x ULN (=< 5 x ULN for subjects with liver involvement of their cancer) obtained =<14 days prior to randomization
- Creatinine within institutional limits of normal OR creatinine clearance >= 60 mL/min/1.73 m^2 for patients with creatinine levels above institutional normal obtained =<14 days prior to randomization
- Urinary protein =< 1+ obtained =<14 days prior to randomization
- Patients discovered to have >= 2+ proteinuria must have a spot urine protein:creatinine ratio (UPCR) < 1.0
- **Partial thromboplastin time (PTT) =< 1 x institutional ULN and international normalized ratio (INR) =< 1.5 , unless participant is on full dose anticoagulation therapy obtained =<14 days prior to randomization; patients on full-dose anticoagulation are eligible if the following criteria are met:**
- Patient has an in-range INR (usually 2-3) on a stable dose of warfarin or other anticoagulant =< 14 days or is on a stable dose of low molecular weight heparin
- Patient has no active bleeding or pathological condition that carries a high risk of bleeding (i.e., tumor involving major vessels or known varices)
- Patients receiving anti-platelet agents are eligible; in addition, patients who are on daily prophylactic aspirin or anticoagulation for atrial fibrillation are eligible
- Life expectancy > 3 months
- Provide informed written consent
- Willing to provide blood samples for mandatory correlative and research purposes
- Willing to provide tissue and blood samples for mandatory banking purposes
- Any major surgery or open biopsy completed >= 4 weeks prior to randomization
- Any minor surgery or core biopsy completed >= 1 week prior to randomization and patient must have fully recovered from the procedure; Note: insertion of a vascular access device is not considered major or minor surgery

Exclusion Criteria:

- Presence of a RAS mutation in exons 2, 3, or 4 of KRAS or NRAS (patients with mutations in exons 2, 3, or 4 of KRAS and/or NRAS are excluded)
- Prior treatment with cetuximab or panitumumab
- Prior intolerance to irinotecan and/or bevacizumab despite dose reduction
- Known or suspected brain or central nervous system (CNS) metastases, or carcinomatous meningitis
- Active, uncontrolled infection, including hepatitis B, hepatitis C
- Concurrent anti-cancer therapy, including chemotherapy agents, targeted agents, or biological agents not otherwise specified in this protocol
- Anti-cancer therapy =< 14 days prior to randomization
- Prior radiotherapy to > 25% of bone marrow; Note: standard rectal cancer chemoradiation will not exclude subject from study protocol
- Radiation therapy =< 2 weeks prior to randomization
- **Any of the following:**
- Pregnant women
- Nursing women
- Men or women of childbearing potential who are unwilling to employ adequate contraception
- Co-morbid systemic illnesses or other severe concurrent disease, history of any psychiatric or addictive disorder, or laboratory abnormality, which, in the judgment of the investigator, would make the patient inappropriate for entry into this study or interfere significantly with the proper assessment of safety and toxicity of the prescribed regimens

- Patients known to be human immunodeficiency virus (HIV) positive
- Uncontrolled intercurrent illness including, but not limited to, ongoing or active infection, symptomatic congestive heart failure, unstable angina pectoris, cardiac arrhythmia, symptomatic pulmonary fibrosis or interstitial pneumonitis, or psychiatric illness/social situations that, in the opinion of the investigator, may increase the risks associated with study participation or study treatment, or may interfere with the conduct of the study or the interpretation of the study results
- Receiving any other investigational agent which would be considered as a treatment for the primary neoplasm
- Other active malignancy =< 3 years prior to registration; EXCEPTIONS: non-melanoma skin cancer, prostatic intraepithelial neoplasia without evidence of prostate cancer, lobular carcinoma in situ in one breast, or carcinoma-in-situ of the cervix that has been treated
- History of prior malignancy for which patient is receiving other specific treatment for their cancer
- History of allergic reactions attributed to compounds of similar chemical or biologic composition to irinotecan, cetuximab, and/or bevacizumab that led to discontinuation of those agents
- Significant history of bleeding events or pre-existing bleeding diathesis =< 6 months of randomization (unless the source of bleeding has been resected)
- History of gastrointestinal perforation =< 12 months prior to randomization
- Predisposing colonic or small bowel disorders in which the symptoms are uncontrolled as indicated by baseline pattern of > 3 loose stools daily in subjects without a colostomy or ileostomy; subjects with a colostomy or ileostomy may be entered at investigator discretion
- Arterial thrombotic events =< 6 months prior to randomization; Note: this includes transient ischemic attack (TIA), cerebrovascular accident (CVA), unstable angina or angina requiring surgical or medical intervention in the past 6 months, or myocardial infarction (MI)
- Clinically significant peripheral artery disease (e.g., claudication with < 1 block) or any other arterial thrombotic event
- Serious or non-healing wound, ulcer, or bone fracture
- History of hypertension not well-controlled (>= 160/90) even though on a regimen of anti-hypertensive therapy
- Evidence of Gilbert?s syndrome or known homozygosity for the UGT1A1

28 allele (special screening not required)

- ▤ **Sex/Gender**

  All

- ▤ **Ages**

  18 Years to N/A

- ▤ **Accepts Healthy Volunteers**

  No

Copper Cu 64 Anti-CEA Monoclonal Antibody M5A PET in Diagnosing Patients With CEA Positive Cancer

Study ID:

NCT02293954

Sponsor:

City of Hope Medical Center

Information provided by (Responsible Party):

City of Hope Medical Center (City of Hope Medical Center)

Tracking Information

- ▤ **First Submitted Date**

  October 9, 2014

- ▤ **Start Date**

  June 8, 2015

- ▤ **Primary Completion Date**

  June 2018

- ▤ **Last Update Posted Date**

  October 31, 2017

- ▤ **Current Primary Outcome Measures**

  Efficacy of each modality in locating cancer in each of four regions (primary, hepatic, extra-hepatic abdominal, and extra-abdominal) using lesion analysis[Time Frame: Up to day 2]

  For lesion analysis, the efficacy of each modality will be evaluated where a successful outcome will be defined as the ability of at least one known tumor identified by conventional imaging modalities to be imaged using the M5A antibody. Using the standard statistical formulas, the number of true positives, false positives, true negatives, and false negatives, as well as the sensitivity and corresponding 95% confidence interval will be estimated using the method of Lee and Dubin or Rao and Scott, which accounts for the correlation between lesions within in same subject.

Efficacy of each modality in locating cancer in each of four regions (primary, hepatic, extra-hepatic abdominal, and extra-abdominal) using region analysis[Time Frame: Up to day 2]

For region analysis, a successful outcome will be defined as the identification of suspicious tissue within a region. Using the standard statistical formulas, the number of true positives, false positives, true negatives, and false negatives, as well as the sensitivity and corresponding 95% confidence interval will be estimated using the method of Lee and Dubin or Rao and Scott, which accounts for the correlation between lesions within in same subject.

Pharmacokinetic parameters of copper Cu 64 anti-CEA monoclonal antibody M5A[Time Frame: Pre-dose, 30 minutes, and 1, 2, and 3-4 hours post start of infusion]

Blood samples will be drawn at various time points to construct the blood activity curve. Urine data will also be included in our analyses to check the whole body clearance curves. A computer pharmacokinetic model containing 5 compartments including blood, liver, residual body, urine and feces will be used to analyze time activity data. Residence times for various organs will be calculated from this pharmacokinetic model and/or uptake data. Different residence times for different isotopes, e.g. 64Cu, will be calculated by adjusting for physical decay. These times are then substituted into the OLINDA program.

Immunogenicity properties of copper Cu 64 anti-CEA monoclonal antibody M5A[Time Frame: Up to 3 months]

The patient's serum samples are evaluated in both a bridging radioimmunoassay and an HPLC assay. The sera are incubated with the appropriate radiolabeled M5A and then analyzed by HPLC size exclusion chromatography on a Superose 6 HR column.

Current Secondary Outcome Measures

Incidence of adverse events graded using the National Cancer Institute Common Terminology Criteria for Adverse Events version 4.03[Time Frame: Up to 3 months]

Safety data will be displayed and abnormal laboratory values flagged. The frequency of adverse events will be tabulated by body system.

Descriptive Information

Offical Title

Pilot Study: Detection of Carcinomas Using 64Cu-Labeled M5A Antibody to Carcinoembryonic Antigen (CEA)

Brief Summary

This pilot clinical trial studies copper Cu 64 anti-carcinoembryonic antigen (CEA) monoclonal antibody M5A positron emission tomography (PET) in diagnosing patients with CEA positive cancer. Diagnostic procedures, such as copper Cu 64 anti-CEA monoclonal antibody M5A PET, may help find and diagnose CEA positive cancer that may not be detected by standard diagnostic methods.

Detailed Description

PRIMARY OBJECTIVES:

I. To determine the ability of 64Cu labeled M5A antibody (copper Cu 64 anti-CEA monoclonal antibody M5A) to localize CEA positive cancers (such as gastrointestinal, lung, medullary thyroid and breast cancers), as determined by PET imaging.

SECONDARY OBJECTIVES:

I. To characterize the frequency of titer of the human anti-human antibody (HAHA) response to 64Cu labeled M5A antibody.

II. To determine the safety of administration of 64Cu labeled M5A antibody.

OUTLINE:

Patients receive copper Cu 64 anti-CEA monoclonal antibody M5A intravenously (IV) on day 0 and then undergo PET on day 1 and day 2.

After completion of study, patients are followed up at 1 and 3 months.

Study Type

Interventional

Study Phase

N/A

Condition

- Breast Cancer
- Colon Cancer
- Extrahepatic Bile Duct Cancer
- Gallbladder Cancer

- Gastrointestinal Cancer
- Liver and Intrahepatic Biliary Tract Cancer
- Lung Cancer
- Metastatic Cancer
- Pancreatic Cancer
- Rectal Cancer
- Thyroid Gland Medullary Carcinoma
- Unspecified Adult Solid Tumor, Protocol Specific

Intervention

Procedure: radionuclide imaging
  Given copper Cu 64 anti-CEA monoclonal antibody M5A IV

Other Names:
  radionuclide scanning

  Procedure: positron emission tomography

  Undergo PET

Other Names:
  FDG-PET

  PET

  PET scan

  tomography, emission computed

  Other: laboratory biomarker analysis

  Correlative studies

Other: pharmacological study
  Correlative studies

Other Names:
  pharmacological studies

Drug: Cu 64 anti-CEA monoclonal antibody M5A IV
  Cu 64 anti-CEA monoclonal antibody M5A IV

Study Arms

Experimental: Diagnostic (copper Cu 64 anti-CEA monoclonal antibody M5A PET)
  Patients receive copper Cu 64 anti-CEA monoclonal antibody M5A IV on day 0 and then undergo PET on day 1 and day 2.

Recruitment Information

Recruitment Status
Recruiting

Estimated Enrollment
20

Completion Date
June 2018

Primary Completion Date
June 2018

Eligibility Criteria

Inclusion Criteria:
- Patients must have histologically confirmed primary or metastatic cancer; if biopsies were performed at an outside facility, the histology must be reviewed and confirmed by the Department of Pathology at the City of Hope
- Patients must have tumors that produce CEA as documented by a current or past history of an elevated serum CEA above the institutional limit of normal; NOTE: Patients with colorectal cancer are exempt from this requirement since > 95% are CEA positive
- Women of child-bearing potential and men must agree to use adequate contraception (hormonal or barrier method of birth control or abstinence) prior to study entry and for six months following duration of study participation; should a woman become pregnant or suspect that she is pregnant while participating on the trial, she should inform her treating physician immediately
- Patients must have a known site of disease; please note, for patients undergoing neoadjuvant therapy, this requirement must be met retrospectively prior to the start of neoadjuvant therapy; patients who are in radiological/clinical remission after neoadjuvant therapy, prior to infusion of radiolabeled antibody, are still eligible

- Although not mandated by the protocol, the results of the CT scan and labs (complete blood count [CBC], comprehensive metabolic panel [CMP]) that are performed as part of the standard work up should be available and should have been done within 2 months prior to study entry
- All subjects must have the ability to understand and the willingness to sign a written informed consent
- Prior therapy (chemotherapy, immunotherapy, radiotherapy) must be completed at least 2 weeks prior to infusion of radiolabeled antibody

Exclusion Criteria:

- Patients should not have any uncontrolled illness including ongoing or active infection
- History of allergic reactions attributed to compounds of similar chemical or biologic composition to copper Cu 64 anti-CEA monoclonal antibody M5A (64Cu-M5A)
- Patients must not have received prior chemotherapy or radiation for >= 2 weeks before study enrollment
- Pregnant women are excluded from this study; breastfeeding should be discontinued is the mother is treated with 54Cu-m5A
- Any patient who has had exposure to mouse or chimeric (human/mouse) immunoglobulin and has antibody to the M5A
- Subjects, who in the opinion of the investigator, may not be able to comply with the safety monitoring requirements of the study

Sex/Gender

All

Ages

18 Years to N/A

Accepts Healthy Volunteers

No

Pembrolizumab and Ziv-aflibercept in Treating Patients With Advanced Solid Tumors

Study ID:

NCT02298959

Sponsor:

National Cancer Institute (NCI)

Information provided by (Responsible Party):

National Cancer Institute (NCI) (National Cancer Institute (NCI))

Tracking Information

First Submitted Date

November 21, 2014

Start Date

March 13, 2015

Primary Completion Date

December 31, 2018

Last Update Posted Date

December 12, 2017

Current Primary Outcome Measures

Recommended combination dose of ziv-aflibercept and pembrolizumab, assessed by dose-limiting toxicities[Time Frame: 4 weeks]

Safety will be evaluated for all treated patients using the National Cancer Institute Common Terminology Criteria for Adverse Events version 4.0. All adverse events recorded during the trial will be summarized and presented by dose level. For patients enrolled in the dose expansion phase of the trial, adverse events summaries will also be summarized according to disease cohort. The proportion of patients with grade-3 or higher adverse events will be presented with 90% exact binomial confidence interval.

Current Secondary Outcome Measures

Objective response rate (ORR)[Time Frame: Between the date of first dose of trial therapy and the date of objectively documented disease progression or cessation of trial therapy, whichever occurs first, assessed up to 12 weeks]

The ORR will be the proportion of patients achieving complete or partial response as their best response to therapy. The analysis will be descriptive and will be used to assess for early indications of efficacy. Will be summarized by disease type and in the aggregate, if appropriate. ORR will be estimated and will be summarized with 90% confidence intervals estimated using exact binomial methods.

Overall survival[Time Frame: Time from start of trial treatment to death from any cause, assessed up to 12 months]

> The analysis will be descriptive and will be used to assess for early indications of efficacy. Will be summarized by disease type and in the aggregate, if appropriate. Will be summarized using the product-limit method of Kaplan-Meier; 90% confidence intervals will be based on log(-log[outcome]) methodology.

Progression-free survival[Time Frame: Time from start of trial treatment until objective disease progression (per RECIST) or death, whichever occurs first, assessed up to 6 months]

> The analysis will be descriptive and will be used to assess for early indications of efficacy. Will be summarized by disease type and in the aggregate, if appropriate. Will be summarized using the product-limit method of Kaplan-Meier; 90% confidence intervals will be based on log(-log[outcome]) methodology.

Time-to-progression[Time Frame: Time interval between the dates of the start of trial treatment and first documentation of progressive disease, assessed up to 12 weeks]

> The analysis will be descriptive and will be used to assess for early indications of efficacy. Will be summarized by disease type and in the aggregate, if appropriate. Will be summarized using the product-limit method of Kaplan-Meier; 90% confidence intervals will be based on log(-log[outcome]) methodology.

Descriptive Information

▥ Offical Title

A Phase 1 Trial of MK-3475 Plus Ziv-Aflibercept in Patients With Advanced Solid Tumors

▥ Brief Summary

This phase I trial studies the side effects and best dose of ziv-aflibercept when given together with pembrolizumab in treating patients with solid tumors that have spread to other places in the body. Ziv-afibercept works by decreasing blood and nutrient supply to the tumor, which may result in shrinking the tumor. Monoclonal antibodies, such as pembrolizumab, may block tumor growth in different ways by targeting certain cells. Giving ziv-aflibercept together with pembrolizumab may be a better treatment for patients with advanced solid tumors.

▥ Detailed Description

PRIMARY OBJECTIVES:

I. To determine the safety, tolerability and recommended phase II dosing for the combination of ziv-aflibercept plus MK-3475 (pembrolizumab) in patients with unresectable stage III or stage IV melanoma, renal cell cancer, ovarian cancer, or colorectal cancer.

SECONDARY OBJECTIVES:

I. To obtain preliminary estimates of progression-free survival at 6 months. II. To obtain preliminary estimates of the rate of 1-year overall survival. III. To obtain preliminary estimates of the response rate. IV. To obtain preliminary estimates of time to progression. V. To perform a pilot assessment of positron emission tomography (PET) response versus Response Evaluation Criteria in Solid Tumors (RECIST) versus immune-related response criteria (irRC) criteria.

VI. To perform correlative sciences that provide information regarding the mechanisms of action for this combination treatment.

OUTLINE: This is a dose-escalation study of ziv-aflibercept.

Patients receive pembrolizumab intravenously (IV) over approximately 30 minutes and ziv-aflibercept IV over 1-2 hours on day 1. Courses repeat every 2 weeks for up to 2 years in the absence of disease progression or unacceptable toxicity.

After completion of study treatment, patients are followed up for at least 12 weeks.

▥ Study Type

Interventional

▥ Study Phase

Phase 1

▥ Condition

- Adult Solid Neoplasm
- Metastatic Melanoma
- Metastatic Renal Cell Cancer
- Recurrent Colorectal Carcinoma
- Recurrent Melanoma
- Recurrent Ovarian Carcinoma
- Recurrent Renal Cell Carcinoma
- Stage IV Ovarian Cancer AJCC v6 and v7
- Stage IVA Colorectal Cancer AJCC v7
- Stage IVB Colorectal Cancer AJCC v7

Intervention

Other: Laboratory Biomarker Analysis

Correlative studies

Biological: Pembrolizumab

Given IV

Other Names:

Keytruda

Lambrolizumab

MK-3475

SCH 900475

Biological: Ziv-Aflibercept

Given IV

Other Names:

AFLIBERCEPT

AVE0005

Eylea

vascular endothelial growth factor trap

VEGF Trap

VEGF Trap R1R2

VEGF-Trap

Zaltrap

Study Arms

Experimental: Treatment (pembrolizumab and ziv-aflibercept)

Patients receive pembrolizumab IV over approximately 30 minutes and ziv-aflibercept IV over 1-2 hours on day 1. Courses repeat every 2 weeks for up to 2 years in the absence of disease progression or unacceptable toxicity.

Recruitment Information

Recruitment Status

Recruiting

Estimated Enrollment

36

Completion Date

N/A

Primary Completion Date

December 31, 2018

Eligibility Criteria

Inclusion Criteria:

- In dose escalation, patients must have histologically or cytologically confirmed metastatic disease from any solid tumor; in dose expansion, patients must have histologically or cytologically confirmed metastatic melanoma, renal cell carcinoma, ovarian cancer, or colorectal cancer
- Renal cell patients must have had at least one prior vascular endothelial growth factor (VEGF) tyrosine kinase inhibitor (TKI)
- Ovarian cancer patients must be resistant to platinum therapy; therapy (i.e. within 6 months of last platinum therapy); patients who received greater than two prior platinum containing regimens will not be eligible
- Patients with colorectal cancer should have failed at least one oxaliplatin-containing regimen
- No more than two prior therapies for metastatic disease
- Eastern Cooperative Oncology Group (ECOG) performance status =< 1 (Karnofsky >= 70%)
- Estimated life expectancy of greater than 6 months
- Leukocytes >= 2,000/mcL
- Absolute neutrophil count >= 1,500/mcL
- Platelets >= 100,000/mcL
- Hemoglobin >= 9 g/dL OR >= 5.6 mmol/L
- Serum total bilirubin =< 1.5 X upper limit of normal (ULN) or direct bilirubin =< ULN for patients with total bilirubin levels > 1.5 ULN

- Aspartate aminotransferase (AST)(serum glutamic oxaloacetic transaminase [SGOT])/alanine aminotransferase (ALT)(serum glutamate pyruvate transaminase [SGPT]) =< 2.5 × institutional ULN OR =< 5 X ULN for patients with liver metastases
- Serum creatinine =< 1.5 X ULN or measured or calculated creatinine clearance (CrCl) >= 60 mL/min for subject with creatinine levels > 1.5 X institutional ULN (glomerular filtration rate [GFR] can also be used in place of creatinine or CrCl); creatinine clearance should be calculated per institutional standard
- International normalized ratio (INR) or prothrombin time (PT) =< 1.5 X ULN unless subject is receiving anticoagulant therapy not requiring laboratory monitoring as long as PT or partial thromboplastin time (PTT) is within therapeutic range of intended use of anticoagulants; therapeutic Coumadin is not acceptable
- Activated partial thromboplastin time (aPTT) =< 1.5 X ULN unless subject is receiving anticoagulant therapy as long as PT or PTT is within therapeutic range of intended use of anticoagulants
- Urine protein-creatinine ratio (UPCR) =< 1 on spot urinalysis or protein =< 500 mg/24 hour urine
- Archival tissue must be available or newly obtained core or excisional biopsy of a tumor lesion
- Patients must have measurable disease based on RECIST 1.1
- Women of child-bearing potential and men must agree to use adequate contraception (hormonal or barrier method of birth control; abstinence) prior to study entry and for the duration of study participation; patients should continue contraceptive measures for 6 months from the last dose of all study medications
- Female patients of childbearing potential should have a negative urine or serum pregnancy test within 24 hours prior to receiving the first dose of study medication; if the urine test is positive or cannot be confirmed as negative, a serum pregnancy test will be required
- Female patients of childbearing potential should be willing to use 2 methods of birth control or be surgically sterile, or abstain from heterosexual activity for the course of the study through 120 days after the last dose of study medication; patients of childbearing potential are those who have not been surgically sterilized or have not been free from menses for > 1 year
- Should a woman become pregnant or suspect she is pregnant while she is participating in this study, she should inform her treating physician immediately; men treated or enrolled on this protocol must also agree to use adequate contraception prior to the study, for the duration of study participation, and 4 months after completion of MK 3475 and ziv-aflibercept administrations
- Ability to understand and the willingness to sign a written informed consent document

Exclusion Criteria:

- Patients who have had chemotherapy, targeted small molecule therapy, or radiotherapy within 4 weeks (6 weeks for nitrosoureas or mitomycin C) prior to entering the study or those who have not recovered from adverse events due to agents administered more than 4 weeks earlier
- Note: patients with =< grade 2 neuropathy are an exception to this criterion and may qualify for the study
- Note: if patients received major surgery, they must have recovered adequately from the toxicity and/or complications from the intervention prior to starting therapy
- Patients who are currently participating in or have participated in a study of an investigational agent or using an investigational device within 4 weeks of the first dose of treatment
- Has a diagnosis of immunodeficiency or is receiving systemic steroid therapy or any other form of immunosuppressive therapy within 7 days prior to the first dose of trial treatment
- Has had a prior monoclonal antibody within 4 weeks prior to study day 1 or who has not recovered (i.e., =< grade 1 or at baseline) from adverse events (AEs) due to agents administered more than 4 weeks earlier
- Has a known additional malignancy that is progressing or requires active treatment; exceptions include basal cell carcinoma of the skin, squamous cell carcinoma of the skin, or in situ cervical cancer that has undergone potentially curative therapy
- Lesions suspected to be at higher-risk for bleeding such as bowel involvement with tumor that invades into the bowel wall or involves the intraluminal component of bowel by imaging or direct visualization or central pulmonary lesions
- Ulcerated skin lesions
- Full anti-coagulant therapy Coumadin; patients may be receiving therapeutic Lovenox, Fragmin, or other heparin product that does not require laboratory monitoring
- Poorly-controlled hypertension as defined blood pressure (BP) > 150/100 mmHg, or systolic (S) BP > 180 mmHg when diastolic (D) BP < 90 mmHg, on at least 2 repeated determinations on separate days within 3 months prior to study enrollment
- Pregnant or nursing women
- Patients with known brain metastases should be excluded from this clinical trial
- Patients with carcinomatous meningitis should also be excluded
- Patients with previously treated brain metastases may participate provided they are stable (without evidence of progression by imaging for at least 3 months prior to the first dose of trial treatment and any neurologic symptoms have returned to baseline), have no evidence of new or enlarging brain metastases, and are not using steroids for at least 7 days prior to trial treatment
- History of allergic reactions attributed to compounds of similar chemical or biologic composition to MK-3475 and ziv-aflibercept
- Has an active autoimmune disease requiring systemic treatment within the past 3 months or a documented history of clinically severe autoimmune disease, or a syndrome that requires systemic steroids or immunosuppressive agents; patients with vitiligo or resolved childhood asthma/atopy would be an exception to this rule; patients that require intermittent use of bronchodilators or local steroid injections would not be excluded from the study; patients with hypothyroidism stable on hormone replacement or Sjogren's syndrome will not be excluded from the study

- Has a history or current evidence of any condition, therapy, or laboratory abnormality that might confound the results of the trial, interfere with the patient's participation for the full duration of the trial, or is not in the best interest of the patient to participate, in the opinion of the treating investigator
- Has known psychiatric or substance abuse disorders that would interfere with cooperation with the requirements of the trial
- Has received prior therapy with an anti-programmed cell death-1 (PD-1), anti-programmed death-ligand 1 (PD-L1), anti-programmed cell death 1 ligand 2 (PD-L2), anti-cluster of differentiation 137 (CD137), ziv-aflibercept or anti-cytotoxic T-lymphocyte-associated protein 4 (CTLA-4) antibody (including ipilimumab or any other antibody or drug specifically targeting T-cell co-stimulation or checkpoint pathways)(prior treatment with bevacizumab is not an exclusion criteria)
- Uncontrolled intercurrent illness including, but not limited to, ongoing or active infection, interstitial lung disease or active, non-infectious pneumonitis, symptomatic congestive heart failure, unstable angina pectoris, cardiac arrhythmia, or psychiatric illness/social situations that would limit compliance with study requirements
- If pregnant or breastfeeding, or expecting to conceive or father children within the projected duration of the trial, starting with the pre-screening or screening visit through 120 days after the last dose of trial treatment; pregnant women are excluded from this study; breastfeeding should be discontinued if the mother is treated with MK-3475
- Men and non-pregnant, non-breast-feeding women may be enrolled if they are willing to use 2 methods of birth control or are considered highly unlikely to conceive; highly unlikely to conceive is defined as 1) surgically sterilized, or 2) postmenopausal (a woman who is >= 45 years of age and has not had menses for greater than 2 years will be considered postmenopausal), or 3) not heterosexually active for the duration of the study; the two birth control methods can be barrier method or a barrier method plus a hormonal method to prevent pregnancy; patients should start using birth control from study visit 1 throughout the study period up to 120 days after the last dose of study therapy; the following are considered adequate barrier methods of contraception: diaphragm, condom (by the partner), copper intrauterine device, sponge, or spermicide; appropriate hormonal contraceptives will include any registered and marketed contraceptive agent that contains an estrogen and/or a progestational agent (including oral, subcutaneous, intrauterine, or intramuscular agents); patients should continue contraceptive measures for 6 months from the last dose of all study medications
- **Patients who are human immunodeficiency virus (HIV) positive may participate if they meet the following eligibility requirements:**
- They must be stable on their anti-retroviral regimen, and they must be healthy from an HIV perspective
- They must have a cluster of differentiation (CD)4 count of greater than 250 cells/mcL
- They must not be receiving prophylactic therapy for an opportunistic infection
- Has known active hepatitis B (e.g., hepatitis B surface antigen [HBsAg] reactive) or hepatitis C (e.g., hepatitis C virus [HCV] ribonucleic acid [RNA] [qualitative] is detected)
- Has received a live vaccine within 30 days prior to the first dose of trial treatment
- History within 6 months prior to treatment of myocardial infarction, severe/unstable angina pectoris, coronary artery bypass graft (CABG), New York Heart Association (NYHA) class III or IV congestive heart failure (CHF), stroke or transient ischemic attack (TIA)
- History within 3 months prior to treatment of grade 3-4 gastrointestinal (GI) bleeding/hemorrhage, treatment resistant peptic ulcer disease, erosive esophagitis or gastritis, infectious or inflammatory bowel disease, diverticulitis, pulmonary embolus, or other uncontrolled thromboembolic event
- Patients who are less than 4 weeks post-operative (op) after major surgery

Sex/Gender

All

Ages

18 Years to N/A

Accepts Healthy Volunteers

No

Trial of Active Immunotherapy With OBI-833 (Globo H-CRM197) in Advanced/Metastatic Gastric, Lung, Colorectal or Breast Cancer Subjects

Study ID:
NCT02310464

Sponsor:
OBI Pharma, Inc

Information provided by (Responsible Party):
OBI Pharma, Inc (OBI Pharma, Inc)

Tracking Information

First Submitted Date

December 2, 2014

Start Date

December 2015

Current Primary Outcome Measures

Safety and tolerability assessed by adverse events, changes in laboratory values, and changes in vital signs.[Time Frame: 36 weeks]

Primary Completion Date

December 2018

Last Update Posted Date

January 11, 2018

Descriptive Information

Offical Title

An Open-Label Study to Assess the Safety, Tolerability, and Efficacy of Active Immunotherapy With Dose Escalation and Cohort Expansion of OBI-833 (Globo H-CRM197) in Advanced/Metastatic Gastric, Lung, Colorectal, or Breast Cancer Subjects

Brief Summary

The purpose of this clinical study is to assess the safety and tolerability and efficacy of active immunotherapy with dose escalation and cohort expansion of OBI-833 in advanced/metastatic gastric, lung, colorectal, or breast cancer subjects.

Study Type

Interventional

Study Phase

Phase 1

Condition

- Metastatic Gastric Cancer
- Metastatic Breast Cancer
- Metastatic Colorectal Cancer
- Metastatic Lung Cancer

Intervention

Drug: OBI-833/OBI-821

Study Arms

Experimental: Dose escalation

Each subject will be given a total of 10 doses of OBI-833/OBI-821 subcutaneously at weeks 1,2,3,4,6,8,12,16,20,and 24 (Visits 1,2,3,4,5,6,7,8,9 and 10, respectively). Post treatment, subjects will be continually evaluated for safety and immune response every 4 weeks until the end of study, which is 12 weeks after the last dose, i.e., week 36. Subsequently, subjects will be followed for survival every 8 weeks up to 12 months after the end of study.

Experimental: Cohort expansion phase

Each subject will be given OBI-833/OBI-821 at Weeks 1, 2, 3, 4, 6, 8, 12, 16, 20, 24, and every 8 weeks thereafter (Visits 1, 2, 3, 4, 5, 6, 7, 8, 9, 10, and every 8 weeks thereafter) until disease progression. For the subjects discontinued treatment because of disease progression, subjects will be continually evaluated for safety and immune response every 8 weeks until the end of the study, which is 24 weeks after the last dose.

Recruitment Information

Recruitment Status

Recruiting

Estimated Enrollment

25

Eligibility Criteria

Inclusion Criteria:

1. Subjects ≥21 years of age

2. Dose escalation phase: Histologically or cytologically confirmed diagnosis of gastric, lung, colorectal or breast cancer on file Cohort expansion phase: Histologically or cytologically confirmed diagnosis of Globo H-positive NSCLC

3. Dose escalation: Subjects with recurrent or metastatic incurable disease that failed to respond to at least one line of anticancer standard therapy and for which standard treatment is no longer effective or tolerable.

Completion Date

December 2019

Primary Completion Date

December 2018

Cohort expansion phase: Subjects with recurrent or metastatic NSCLC who have achieved stable disease (SD), or partial response (PR) status after at least 1 regimen of anticancer therapy (i.e., chemotherapy, or targeted therapy, or PD-1/PD-L1 antagonists either alone or in combination) , and there are no standard treatments available except permitted Target or PD-1/PD-L1 therapies

4. Measurable disease (i.e., present with at least one measurable lesion per RECIST, version 1.1.

5. Dose Escalation Phase: No known central nervous system (CNS) metastases or neurological symptoms possibly related to active CNS metastasis in Dose Escalation Phase.

Cohort Expansion Phase: Subjects with asymptomatic CNS metastases for at least four weeks before study drug treatment

6. Performance status: ECOG ≤ 1

- 7. Organ Function Requirements Subjects must have adequate organ functions as defined below:

AST/ALT ≤ 3X ULN (upper limit of normal) AST/ALT ≤ 5X ULN [with underlying liver metastasis] Total bilirubin ≤ 2.0 X ULN Serum creatinine ≤ 1.5X ULN ANC ≥ 1500 /µL Platelets > 100,000/µL

8. Subjects of child-bearing potential must agree to use acceptable contraceptive methods during treatment and until the end of the study. Subject not of childbearing potential (i.e., permanently sterilized, postmenopausal) can be included in study. Postmenopausal is defined as 12 months with no menses without an alternative medical cause.

9. Ability to understand and the willingness to sign a written informed consent document according to institutional guidelines.

Exclusion Criteria:

1. Patients who have not received standard chemotherapy, hormonal or targeted therapy for their underlying advanced/metastatic cancer.

2. Subjects who are pregnant or breast-feeding at entry.

3. Subjects with splenectomy.

4. Subjects with known or clinically manifest, symptomatic CNS metastases in Dose Escalation Phase.

5. Subjects with HIV infection, active hepatitis B infection or active hepatitis C infection.

6. Subjects with any autoimmune disorders requiring iv/oral steroids or immunosuppressive or immunomodulatory therapies.

- e.g., Type 1 juvenile onset diabetes mellitus, antibody positive for rheumatoid arthritis, Grave's disease, Hashimoto's thyroiditis, lupus, scleroderma, systemic vasculitis, hemolytic anemia, immune mediated thrombocytopenia, etc.

7. Subjects with any known uncontrolled inter-current illness including ongoing or active infections, symptomatic congestive heart failure (NYHA>2), unstable angina pectoris, cardiac arrhythmia, or psychiatric illness/social situations that would limit compliance with study requirements.

8. Dose escalation phase: Subjects with any of the following MEDICATIONS within 4 weeks prior to IP treatment, except permitted therapies as listed in section 7.1:

- Chemotherapeutic Agent
- Immunotherapy [mAbs, Interferons, Cytokines (except GCSF)]
- Immunosuppressants (e.g., cyclosporin, rapamycin, tacrolimus, rituximab, alemtuzumab, natalizumab, etc.).
- IV/oral steroids except single prophylactic use in CT/MRI scan or other one-time use in approved indications. The interval between IV/oral steroids administration and first dose of OBI-833/OBI-821 must be more than pharmacological duration or 5 half-lives of administered steroids, whichever is the longer. Uses of inhaled and topical use of steroids are allowed.
- Another investigational drug

Cohort Expansion Phase: Subjects with any of the following MEDICATIONS within 4 weeks prior to IP treatment, except permitted therapies:

- Chemotherapeutic Agent
- Immunotherapy [Interferons, Cytokines] (except PD-1/PD-L1 antagonists)
- Immunosuppressants (e.g., cyclosporin, rapamycin, tacrolimus, rituximab, alemtuzumab, natalizumab, etc.).
- IV/oral steroids except single prophylactic use in CT/MRI scan or other one-time use in approved indications. The interval between IV/oral steroids administration and first dose of OBI-833/OBI-821 must be more than pharmacological duration or 5 half-lives of administered steroids, whichever is longer. Uses of inhaled and topical steroids are allowed.
- Another investigational drug

9. Subjects with pleural effusions and/or ascites, due to malignancy, requiring paracentesis every 2 weeks or more frequently.

10. Subjects with any known severe allergies (e.g., anaphylaxis) to any active or inactive ingredients in the study drugs.

▨ Sex/Gender

All

▨ Ages

21 Years to N/A

▨ Accepts Healthy Volunteers

No

Vorinostat Plus Hydroxychloroquine Versus Regorafenib in Colorectal Cancer

Study ID:

NCT02316340

Sponsor:

The University of Texas Health Science Center at San Antonio

Information provided by (Responsible Party):

The University of Texas Health Science Center at San Antonio (The University of Texas Health Science Center at San Antonio)

Tracking Information

■ **First Submitted Date**

December 9, 2014

■ **Start Date**

February 2015

■ **Current Primary Outcome Measures**

Efficacy based on progression free survival of vorinostat and hydroxychloroquine compared to Regorafenib[Time Frame: Every 8 weeks]

 CT Scan

■ **Primary Completion Date**

January 2018

■ **Last Update Posted Date**

October 11, 2017

Descriptive Information

■ **Offical Title**

Modulation of Autophagy: A Clinical Study of Vorinostat Plus Hydroxychloroquine Versus Regorafenib in Refractory Metastatic Colorectal Cancer (mCRC) Patients (CTMS# 14-2015)

■ **Brief Summary**

This will be a randomized phase II clinical trial of patients with histologic documentation of metastatic colorectal cancer, who have received local and currently approved standard therapies, excluding RGF.

■ **Detailed Description**

The investigators will give VOR 400 mg PO daily and HCQ 600 mg PO daily in 4-week cycles. Patients will require imaging up to 6 weeks prior to enrollment and will be assessed for measureable evidence of mCRC. This will be a randomized, controlled phase II clinical trial of patients with histological documentation of metastatic colorectal cancer, who have received locally and currently approved standard therapies, excluding RGF. Patients will be randomized 1:1 to RGF or VOR/HCQ (see schema below). Also, crossover is optional after first progression on the initial therapy, and based on physician discretion and in the best interest of the patient. If crossover is not done, then the patient will be off study and can go on to receive other treatments.

■ **Study Type**

Interventional

■ **Study Phase**

Phase 2

■ **Condition**

• Colorectal Cancer

■ **Intervention**

Drug: Vorinostat

 400mg by mouth daily

Other Names:

 Zolinza

 SAHA

VOR

Drug: Hydroxychloroquine

600mg by mouth daily

Other Names:

HCQ

plaquenil

Drug: Regorafenib

160 mg by mouth daily

Other Names:

Stivarga

RGF

Study Arms

- Experimental: Study Arm VOR with HCQ
  Patients will be given vorinostat 400 mg daily and hydroxychloroquine 600 mg daily in 4 week cycles.

- Active Comparator: Control Arm Regorafenib
  Patients will be given oral RGF 160 mg daily for 3 weeks in 4 week cycles.

Recruitment Information

Recruitment Status

Recruiting

Estimated Enrollment

76

Completion Date

January 2018

Primary Completion Date

January 2018

Eligibility Criteria

Inclusion Criteria:

- Histological documentation of metastatic colorectal cancer (mCRC)
- ECOG performance status of 0-2
- Radiographical documentation of metastatic disease with imaging up to 6 weeks prior to enrollment
- Patients with mCRC must have been previously treated with irinotecan and/or oxaliplatin and/or VEGF/EGFR therapy or intolerant to these agents
- Documentation of K-Ras mutational status
- Adequate hematologic, renal and liver function (i.e. absolute neutrophil count > 1000/mm3, platelets > 75,000/mm3); creatinine < 2 times the upper limits of normal (ULN) total bilirubin < 1.5 mg/dl, ALT and AST< 3 times above the ULN, ALT and AST can be < 5 times ULN if patients have hepatic involvement.
- Able to provide written informed consent
- Patients with the potential for pregnancy or impregnating their partner must agree to follow acceptable birth control methods to avoid conception. Women of childbearing potential must have a negative pregnancy test within 72 hours prior to receiving the investigational product
- Tumor blocks available from previous surgery/biopsy, or if not available, patients willing to have biopsy

Exclusion Criteria:

- Patients receiving prior therapy with RGF, VOR, and/or HCQ
- Patients with uncontrolled brain metastases. Patients with brain metastases must be asymptomatic and off corticosteroids for at least one week
- Due to risk of disease exacerbation, patients with porphyria are not eligible
- Due to risk of disease exacerbation, patients with psoriasis are ineligible unless the disease is well controlled, and they are under the care of a specialist for the disorder who agrees to monitor the patient for exacerbations
- Patients with previously documented macular degeneration or diabetic retinopathy
- Patients who have had chemotherapy or radiotherapy within 2 weeks (6 weeks for nitrosoureas or mitomycin C) prior to entering the study. For targeted therapies, patients will need to clear for 5 half-lives
- Patients may not be receiving any other investigational agents
- Patients should not have taken valproic acid or another histone deacetylase inhibitor for at least 2 weeks prior to enrollment
- History of allergic reactions attributed to compounds of similar chemical or biologic composition to VOR or HCQ
- Uncontrolled intercurrent illness including, but not limited to, ongoing or active infection, symptomatic congestive heart

failure, unstable angina pectoris, cardiac arrhythmia, or psychiatric illness/social situations that would limit compliance with study requirements

- Major surgery or significant traumatic injury occurring within 21 days prior to treatment
- QTc > 500 ms at baseline (average of 3 determinations at 10 minutes interval)
- Gastrointestinal tract disease resulting in an inability to take oral medication or a requirement for IV alimentation, prior surgical procedures affecting absorption, or active peptic ulcer disease. Patients with NG-tube, J-tube, or G-tube will not be allowed to participate
- Pregnant women are excluded from this study because vorinostat has the potential for teratogenic or abortifacient effects. For this reason, women of childbearing potential and men must also agree to use adequate contraception (hormonal or barrier method of birth control) prior to study entry and for the duration of study participation
- Should a woman become pregnant or suspect she is pregnant while participating in this study, she should inform her treating physician immediately. Because there is an unknown but potential risk for adverse events in nursing infants secondary to treatment of the mother with vorinostat, breastfeeding should be discontinued
- Informed Consent No study specific procedures will be performed without a written and signed informed consent document. Patients who do not demonstrate the ability to understand or the willingness to sign the written informed consent document will be excluded from study entry

▧ Sex/Gender

All

▧ Ages

18 Years to N/A

▧ Accepts Healthy Volunteers

No

▧ Contacts

Epp Goodwin   210-450-5798   CTRCReferral@uthscsa.edu

A Study of the Safety, Tolerability, and Efficacy of Epacadostat Administered in Combination With Nivolumab in Select Advanced Cancers (ECHO-204)

Study ID:
NCT02327078

Sponsor:
Incyte Corporation

Information provided by (Responsible Party):
Incyte Corporation (Incyte Corporation)

Tracking Information

▧ First Submitted Date
December 1, 2014

▧ Primary Completion Date
April 2020

▧ Start Date
November 2014

▧ Last Update Posted Date
January 17, 2018

▧ Current Primary Outcome Measures

Phase 1, Part 1: Safety and tolerability of epacadostat and nivolumab assessed by number of subjects with dose limiting toxicities (DLTs)[Time Frame: 42 days]

Phase 1, Part 2: Safety and tolerability of epacadostat administered in combination with nivolumab and chemotherapy regimen assessed by number of subjects with DLTs[Time Frame: 42 days]

Phase 1, Part 1 and 2: Safety assessed by the frequency of adverse events, serious adverse events, and deaths[Time Frame: Assessed through 100 days after the end of treatment, estimated to be up to 18 months per subject.]

Phase 2: Objective response rate (ORR) per Response Evaluation Criteria in Solid Tumors (RECIST) v1.1 for subjects with solid tumors and per Cheson criteria for subjects with DLBCL[Time Frame: Response is assessed every 8 weeks for the duration of study participation.]

Phase 2: Progression free survival (PFS)[Time Frame: Response is assessed every 8 weeks for the duration of study participation.]

Phase 2: Overall survival (OS)[Time Frame: Subjects will be followed-up for survival every 12 weeks for duration of study participation.]

Current Secondary Outcome Measures

Phase 1, Part 1: ORR per RECIST v1.1 and mRECIST for subjects with solid tumors; per Cheson and mCheson criteria for subjects with B-cell NHL; and per RANO and mRANO criteria for subjects with GBM[Time Frame: Response will be assessed every 8 weeks during study participation which is estimated to be up to 18 months.]

Phase 1, Part 2: ORR per RECIST v1.1 and modified RECIST for subjects with advanced or metastatic SCCHN and advanced or metastatic NSCLC[Time Frame: Response will be assessed every 8 weeks during study participation which is estimated to be up to 18 months.]

Phase 1, Part 2: Duration of response (DOR) for subjects with advanced or metastatic SCCHN and advanced or metastatic NSCLC[Time Frame: Response will be assessed every 8 weeks during study participation which is estimated to be up to 18 months.]

Phase 1, Part 2: PFS for subjects with advanced or metastatic SCCHN and advanced or metastatic NSCLC[Time Frame: Response will be assessed every 8 weeks during study participation which is estimated to be up to 18 months.]

Phase 2: Duration of response (DOR)[Time Frame: Response will be assessed every 8 weeks during study participation which is estimated to be up to 42 months.]

Phase 2: Duration of disease control, defined as CR, PR, and stable disease (SD)[Time Frame: Response will be assessed every 8 weeks during study participation which is estimated to be up to 42 months.]

Phase 2: Safety and tolerability measured by the frequency of adverse events (AEs), serious adverse events (SAEs), and deaths[Time Frame: AEs are assessed for the duration of the study participation which is estimated to be up to 18 months for Phase 1 and up to 42 months for Phase 2.]

Descriptive Information

Offical Title

A Phase 1/2 Study of the Safety, Tolerability, and Efficacy of Epacadostat Administered in Combination With Nivolumab in Select Advanced Cancers (ECHO-204)

Brief Summary

This is a Phase 1/2, open label study. Phase 1 consists of 2 parts. Part 1 is a dose-escalation assessment of the safety and tolerability of epacadostat administered with nivolumab in subjects with select advanced solid tumors and lymphomas. Part 2 will evaluate the safety and tolerability of epacadostat in combination with nivolumab and chemotherapy in subjects with squamous cell carcinoma of head and neck (SCCHN) and non-small cell lung cancer (NSCLC).

Phase 2 will include expansion cohorts in 7 tumor types, including melanoma, NSCLC, SCCHN, colorectal cancer, ovarian cancer, glioblastoma and diffuse large B-cell lymphoma (DLBCL).

Study Type

Interventional

Study Phase

Phase 1/Phase 2

Condition

- I/O naïve Melanoma (MEL)
- I/O Relapsed MEL
- I/O Refractory MEL
- Carcinoma, Non-Small-Cell Lung
- CRC (Colorectal Cancer)
- HNSCC (Head and Neck Squamous Cell Cancer
- Ovarian Cancer
- B Cell NHL Including DLBCL
- Hodgkin Lymphona (B-cell Malignancies)
- Glioblastoma

Intervention

Drug: Nivolumab (Phase 1)

specified dose and dosing schedule

Drug: Epacadostat (Phase 1)

oral twice daily continuous at the protocol-defined dose

Drug: Chemotherapy (Phase 1)

Specified dose on specified days

Drug: Nivolumab (Phase 2)
specified dose and dosing schedule

Drug: Epacadostat (Phase 2)
oral twice daily continuous at the protocol-defined dose

■ Study Arms

Experimental: (Phase 1, Part 1) : Nivolumab + Epacadostat
Experimental: (Phase 2): Nivolumab + Epacadostat
Experimental: (Phase 1, Part 2): Nivolumab + Epacadostat + Chemotherapy

Recruitment Information

■ **Recruitment Status**

Recruiting

■ **Estimated Enrollment**

485

■ **Completion Date**

October 2020

■ **Primary Completion Date**

April 2020

■ **Eligibility Criteria**

Inclusion Criteria:

- Male or female subjects, age 18 years or older
- Subjects with histologically or cytologically confirmed NSCLC, MEL, CRC, SCCHN, ovarian cancer, recurrent B cell NHL or HL, or glioblastoma
- Presence of measurable disease by RECIST v1.1 for solid tumors or Cheson criteria for B cell NHL (including DLBCL) or HL. For subjects with glioblastoma, presence of measurable disease is not required.
- Eastern Cooperative Oncology Group (ECOG) performance status 0 to 1
- Fresh baseline tumor biopsies (defined as a biopsy specimen taken since completion of the most recent prior chemotherapy regimen) are required for all cohorts except glioblastoma

Exclusion Criteria:

- Laboratory and medical history parameters not within Protocol-defined range
- Currently pregnant or breastfeeding
- Subjects who have received prior immune checkpoint inhibitors or an IDO inhibitor (except select Phase 2 cohorts evaluating I/O relapsed or I/O refractory MEL). Subjects who have received experimental vaccines or other immune therapies should be discussed with the medical monitor to confirm eligibility
- Untreated central nervous system (CNS) metastases or CNS metastases that have progressed
- Subjects with any active or inactive autoimmune process
- Evidence of interstitial lung disease or active, noninfectious pneumonitis
- Subjects with any active or inactive autoimmune process
- Ocular MEL

■ **Sex/Gender**

All

■ **Ages**

18 Years to N/A

■ **Accepts Healthy Volunteers**

No

■ **Contacts**

Incyte Call Center   1-855-463-3463

Increased Frequency of AlloStim® Immunotherapy Dosing in Combination With Cryoablation in Metastatic Colorectal Cancer

Study ID:

NCT02380443

Sponsor:

Immunovative Therapies, Ltd.

Information provided by (Responsible Party):

Immunovative Therapies, Ltd. (Immunovative Therapies, Ltd.)

Tracking Information

▥ **First Submitted Date**

March 2, 2015

▥ **Primary Completion Date**

October 2017

▥ **Start Date**

September 2016

▥ **Last Update Posted Date**

October 21, 2016

▥ **Current Primary Outcome Measures**

To determine the safety of increased frequency of dosing (Part 1) (whether a Dose Limiting Toxicity (DLT) has occurred)[Time Frame: Window is defined from baseline until 28 days after the last dose administration ("Safety Evaluation Period")]

Three patients are enrolled at each frequency schedule in the absence of dose limiting toxicity (DLT).Two types of toxicity are assessed for determination of whether a Dose Limiting Toxicity (DLT) has occurred. An acute dose limiting toxicity (ADLT) is assessed within 48h of a dose administration. Cumulative dose limiting toxicity (CDLT) is assessed during the complete Safety Evaluation Period.

To evaluate the anti-tumor effect of AlloStim combined with cryoablation at the new proposed dose and frequency schedule (Part 2)[Time Frame: 28 days after last dose administration]

Subjects at the new proposed dose and frequency schedule will be monitored for radiological, pathological and immunological response

▥ **Current Secondary Outcome Measures**

To assess change from baseline in Health-Related Quality of Life (HRQoL)[Time Frame: From enrollment to 28 days after last dose administration]

Health-Related Quality of Life (HRQoL) will be measured using the European Organization for Research and Treatment of Cancer (EORTC) Quality of Life Questionnaire (QLQ-C30)

Descriptive Information

▥ **Offical Title**

In-Situ Cancer Vaccine: Phase I/IIb, Open-Label Study to Assess the Safety of AlloStim® Immunotherapy in Combination With Cryoablation as Third Line Therapy for Metastatic Colorectal Cancer

▥ **Brief Summary**

This is a single center, open label dose frequency escalation study of InSituVax personalized anti-tumor vaccine protocol combining the cryoablation of a selected metastatic lesion with intra-lesional immunotherapy with AlloStim®. The in-situ (in the body) cancer vaccine step combines killing a single metastatic tumor lesion by use of cryoablation in order to cause the release of tumor-specific markers to the immune system and then injecting bioengineered allogeneic immune cells (AlloStim®) into the lesion as an adjuvant in order to modulate the immune response and educate the immune system to kill other tumor cells where ever they reside in the body.

▥ **Detailed Description**

Colorectal cancer (CRC) ranks as the third most common cancer worldwide. Metastasis is the main reason of death in CRC patients. The current drugs used to treat colorectal cancer provide important treatment options for patients, their limitations including drug resistance, poor efficacy and severe side effects. Development of new therapeutic strategies for KRAS mutant as well as BRAF mutant tumors are therefore highly needed in order to offer a new category of drug (immunotherapy). This study targets the population of mCRC patients that have progressed after two lines of chemotherapy and are not eligible for targeted therapies. The study will assess six different dosing schedules. A standard 3 plus 3 study design will be used. The starting frequency for each dosing schedule will be escalated in subsequent groups of patients. The study will evaluate safety of increased frequency of AlloStim® dosing and anti-tumor effect of the new proposed dose and frequency schedule.

- ■ **Study Type**

  Interventional

- ■ **Study Phase**

  Phase 2

- ■ **Condition**

  - Colorectal Cancer Metastatic

- ■ **Intervention**

  Biological: AlloStim

  AlloStim is an activated living CD4+ Th1 memory cell derived from the blood of normal blood donors and intentionally mismatched to the recipient. AlloStim is bioengineered to express high levels of Type 1 inflammatory cytokines (such as interferon-gamma, TNF-alpha, GM-CSF) and immunomodulatory molecules such as CD40L. AlloStim has CD3/CD28-coated microbeads attached to assure activation upon infusion.

  Other Names:

  InSituVax

  Procedure: Cryoablation

  Percutaneous partial cryoablation of a single metastatic tumor lesion in the liver. The procedure is conducted under CT or ultrasound image-guidance

- ■ **Study Arms**

  Experimental: Dosing Schedule A

  The priming step with ID injections of AlloStim on Days 0, 7, and 14

  The vaccination step with cryoablation and IT (intratumoral) injection of AlloStim on Day 21

  The activation step with IV infusion of AlloStim on Day 28

  The booster step with two IV booster infusions of AlloStim on Days 56 and 84

  Protocol follow-up procedures continue until day 112. Efficacy evaluation will continue monthly for each subject until death or loss to follow-up

  Experimental: Dosing Schedule B

  The priming step with ID injections of AlloStim on Days 0, 3 and days 7 and 10

  The vaccination step with cryoablation and IT (intratumoral) injection of AlloStim on Day 14

  The activation step with IV infusion of AlloStim on Day 21

  The booster step with two IV booster infusions of AlloStim on Days 49 and 77

  Protocol follow-up procedures continue until day 105. Efficacy evaluation will continue monthly for each subject until death or loss to follow-up

  Experimental: Dosing Schedule C

  The priming step with ID injections of AlloStim on Days 0, 3 and days 7 and 10

  The vaccination step with cryoablation and IT (intratumoral) injection of AlloStim on Day 14 and an additional IT injection of AlloStim on Day 17

  The activation step with IV infusion of AlloStim on Day 21

  The booster step with two IV booster infusions of AlloStim on Days 49 and 77

  Protocol follow-up procedures continue until day 105. Efficacy evaluation will continue monthly for each subject until death or loss to follow-up

  Experimental: Dosing Schedule D

  The priming step with ID and IV injections of AlloStim on Days 0, 3 and days 7 and 10

  The vaccination step with cryoablation and IT injection of AlloStim on Day 14

  The activation step with IV infusion of AlloStim on Day 21

  The booster step with two IV booster infusions of AlloStim on Days 49 and 77

  Protocol follow-up procedures continue until day 105. Efficacy evaluation will continue monthly for each subject until death or loss to follow-up

  Experimental: Dosing Schedule E

  The priming step with ID and IV injections of AlloStim on Days 0, 3 and days 7 and 10

The vaccination step with cryoablation and IT and IV injections of AlloStim on Day 14

The activation step with IV infusion of AlloStim on Day 21

The booster step with two IV booster infusions of AlloStim on Days 49 and 77

Protocol follow-up procedures continue until day 105. Efficacy evaluation will continue monthly for each subject until death or loss to follow-up

Experimental: Dosing Schedule F

The priming step with ID and IV injections of AlloStim on Days 0, 3 and days 7 and 10

The vaccination step with cryoablation and IT injection of AlloStim on Day 14 and IV injection of AlloStim on Day 17

The activation step with IV infusion of AlloStim on Day 21

The booster step with two IV booster infusions of AlloStim on Days 49 and 77

Protocol follow-up procedures continue until day 105. Efficacy evaluation will continue monthly for each subject until death or loss to follow-up

Publications

(Includes publications given by the data provider as well as publications identified by ClinicalTrials.gov Identifier (NCT Number) in Medline.)Epple LM, Bemis LT, Cavanaugh RP, Skope A, Mayer-Sonnenfeld T, Frank C, Olver CS, Lencioni AM, Dusto NL, Tal A, Har-Noy M, Lillehei KO, Katsanis E, Graner MW. Prolonged remission of advanced bronchoalveolar adenocarcinoma in a dog treated with autologous, tumour-derived chaperone-rich cell lysate (CRCL) vaccine. Int J Hyperthermia. 2013 Aug;29(5):390-8. doi: 10.3109/02656736.2013.800997. Epub 2013 Jun 20. (https://www.ncbi.nlm.nih.gov/pubmed/23786302)

Mayer-Sonnenfeld T, Har-Noy M, Lillehei KO, Graner MW. Proteomic analyses of different human tumour-derived chaperone-rich cell lysate (CRCL) anti-cancer vaccines reveal antigen content and strong similarities amongst the vaccines along with a basis for CRCL's unique structure: CRCL vaccine proteome leads to unique structure. Int J Hyperthermia. 2013 Sep;29(6):520-7. doi: 10.3109/02656736.2013.796529. Epub 2013 Jun 4. (https://www.ncbi.nlm.nih.gov/pubmed/23734882)

LaCasse CJ, Janikashvili N, Larmonier CB, Alizadeh D, Hanke N, Kartchner J, Situ E, Centuori S, Har-Noy M, Bonnotte B, Katsanis E, Larmonier N. Th-1 lymphocytes induce dendritic cell tumor killing activity by an IFN-γ-dependent mechanism. J Immunol. 2011 Dec 15;187(12):6310-7. doi: 10.4049/jimmunol.1101812. Epub 2011 Nov 9. (https://www.ncbi.nlm.nih.gov/pubmed/22075702)

Janikashvili N, LaCasse CJ, Larmonier C, Trad M, Herrell A, Bustamante S, Bonnotte B, Har-Noy M, Larmonier N, Katsanis E. Allogeneic effector/memory Th-1 cells impair FoxP3+ regulatory T lymphocytes and synergize with chaperone-rich cell lysate vaccine to treat leukemia. Blood. 2011 Feb 3;117(5):1555-64. doi: 10.1182/blood-2010-06-288621. Epub 2010 Dec 1. (https://www.ncbi.nlm.nih.gov/pubmed/21123824)

Har-Noy M, Zeira M, Weiss L, Fingerut E, Or R, Slavin S. Allogeneic CD3/CD28 cross-linked Th1 memory cells provide potent adjuvant effects for active immunotherapy of leukemia/lymphoma. Leuk Res. 2009 Apr;33(4):525-38. doi: 10.1016/j.leukres.2008.08.017. Epub 2008 Oct 1. (https://www.ncbi.nlm.nih.gov/pubmed/18834631)

Har-Noy M, Zeira M, Weiss L, Slavin S. Completely mismatched allogeneic CD3/CD28 cross-linked Th1 memory cells elicit anti-leukemia effects in unconditioned hosts without GVHD toxicity. Leuk Res. 2008 Dec;32(12):1903-13. doi: 10.1016/j.leukres.2008.05.007. Epub 2008 Jun 18. (https://www.ncbi.nlm.nih.gov/pubmed/18565579)

Har-Noy M, Slavin S. The anti-tumor effect of allogeneic bone marrow/stem cell transplant without graft vs. host disease toxicity and without a matched donor requirement? Med Hypotheses. 2008;70(6):1186-92. Epub 2007 Dec 3. (https://www.ncbi.nlm.nih.gov/pubmed/18054441)

Zeng Y, Stokes J, Hahn S, Hoffman E, Katsanis E. Activated MHC-mismatched T helper-1 lymphocyte infusion enhances GvL with limited GvHD. Bone Marrow Transplant. 2014 Aug;49(8):1076-83. doi: 10.1038/bmt.2014.91. Epub 2014 Apr 28. (https://www.ncbi.nlm.nih.gov/pubmed/24777185)

Recruitment Information

Recruitment Status

Recruiting

Estimated Enrollment

18

Completion Date

February 2018

Primary Completion Date

October 2017

Eligibility Criteria

Inclusion Criteria:

1. Adult males and female subjects aged 18-80 years at screening visit

2. Pathologically confirmed diagnosis of colorectal adenocarcinoma

3. Presenting with metastatic disease:

- Primary can be intact or previously resected
- Metastatic lesion(s) in liver must be non-resectable
- Extrahepatic disease acceptable

4. At least one liver lesion able to be visualized by ultrasound and determined to be safely assessable for percutaneous cryoablation

5. Previous treatment failure of two previous lines of active systemic chemotherapy:

- Previous chemotherapy must have included an oxaliplatin-containing (e.g. FOLFOX) and an irinotecan-containing (e.g. FOLFIRI) regimen
- with or without bevacizumab
- administered in adjuvant setting or for treatment of metastatic disease
- If KRAS wild type, must have at least one prior anti-EGFR therapy
- Treatment failure can be due to disease progression or toxicity
- Disease progression on second line therapy must be documented radiologically and must have occurred during or within 30 days following the last administration of treatment for metastatic disease

6. ECOG performance score: 0-1

7. Adequate hematological function:

- Absolute granulocyte count ≥ 1,200/mm3
- Platelet count ≥ 100,000/mm3
- PT/INR ≤ 1.5 or correctable to <1.5 at time of interventional procedures
- Hemoglobin ≥ 9 g/dL (may be corrected by transfusion)

8. Adequate Organ Function:

- Creatinine ≤ 1.5 mg/dL
- Total bilirubin ≤ 1.5 times upper limit of normal (ULN)
- Alkaline phosphatase ≤ 2.5 times ULN
- Aspartate aminotransferase (AST) or (SGOT) ≤ 2.5 times ULN
- Alanine aminotransferase (ALT) or (SGPT) ≤ 2.5 times ULN

9. EKG without clinically relevant abnormalities

10. Female subjects: Not pregnant or lactating

11. Patients with child bearing potential must agree to use adequate contraception

12. Study specific informed consent in the native language of the subject.

Exclusion Criteria:

1. Bowel obstruction or high risk for obstruction

2. Moderate or severe ascites requiring medical intervention

3. Clinical evidence or radiological evidence of brain metastasis or leptomeningeal involvement

4. Symptomatic asthma or COPD

5. Pulmonary lymphangitis or symptomatic pleural effusion (grade ≥ 2) that results in pulmonary dysfunction requiring active treatment or oxygen saturation <92% on room air

6. Bevacizumab (Avastin®) treatment within 6 weeks of scheduled cryoablation procedure

7. Regorafenib prior to the Study Period

8. Taking anticoagulant medication for concomitant medical condition (unless can be safely discontinued for invasive cryoablation, biopsy and intratumoral injection procedures)

9. Prior allogeneic bone marrow/stem cell or solid organ transplant

10. Chronic use (> 2 weeks) of greater than physiologic doses of a corticosteroid agent (dose equivalent to > 5 mg/day of prednisone) within 30 days of the first day of study drug treatment

- Topical corticosteroids are permitted

11. Prior diagnosis of an active autoimmune disease (e.g., rheumatoid arthritis, multiple sclerosis, autoimmune thyroid disease, uveitis). Well controlled Type I diabetes allowed

12. Prior experimental therapy

13. History of blood transfusion reactions

14. Known allergy to bovine products

15. Progressive viral or bacterial infection

- All infections must be resolved and the subject must remain afebrile for seven days without antibiotics prior to being placed on study

16. Cardiac disease of symptomatic nature

17. History of HIV positivity or AIDS

18. Concurrent medication known to interfere with platelet function or coagulation (e.g., aspirin, ibuprofen, clopidogrel, or warfarin) unless such medications can be discontinued for an appropriate time period based on the drug half-life and known activity (e.g., aspirin for 7 days) prior to cryoablation and biopsy procedures

19. History of severe hypersensitivity to monoclonal antibody drugs or any contraindication to any of the study drugs

20. Psychiatric or addictive disorders or other condition that, in the opinion of the investigator, would preclude study

participation.

21. Subjects that lack ability to provide consent for themselves

■ Sex/Gender

All

■ Ages

18 Years to 80 Years

■ Accepts Healthy Volunteers

No

■ Contacts

Andrea Horstman   1-480-440-7458   BMDACCResearch@bannerhealth.com
Thu Bui, M.A.   1-619-227-4872   thu@immunovative.com

Ropidoxuridine in Treating Patients With Advanced Gastrointestinal Cancer Undergoing Radiation Therapy

Study ID:
NCT02381561

Sponsor:
National Cancer Institute (NCI)

Information provided by (Responsible Party):
National Cancer Institute (NCI) (National Cancer Institute (NCI))

Tracking Information

■ First Submitted Date
March 5, 2015

■ Start Date
February 1, 2016

■ Primary Completion Date
August 1, 2018

■ Last Update Posted Date
January 3, 2018

■ Current Primary Outcome Measures

Maximum tolerated dose (MTD) defined as the dose below which 2 or more of 6 patients experience dose-limiting toxicity[Time Frame: Up to 28 days]

■ Current Secondary Outcome Measures

%iododeoxyuridine (IUdR)-deoxyribonucleic acid (DNA) incorporation in peripheral (circulating) granulocytes[Time Frame: Up to 4 weeks after completion of study treatment]

Correlate %IUdR-DNA incorporation in human GI tumor biopsies in the proposed phase I and PK clinical trial in GI cancer patients receiving palliative abdominal and/or pelvic RT by linear regression.

%iododeoxyuridine (IUdR)-deoxyribonucleic acid (DNA) incorporation in tumor biopsies[Time Frame: Up to 2 weeks]

Correlate %IUdR-DNA incorporation in human gastrointestinal (GI) tumor biopsies in the proposed phase I and pharmacokinetic (PK) clinical trial in GI cancer patients receiving palliative abdominal and/or pelvic radiation therapy (RT) by linear regression.

Pharmacokinetic (PK) incorporation in peripheral (circulating) granulocytes[Time Frame: Days 1, 15 and 22 before drug administration, 30, 60, 120, and 240 minutes (and 24 hours on day 1 only) following drug administration]

Correlate %IUdR-DNA incorporation in human GI tumor biopsies in the proposed phase I and PK clinical trial in GI cancer patients receiving palliative abdominal and/or pelvic RT by linear regression.

Pharmacokinetic (PK) incorporation in tumor biopsies[Time Frame: Days 1, 15 and 22 before drug administration, at 30, 60, 120, and 240 minutes (and 24 hours on day 1 only) following drug administration]

Correlate %IUdR-DNA incorporation in human GI tumor biopsies in the proposed phase I and PK clinical trial in GI cancer patients receiving palliative abdominal and/or pelvic RT by linear regression.

Tumor response relationship to the %iododeoxyuridine (IUdR)-deoxyribonucleic acid (DNA) incorporation using Response Evaluation Criteria in Solid Tumors (RECIST) criteria based on high-pressure liquid chromatography (HPLC) and flow cytometry measurements[Time Frame: Day 8]

Tumor response is the dependent variable and can be binomial (i.e. response versus [vs.] no response) or multinomial (i.e. complete response, partial response, stable disease or progressive disease) and the %IUdR-DNA incorporation is the independent variable.

Descriptive Information

▣ Offical Title

- Phase I and Pharmacology Study of Oral 5-Iodo-2-Pyrimidinone-2'Deoxyribose (IPdR) as a Prodrug for IUdR-Mediated Tumor Radiosensitization in Gastrointestinal Cancers

▣ Brief Summary

This phase I trial studies the side effects and best dose of ropidoxuridine in treating patients with gastrointestinal cancer that has spread to other places in the body and usually cannot be cured or controlled with treatment undergoing radiation therapy. Ropidoxuridine may help radiation therapy work better by making tumor cells more sensitive to the radiation therapy.

▣ Detailed Description

PRIMARY OBJECTIVES:

I. To conduct a phase I dose escalation trial, to determine the safety and the maximum tolerated dose (MTD), of oral (po) IPdR (ropidoxuridine) given daily for 28 consecutive days with concurrent intensity-modulated radiation therapy (IMRT) in patients with advanced gastrointestinal cancers treated with palliative radiation.

SECONDARY OBJECTIVES:

I. To observe and record anti-tumor activity. II. To establish the pharmacokinetics of daily po dosing of IPdR x 28 days. III. To assess, for patients treated at the MTD, for biochemical evidence of IPdR effect in normal tissue (circulating granulocytes) and tumor tissue (in patients with accessible tumor tissue) by measuring %iododeoxyuridine (IUdR)-deoxyribonucleic acid (DNA) cellular incorporation by flow cytometry and high-pressure liquid chromatography (HPLC) analyses.

IV. To assess the use of %IUdR-DNA cellular incorporation (measured by the investigational laboratory assays of flow cytometry and HPLC) as an exploratory biomarker of IPdR for the following effects: the %IUdR-DNA tumor cell incorporation from day 8 tumor biopsies in gastrointestinal (GI) cancer patients receiving MTD doses of IPdR as an exploratory biomarker of tumor radiosensitization using Response Evaluation Criteria in Solid Tumors (RECIST) criteria.

V. To assess the use of %IUdR-DNA cellular incorporation (measured by the investigational laboratory assays of flow cytometry and HPLC) as an exploratory biomarker of IPdR for the following effects: the %IUdR-DNA cellular incorporation in patients' circulating granulocytes taken weekly during the 28-day IPdR MTD dose, on day 29, and week 8 as an exploratory biomarker of IPdR systemic toxicities to bone marrow as measured by complete blood count (CBC)/differential values.

OUTLINE: This is a dose-escalation study of ropidoxuridine.

Beginning 30 minutes to 2 hours before radiation therapy, patients receive ropidoxuridine PO once daily (QD) on days 1-28 in the absence of disease progression or unacceptable toxicity. Beginning on day 8, patients undergo IMRT 5 days a week for 3 weeks in the absence of disease progression or unacceptable toxicity.

After completion of study treatment, patients are followed up for 4 weeks.

▣ Study Type

Interventional

▣ Study Phase

Phase 1

▣ Condition

- Bile Duct Carcinoma
- Stage II Esophageal Cancer AJCC v7
- Stage II Pancreatic Cancer AJCC v6 and v7
- Stage IIA Esophageal Cancer AJCC v7
- Stage IIA Pancreatic Cancer AJCC v6 and v7
- Stage IIB Esophageal Cancer AJCC v7
- Stage IIB Pancreatic Cancer AJCC v6 and v7
- Stage III Colon Cancer AJCC v7
- Stage III Esophageal Cancer AJCC v7
- Stage III Gastric Cancer AJCC v7
- Stage III Liver Cancer
- Stage III Pancreatic Cancer AJCC v6 and v7
- Stage III Rectal Cancer AJCC v7
- Stage III Small Intestinal Cancer AJCC v7
- Stage IIIA Colon Cancer AJCC v7
- Stage IIIA Esophageal Cancer AJCC v7

- Stage IIIA Gastric Cancer AJCC v7
- Stage IIIA Rectal Cancer AJCC v7
- Stage IIIA Small Intestinal Cancer AJCC v7
- Stage IIIB Colon Cancer AJCC v7
- Stage IIIB Esophageal Cancer AJCC v7
- Stage IIIB Gastric Cancer AJCC v7
- Stage IIIB Rectal Cancer AJCC v7
- Stage IIIB Small Intestinal Cancer AJCC v7
- Stage IIIC Colon Cancer AJCC v7
- Stage IIIC Esophageal Cancer AJCC v7
- Stage IIIC Gastric Cancer AJCC v7
- Stage IIIC Rectal Cancer AJCC v7
- Stage IV Colon Cancer AJCC v7
- Stage IV Esophageal Cancer AJCC v7
- Stage IV Gastric Cancer AJCC v7
- Stage IV Liver Cancer
- Stage IV Pancreatic Cancer AJCC v6 and v7
- Stage IV Rectal Cancer AJCC v7
- Stage IV Small Intestinal Cancer AJCC v7
- Stage IVA Colon Cancer AJCC v7
- Stage IVA Liver Cancer
- Stage IVA Rectal Cancer AJCC v7
- Stage IVB Colon Cancer AJCC v7
- Stage IVB Liver Cancer
- Stage IVB Rectal Cancer AJCC v7

Intervention

Radiation: Intensity-Modulated Radiation Therapy
Undergo IMRT

Other Names:

IMRT

Intensity Modulated RT

Intensity-Modulated Radiotherapy

Other: Laboratory Biomarker Analysis

Correlative studies

Other: Pharmacological Study

Correlative studies

Drug: Ropidoxuridine
Given PO

Other Names:

5-Iodo-2-pyrimidinone 2' deoxyribonucleoside

5-Iodo-2-pyrimidinone-2'-deoxyribose

IPdR

Study Arms

Experimental: Treatment (ropidoxuridine, IMRT)

Beginning 30 minutes to 2 hours before radiation therapy, patients receive ropidoxuridine PO QD on days 1-28 in the absence of disease progression or unacceptable toxicity. Beginning on day 8, patients undergo IMRT 5 days a week for 3 weeks in the absence of disease progression or unacceptable toxicity.

Recruitment Information

Recruitment Status

Recruiting

Estimated Enrollment

30

Completion Date

N/A

Primary Completion Date

August 1, 2018

Eligibility Criteria

Inclusion Criteria:

- Patients must have histologically or cytologically confirmed advanced, incurable cancers of the esophagus, liver, stomach, small bowel, pancreas, bile duct, colon or rectum and be eligible to receive chest, abdominal and/or pelvic radiation therapy (RT) for palliation; documentation of this is required in physician note; concomitant systemic therapy is not allowed during administration of palliative RT; palliative RT can be considered for advanced primary tumors or metastatic disease as above
- Patients must not have received systemic chemotherapy for at least 4 weeks, and must not have received prior radiation therapy to the tumor site being irradiated on this study
- Eastern Cooperative Oncology Group (ECOG) performance status =< 2 (Karnofsky >= 60%)
- Life expectancy of greater than 12 weeks
- Leukocytes >= 3,000/mcL
- Absolute neutrophil count >= 1,500/mcL
- Platelets >= 100,000/mcL
- Total bilirubin within normal institutional limits
- Aspartate aminotransferase (AST) (serum glutamic oxaloacetic transaminase [SGOT])/alanine aminotransferase (ALT) (serum glutamate pyruvate transaminase [SGPT]) =< 2.5 x institutional upper limit of normal
- Creatinine within normal institutional limits OR creatinine clearance >= 60 mL/min/1.73 m^2 for patients with creatinine levels above institutional normal
- Women of child-bearing potential and men must agree to use adequate contraception (hormonal or barrier method of birth control; abstinence) prior to study entry and for the duration of study participation; should a woman become pregnant or suspect she is pregnant while she or her partner is participating in this study, she should inform her treating physician immediately; men and women treated or enrolled on this protocol must also agree to use adequate contraception prior to the study, for the duration of study participation, and 4 months after completion of IPdR administration
- Ability to understand and the willingness to sign a written informed consent document
- Human immunodeficiency virus (HIV) positive (+) patients with cluster of differentiation 4 (CD4) counts >= 250 cells/mm^3 on anti-viral therapy
- Women of child-bearing potential must have a negative pregnancy test

Exclusion Criteria:

- Patients who have had chemotherapy or radiotherapy within 4 weeks (6 weeks for nitrosoureas or mitomycin C) prior to entering the study or those who have not recovered from adverse events due to agents administered more than 4 weeks earlier
- Patients who are receiving any other investigational agents
- Patients with known brain metastases should be excluded from this clinical trial
- History of allergic reactions attributed to compounds of similar chemical or biologic composition to IPdR
- Uncontrolled intercurrent illness including, but not limited to, ongoing or active infection, symptomatic congestive heart failure, unstable angina pectoris, cardiac arrhythmia, or psychiatric illness/social situations that would limit compliance with study requirements
- Pregnant women are excluded from this study; breastfeeding should be discontinued if the mother is treated with IPdR

Sex/Gender

All

Ages

18 Years to N/A

Accepts Healthy Volunteers

No

INC280 Combined With Bevacizumab in Patients With Glioblastoma Multiforme

Study ID:

NCT02386826

Sponsor:

SCRI Development Innovations, LLC

Information provided by (Responsible Party):

SCRI Development Innovations, LLC (SCRI Development Innovations, LLC)

Tracking Information

■ **First Submitted Date**

March 6, 2015

■ **Start Date**

September 22, 2015

■ **Primary Completion Date**

September 2018

■ **Last Update Posted Date**

May 12, 2017

■ **Current Primary Outcome Measures**

Maximum Tolerated Dose (MTD) of INC280[Time Frame: weekly for 4 weeks]

> The MTD of INC280 to be administered with standard dose bevacizumab is determined as the highest dose at which ≤1 of 6 patients experiences a dose limiting toxicity (DLT) during one cycle (28 days) of therapy, assessed by National Cancer Institute Common Terminology Criteria for Adverse Events (NCI CTCAE) v. 4.0.3

■ **Current Secondary Outcome Measures**

Progression-free Survival[Time Frame: every 8 weeks until treatment discontinuation, expected average of 6 months]

> Progression-free survival is measured from Day 1 of study drug administration to disease progression or death on study. Disease progression is assessed by Response Assessment in Neuro-Oncology (RANO) criteria.

Overall Response Rate[Time Frame: Every 8 weeks up to 6 months]

> Defined as the proportion of patients with confirmed complete response or partial response (CR or PR) assessed according to RANO criteria. CR=complete disappearance of all measurable and non-measurable disease sustained for at least 4 weeks. PR=≥ 50% decrease compared with baseline in the sum of products of perpendicular diameters of all measurable enhancing lesions sustained for at least 4 weeks.

Descriptive Information

■ **Offical Title**

Phase Ib Study Evaluating the c-Met Inhibitor INC280 in Combination With Bevacizumab in Patients With Glioblastoma Multiforme (GBM)

■ **Brief Summary**

The purpose of this study is to determine whether the combination of two agents, INC280 and bevacizumab, is safe and effective when administered to patients with Glioblastoma Multiforme (GBM) who have progressed after receiving prior therapy or who have unresectable GBM.

■ **Detailed Description**

Despite recent advances, glioblastoma multiforme (GBM) remains an incurable malignancy with a short expected survival. c-MET signalling promotes invasive growth and has been described in various cancers. INC280 is a highly potent and selective c-MET inhibitor which also penetrates the blood-brain barrier. In this open-label, multicenter Phase 1b study, investigators determined the optimal dose of the INC280/bevacizumab combination to administer to patients. Enrollment has now expanded in order to treat 3 cohorts of GBM patients: those who progressed after ≥ first-line standard therapy, those who progressed after ≥ second-line therapy with INC280/bevacizumab, and those with unresectable GBM.

■ **Study Type**

Interventional

■ **Study Phase**

Phase 1

■ **Condition**

- Glioblastoma Multiforme
- Gliosarcoma
- Colorectal Cancer
- Renal Cell Carcinoma

■ **Intervention**

Drug: INC280

> **Dose Escalation: INC280 by mouth (PO) twice daily for 28 days according to the following schedule until the maximum tolerated dose (MTD) is determined:**
>
> Dose Level 1 (starting dose): 200 mg (divided dose of 100 mg twice per day) Dose Level 2: 400 mg (divided dose of 200 mg

twice per day) Dose Level 3: 800 mg (divided dose of 400 mg twice per day)

Dose Expansion: INC280 PO twice daily at the MTD determined in the dose escalation phase

Other Names:

INCB28060

Biological: bevacizumab

bevacizumab: 10 mg/kg IV every 2 weeks. Patients with unresectable GBM will be given 15 mg/kg IV every 4 weeks.

Other Names:

Avastin

Study Arms

Experimental: INC280 + Bevacizumab

Dose Escalation: 18 GBM patients received bevacizumab 10 mg/kg intravenously (IV) once every 2 weeks in combination with INC280 given by mouth (PO) starting at 100 mg twice daily and escalating on a 3+3 escalation pattern until the maximum tolerated dose (MTD) was determined.

Dose Expansion: Up to 45 GBM patients enrolled in 3 Cohorts:

Cohort A: 20 GBM patients progressed during or after standard 1st-line therapy; Cohort B: 15 GBM patients progressed during or after 2nd-line bevacizumab therapy; Cohort C: 10 unresectable GBM patients.

INC280: PO twice daily at the MTD. Bevacizumab: 10 mg/kg IV once every 2 weeks for Cohorts A and B; 15 mg/kg IV every 4 weeks for Cohort C Treatment cycles will be repeated every 28 days (4 weeks).

Recruitment Information

Recruitment Status

Recruiting

Estimated Enrollment

63

Completion Date

November 2019

Primary Completion Date

September 2018

Eligibility Criteria

Inclusion Criteria:

KEY POINTS:

1. Dose Escalation Phase: Histologic diagnosis of GBM or gliosarcoma. Progressed during or after standard 1st-line therapy for GBM. Patients scheduled to undergo a repeat primary surgical resection are also eligible. Measurable disease as measured by RANO (Response Assessment in Neuro-Oncology) criteria.

2. Dose Expansion Phase:

Cohort A: Histologic diagnosis of GBM. Patients should have progressed during or after standard 1st-line therapy. Patients scheduled to undergo a repeat primary surgical resection are also eligible. Measurable disease as measured by RANO criteria.

At least 5 patients must have an alteration of MET [as assessed by fluorescence in situ hybridization (FISH) (c-MET/centromere ratio ≥2, or c-MET gene copy number ≥ 5) or RT-PCR or Met immunohistochemistry (IHC) score of 2-3+ or a mutation].

Cohort B: Histologic diagnosis of GBM patients who have progressed during or after 2nd-line therapy with bevacizumab or a bevacizumab-based regimen. Measurable disease according to RANO criteria.

Cohort C: Histologic diagnosis of GBM by stereotactic biopsy in patients with unresectable brain tumors.

3. Eastern Cooperative Oncology Group (ECOG) Performance Status score of 0-2 or Karnofsky Performance Scale (KPS) of at least 70%.

4. Adequate hematologic, renal and liver function

5. Life expectancy ≥ 3 months

6. Availability of archived tumor samples and/or willingness to provide tissue samples if resection is done. (Fresh tissue biopsy is not required if archival tissue is not available.)

Exclusion Criteria:

1. Prior treatment with bevacizumab for GBM patients eligible for Cohorts A and C. (Prior treatment with bevacizumab is permitted for GBM patients eligible for Cohort B only.)

2. Most recent chemotherapy ≤ 21 days to the start of treatment and ≥ Grade 2 chemotherapy-related side effects with the exception of alopecia.

3. Use of any investigational drug ≤ 21 days to the start of treatment or 5 half-lives (whichever is shorter) prior to the first dose of INC280 with bevacizumab. For study drugs for which 5 half-lives is ≤ 21 days, a minimum of 10 days between termination of the study drug and the start of treatment is required.

4. Uncontrolled seizures (Patients with a history of seizures are eligible if they are currently without seizures on a stable dose of anti-epileptic drugs for 14 days prior to enrollment.)

5. History of uncontrolled hereditary or acquired bleeding or thrombotic disorders.

6. Major surgery ≤ 28 days to the start of treatment, or subcutaneous venous access device placement ≤ 7 days to the start of treatment

7. A serious non healing wound, ulcer, or bone fracture ≤ 28 days to the start of treatment

8. Wide field radiotherapy (including therapeutic radioisotopes such as strontium 89) administered ≤ 28 days or limited field radiation for palliation ≤ 7 days prior to starting study drug or has not recovered from side effects of such therapy.

9. Leptomeningeal metastases or spinal cord compression due to disease.

10. Women of child-bearing potential.

11. Receiving drugs known to be strong inhibitors or inducers of CYP3A4 and cannot be discontinued 7 days prior to the start of INC280 treatment and during the course of the study, or medications that are known CYP3A4, CYP1A2, CYP2C8, CYP2C9 or CYP2C19 substrates with narrow therapeutic index, and cannot be discontinued during the course of the study.

12. Treatment with proton pump inhibitors within three days prior to study entry.

13. Cardiac disease currently or less than 6 months from baseline screening

14. Inadequately controlled hypertension (i.e., systolic blood pressure [SBP] >180 mmHg or diastolic blood pressure (DBP) >100 mmHg) (patients with values above these levels must have their blood pressure (BP) controlled with medication prior to starting treatment).

15. Currently receiving treatment with therapeutic doses of warfarin sodium. Low molecular weight heparin is allowed.

Sex/Gender

All

Ages

18 Years to N/A

Accepts Healthy Volunteers

No

Contacts

Sarah Cannon Research Institute   1-877-691-7274   asksarah@scresearch.net

Safety, Immunogenicity and Pharmacokinetics of SYN004 in Patients With Solid Tumors

Study ID:

NCT02391727

Sponsor:

Synermore Biologics Co., Ltd.

Information provided by (Responsible Party):

Synermore Biologics Co., Ltd. (Synermore Biologics Co., Ltd.)

Tracking Information

First Submitted Date

March 9, 2015

Start Date

May 2015

Primary Completion Date

September 2018

Last Update Posted Date

January 10, 2018

Current Primary Outcome Measures

Number of patients with adverse events[Time Frame: 28 days of last SYN004 Administration]
    cutaneous toxicity, hypersensitivity

Current Secondary Outcome Measures

maximum plasma concentration (Cmax)[Time Frame: 84 days]
    Cmax will be determined using noncompartmental methods for SYN004

time to Cmax (Tmax)[Time Frame: 84 days]
    Tmax will be determined using noncompartmental methods for SYN004

elimination rate constant (λz)[Time Frame: 84 days]

λz will be determined using noncompartmental methods for SYN004

elimination half-life (t½)[Time Frame: 84 days]

t½ will be determined using noncompartmental methods for SYN004

mean residence time (MRT)[Time Frame: 84 days]

MRT will be determined using noncompartmental methods for SYN004

area under the plasma concentration vs. time curve from 0 (initiation of infusion) to the time of the last detectable concentration (AUC0-t), AUC from time 0 extrapolated to infinity (AUC0-∞)[Time Frame: 84 days]

AUC0-t and AUC0-∞ will be determined using noncompartmental methods for SYN004

systemic clearance (CL)[Time Frame: 84 days]

CL will be determined using noncompartmental methods for SYN004

volume of distribution in the terminal phase (Vdβ), and estimated steady-state volume of distribution (VSS)[Time Frame: 84 days]

Vdβ and VSS will be determined using noncompartmental methods for SYN004

anti-cancer activity[Time Frame: 84 days]

Measurement of objective response (OR), durability of objective response (DOR), and progression-free survival (PFS). The number and proportion of subjects who achieve objective tumor response (complete response [CR], partial response [PR], and CR+PR) or stable disease (SD) using Response Evaluation Criteria in Solid Tumors (RECIST) version 1.1, according to local radiological assessments from date of first administration of the investigational product to the end of the study treatment.

Descriptive Information

▣ Offical Title

A Phase 1, Multi-center, Open-Label Dose Escalation Study of SYN004 in Patients With Solid Tumors to Evaluate the Safety, Immunogenicity and Pharmacokinetics of SYN004 Following Administration of Eight Intravenous Doses

▣ Brief Summary

A first-in-human evaluation of SYN004, a monoclonal antibody that binds to the EGF receptor on cancer cells. Cetuximab, a marketed antibody, has been shown to be effective by inhibiting the growth of cancer cells thereby prolonging the life of patients who have received it. SYN004 is a closely related monoclonal antibody also binds to the EGF receptor in the same way. SYN004 might also inhibit cancer cells and prolong life but has been engineered to avoid some of the hypersensitivity reactions known to provoked by cetuximab.

▣ Detailed Description

Study Design:

In this open-label, dose escalation study, subjects will receive a single IV loading dose of SYN004 on Day 1 of the first treatment week, followed by up to 7 fixed weekly doses of SYN004. Subjects will be assigned to loading and fixed doses by dose group.

Each dose group will comprise 3 subjects and may be expanded to 6 subjects. Subjects will enter dose groups in the order in which they are enrolled. There will be no intra-subject dose adjustments.

Only 1 subject in a cohort may receive the loading dose of SYN004 on any given day; at least 1 day must elapse before the next subject in the cohort receives the loading dose.

Study SYN004-001 Dose Matrix. Three initial subjects will be enrolled followed by an additional three if specified by protocol. Dose levels are specified below.

Group 1: Loading dose: 100 mg/m2; Weekly Dose: 62.5 mg/m2. Group 2: Loading dose: 200 mg/m2; Weekly Dose: 125 mg/m2. Group 3: Loading dose: 400 mg/m2; Weekly Dose: 250 mg/m2.

After each dose of IV SYN004, subjects will be observed in the clinic for 12 hours. After the loading dose, subjects will undergo safety evaluations on Days 2, 3 and 5. Safety evaluation will also be performed on Day 1 (pre-treatment) and Day 3 of each fixed dose treatment week.

Dose-limiting toxicities (DLTs) are defined as any Grade ≥3 AE assessed by the investigator or Medical Monitor, with agreement of the Safety Review Board (SRB), as related to SYN004. Subjects with DLTs will be withdrawn from treatment. If 2 or more subjects in a dose group experience DLTs, or one subject in a dose group experiences a Grade ≥3 infusion reaction, all subjects in that dose group will be withdrawn from treatment.

Subjects in the dose groups are considered evaluable for dose escalation decisions if they receive at least 4 doses of SYN004, or discontinue SYN004 because of a DLT.

Subjects who withdraw or are terminated per protocol before receiving 4 doses of SYN004 will be replaced.

For subjects who receive at least 4 doses of SYN004, End of Study CT scans for RECIST (version 1.1) evaluation will be performed six (6) days following the final SYN004 treatment.

There will be a 28-day safety monitoring period following the final dose of SYN004 for all subjects in the study. All subjects will attend an End-of-Study Visit 28 days after the final dose of SYN004.

Subjects who complete Cycles 1 and 2, who have evidence of improvement per RECIST 1.1 (i.e., findings of complete or partial response per RECIST 1.1) and meet the other eligibility criteria will be offered up to 3 additional treatment cycles (i.e., up to 12 additional weekly doses) of SYN004 in the SYN004-001 Extension Study. During the Extension Study, subjects will receive the same fixed dose of SYN004 they received in Cycles 1 and 2.

Dose escalation will proceed according to a standard 3+3 study design.

Study Type

Interventional

Study Phase

Phase 1

Condition

- Colon Cancer, Breast Cancer, Cancer of the Head and Neck

Intervention

Biological: SYN004

subjects who have received effective treatment for their cancers are eligible

Study Arms

Other: SYN004

open label study

Recruitment Information

Recruitment Status

Recruiting

Completion Date

September 2018

Estimated Enrollment

18

Primary Completion Date

September 2018

Eligibility Criteria

Inclusion Criteria:

Note: No waivers of the study inclusion or exclusion criteria will be granted.

1. Diagnosis of a solid tumor for which the accepted standard of care includedsa licensed anti-EGFR therapy;

2. Tumor progression in patients with RAS wild type metastatic colorectal cancer irrespective of their exposure to licensed anti-EGFR therapy including anti-EGFR antibodies; OR Tumor progression in patients with metastatic colorectal cancer refractory to cetuximab or panitumumab or other anti-EGFR antibodies OR Tumor progression in patients with EGFR-mutated non-small cell lung cancer (NSCLC) who have refused therapy.

OR Tumor progression or recurrence in patients with squamous cell carcinoma of the head and neck irrespective of their exposure to licensed anti-EGFR therapy including anti-EGFR antibodies.

OR Patients with locally advanced or metastatic colorectal carcinoma who have

1. relapsed after standard of care treatment,

2. proved refractory to standard of care treatment

3. refused standard of care treatment

4. been found to be medically unsuitable for standard of care treatment

3. Completion of written informed consent procedure;

4. Male or female subjects over 17 years of age

5. Life expectancy of at least 3 months;

6. Eastern Cooperative Oncology Group (ECOG) Performance Status of 0 to 2;

7. At least one measureable non-irradiated site of disease according to Response Evaluation Criteria in Solid Tumors (RECIST) version 1.1;

8. Adequate bone marrow function, with absolute neutrophil count (ANC) >1,500/mm3, platelet count >100,000/mm3, and hemoglobin > 10 g/mm3;

9. Adequate liver function, with bilirubin <1.5 x the upper limit of the normal range (ULN), aspartate aminotransferase (AST) and alanine aminotransferase (ALT) <2.5 x the ULN;

10. Adequate renal function, with serum creatinine <1.5 mg/dL;

11. Adequate cardiac function, with left ventricular ejection fraction (LVEF) ≥50%, normal electrocardiogram, and absence of significant cardiac disease;

12. In women of childbearing potential (defined as women of reproductive capacity who are pre-menopausal or within 12 months of cessation of menses): negative serum pregnancy test and use of an acceptable non-hormonal method of contraception;

13. Ability to communicate with the investigator, and understand and comply with the requirements of the protocol;

14. Agrees to notify the investigator when deviating from the protocol requirements with regard to concomitant medications;

15. Agrees to stay in contact with the study site for the duration of the study and to provide updated contact information as necessary, and has no current plans to move from the study area for the duration of the study.

Exclusion Criteria:

1. Participation in a study of an investigational agent or use of an investigational device at the time of screening or within 4 weeks of enrollment;

2. Receipt of treatment with a monoclonal antibody (mAb) within 4 weeks of enrollment or not recovered from an adverse event (i.e., event is >Grade 1 or subject has not returned to baseline) due to treatment with a mAb administered >4 weeks before enrollment;

3. Receipt of chemotherapy, targeted small molecule therapy, or radiation therapy within 2 weeks prior to enrollment, or not recovered from an adverse event (i.e., event is >Grade 1 or subject has not returned to baseline) due to a previously-administered agent;

4. Major surgical procedure or significant traumatic injury within 4 weeks prior to screening;

5. Diagnosis of an additional malignancy that is progressing and requires treatment; exceptions include basal cell carcinoma of the skin, squamous cell carcinoma of the skin, and in situ cervical cancer that has undergone potentially curative therapy;

6. Active autoimmune disease requiring systemic treatment within the past 3 months, or a documented history of severe autoimmune disease, or a syndrome that requires systemic steroids or immunosuppressive agents (subjects with vitiligo or resolved childhood asthma/atopy are allowed);

7. Diagnosis of an immune deficiency;

8. Receipt of systemic steroids or any form of immunosuppressive therapy within 7 days prior to enrollment, with the following exceptions:

1. Stable doses of topical, ocular, intranasal or inhaled corticosteroids

2. Doses of systemic steroids that, in the opinion of the investigator, are pysiologic replacement doses

3. Systemic steroids as prophylactic treatment for subjects with allergy to contrast media

4. Non-absorbed intra-articular steroid injections

5. Systemic corticosteroids required for control of infusion reactions or AEs if doses have been tapered to <10 mg prednisone or equivalent for 2 weeks prior to the first study treatment

9. Evidence of interstitial lung disease or active, non-infectious pneumonitis;

10. Active infection requiring systemic therapy;

11. History of cerebrovascular accident, transient ischemic attack, or subarachnoid hemorrhage within 6 months prior to screening;

12. Active hepatitis B (i.e., hepatitis B surface antigen [HBsAg] positive) or hepatitis C (i.e., hepatitis C virus [HCV] ribonucleic acid [RNA; qualitative] is detected);

13. Serious non-healing wound, ulcer, or bone fracture;

14. Any severe or uncontrolled medical condition or other condition that could affect participation in the study;

15. Any current medical, psychiatric, occupational, or substance abuse problems that, in the opinion of the investigator, will make it unlikely that the subject will comply with the protocol.

▧ Sex/Gender

All

▧ Ages

18 Years to 70 Years

▧ Accepts Healthy Volunteers

No

▧ Contacts

David Jabs   1-919-972-7143   djabs@novellaclinical.com
Valentina Conant, MS   1-919-972-7225   vconant@novellaclinical.com

Ph1b/2 Dose-Escalation Study of Entinostat With Pembrolizumab in NSCLC With Expansion Cohorts in NSCLC, Melanoma, and Colorectal Cancer

Study ID:

NCT02437136

Sponsor:

Syndax Pharmaceuticals

Information provided by (Responsible Party):

Syndax Pharmaceuticals (Syndax Pharmaceuticals)

Tracking Information

▨ **First Submitted Date**

April 27, 2015

▨ **Start Date**

July 2015

▨ **Primary Completion Date**

October 2017

▨ **Last Update Posted Date**

September 21, 2017

▨ **Current Primary Outcome Measures**

Number of Participants taking 3mg entinostat weekly with Adverse Events as a Measure of Safety and Tolerability[Time Frame: In approximately 3-4 months after 3-6 patients have enrolled and been on study for 1 cycle]

> Ph 1 Dose Escalation All patients within each dose escalation cohort are to complete C1, have safety assessments performed through C2D1, and be assessed for DLT before enrollment of the next cohort may commence.

Number of Participants taking 5mg entinostat weekly with Adverse Events as a Measure of Safety and Tolerability[Time Frame: In approximately 6-8 months after 3-6 patients have enrolled and been on study for 1 cycle]

> Ph 1 Dose Escalation All patients within each dose escalation cohort are to complete C1, have safety assessments performed through C2D1, and be assessed for DLT before enrollment of the next cohort may commence.

Overall Response Rate using irRECIST for Phase 2 Dose and Schedule for Cohort 1 Stage 1 (NSCLC)[Time Frame: In approximately 1 year]

> Cohort 1 Stage 1: If enough patients achieve an objective response (CR or PR), enrollment will continue into the second stage.

Overall Response Rate using irRECIST for Phase 2 Dose and Schedule for Cohort 2 Stage 1 (NSCLC pre-treated)[Time Frame: In approximately 1 year]

> Cohort 2 Stage 1: If enough patients achieve an objective response, then enrollment will continue into the second stage.

Overall Response Rate using irRECIST for Phase 2 Dose and Schedule for Cohort 3 Stage 1 (Melanoma pre-treated)[Time Frame: In approximately 1 year]

> Cohort 3 Stage 1: If enough patients achieve an objective response, then enrollment will continue into the second stage.

Overall Response Rate using irRECIST for Phase 2 Dose and Schedule for Cohort 1 Stage 2 (NSCLC)[Time Frame: In approximately 2 years]

> Cohort 1 Stage 2: If enough patients achieve a CR or PR than the true ORR for the combination therapy.

Overall Response Rate using irRECIST for Phase 2 Dose and Schedule for Cohort 2 Stage 2 (NSCLC pre-treated)[Time Frame: In approximately 2 years]

> Cohort 2 Stage 2: IIf enough patients achieve a CR or PR than the true ORR for the combination therapy.

Overall Response Rate using irRECIST for Phase 2 Dose and Schedule for Cohort 3 Stage 2 (Melanoma pre-treated)[Time Frame: In approximately 2 years]

> Measured by Overall Response Rate using irRECIST.

> Cohort 3 Stage 2: If enough patients achieve a CR or PR than the true ORR for the combination therapy.

▨ **Current Secondary Outcome Measures**

Clinical Benefit Rate (CBR)[Time Frame: At 6 months of treatment for each of the 3 Dose Escalation (Ph 2 cohorts) as applicable]

> CBR is Complete Response + Partial Response + Stable Disease for each patient after 6 months of study treatment

Progression-free survival (PFS) @ 6mo[Time Frame: At 6 months of treatment for each of the 3 Dose Escalation (Ph 2 cohorts) as applicable]

> PFS status in each patient after 6 months of study treatment. PFS is defined as the number of months from the date of the first dose of study drug to the earliest of documented PD or death due to any cause without prior progression.

Progression-free survival (PFS)[Time Frame: In approximately 3 years]

PFS status in each patient. PFS is defined as the number of months from the date of the first dose of study drug to the earliest of documented PD or death due to any cause without prior progression.

Overall survival (OS)[Time Frame: In approximately 3 years]

OS status in each patient. OS is defined as the number of months from the first dose of study drug to the date of death due to any cause.

Duration of Response (DOR)[Time Frame: In approximately 3 years]

DOR will be calculated for patients who achieve a CR or PR and is defined as the number of months from the start date of the response (and subsequently confirmed) to the first date that recurrent disease or PD is documented.

Time to Response (TTR)[Time Frame: In approximately 3 years]

TTR status in each patient.

Descriptive Information

▣ Offical Title

A Phase 1b/2, Open-label, Dose Escalation Study of Entinostat in Combination With Pembrolizumab in Patients With Non-small Cell Lung Cancer, With Expansion Cohorts in Patients With Non-small Cell Lung Cancer, Melanoma, and Mismatch Repair-Proficient Colorectal Cancer

▣ Brief Summary

The purpose of this study is to determine the safety and tolerability of entinostat used in combination with pembrolizumab in patients with Non-small Cell Lung Cancer. Additionally the purpose of the study is to assess how effective entinostat and pembrolizumab are in combination in patients with Non-small Cell Lung Cancer, Melanoma, and Mismatch-Repair Proficient Colorectal Cancer

▣ Detailed Description

SNDX-275-0601 is an open-label, Phase 1b/2 study evaluating the combination of entinostat plus pembrolizumab in patients with advanced metastatic or recurrent NSCLC or melanoma or mismatch repair-proficient colorectal cancer. The study has 2 phases, a Dose Escalation/Confirmation Phase (Phase 1b) and an Expansion Phase (Phase 2). An additional cohort (Entinostat Monotherapy Immune Correlate [EMIC] Cohort) evaluating single agent entinostat for 2 weeks followed by the combination will also be evaluated in patients with NSCLC in the Phase 2 expansion phase.

Toxicities will be assessed by the Investigator using the United States (US) National Cancer Institute (NCI) Common Terminology Criteria for Adverse Events (CTCAE), version 4.03.

Dose Confirmation: The prospective MTD/RP2D identified in the Dose Escalation Phase will be confirmed in 9 patients in Dose Confirmation Cohort(s) to obtain additional AE, immune correlate, and anti-tumor activity data on entinostat in combination.

Phase 2 (Expansion): In the Expansion Phase, entinostat in combination will be evaluated using the RP2D identified in the Dose Escalation/Confirmation Phase. Up to 3 Expansion Cohorts consisting of distinct subsets of patients with solid tumor cancers may be explored. Expansion cohorts may include:

1. Cohort 1: NSCLC

2. Cohort 2: Patients with NSCLC (any histology) who have previously been treated and responded and then progressed on either a PD-1 or PD-L1-blocking antibody

3. Cohort 3: Patients with melanoma who have previously been treated with and unequivocally progressed on either a PD-1 or PD-L1-blocking antibody

4. Cohort 4: Patients with CRC (mismatch repair-proficient) who have not been previously treated with a PD-1 or PD-L1 blocking antibody

EMIC Cohort: 15 NSCLC patients Stage 2 of Cohort 1 will be randomly assigned to participate.

▣ Study Type

Interventional

▣ Study Phase

Phase 1/Phase 2

▣ Condition

- Non-Small Cell Lung Cancer
- Melanoma
- Mismatch Repair-Proficient Colorectal Cancer

▣ Intervention

Drug: entinostat

An orally available histone deacetylases inhibitor (HDACs)

Other Names:

SNDX-275

MS-275

Drug: pembrolizumab

A selective humanized monoclonal antibody (mAb)

Other Names:

Keytruda

MK-3475

SCH 900475

Study Arms

Experimental: Ph 2 NSCLC (squamous or adeno)

Cohort 1: Patients with Non-Small Cell Lung Cancer, with squamous cell or adenocarcinoma histology who have not been treated with a PD-1 or PD-L-1 blocking antibody (entinostat + pembrolizumab)

Experimental: Ph 2 NSCLC pre-treated PD-1/LD-L1

Cohort 2: Patients with NSCLC (any histology) who have previously been treated with and unequivocally progressed on either a PD-1 or PD-L1-blocking antibody (entinostat + pembrolizumab)

Experimental: Ph 2 Melanoma pre-treated PD-1/PD-L1

Cohort 3: Patients with melanoma who have previously been treated with and unequivocally progressed on either a PD-1 or PD-L1-blocking antibody (entinostat + pembrolizumab)

Experimental: Ph 2 Mismatch Repair-Proficient CRC

Cohort 4: Patients with CRC (mismatch repair-proficient) who have not been previously treated with a PD-1 or PD-L1 blocking antibody

Publications

(Includes publications given by the data provider as well as publications identified by ClinicalTrials.gov Identifier (NCT Number) in Medline.)Simon R. Optimal two-stage designs for phase II clinical trials. Control Clin Trials. 1989 Mar;10(1):1-10. (https://www.ncbi.nlm.nih.gov/pubmed/2702835)

Recruitment Information

Recruitment Status

Recruiting

Estimated Enrollment

202

Completion Date

October 2019

Primary Completion Date

October 2017

Eligibility Criteria

Inclusion Criteria:

Patients with NSCLC:

- 1. Has histologicallyor pathologically-confirmed recurrent/metastatic NSCLC.

2. If has adenocarcinoma, required to have previously been tested for anaplastic lymphoma kinase (ALK) rearrangements and epidermal growth factor receptor (EGFR) mutations, with results available for collection in this study, and, if positive, has been treated with prior EGFR or ALK therapy.

3. Received at least 1 chemotherapeutic regimen in the advanced/metastatic setting and experienced documented, unequivocal progressive disease by either RECIST 1.1 or clinical assessment.

4. Patients with NSCLC enrolled in Cohort 1 of the Expansion Phase should not have been previously treated with a PD-1/PD-L1-blocking antibody

Patients in Expansion Phase, Cohorts 2 and 3

5. Previously treated with a PD-1/PD-L1-blocking antibody and experienced experienced documented, unequivocal radiographic progression of disease by irRECIST, or similar criteria during or within 12 weeks after last dose of such treatment. Patients must have received at least 6 weeks of PD-1/PD-L1 therapy for Cohort 3.

Patients with Melanoma:

- 6. In addition to having been previously treated with a PD-1/PD-L1-blocking antibody (inclusion #5), has a histologicallyor cytologically-confirmed diagnosis of unresectable or metastatic melanoma and experienced unequivocal progressive disease during treatment with a BRAF inhibitor if BRAF V600 mutation-positive. Treatment with BRAF inhibitor may occur AFTER treatment with the checkpoint inhibitor.

Patients in Expansion Phase, Cohort 4 (Colorectal Cancer)

7. Received at least 1 chemotherapeutic regimen in the advanced/metastatic setting and experienced documented, unequivocal progressive disease by either RECIST 1.1 or clinical assessment. Must have documented mismatch repair-proficient colon cancer as determined by either immunohistochemistry for mismatch repair proteins or PCR-based functional microsatellite instability.

Patients with colorectal cancer enrolled in Cohort 4 should not have been previously treated with a PD-1/PD-L1-blocking antibody (i.e., pembrolizumab, nivolumab, MEDI36MEDI4376, or GNE PDL1 [MPDL3280A])

All Patients

8. Aged 18 years or older on the day written informed consent is given.

9. If has brain metastases, must have stable neurologic status following local therapy for at least 4 weeks without the use of steroids or on stable or decreasing dose of ≤10 mg daily prednisone (or equivalent), and must be without neurologic dysfunction that would confound the evaluation of neurologic and other AEs.

10. Evidence of locally recurrent or metastatic disease based on imaging studies within 28 days before the first study drug dose:

- At least 1 measurable lesion ≥20 mm by conventional techniques or ≥10 mm by spiral CT scan or MRI, with the last imaging performed within 28 days before the first study drug dose. If there is only 1 measurable lesion and it is located in previously irradiated field, it must have demonstrated unequivocal progression according to RECIST, version 1.1.

11. If receiving radiation therapy, has a 2-week washout period following completion of the treatment prior to receiving the first study drug dose and continues to have at least 1 measureable lesion, per above criterion.

12. ECOG performance status of 0 or 1.

13. Has acceptable, applicable laboratory parameters.

14. Female subjects must not be pregnant.

15. If male, agrees to use an adequate method of contraception

15. Experienced resolution of toxic effect(s) of the most recent prior chemotherapy to Grade 1 or less (except alopecia). If patient underwent major surgery or radiation therapy of >30 Gy, they must have recovered from the toxicity and/or complications from the intervention.

17. Willing to have fresh tumor samples collected during screening and at other time points designated as mandatory, per the Schedule of Study Assessments.

18. Able to understand and give written informed consent and comply with study procedures.

Exclusion Criteria:

Patients meeting any of the following criteria are not eligible for study participation:

1. Diagnosis of immunodeficiency or receiving systemic steroid therapy or any other form of immunosuppressive therapy within 7 days prior to the first dose of study drug. The use of physiologic doses of corticosteroids may be approved after consultation with the Sponsor.

2. Active autoimmune disease that has required systemic treatment in past 2 years (i.e., with disease modifying agents, corticosteroids, or immunosuppressive drugs). Replacement therapy (e.g., thyroxine, insulin, or physiologic corticosteroid replacement therapy for adrenal or pituitary insufficiency) is not considered a form of systemic treatment.

3. History of interstitial lung disease (ILD).

4. Allergy to benzamide or inactive components of entinostat.

5. History of allergies to any active or inactive ingredients of pembrolizumab or severe hypersensitivity (>= Grade 3) to pembroluzumab.

6. History or current evidence of any condition, therapy, or laboratory abnormality that might confound the results of the study, interfere with the patient's participation for the full duration of the study, or is not in the best interest of the patient to participate, in the opinion of the treating Investigator, including, but not limited to:

- Myocardial infarction or arterial thromboembolic events within 6 months prior to baseline or severe or unstable angina, New York Heart Association (NYHA) Class III or IV disease, or a QTc interval > 470 msec.

- Uncontrolled heart failure or hypertension, uncontrolled diabetes mellitus, or uncontrolled systemic infection.

- Another known additional malignancy that is progressing or requires active treatment (excluding adequately treated basal cell carcinoma, squamous cell of the skin, cervical intraepithelial neoplasia [CIN]/cervical carcinoma in situ or melanoma in situ, or ductal carinoma in situ of the breast). Prior history of other cancer is allowed, as long as there is no active disease within the prior 5 years.

- Has a history of (non-infectious) pneumonitis that required steroids or current pneumonitis.

- Active infection requiring systemic therapy.

- Known active central nervous system (CNS) metastases and/or carcinomatous meningitis.

Note: Patients with previously treated brain metastases may participate provided they are stable (without evidence of progression by imaging [using the identical imaging modality for each assessment, either MRI or CT scan] for at least 4 weeks prior to the first dose of study drug and any neurologic symptoms have returned to baseline), have no evidence of new or enlarging brain metastases, and are not using steroids for at least 2 weeks prior to the first dose of study drug or are on stable or decreasing dose of ≤10 mg daily prednisone (or equivalent). This exception does not include carcinomatous meningitis which is excluded regardless of clinical stability.

7. Known psychiatric or substance abuse disorders that would interfere with cooperation with the requirements of the study.

8. Currently participating and receiving study therapy or has participated in a study of an investigational agent and received study therapy or used an investigational device within 4 weeks of the first dose of treatment.

9. Received a live virus vaccination within 30 days of the first dose of treatment.

10. Prior anti-cancer monoclonal antibody (mAb) within 4 weeks prior to baseline or who has not recovered (i.e., ≤Grade 1 or at baseline) from AEs due to agents administered more than 4 weeks earlier.

11. Prior chemotherapy, targeted small molecule therapy, or radiation therapy within 2 weeks prior to study baseline or who has not recovered (i.e., ≤Grade 1 or at baseline) from AEs due to a previously administered agent.

Note: Patients with ≤Grade 2 neuropathy or ≤Grade 2 alopecia are an exception to this criterion and may qualify for the study.

Note: If patient underwent major surgery, they must have recovered adequately from the toxicity and/or complications from the intervention prior to starting therapy.

12. Received transfusion of blood products (including platelets or red blood cells) or administration of colony stimulating factors (including granulocyte-colony stimulating factor [G-CSF], granulocyte macrophage-colony stimulating factor [GM-CSF], or recombinant erythropoietin) within 4 weeks prior to the first dose of study drug.

13. Currently receiving treatment with any other agent listed on the prohibited medication list such as valproic acid, or other systemic cancer agents within 14 days of the first dose of treatment.

14. If female, is pregnant, breastfeeding, or expecting to conceive, or if male, expect to father children within the projected duration of the study, starting with the screening visit through 120 days after the last dose of study drug.

15. Known history of human immunodeficiency virus (HIV) (HIV 1/2 antibodies).

16. Known active hepatitis B (e.g., hepatitis B surface antigen-reactive) or hepatitis C (e.g., hepatitis C virus ribonucleic acid [qualitative]).

17. For CRC expansion cohort, no prior history of malignant bowel obstruction requiring hospitalization in the 6 months prior to enrollment

18. For the CRC expansion cohort, no history of uncontrolled ascites, defined as symptomatic ascites and/or repeated paracenteses for symptom control in the past 3 months

Sex/Gender

All

Ages

18 Years to N/A

Accepts Healthy Volunteers

No

Contacts

Jeannette Hasapidis   781-419-1404   jhasapidis@syndax.com
Susan Brouwer   781-419-1401   sbrouwer@syndax.com

A Multicenter Study of Active Specific Immunotherapy With OncoVax® in Patients With Stage II Colon Cancer

Study ID:
NCT02448173

Sponsor:
Vaccinogen Inc

Information provided by (Responsible Party):

Vaccinogen Inc (Vaccinogen Inc)

Tracking Information

First Submitted Date
May 6, 2015

Start Date
May 2015

Primary Completion Date
July 2020

Last Update Posted Date
July 27, 2015

Current Primary Outcome Measures

Disease-Free Survival[Time Frame: Up to Five years]
    Defined as time from randomization to the date of the first objective test confirming tumor recurrence or death due to any cause

Current Secondary Outcome Measures

Overall Survival[Time Frame: Up to Five Years]
    Defined as the time from randomization to death due to any cause

Recurrence-Free Interval[Time Frame: Up to Five Years]
Defined as the time from randomization to the first objective test confirming tumor recurrence

Descriptive Information

▨ Offical Title

A Randomized Multicenter Study of Active Specific Immunotherapy With OncoVax® in Patients With Stage II Colon Cancer

▨ Brief Summary

OncoVAX® is the first cancer vaccine that both prevents cancer recurrence and addresses the diversity of cancer cells. In this pivotal randomized, multicenter Phase IIIb study in patients with Stage II colon cancer, OncoVAX is designed to use a patient's own cancer cells to mobilize the body's immune system to prevent the return of colon cancer following surgery.

▨ Detailed Description

OncoVAX is an active specific immunotherapeutic (ASI) stimulating a patient's immune response to autologous (patient-specific) tumor cells. It is comprised of sterile, live but non-dividing tumor cells obtained following standard-of-care surgical tumor resection for Stage II colon cancer. Within 35 days following surgery, patients are immunized with OncoVAX to prevent disease recurrence, which is incurable and occurs in up to 35% of patients. Patients are given three vaccinations once per week for three weeks, followed by a booster vaccination after six months. A previously completed Phase III trial published in The Lancet showed that OncoVAX cut the risk of recurrence by 61% in **patients with Stage II colon cancer. The primary endpoint is Disease-Free Survival:** defined as the time from curative surgery to the objective test confirming tumor recurrence or death due to any cause. The secondary endpoints are Overall Survival and Recurrence-Free-Interval. An interim analysis will be performed at a significance level of 0.005 once 2/3 of anticipated events have occurred, resulting in a significance level of 0.0483 at the end of the study. A total of 550 patients is planned, randomized 1:1 to receive OncoVAX® plus surgery (n=275) or surgery alone (n=275).

▨ Study Type

Interventional

▨ Study Phase

Phase 3

▨ Condition

- Stage II Colon Cancer

▨ Intervention

Biological: OncoVAX and Surgery

OncoVAX is comprised of sterile, live but non-dividing tumor cells obtained following standard-of-care surgical tumor resection for Stage II colon cancer

Procedure: Surgery

Surgical resection of Stage II colon cancer

▨ Study Arms

Experimental: OncoVAX and Surgery

Autologous Specific Immunotherapy given intradermally following surgical resection of Stage II colon cancer

Active Comparator: Surgery

Surgical resection of Stage II colon cancer

Recruitment Information

▨ Recruitment Status

Recruiting

▨ Estimated Enrollment

550

Completion Date

July 2022

Primary Completion Date

July 2020

Eligibility Criteria

Inclusion Criteria:

- Patients must have Stage II (IIA = T3N0M0, IIB = T4aN0M0, IIC = T4bN0M0) disease.
- Patients must have undergone curative resection and have no evidence of residual or metastatic disease.
- Following curative resection patients must have a CEA within normal limits. If elevated prior to resection, it must return to normal within 21 days post surgery and prior to randomization.

Exclusion Criteria:

- Patients with prior radiation therapy or chemotherapy or a prior malignancy of any type will be excluded. However, subjects with prior, curatively-treated squamous cell or basal cell carcinoma of the skin or carcinoma in situ of the cervix will be eligible for participation in this study.
- Patients with more than one malignant primary colon cancer will be excluded.

Sex/Gender

All

Ages

18 Years to N/A

Accepts Healthy Volunteers

No

Contacts

Rachel L Hoover, MS, MBA   410-387-4000   rhoover@vaccinogeninc.com
LaTonjia S Wallace, MS, MBA   410-387-4000

NCI-MATCH: Targeted Therapy Directed by Genetic Testing in Treating Patients With Advanced Refractory Solid Tumors, Lymphomas, or Multiple Myeloma

Study ID:

NCT02465060

Sponsor:

National Cancer Institute (NCI)

Information provided by (Responsible Party):

National Cancer Institute (NCI) (National Cancer Institute (NCI))

Tracking Information

First Submitted Date

June 3, 2015

Primary Completion Date

June 30, 2022

Start Date

August 12, 2015

Last Update Posted Date

February 12, 2018

Current Primary Outcome Measures

Objective response rate, defined as the percentage of patients whose tumors have a complete or partial response to treatment[Time Frame: Up to 3 years]

Objective response rate is defined consistent with Response Evaluation Criteria in Solid Tumors version 1.1 criteria for solid tumors, the Cheson (2014) criteria for lymphoma patients, and the Response Assessment in Neuro-Oncology criteria for glioblastoma patients. For each treatment arm, 80% two-sided confidence intervals will be calculated.

Current Secondary Outcome Measures

Overall survival, evaluated specifically for each drug (or step)[Time Frame: From registration onto that step until death, or censored at the date of last contact, assessed up to 3 years]

Overall survival will be estimated using the Kaplan-Meier method.

Progression free survival[Time Frame: From entry onto that step until determination of disease progression or death from any cause, censored at the date of last disease assessment for patients who have not progressed, assessed at 6 months]

Progression free survival will be estimated using the Kaplan-Meier method. For each treatment arm, 80% two-sided confidence intervals will be calculated.

Time to progression[Time Frame: From entry to that step until determination of disease progression or death due to disease, censored at the date of last disease assessment for patients who have not progressed, assessed up to 3 years]

Time to progression will be estimated using the Kaplan-Meier method.

Descriptive Information

▨ Offical Title

Molecular Analysis for Therapy Choice (MATCH)

▨ Brief Summary

This phase II trial studies how well treatment that is directed by genetic testing works in patients with solid tumors or lymphomas that have progressed following at least one line of standard treatment or for which no agreed upon treatment approach exists. Genetic tests look at the unique genetic material (genes) of patients' tumor cells. Patients with genetic abnormalities (such as mutations, amplifications, or translocations) may benefit more from treatment which targets their tumor's particular genetic abnormality. Identifying these genetic abnormalities first may help doctors plan better treatment for patients with solid tumors, lymphomas, or multiple myeloma.

▨ Detailed Description

PRIMARY OBJECTIVES:

I. To evaluate the proportion of patients with objective response (OR) to targeted study agent(s) in patients with advanced refractory cancers/lymphomas/multiple myeloma.

SECONDARY OBJECTIVES:

I. To evaluate the proportion of patients alive and progression free at 6 months of treatment with targeted study agent in patients with advanced refractory cancers/lymphomas/multiple myeloma.

II. To evaluate time until death or disease progression. III. To identify potential predictive biomarkers beyond the genomic alteration by which treatment is assigned or resistance mechanisms using additional genomic, ribonucleic acid (RNA), protein and imaging-based assessment platforms.

- IV. To assess whether radiomic phenotypes obtained from pre-treatment imaging and changes from prethrough post-therapy imaging can predict objective response and progression free survival and to evaluate the association between pre-treatment radiomic phenotypes and targeted gene mutation patterns of tumor biopsy specimens.

OUTLINE:

STEP 0 (Screening): Patients undergo biopsy along with molecular characterization of the biopsy material for specific, pre-defined mutations, amplifications, or translocations of interest via tumor sequencing and immunohistochemistry. Consenting patients also undergo collection of blood samples for research purposes.

STEPS 1, 3, 5, 7 (Treatment): Patients are assigned to 1 of 30 treatment subprotocols based on molecularly-defined subgroup. (See Arms Section)

STEPS 2, 4, 6 (Screening): Patients experiencing disease progression on the prior Step treatment or who could not tolerate the assigned treatment undergo review of their previous biopsy results to determine if another treatment is available or undergo another biopsy. Patients may have a maximum of 2 screening biopsies and 2 treatments per biopsy.

STEP 8 (Optional Research): Consenting patients undergo end-of-treatment biopsy and collection of blood samples for research purposes.

After completion of study treatment, patients are followed up every 3 months for 2 years and then every 6 months for 1 year.

▨ Study Type

Interventional

▨ Study Phase

Phase 2

▨ Condition

- Advanced Malignant Solid Neoplasm
- Bladder Carcinoma
- Breast Carcinoma
- Cervical Carcinoma
- Colon Carcinoma
- Colorectal Carcinoma
- Endometrial Carcinoma
- Esophageal Carcinoma

- Gastric Carcinoma
- Glioma
- Head and Neck Carcinoma
- Kidney Carcinoma
- Liver and Intrahepatic Bile Duct Carcinoma
- Lung Carcinoma
- Lymphoma
- Malignant Uterine Neoplasm
- Melanoma
- Ovarian Carcinoma
- Pancreatic Carcinoma
- Plasma Cell Myeloma
- Prostate Carcinoma
- Rectal Carcinoma
- Recurrent Bladder Carcinoma
- Recurrent Breast Carcinoma
- Recurrent Cervical Carcinoma
- Recurrent Colon Carcinoma
- Recurrent Colorectal Carcinoma
- Recurrent Esophageal Carcinoma
- Recurrent Gastric Carcinoma
- Recurrent Glioma
- Recurrent Head and Neck Carcinoma
- Recurrent Liver Carcinoma
- Recurrent Lung Carcinoma
- Recurrent Lymphoma
- Recurrent Malignant Solid Neoplasm
- Recurrent Melanoma
- Recurrent Ovarian Carcinoma
- Recurrent Pancreatic Carcinoma
- Recurrent Plasma Cell Myeloma
- Recurrent Prostate Carcinoma
- Recurrent Rectal Carcinoma
- Recurrent Skin Carcinoma
- Recurrent Thyroid Gland Carcinoma
- Recurrent Uterine Corpus Carcinoma
- Refractory Lymphoma
- Refractory Malignant Solid Neoplasm
- Refractory Plasma Cell Myeloma
- Skin Carcinoma
- Thyroid Gland Carcinoma
- Uterine Corpus Cancer

Intervention

Drug: Afatinib
  Given PO

Other Names:
  BIBW 2992

  Drug: Binimetinib

  Given PO

Other Names:
  ARRY-162

  ARRY-438162

MEK162

Drug: Capivasertib

Given PO

Other Names:

AZD5363

Drug: Crizotinib

Given PO

Other Names:

MET Tyrosine Kinase Inhibitor PF-02341066

PF-02341066

PF-2341066

Xalkori

Other: Cytology Specimen Collection Procedure
Optional correlative studies

Other Names:

Cytologic Sampling

Drug: Dabrafenib
Given PO

Other Names:

BRAF Inhibitor GSK2118436

GSK-2118436A

GSK2118436

Drug: Dasatinib
Given PO

Other Names:

BMS-354825

Sprycel

Drug: Defactinib
Given PO

Drug: FGFR Inhibitor AZD4547
Given PO

Other Names:

AZD4547

Other: Laboratory Biomarker Analysis
Undergo molecular analysis

Drug: Larotrectinib
Given PO

Other Names:

ARRY 470

LOXO 101

LOXO-101

Biological: Nivolumab
Given IV

Other Names:

BMS-936558

MDX-1106

NIVO

ONO-4538

Opdivo

Drug: Osimertinib
Given PO

Other Names:
AZD-9291

AZD9291

Mereletinib

Tagrisso

Drug: Palbociclib
Given PO

Other Names:
Ibrance

PD-0332991

PD-332991

Biological: Pertuzumab
Given IV

Other Names:
2C4

2C4 Antibody

MoAb 2C4

Monoclonal Antibody 2C4

Perjeta

rhuMAb2C4

RO4368451

Drug: PI3K-beta Inhibitor GSK2636771
Given PO

Other Names:
GSK2636771

Drug: Sapanisertib
Given PO

Other Names:
INK-128

INK128

MLN-0128

MLN0128

TAK-228

Drug: Sunitinib Malate
Given PO

Other Names:
SU011248

SU11248

sunitinib

Sutent

Drug: Taselisib
Given PO

Other Names:

GDC-0032

Drug: Trametinib

Given PO

Other Names:

GSK1120212

JTP-74057

MEK Inhibitor GSK1120212

Mekinist

Biological: Trastuzumab Emtansine

Given IV

Other Names:

Ado Trastuzumab Emtansine

ADO-TRASTUZUMAB EMTANSINE

Kadcyla

PRO132365

RO5304020

T-DM1

Trastuzumab-DM1

Trastuzumab-MCC-DM1

Trastuzumab-MCC-DM1 Antibody-Drug Conjugate

Trastuzumab-MCC-DM1 Immunoconjugate

Drug: Vismodegib

Given PO

Other Names:

Erivedge

GDC-0449

Hedgehog Antagonist GDC-0449

Drug: WEE1 Inhibitor AZD1775

Given PO

Other Names:

AZD-1775

AZD1775

MK-1775

MK1775

Study Arms

Experimental: Subprotocol A (EGFR activating mutation)

Patients with EGFR activating mutation receive afatinib orally (PO) once daily (QD) on days 1-28. Courses repeat every 28 days in the absence of disease progression or unacceptable toxicity.

Experimental: Subprotocol B (HER2 activating mutation)

Patients with HER2 activating mutation receive afatinib PO QD on days 1-28. Courses repeat every 28 days in the absence of disease progression or unacceptable toxicity.

Experimental: Subprotocol C1 (MET amplification)

Patients with MET amplification receive crizotinib PO BID on days 1-28. Courses repeat every 28 days in the absence of disease progression or unacceptable toxicity.

Experimental: Subprotocol C2 (MET exon 14 deletion)

Patients with MET exon 14 deletion receive crizotinib PO BID on days 1-28. Courses repeat every 28 days in the absence of disease progression or unacceptable toxicity.

Experimental: Subprotocol E (EGFR T790M or rare activating mutation)

Patients with EGFR T790M or rare activating mutation receive osimertinib PO QD on days 1-28. Courses repeat every 28 days in the absence of disease progression or unacceptable toxicity.

Experimental: Subprotocol F (ALK translocation)

Patients with ALK translocation receive crizotinib PO twice daily (BID) on days 1-28. Courses repeat every 28 days in the absence of disease progression or unacceptable toxicity.

Experimental: Subprotocol G (ROS1 translocation or inversion)

Patients with ROS1 translocation or inversion receive crizotinib PO BID on days 1-28. Courses repeat every 28 days in the absence of disease progression or unacceptable toxicity.

Experimental: Subprotocol H (BRAF V600E/R/K/D mutation)

Patients with BRAF V600E/R/K/D mutation receive dabrafenib PO BID and trametinib PO QD on days 1-28. Courses repeat every 28 days in the absence of disease progression or unacceptable toxicity.

Experimental: Subprotocol I (PIK3CA mutation)

Patients with PIK3CA mutation without RAS mutation or PTEN loss receive taselisib PO QD on days 1-28. Courses repeat every 28 days in the absence of disease progression or unacceptable toxicity.

Experimental: Subprotocol J (HER2 amplification >= 7 copy numbers)

Patients with HER2 amplification >= 7 copy numbers receive pertuzumab IV over 30-60 minutes and trastuzumab emtansine IV over 30 minutes on day 1. Courses repeat every 3 weeks in the absence of disease progression or unacceptable toxicity.

Experimental: Subprotocol L (mTOR mutation)

Patients with mTOR mutation receive sapanisertib PO daily on days 1-28. Courses repeat every 3 weeks in the absence of disease progression or unacceptable toxicity.

Experimental: Subprotocol M (TSC1 or TSC2 mutation)

Patients with TSC1 or TSC2 mutation receive sapanisertib PO daily on days 1-28. Courses repeat every 3 weeks in the absence of disease progression or unacceptable toxicity.

Experimental: Subprotocol N (PTEN mutation or deletion and PTEN expression)

Patients with PTEN mutation or deletion and PTEN expression receive PI3K-beta inhibitor GSK2636771 PO QD on days 1-28. Courses repeat every 28 days in the absence of disease progression or unacceptable toxicity.

Experimental: Subprotocol P (PTEN loss)

Patients with PTEN loss receive PI3K-beta inhibitor GSK2636771 PO QD on days 1-28. Courses repeat every 28 days in the absence of disease progression or unacceptable toxicity.

Experimental: Subprotocol Q (HER2 amplification)

Patients with HER2 amplification receive trastuzumab emtansine intravenously (IV) over 30-90 minutes on day 1. Courses repeat every 21 days in the absence of disease progression or unacceptable toxicity.

Experimental: Subprotocol R (BRAF fusion or BRAF non-V600 mutation)

Patients with BRAF fusion or BRAF non-V600 mutation receive trametinib PO QD on days 1-28. Courses repeat every 28 days in the absence of disease progression or unacceptable toxicity.

Experimental: Subprotocol S1 (NF1 mutation)

Patients with NF1 mutation receive trametinib PO QD on days 1-28. Courses repeat every 28 days in the absence of disease progression or unacceptable toxicity.

Experimental: Subprotocol S2 (GNAQ or GNA11 mutation)

Patients with GNAQ or GNA11 mutation receive trametinib PO QD on days 1-28. Courses repeat every 28 days in the absence of disease progression or unacceptable toxicity.

Experimental: Subprotocol T (SMO or PTCH1 mutation)

Patients with SMO or PTCH1 mutation receive vismodegib PO QD on days 1-28. Courses repeat every 28 days in the absence of disease progression or unacceptable toxicity.

Experimental: Subprotocol U (NF2 inactivating mutation)

Patients with NF2 inactivating mutation receive defactinib PO BID on days 1-28. Courses repeat every 28 days in the absence of disease progression or unacceptable toxicity.

Experimental: Subprotocol V (cKIT exon 9, 11, 13, or 14 mutation)

Patients with cKIT exon 9, 11, 13, or 14 mutation receive sunitinib malate PO QD for 4 weeks. Courses repeat every 6 weeks in the absence of disease progression or unacceptable toxicity.

Experimental: Subprotocol W (FGFR pathway aberrations)

Patients with FGFR1-3 mutation or translocation receive FGFR Inhibitor AZD4547 PO BID on days 1-28. Courses repeat every 28 days in the absence of disease progression or unacceptable toxicity.

Experimental: Subprotocol X (DDR2 S768R, I638F, or L239R mutation)

Patients with DDR2 S768R, I638F, or L239R mutation receive dasatinib PO QD on days 1-28. Courses repeat every 28 days in the absence of disease progression or unacceptable toxicity.

Experimental: Subprotocol Y (Akt mutation)

Patients with Akt mutation receive Akt inhibitor AZD5363 PO BID on days 1-4, 8-11, 15-18, and 22-25. Courses repeat every 28 days in the absence of disease progression or unacceptable toxicity.

Experimental: Subprotocol Z1A (NRAS mutation in codon 12, 13, or 61)

Patients with NRAS mutation in codon 12, 13, or 61 receive binimetinib PO BID on days 1-28. Courses repeat every 28 days in the absence of disease progression or unacceptable toxicity.

Experimental: Subprotocol Z1B (CCND1, 2, or 3 amplification with Rb by IHC)

Patients with CCND1, 2, or 3 amplification that have tumor Rb expression by IHC receive palbociclib PO QD for 21 days. Courses repeat every 28 days in the absence of disease progression or unacceptable toxicity.

Experimental: Subprotocol Z1C (CDK4 or CDK6 amplification and Rb protein)

Patients with CDK4 or CDK6 amplification and tumor Rb protein receive palbociclib PO QD on days 1-21. Courses repeat every 28 days in the absence of disease progression or unacceptable toxicity.

Experimental: Subprotocol Z1D (Loss of MLH1 or MSH2 by IHC)

Patients with mismatch repair deficiency (loss of MLH1 or MSH2 by IHC) receive nivolumab IV over 60 minutes on days 1 and 15 for 4 courses and then on day 1 every 28 days. Courses repeat every 28 days in the absence of disease progression or unacceptable toxicity.

Experimental: Subprotocol Z1E (NTRK1, NTRK2 or NTRK3 gene fusion)

Patients with NTRK1, NTRK2, or NTRK3 gene fusion receive trk inhibitor LOXO-101 PO BID on days 1-28. Courses repeat every 28 days in the absence of disease progression or unacceptable toxicity.

Experimental: Subprotocol Z1I (BRCA1 or BRCA2 gene mutation)

Patients with BRCA1 or BRCA2 gene mutation receive WEE1 inhibitor AZD1775 PO QD for 5 days for 2 weeks. Courses repeat every 21 days in the absence of disease progression or unacceptable toxicity.

Recruitment Information

▦ Recruitment Status

Recruiting

▦ Estimated Enrollment

6452

▦ Completion Date

June 30, 2022

▦ Primary Completion Date

June 30, 2022

▦ Eligibility Criteria

Inclusion Criteria:

- **Women of childbearing potential must have a negative serum pregnancy test within 2 weeks prior to registration; patients that are pregnant or breast feeding are excluded; a female of childbearing potential is any woman, regardless of sexual orientation or whether they have undergone tubal ligation, who meets the following criteria:**
- Has not undergone a hysterectomy or bilateral oophorectomy; or
- Has not been naturally postmenopausal for at least 24 consecutive months (i.e., has had menses at any time in the preceding 24 consecutive months)
- Women of childbearing potential and men must agree to use adequate contraception (hormonal or barrier method of birth control; abstinence) prior to study entry, for the duration of study participation, and for 4 months after completion of study; should a woman become pregnant or suspect while she or her partner is participating in this study, she should inform her treating physician immediately
- **Patients must have histologically documented solid tumors or histologically confirmed diagnosis of lymphoma or multiple myeloma requiring therapy and meet one of the following criteria:**
- Patients must have progressed following at least one line of standard systemic therapy and there must not be other approval/ standard therapy available that has been shown to prolong overall survival (i.e. in a randomized trial against another standard treatment or by comparison to historical controls); patients who cannot receive other standard therapy that has been shown to prolong overall survival due to medical issues will be eligible, if other eligibility criteria are met; if the patient is currently receiving therapy, the clinician must have assessed that the current therapy is no longer benefitting the patient prior to enrolling on MATCH, regardless of whether it is considered standard OR
- Patients for whose disease no standard treatment exists that has been shown to prolong overall survival
- NOTE: No other prior malignancy is allowed except for the following: adequately treated basal cell or squamous cell skin cancer; in situ cervical cancer; adequately treated stage I or II cancer from which the patient is currently in complete remission; any other cancer from which the patient has been disease-free for 5 years
- Patients must have measurable disease
- **Patients must meet one of the following criteria:**

- Patients must have tumor amenable to image guided or direct vision biopsy and be willing and able to undergo a tumor biopsy for molecular profiling; patients with multiple myeloma other than plasmacytomas are to have a bone marrow aspirate to obtain tumor cells; biopsy must not be considered to be more than minimal risk to the patient
- NOTE: Registration to screening steps (Step 0, 2, 4, 6) must occur after stopping prior therapy; there is no specific duration for which patients must be off treatment prior to registration to the relevant screening step (and subsequently, the biopsy), as long as all other eligibility criteria are met OR
- Patient will be undergoing a procedure due to medical necessity during which the tissue may be collected
- NOTE: Registration to screening steps (Step 0, 2, 4, 6) must occur after stopping prior therapy; there is no specific duration for which patients must be off treatment prior to registration to the relevant screening step (and subsequently, the biopsy), as long as all other eligibility criteria are met OR
- **Formalin-fixed paraffin-embedded tumor tissue block(s) are available for submission following pre-registration (not applicable for bone marrow aspirate specimens); criteria for the submission of formalin-fixed paraffin-embedded (FFPE) tissue are:**
- Tissue must have been collected within 6 months prior to pre-registration to Step 0
- **Patient may receive treatment after tissue collection; however, lack of response must be documented prior to Step 1; the following restrictions apply:**
- Enrollment onto another investigational study is not permitted
- Intervening therapy that constitutes a new, molecularly targeted therapy is not permitted; please note, immunotherapy is not considered molecularly targeted
- Continuation of an agent/regimen for which disease progression has been observed prior to biopsy is permitted, including targeted therapy
- A new immunotherapy regimen is permitted; but, lack of response must also be documented prior to registration to Step 0
- Formalin-fixed paraffin-embedded tumor tissue block(s) must meet the minimum requirements OR
- **Results from one of the designated outside laboratories indicate a "rare variant" that is an actionable mutation of interest (aMOI) for specific designated rare variant subprotocols; the following requirements apply:**
- The outside laboratory notified the site that patient may be a potential candidate for MATCH due to a detected "rare variant"
- Patients with an applicable "rare variant" must be able to meet the eligibility criteria for the appropriate subprotocols within 4 weeks following entry on the EAY131 Step 0 screening step
- Registration to Step 0 must occur after stopping prior systemic anti-cancer therapy; there is no specific duration for which patients must be off treatment prior to registration to Step 0, as long as all eligibility criteria are met
- NOTE: Other potential aMOIs that would be eligibility criteria for NON RARE arms, as determined by the above laboratories, are not applicable for direct treatment assignment on MATCH
- NOTE: Tumor tissue for the confirmation of "rare variant" by the MATCH assay is to be submitted, preferably from the same time of collection as that evaluated by the designated outside laboratory
- Patient must not require the use of full dose coumarin-derivative anticoagulants such as warfarin; low molecular weight heparin is permitted for prophylactic or therapeutic use; factor X inhibitors are permitted
- NOTE: Warfarin may not be started while enrolled in the EAY131 study
- Stopping the anticoagulation for biopsy should be per site standard operating procedure (SOP)
- Patients must have Eastern Cooperative Oncology Group (ECOG) performance status =< 1 and a life expectancy of at least 3 months
- Patients must not currently be receiving any other investigational agents
- **Patients must not have any uncontrolled intercurrent illness including, but not limited to:**
- Symptomatic congestive heart failure (New York Heart Association [NYHA] classification of III/IV)
- Unstable angina pectoris or coronary angioplasty, or stenting within 6 months prior to registration to Step 0, 2, 4, 6
- Cardiac arrhythmia (ongoing cardiac dysrhythmias of National Cancer Institute [NCI] Common Terminology Criteria for Adverse Events [CTCAE] version [v]4 grade >= 2)
- Psychiatric illness/social situations that would limit compliance with study requirements
- Intra-cardiac defibrillators
- Known cardiac metastases
- Abnormal cardiac valve morphology (>= grade 2) documented by echocardiogram (ECHO) (as clinically indicated); (subjects with grade 1 abnormalities [i.e., mild regurgitation/stenosis] can be entered on study); subjects with moderate valvular thickening should not be entered on study
- NOTE: To receive an agent, patient must not have any uncontrolled intercurrent illness such as ongoing or active infection; patients with infections unlikely to be resolved within 2 weeks following screening should not be considered for the trial
- Patients must be able to swallow tablets or capsules; a patient with any gastrointestinal disease that would impair ability to swallow, retain, or absorb drug is not eligible
- **Patients who are human immunodeficiency virus (HIV)-positive are eligible if:**
- CD4+ cell count greater or equal to 250 cells/mm^3
- If patient is on antiretroviral therapy, there must be minimal interactions or overlapping toxicity of the antiretroviral therapy with the experimental cancer treatment; for experimental cancer therapeutics with CYP3A/4 interactions, protease inhibitor

therapy is disallowed; suggested regimens to replace protease inhibitor therapy include dolutegravir given with tenofovir/emtricitabine; raltegravir given with tenofovir and emtricitabine; once daily combinations that use pharmacologic boosters may not be used

- No history of non-malignancy acquired immune deficiency syndrome (AIDS)-defining conditions other than historical low CD4+ cell counts

- Probable long-term survival with HIV if cancer were not present

- Any prior therapy, radiotherapy (except palliative radiation therapy of 30 gray [Gy] or less), or major surgery must have been completed >= 4 weeks prior to start of treatment; all adverse events due to prior therapy have resolved to a grade 1 or better (except alopecia and lymphopenia) by start of treatment; palliative radiation therapy must have been completed at least 2 weeks prior to start of treatment; the radiotherapy must not be to a lesion that is included as measurable disease

- NOTE: Prostate cancer patients may continue their luteinizing hormone-releasing hormone (LHRH) agonist

- NOTE: Patients may receive non-protocol treatment after biopsy (if clinically indicated) until they receive notification of results; however, lack of response must be documented prior to registration to Step 1; new non-protocol treatment will NOT be permitted as intervening therapy after registration to Step 0; the decision to stop the intervening non-protocol treatment will be left up to the treating physician if patient has an aMOI; however, patients will need to be off such therapy for at least 4 weeks before receiving any MATCH protocol treatment

- NOTE: For patients entering the study via a designated outside laboratory, no intervening systemic non-protocol treatment is permitted after Step 0 registration; all other eligibility requirements still apply to these patients, including the washouts for prior therapy noted above in this section, the time restrictions outlined, and the eligibility criteria for the intended subprotocol

- Patients with brain metastases or primary brain tumors must have completed treatment, surgery or radiation therapy >= 4 weeks prior to start of treatment

- Patients must have discontinued steroids >= 1 week prior to registration to Step 0 and remain off steroids thereafter, except as permitted (see below); patients with glioblastoma (GBM) must have been on stable dose of steroids, or be off steroids, for one week prior to registration to treatment (Step 1, 3, 5, 7)

- **NOTE: The following steroids are permitted (low dose steroid use is defined as prednisone 10 mg daily or less, or bioequivalent dose of other corticosteroid):**

- Temporary steroid use for computed tomography (CT) imaging in setting of contrast allergy

- Low dose steroid use for appetite

- Chronic inhaled steroid use

- Steroid injections for joint disease

- Stable dose of replacement steroid for adrenal insufficiency or low doses for non-malignant disease

- Topical steroid

- Steroids required to manage toxicity related to study treatment, as described in the subprotocols

- Steroids required as preor post-chemotherapy medication for acceptable intervening chemotherapy

- NOTE: Steroids must be completed alongside last dose of chemotherapy

- Leukocytes >= 3,000/mcL

- Absolute neutrophil count >= 1,500/mcL

- Platelets >= 100,000/mcL

- NOTE: Patients with documented bone marrow involvement by lymphoma are not required to meet the above hematologic parameters, but must have a platelet count of at least 75,000/mcL and neutrophil count of at least 1,000/mcL

- Total bilirubin =< 1.5 X institutional upper limit of normal (ULN) (unless documented Gilbert's syndrome, for which bilirubin =< 3 x institutional ULN is permitted)

- Aspartate aminotransferase (AST) (serum glutamic oxaloacetic transaminase [SGOT])/alanine aminotransferase (ALT) (serum glutamate pyruvate transaminase [SGPT]) =< 2.5 X institutional ULN (up to 5 times ULN in presence of liver metastases)

- Creatinine clearance >= 45 mL/min/1.73 m^2 for patients with creatinine levels above institutional normal

- **Patients must have an electrocardiogram (ECG) within 8 weeks prior to registration to screening step and must meet the following cardiac criteria:**

- Resting corrected QT interval (QTc) =< 480 msec

- NOTE: If the first recorded QTc exceeds 480 msec, two additional, consecutive ECGs are required and must result in a mean resting QTc =< 480 msec; it is recommended that there are 10-minute (+/5 minutes) breaks between the ECGs

- The following only need to be assessed if the mean QTc > 480 msec

- Check potassium and magnesium serum levels

- Correct any identified hypokalemia and/or hypomagnesemia and may repeat ECG to confirm exclusion of patient due to QTc

- For patients with heart rate (HR) 60-100 beats per minute (bpm), no manual read of QTc is required

- For patients with baseline HR < 60 or > 100 bpm, manual read of QT by trained personnel is required, with Fridericia correction applied to determine QTc

- Patient must not have hypokalemia (value < institutional lower limit of normal)

- No factors that increase the risk of QTc prolongation or risk of arrhythmic events such as heart failure, congenital long QT syndrome, family history of long QT syndrome or unexplained sudden death under 40 years of age or any concomitant medication known to prolong the QT interval

- NOTE: Patient must be taken off prohibited medication prior to registration to the screening step (Step 0, 2, 4, 6) and remain off these medications thereafter, unless permitted on a subprotocol for the management of treatment related toxicity; patient must be off the drug for at least 5 half-lives prior to registration to the treatment step (Step 1, 3, 5, 7); the medication half-life can be found in the package insert for Food and Drug Administration (FDA) approved drugs

▧ **Sex/Gender**

All

▧ **Ages**

18 Years to N/A

▧ **Accepts Healthy Volunteers**

No

Regorafenib in Metastatic Colorectal Cancer

Study ID:

NCT02466009

Sponsor:

University of Rochester

Information provided by (Responsible Party):

University of Rochester (University of Rochester)

Tracking Information

▧ **First Submitted Date**

April 9, 2015

▧ **Start Date**

March 2015

▧ **Primary Completion Date**

July 2018

▧ **Last Update Posted Date**

August 24, 2017

▧ **Current Primary Outcome Measures**

Number of subjects who experience grade 3-5 toxicity as a measure of safety and tolerability.[Time Frame: From the date of study entry until 30 days after the last dose of study treatment.]

▧ **Current Secondary Outcome Measures**

Number of subjects who respond to study treatment.[Time Frame: From the date of completion of three cycles of treatment until the date of progression of disease as determined by restaging scans up to 2 years.]

Association of adverse events with the Comprehensive Geriatric Assessments.[Time Frame: From the date of study entry until 30 days after the last dose of study treatment.]

Subject's quality of life as assessed by the Comprehensive Geriatric Assessment form while receiving study treatment.[Time Frame: From the date of study entry until 30 days after the last dose of study treatment.]

Descriptive Information

▧ **Offical Title**

Regorafenib in Adults 70 Years or Older With Metastatic Colorectal Cancer: A Phase II Study

▧ **Brief Summary**

The purpose of the study is to measure high grade (3-5) toxicity of regorafenib and to monitor the impact of treatment with regorafenib on the quality of life in older adults with metastatic colorectal cancer.

▧ **Detailed Description**

Subjects will be asked to participate in the study because they are aged 70 or older and require treatment for colorectal cancer that has spread to other parts of the body and has not gotten better with other treatment. Subjects will undergo some initial tests to ensure that they meet all criteria necessary to participate in the study. Once the subject has completed initial testing and meets eligibility criteria, the subject will begin treatment with 120 mg of regorafenib (3 tablets) each day for 21 days (3 weeks) in a 28 day cycle (4 weeks). After the first cycle, the doctor will discuss the possibility of increasing the dose to 160 mg (4 tablets) each day for 21 days (3 weeks) in a 28 day cycle (4 weeks) based on the subjects health status. During the study, assessments will be performed to monitor the subjects tolerance and response to the treatment. Regorafenib will continue as long as the subject is tolerating the treatment and the subjects colorectal cancer is either responding to treatment or remains stable.

■ **Study Type**

Interventional

■ **Study Phase**

Phase 2

■ **Condition**

- Metastatic Colorectal Cancer

■ **Intervention**

Drug: Regorafenib

Regorafenib 120 mg (3 tablets) each day for 21 days of a 28 day cycle with the possibility of an increase in the dose to 160 mg (4 tablets).

Other Names:

Stivarga

■ **Study Arms**

Experimental: Regorafenib

120 mg qd, 3 weeks on/1 week off (each cycle is 28 days)

Three 40 mg tablets should be taken in the morning with approximately 8 fluid ounces (240 mL) of water after a low-fat (< 30% fat) breakfast.

Recruitment Information

■ **Recruitment Status**

Recruiting

■ **Estimated Enrollment**

60

■ **Completion Date**

July 2018

■ **Primary Completion Date**

July 2018

■ **Eligibility Criteria**

Inclusion Criteria:

- Histologically confirmed colorectal adenocarcinoma
- Measurable metastatic disease.
- Age +/> 70
- Progression on standard therapy, not a candidate for further chemotherapy or patient declines other options
- Life expectancy >/= 12 weeks
- Able to understand and willing to sign written informed consent.
- Laboratory requirements:
- Total bili ≤ 1.5 x upper limit or normal
- Alanine aminotransferase & Asparate aminotransferase ≤ 2.5 x upper limit or normal
- Serum creatinine ≤ 1.5 x upper limit or normal
- International normalized ratio/prothrombin time ≤ 1.5 x upper limit or normal
- Platelet count ≥ 100,000, hemoglobin ≥ 9 g/dL
- Absolute neutrophil count ≥ 1,500. Blood transfusion to meet the inclusion criteria not be allowed.
- Glomerular filtration rate ≥ 60 ml/min
- Subjects of childbearing potential must agree to use adequate contraception beginning at the signing informed consent form until at least 3 months after the last dose of study drug.
- Must be able to swallow and retain oral medications

Exclusion Criteria:

- Currently receiving other systemic therapy for metastatic colorectal cancer
- Previous assignment to treatment during this study. Subjects permanently withdrawn from study participation will not be allowed to re-enter study.
- Uncontrolled hypertension despite optimal medical management
- Active or clinically significant cardiac disease.
- Evidence or history of bleeding diathesis or coagulopathy
- Any hemorrhage or bleeding event ≥ grade 3 within 4 weeks.
- Subjects with thrombotic, embolic, venous, or arterial events, such as cerebrovascular accident, deep vein thrombosis or

pulmonary embolus within 6 months of informed consent
- History of other active malignancy within past 2 years.
- Patients with phaeochromocytoma
- Known history of human immunodeficiency virus infection or current chronic/active hepatitis B or C infection.
- Ongoing infection > grade 2
- Symptomatic metastatic brain or meningeal tumors
- Presence of non-healing wound, non-healing ulcer, or bone fracture
- Renal failure requiring hemoor peritoneal dialysis
- Dehydration ≥ grade 1
- Patients with seizure disorder requiring medication
- Persistent proteinuria ≥ grade 3 Interstitial lung disease with ongoing signs and symptoms at the time of informed consent
- Pleural effusion or ascites that causes respiratory compromise, grade 2 dyspnea
- History of organ allograft including corneal transplant
- Known or suspected allergy or hypersensitivity to the study drug
- Any malabsorption condition
- Any condition which makes the subject unsuitable for trial participation
- Substance abuse, medical, psychological, or social conditions that may interfere with the subject's participation in the study.

■ **Sex/Gender**

All

■ **Ages**

70 Years to N/A

■ **Accepts Healthy Volunteers**

No

■ **Contacts**

Mohamed Tejani, MD   585-275-5863   mohamed   tejani@urmc.rochester.edu
Supriya Mohile, MD   585-275-5863   supriya   mohile@urmc.rochester.edu

Phase I/II Study of the Anti-Programmed Death Ligand-1 Antibody MEDI4736 in Combination With Olaparib and/or Cediranib for Advanced Solid Tumors and Advanced or Recurrent Ovarian, Triple Negative Breast, Lung, Prostate and Colorectal Cancers

Study ID:

NCT02484404

Sponsor:

National Cancer Institute (NCI)

Information provided by (Responsible Party):

National Institutes of Health Clinical Center (CC) (National Cancer Institute (NCI))

Tracking Information

■ **First Submitted Date**

June 25, 2015

■ **Start Date**

June 8, 2015

■ **Primary Completion Date**

December 14, 2018

■ **Last Update Posted Date**

October 19, 2017

Ph I Determine the recommended phase II dose (RP2D) and the safety of doublet therapies of MEDI4736/olaparib (MEDI-O) and MEDI4736/cediranib (MEDI-C) in patients with advanced solid tumors[Time Frame: 28 Days]

Ph II Determine overall response rate of MED-O and MEDI-C in patients with recurrent ovarian cancer[Time Frame: Every 4 wks for Toxicity and every 8 wks for response]

Descriptive Information

■ Offical Title

Phase I/II Study of the Anti-Programmed Death Ligand-1 Antibody MEDI4736 in Combination With Olaparib and/or Cediranib for Advanced Solid Tumors and Advanced or Recurrent Ovarian, Triple Negative Breast, Lung, Prostate and Colorectal Cancers

■ Brief Summary

Background:

- MEDI4736 is a drug that may help people s immune systems respond to and kill cancer cells. Olaparib is a drug that may inhibit repairing DNA damage of cancer cells. Cediranib is a drug that may stop the blood vessel growth of cancer cells. This study has two components. In the phase 1 component of the study, researchers want to investigate how well participants tolerate the combination of these drugs in treating advanced solid tumors, and in the phase 2 part of this study, researchers want to study if the combination treatments are effective in ovarian cancer.

Objectives:

- Phase 1 part of the study: To determine the safety of the combination of MEDI4736 with the drugs olaparib or cediranib.
- Phase 2 part of the study: To determine how effective this combination is in treating ovarian cancer.

Eligibility:

- Phase 1 part of the study: Adults age 18 or older with advanced or recurrent solid tumors that have no standard treatment.
- Phase 2 part of the study: Adults age 18 or older with advanced or recurrent ovarian cancer that has no standard treatment.

Design:

- Participants will be screened with medical history, physical exam, and blood and urine tests. They will have CT or MRI scans. For these, they will lie in a machine that takes pictures of their bodies.
- Phase 2 part of the study requests the participants to have tumor samples removed.
- Participants will get MEDI4636 through an IV. A small plastic tube will be inserted into a vein. The drug will be given every 2 weeks for 12 months.
- Participants will take olaparib or cediranib by mouth every day.
- Every 28 days will be 1 cycle. For cycle 1, participants will have 2 study visits. All other cycles, they will have 1 visit. At these visits, they will repeat the screening procedures.
- Patients will keep a drug and diarrhea diary.
- Patients on cediranib will monitor their blood pressure and keep a blood pressure diary.
- Participants who can become pregnant, or have a partner who can become pregnant, must practice an effective form of birth control.
- After 12 cycles, participants will have 1-3 months of follow-up.

■ Detailed Description

Background:

- Disruption of the immune checkpoint PD-1/PD-L1 pathway yielded clinical activity in subsets of advanced solid tumors, such as melanoma and lung cancer.
- Olaparib (O), a PARP inhibitor (PARPi), has demonstrated single agent activity in recurrent ovarian cancer (OvCa), and subsets of prostate, triple negative breast or lung cancers.
- Our recent randomized phase 2 study showed that O and cediranib (C), a VEGFR1-3 inhibitor was clinically superior to O alone in platinum-sensitive recurrent OvCa.
- We hypothesize that increased DNA damage by PARP inhibition and/or reduced angiogenesis by VEGFR inhibition will complement the anti-tumor activity of an immune checkpoint nhibitor, MEDI4736, in recurrent OvCa and other solid tumors.

Objectives:

- Phase I: To determine the recommended phase II dose (RP2D) and the safety of doublet herapies (MEDI4736/olaparib [MEDI+O] and MEDI4736/cediranib [MEDI+C]) and triplet therapy (MEDI+O+C) in patients with advanced solid tumors.
- Phase II Cohort 1 OvCa; MEDI+O, MEDI+C and MEDI+O+C arms: To determine clinical efficacy as measured by overall response rate (ORR)
- Phase II Cohort 2 non-small cell lung cancer (NSCLC); MEDI+O and MEDI+C arms: To determine clinical efficacy as measured by progression-free survival (PFS)
- Phase II Cohort 3 small cell lung cancer (SCLC); MEDI+O arm: To determine clinical efficacy as measured by ORR
- Phase II Cohort 4 metastatic castrate-resistant prostate cancer (mCRPC); MEDI+O arm: To determine clinical efficacy as

measured by PFS

- Phase II Cohort 5 triple negative breast cancer (TNBC); MEDI+O arm: To determine clinical efficacy as measured by ORR
- Phase II Cohort 6 colorectal cancer (CRC): C+MEDI arm: To determine clinical efficacy as measured by PFS

Eligibility:

- Phase I: Advanced or recurrent solid tumors with evaluable disease.
- Phase II Cohort 1 MEDI+O, MEDI+C and MEDI+O+C arms: Advanced or recurrent OvCa
- Phase II Cohort 2 MEDI+O and MEDI+C arms: Advanced or recurrent NSCLC
- Phase II Cohort 3 MEDI+O arm: Advanced or recurrent SCLC
- Phase II Cohort 4 MEDI+O arm: mCRPC
- Phase II Cohort 5 MEDI+O arm: Advanced or recurrent TNBC
- Phase II Cohort 6 C+MEDI arm: Advanced or recurrent CRC
- Patients must be off prior chemotherapy, radiation therapy or biologic therapy for at least 3 weeks. mCPRC patients (Cohort 4) may be on hormonal therapy with GnRH agonists/antagonists.
- Adults with ECOG performance status 0-2, and adequate organ and marrow function.

Design:

- Phase I: MEDI+O, MEDI+C and MEDI+O+C will dose escalate simultaneously. MEDI4736 will be administered once every 2 weeks or once every 4 weeks until disease progression. O tablets and C will be given orally on a continuous or intermittent dosing schedule. The DLT period will be one cycle, 28 days. Patients on the 2-week schedule greater than one year will be changed to the 4-week schedule until progression.
- MEDI+O: MEDI4736 (3 mg/kg or 10 mg/kg IV every 2 weeks, or a fixed dose of 1500 mg every 4 weeks) and O tablets (150 mg or 200 mg or 300 mg BID)
- MEDI+C: MEDI4736 (3 mg/kg or 10 mg/kg IV every 2 weeks, or a fixed dose of 1500 mg every 4 weeks) and C (15 mg or 20 mg or 30 mg daily or 5 days/week)
- MEDI+O+C: MEDI4736 (a fixed dose of 1500mg every 4 weeks) with O tablets (200 mg or 300 mg BID) and C (15 mg or 20 mg 5 days/week)
- Phase II Cohort 1 OvCa MEDI+O arm: Patients will be treated with MEDI+O at RP2D (O 300mg tablets bid daily and MEDI4736 at 1500 mg IV every 4 weeks.
- Phase II Cohort 1 OvCa MEDI+C arm: Patients will be treated with MEDI+C at RP2D (C 20mg once a day [5 days on/2 days off] and MEDI4736 at 1500 mg every 4 weeks).
- Phase II Cohort 1 OvCa MEDI+O+C arm: Patients with OvCa (Cohort 1) will be treated with RP2D (O tablets 300mg BID, C 20mg once a day [5 days on/2 days off] and MEDI4736 at 1500 mg every 4 weeks).
- Phase II Cohort 2 NSCLC; MEDI+O arm: Patients will be treated with MEDI+O at RP2D (O 300mg tablets bid daily and MEDI4736 at 1500 mg IV every 4 weeks).
- Phase II Cohort 2 NSCLC; MEDI+C arm: Patients will be treated with MEDI+C at RP2D (C 20mg once a day [5 days on/2 days off] and MEDI4736 at 1500 mg every 4 weeks).
- Phase II Cohort 3 SCLC; MEDI+O arm: Patients will be treated with MEDI+O at RP2D (O 300mg tablets bid daily and MEDI4736 at 1500 mg IV every 4 weeks).
- Phase II Cohort 4 mCRPC; MEDI+O arm: Patients will be treated with MEDI+O at RP2D (O 300mg tablets bid daily and MEDI4736 at 1500 mg IV every 4 weeks).
- Phase II Cohort 5 TNBC; MEDI+O arm: Patients will be treated with MEDI+O at RP2D (O 300mg tablets bid daily and MEDI4736 at 1500 mg IV every 4 weeks).
- Phase II Cohort 6 CRC; C+MEDI arm: Patients in the Cohort 6 will be treated with C 20mg daily alone for 14 days followed by the combination at RP2D (C 20mg once a day [5 days on/2 days off] and MEDI4736 at 1500 mg every 4 weeks).
- Phase II Correlative studies: Research samples including whole blood, CTCs, cell free DNA and plasma will be obtained at pretreatment, prior to cycle 1 day 15, prior to cycle 3 day 1 and at progression. Mandatory baseline core biopsy and two optional biopsies will be obtained.
- Patients will be evaluated for toxicity every 4 weeks by CTCAEv4.0, and for response every two cycles (8 weeks) by RECIST 1.1. Patients with mCRPC (MEDI+O Cohort 4) will be evaluated for response initially at 8 weeks then every 12 weeks using RECIST v1.1 criteria as per the Prostate Cancer Clinical Trials Working Group 2 (PCWG2).

Study Type

Interventional

Study Phase

Phase 1/Phase 2

Condition

- Lung Cancer
- Breast Cancer
- Ovarian Cancer
- Colorectal Cancer

- Prostate Cancer
- Triple Negative Breast Cancer

Intervention

Drug: Olaparib

Olaparib tablets will be given orally on a continuous dosing schedule. The DLT period will be one cycle, 28 days.

MEDI4736 (3mg/kg or 10mg/kg IV) and Olaparib tablets (200 mg or 300 mg BID)

Ph II MEDI4736 + Olaparib at RP2D

Drug: Cediranib

Cediranib will be given orally on a continuous dosing schedule. The DLT period will be one cycle, 28 days.

MEDI4736 (10mg/kg IV) and Cediranib (15 mg or 20 mg or 30 mg daily)

Ph II MEDI4736 + Cediranib at RP2D

Drug: MEDI4736

Ph I MEDI4736 will be administered once every 2 weeks for 12 months.

Study Arms

Experimental: P1 MEDI+O
Ph I MEDI4736 + olaparib dose escalation

Experimental: P1 MEDI+C
Ph I MEDI4736 + cediranib dose escalation

Experimental: P2 MEDI+O
Ph II MEDI4736 + olaparib at RP2D

Experimental: P2 MEDI+C
Ph II MEDI4736 + cediranib at RP2D

Experimental: P1 MEDI+O+C
Ph I MEDI4736 + olaparib + cediranib dose escalation

Experimental: P2 MEDI+O+C
Experimental Ph II MEDI4736 + olaparib + cediranib at RP2D

Recruitment Information

Recruitment Status
Recruiting

Estimated Enrollment
421

Completion Date
December 31, 2019

Primary Completion Date
December 14, 2018

Eligibility Criteria

- **INCLUSION CRITERIA GENERAL:**
- Patients must be at least 18 years of age.
- Patients must have adequately controlled blood pressure on a maximum of three antihypertensive medications.
- **Patients who have the following clinical conditions are considered to be at increased risk for cardiac toxicities. Patients with any cardiac history of the following conditions within 1 year prior to study enrollment are excluded from the study:**
- Prior events including myocardial infarction, pericardial effusion, and myocarditis.
- Prior cardiac arrhythmia including atrial fibrillation and atrial flutter, or requiring concurrent use of drugs or biologics with pro-arrhythmic potential.
- NYHA Class II or greater heart failure.
- If cardiac function assessment is clinically indicated or performed, an LVEF less than normal per institutional guidelines, or <55%, if threshold for normal is not otherwise specified by institutional guidelines.
- QTc prolongation >470 msec or other significant ECG abnormality noted within 14 days of treatment.
- Hypertensive crisis or hypertensive encephalopathy.
- Clinically significant peripheral vascular disease or vascular disease, including rapidly growing aortic aneurysm or abdominal aortic aneurysm >5 cm or aortic dissection.
- Unstable angina.

- Eligibility for patients with asymptomatic and a previous diagnosis of immune or inflammatory colitis, or patients with chronic diarrhea > 1 month without immune or inflammatory colitis is a PI decision on an individual patient basis.
- Patients with a history of cerebrovascular accident or transient ischemic attack within 1 year prior to study enrollment are not eligible.
- Patients with a history of previous clinical diagnosis of tuberculosis are not eligible.
- Patients with a history of auto-immune disease requiring steroid maintenance, or history of primary immunodeficiency are not eligible.
- HIV-positive patients on antiretroviral therapy are ineligible because of potential pharmacokinetic interactions with study drugs.
- HBV-or HCV-positive patients are ineligible because of potential reactivation of hepatitis virus following steroids.
- Patients with a history of allergic reactions attributed to compounds of similar chemical or biologic composition to MEDI4736, olaparib, cediranib, or to other humanized monoclonal antibodies, or a history of anaphylaxis, angioedema, laryngeal edema, serum sickness, or uncontrolled asthma, are not eligible.
- Patients who have had prior immune checkpoint inhibitors, such as MEDI4736 or other PD1 or PD-L1 inhibitors or an anti-CTLA4 therapy are not eligible.
- Pregnant and breastfeeding women are excluded from this study.
- Patients with any other concomitant or prior invasive malignancies are ineligible.

PHASE I STUDY ELIGIBILITY CRITERIA
- Patients must have histologically or cytologically confirmed advanced solid tumor that is refractory to standard treatment or for which no standard treatment exists, with evaluable disease.
- Patients are allowed to have received prior PARP inhibitors (PARPi), and/or anti-angiogenesis therapy. However, patients who were treated with both olaparib and cediranib, either in combination or sequentially are not eligible. For this study, BSI-201 (iniparib) is not considered as PARPi.
- PHASE II MEDI4736 PLUS OLAPARIB OR CEDIRANIB STUDY ELIGIBILITY CRITERIA OVARIAN CANCER
- Patients must have histologically or cytologically confirmed persistent or recurrent ovarian, fallopian tube, or primary peritoneal cancer and have received at least two prior platinum-containing regimens or who are platinum resistant or refractory during or after a first platinum containing regimen.
- Patients must have at least one lesion deemed safe to biopsy and be willing to undergo a mandatory baseline biopsy.
- Patients are allowed to have received prior PARPi, and/or anti-angiogenesis therapy including but not limited to thalidomide, bevacizumab, sunitinib, sorafenib, or other anti-angiogenics. However, patients who were treated with both olaparib and cediranib, either in combination or sequentially are not eligible. For this study, BSI-201 (iniparib) is not considered as PARPi.

PHASE II STUDY MEDI4736 PLUS OLAPARIB ELIGIBILITY CRITERIA TRIPLE NEGATIVE BREAST CANCER
- Patients must have histologically confirmed persistent or recurrent triple-negative breast cancer (TNBC)
- ER/PR/HER2 status needs to be documented either by an outside source or at NCI.
- Documentation of germline BRCA1 and BRCA2 mutation (gBRCAm) status will be required for eligibility.
- Patients must have measurable disease as defined by RECIST v1.1.
- Patients must have at least one lesion deemed safe to biopsy and be willing to undergo a mandatory baseline biopsy.
- Patients who have received more than three lines of prior therapy in the metastatic or recurrent settings are not eligible.
- Patients who have received prior PARPi or immune checkpoint inhibitors are ineligible.
- PHASE II MEDI4736 PLUS OLAPARIB OR CEDIRANIB STUDY ELIGIBILITY CRITERIA NON-SMALL CELL LUNG CANCER
- Histologically or cytologically confirmed advanced NSCLC with at least one prior line of platinum-based chemotherapy (or treatment with EGFR or ALK tyrosine kinase inhibitors if tumors harbor an EGFR-sensitizing mutation or ALK translocation respectively).
- Patients must have measurable disease as defined by RECIST v1.1.
- Patients must have at least one lesion deemed safe to biopsy and be willing to undergo a mandatory baseline biopsy.
- Patients who have received anti-angiogenesis therapy are eligible. However, patients who were treated with cediranib, either in combination or monotherapy are not eligible.
- Patients who have had prior PARPi are not eligible.
- Patients who have received more than three lines of prior therapy in the metastatic or recurrent settings are not eligible.
- Patients with prior history of pneumonitis and/or interstitial lung disease will be excluded.
- PHASE II MEDI4736 PLUS OLAPARIB STUDY ELIGIBILITY CRITERIA SMALL CELL LUNG CANCER
- Histologically or cytologically confirmed SCLC with at least one prior line of platinum-based chemotherapy are eligible. Patients with both platinum-sensitive and platinum-refractory disease will be eligible.
- Patients must have measurable disease as defined by RECIST v1.1.
- Patients must have at least one lesion deemed safe to biopsy and be willing to undergo a mandatory baseline biopsy.
- Patients who have received anti-angiogenesis therapy are eligible. However, patients who were treated with cediranib, either in combination or monotherapy are not eligible.
- Patients who have had prior PARPi are not eligible.

- Patients who have received more than three lines of prior therapy in the metastatic or recurrent settings are not eligible.
- Patients with any other concomitant or prior invasive malignancies are ineligible. Patients with prior history of pneumonitis and/or interstitial lung disease will be excluded.
- PHASE II MEDI4736 PLUS OLAPARIB STUDY ELIGIBILITY CRITERIA METASTATIC CASTRATE-RESISTANT PROSTATE CANCER
- Patients must have metastatic, progressive, castrate resistant prostate cancer (mCRPC).
- All patients must have at least one lesion deemed safe to biopsy and be willing to undergo a mandatory baseline biopsy.
- Patients must have received prior treatment with enzalutamide and/or abiraterone.
- Patients must have undergone bilateral surgical castration or must agree to continue on GnRH agonists/antagonists for the duration of the study.
- Patients who have had treatment with docetaxel for the treatment of metastatic castrate-sensitive prostate cancer within 6 months before the first dose of study treatment are not eligible.
- Patients who have had progression of prostate cancer on prior docetaxel treatment for castrate sensitive disease are ineligible.
- Patients who have had prior treatment with PARPi are not eligible.
- Patients who have received radionuclide treatment within 6 weeks prior to the first dose of the study treatment are not eligible.
- Patients with any other concomitant or prior invasive malignancies are ineligible.
- PHASE II MEDI4736 PLUS CEDIRANIB ELIGIBILITY CRITERIA COLORECTAL CANCER
- Histologically or cytologically confirmed advanced colorectal cancer. Patients must have progressed on, been intolerant of or refused prior oxaliplatin and irinotecan-containing chemotherapeutic regimen, and have disease that is not amenable to potentially curative resection. Patients who have a known KRAS wild type tumor must have progressed, been intolerant of or refused cetuximab or panitumumab-based chemotherapy.
- Patients are allowed to have received prior anti-angiogenesis therapy with the exception of prior cediranib. However, patients must not have received other anti-angiogenesis therap(ies) within 6 months prior to study enrollment.
- Patients must be MSI-stable (or low).
- Patients must have at least one focus of metastatic disease that is amenable to pre-and on-treatment biopsy.
- Patients who were previously treated with cediranib are ineligible.
- Patients with any other concomitant or prior invasive malignancies are ineligible.
- Patients with prior history of pneumonitis and/or interstitial lung disease will be excluded.

Additional eligibility criteria may apply as defined per protocol.

Sex/Gender

All

Ages

18 Years to 99 Years

Accepts Healthy Volunteers

No

Contacts

Irene Ekwede, R.N.   (240) 760-6126   ekwedeib@mail.nih.gov

A Study of Enhancing Response to MK-3475 in Advanced Colorectal Cancer

Study ID:

NCT02512172

Sponsor:

Sidney Kimmel Comprehensive Cancer Center

Information provided by (Responsible Party):

Sidney Kimmel Comprehensive Cancer Center (Sidney Kimmel Comprehensive Cancer Center)

Tracking Information

First Submitted Date

July 2, 2015

Start Date

June 2015

■ **Current Primary Outcome Measures**

Degree of change in tumor infiltrating lymphocytes[Time Frame: 1 year]
Change is determined by the number of CD45NO+ cells per high powered field

Descriptive Information

■ **Offical Title**

A Study of Using Epigenetic Modulators to Enhance Response to MK-3475 in Microsatellite Stable Advanced Colorectal Cancer

■ **Brief Summary**

This study is being done to test the safety and effectiveness of the combination of intravenous (IV) romidepsin and/or oral 5-azacitidine with IV MK-3475 in people with microsatellite stable (MSS) advanced colorectal cancer.

■ **Detailed Description**

- This study is being done to test the safety and effectiveness of the combination of intravenous (IV) romidepsin and/or oral CC 486 with IV MK-3475 in people with microsatellite stable advanced colorectal cancer.
- The use of CC 486 in this research study is investigational. The word "investigational" means that the oral form of CC 486 is not approved for marketing by the U.S. Food and Drug Administration (FDA). Oral CC 486 has only been given to a very small number of people so far, and this combination has never before been given together to people.

Romidepsin has been approved by the FDA for the treatment of cutaneous T-cell lymphoma (blood cancer). It is not approved by the FDA for use in other cancers.

MK-3475 is an antibody. Antibodies are proteins that the immune system uses to fight infection. Researchers have designed MK-3475 to block PD-1. PD-1 is a molecule that can shut down an immune response to infection or a cancer cell. An antibody to PD-1 can stop it from turning off an immune response and may be able to boost the immune system against the cancer.

People with advanced colorectal tumors that are microsatellite stable (MSS) may join this study. Tumors that are MSS positive are not deficient in repair of DNA.

- This is a pilot study that will look at different ways of making MSS colorectal tumors sensitive to MK-3475 by giving 14 or 21 days of an epigenetic agent (oral CC 486 and/or romidepsin).

Participants will be randomly assigned (by chance, like drawing numbers from a hat) to one of three study drug combinations:

- A. Oral CC 486 taken daily for 21 days (and later shortened to 14 days if there are side effects) and IV MK-3475 given every 2 weeks.
- B. IV romidepsin given once weekly for 3 weeks and IV MK-3475 given every 2 weeks C. Oral CC 486 taken daily for 21 days (and later shortened to 14 days if there side effects) and IV romidepsin given every 2 weeks and IV MK-3475 given every 2 weeks.

Each arm is repeated every 28 days and will continue until the point that the study drug are no longer working. It will not be possible to cross over onto another arm if a participant's disease does not respond to the study drugs.

In this study investigators are looking for the following information:

- What effects, good and/or bad, the combination of oral CC 486 and/or romidepsin in combination with MK-3475 has on participants' cancer; and
- If the genetic and chemical make-up of participants' blood and tumor cells play a role in a response to oral CC 486 and/or romidepsin in combination with MK-3475.

■ **Study Type**

Interventional

■ **Study Phase**

Phase 1

■ **Condition**

- Colorectal Cancer

■ **Intervention**

- Drug: Oral CC 486
  Other Names:

  oral azacitidine

  oral aza

  Drug: Romidepsin

Other Names:

Istodax

Drug: MK 3475

Other Names:

pembrolizumab

Study Arms

- Experimental: Oral CC 486 & MK-3475

  Oral CC 486 300 mg days 1-14 or 21 every 28 days + IV MK-3475 200 mg days 1 and 15 every 28 days

  Experimental: Romidepsin & MK-3475

  Romidepsin 14 mg/m2 days 1, 8 and 15 + IV MK-3475 200 mg days 1 and 15 every 28 days

- Experimental: Oral CC 486 & Romidepsin & MK-3475

  Oral CC 486 300 mg days 1-14 or 21 + romidepsin 7 mg/m2 (days 1, 8 and 15) + IV MK-3475 200 mg days 1 and 15 every 28 days.

Recruitment Information

Recruitment Status

Recruiting

Estimated Enrollment

30

Completion Date

June 2018

Primary Completion Date

January 2018

Eligibility Criteria

Inclusion Criteria:

1. Have histologically confirmed microsatellite stable metastatic colorectal cancer and have received at least one line of treatment for metastatic colorectal cancer including fluoropyrimidines, oxaliplatin and/or irinotecan

2. Be willing and able to provide written informed consent/assent for the trial

3. Be 18 years of age on day of signing informed consent

4. Have measurable disease

5. Have biopsiable disease. If biopsy is attempted and unsuccessful (the patient undergoes an invasive procedure), the patient may still be treated

6. Have a performance status of 0 or 1 on the ECOG Performance Scale at study entry

7. Demonstrate adequate organ function

8. Female subject of childbearing potential must have a negative urine or serum pregnancy test within 72 hours prior to receiving the first dose of study medication

9. Female subjects of childbearing potential must be willing to use 2 methods of birth control or be surgically sterile, or abstain from heterosexual activity for the course of the study through 120 days after the last dose of study medication

10. Male subjects must agree to use an adequate method of contraception starting with the first dose of study therapy through 120 days after the last dose of study therapy

11. In patients with liver metastases, there should be <50% involvement of the liver.

12. Patients must have had < 3 prior therapies in the metastatic setting.

Exclusion Criteria:

1. Patients whose tumors have progressed at the first restaging during first line therapy

2. Is currently participating in or has participated in a study of an investigational agent or using an investigational device within 4 weeks of the first dose of treatment

3. Has a diagnosis of immunodeficiency or is receiving systemic steroid therapy or any other form of immunosuppressive therapy within 7 days prior to the first dose of trial treatment

4. Has had a prior monoclonal antibody within 4 weeks prior to study Day 1 or who has not recovered from adverse events due to agents administered more than 4 weeks earlier

5. Has had prior chemotherapy, targeted small molecule therapy, or radiation therapy within 4 weeks (6 weeks for nitrosureas or mitomycin C) prior to study Day 1 or who has not recovered from adverse events due to a previously administered agent

6. Has a known additional malignancy that is progressing or requires active treatment

7. Has known central nervous system (CNS) metastases and/or carcinomatous meningitis

8. Has an active autoimmune disease requiring systemic treatment within the past 3 months or a documented history of clinically severe autoimmune disease, or a syndrome that requires systemic steroids or immunosuppressive agents.

9. Has evidence of interstitial lung disease or active, non-infectious pneumonitis.

10. Has an active infection requiring systemic therapy.

11. Any clinical or radiological ascites or pleural effusions

12. Has a history or current evidence of any condition, therapy, or laboratory abnormality that might confound the results of the trial, interfere with the subject's participation for the full duration of the trial, or is not in the best interest of the subject to participate, in the opinion of the treating investigator

13. Has known psychiatric or substance abuse disorders that would interfere with cooperation with the requirements of the trial

14. Is pregnant or breastfeeding, or expecting to conceive or father children within the projected duration of the trial

15. Has received prior therapy with an anti-PD-1, anti-PD-L1, anti-PD-L2, anti-CD137, anti-OX-40, anti-CD40, or anti-Cytotoxic T-lymphocyte-associated antigen-4 (CTLA-4) antibody (including ipilimumab or any other antibody or drug specifically targeting T-cell co-stimulation or checkpoint pathways). Prior therapies with other immunomodulatory agents must be reviewed by the PI and may be cause for ineligibility

16. Has a known history of Human Immunodeficiency Virus (HIV) (HIV 1/2 antibodies)

17. Has known active Hepatitis B or Hepatitis C

18. Has received a live vaccine within 30 days prior to the first dose of trial treatment

19. Any known cardiac abnormalities

Sex/Gender

All

Ages

18 Years to N/A

Accepts Healthy Volunteers

No

Contacts

Rosalind Walker, RN   410-955-9628   rwalker3@jhmi.edu

Amber-Lynn Mitcheltree, BA   410-502-5327   amiche13@jhmi.edu

Efficacy and Tolerability of Suprep With and Without Simethicone for Routine Colonoscopy for Colorectal Cancer Screening

Study ID:

NCT02523911

Sponsor:

Mercy Medical Center, Des Moines, Iowa

Information provided by (Responsible Party):

Mercy Medical Center, Des Moines, Iowa (Mercy Medical Center, Des Moines, Iowa)

Tracking Information

First Submitted Date

August 12, 2015

Start Date

March 2016

Primary Completion Date

July 2019

Last Update Posted Date

August 29, 2017

Current Primary Outcome Measures

Overall bowel cleansing[Time Frame: During procedure]

To be assessed during removal of the colonoscope during the procedure and blinded endoscopist will score using a written questionnaire

Current Secondary Outcome Measures

Number of patients with adverse effects[Time Frame: Day prior to and day of colonoscopy]

A written patient questionnaire will be used to assess patient acceptability and tolerability by recording any adverse effects experienced, including nausea, vomiting, headache, insomnia, bloating, abdominal pain, abdominal discomfort, abdominal cramps or any others.

Number of patients completing the bowel preparation[Time Frame: Day prior to and day of colonoscopy]

A written patient questionnaire will be used to assess compliance by asking if the total prescribed volume of solution was ingested and by recording number of evacuations.

Descriptive Information

▣ Offical Title

Sodium Sulfate/Potassium Sulfate/Magnesium Sulfate Bowel Preparation With and Without Simethicone for Routine Colonoscopy: A Double-blinded Randomized Controlled Trial

▣ Brief Summary

The purpose of this study is to investigate Suprep bowel preparation, with and without the anti-gas medication simethicone, in terms of efficacy and patient tolerability in the preparation of patients undergoing routine colonoscopy for colorectal cancer screening.

▣ Detailed Description

The study will investigate sodium sulfate/potassium sulfate/magnesium sulfate (Suprep), with and without simethicone, in terms of efficacy and patient tolerability in the preparation of patients undergoing routine colonoscopy. Adult ambulatory outpatients who are scheduled for elective routine colonoscopy for colorectal cancer screening will be recruited to participate in the trial. Patients will be randomized to receive either simethicone or placebo in addition to oral sodium sulfate/potassium sulfate/magnesium sulfate solution (Suprep) and will receive verbal and written instruction on administration of solutions. During colonoscopy, three areas of the colon (right colon, transverse colon, and left colon) will be assessed during removal of the colonoscope for overall colon cleansing, presence of bubbles, and degree of haziness; this will be scored by a blinded endoscopist. A separate written patient questionnaire will be used to assess acceptability and tolerability of the preparation, as well as any adverse events.

▣ Study Type

Interventional

▣ Study Phase

N/A

▣ Condition

- Colorectal Cancer

▣ Intervention

Drug: Simethicone

Patients will be randomized to receive either simethicone or placebo in addition to oral sodium sulfate/potassium sulfate/ magnesium sulfate solution (Suprep), and will be blinded to whether they are in the simethicone arm or the placebo arm of the trial. Simethicone and placebo will be prepared as identically-appearing liquid solution (2.4 mL) with the assistance of a pharmacist. The simethicone or placebo solution will then be assigned to patients according to the randomization scheme and samples will be labeled with patient information prior to distribution. Only the pharmacist will participate in the labeling process and know which patients receive simethicone or placebo; administering staff, nurses, physicians, and patients will be blinded to this.

Other Names:

Gas-X Infant Drops

Infants Gas Relief

Infants Simethicone

Infants' Mylicon

Drug: Placebo

Patients will be randomized to receive either simethicone or placebo in addition to oral sodium sulfate/potassium sulfate/ magnesium sulfate solution (Suprep), and will be blinded to whether they are in the simethicone arm or the placebo arm of the trial. Simethicone and placebo will be prepared as identically-appearing liquid solution (2.4 mL) with the assistance of a pharmacist. The simethicone or placebo solution will then be assigned to patients according to the randomization scheme and samples will be labeled with patient information prior to distribution. Only the pharmacist will participate in the labeling process and know which patients receive simethicone or placebo; administering staff, nurses, physicians, and patients will be blinded to this.

Other Names:

Inert solution

Drug: sodium sulfate/potassium sulfate/magnesium sulfate solution

Both arms will receive sodium sulfate/potassium sulfate/magnesium sulfate solution for bowel preparation

Other Names:

Suprep Bowel Prep Kit

Study Arms

Active Comparator: Simethicone Group

Early in the evening prior to colonoscopy, patients will be instructed to consume one 6 ounce bottle of oral sodium sulfate/potassium sulfate/magnesium sulfate (Suprep) solution (containing sodium sulfate 17.5 grams, potassium sulfate 3.13 grams, and magnesium sulfate 1.6 grams) diluted with 16 ounces of water over one hour. Over the next hour, the patient will be instructed to drink an additional 32 ounces of water. On the day of colonoscopy, the same procedure will be repeated. Patients will take 2.4 mL simethicone in a half glass of water immediately after consuming each dose of the Suprep. All of the bowel preparation solution and required water should be consumed at least 2 hours prior to colonoscopy.

Placebo Comparator: Placebo Group

Early in the evening prior to colonoscopy, patients will be instructed to consume one 6 ounce bottle of oral sodium sulfate/potassium sulfate/magnesium sulfate (Suprep) solution (containing sodium sulfate 17.5 grams, potassium sulfate 3.13 grams, and magnesium sulfate 1.6 grams) diluted with 16 ounces of water over one hour. Over the next hour, the patient will be instructed to drink an additional 32 ounces of water. On the day of colonoscopy, the same procedure will be repeated. Patients will take 2.4 mL of placebo (identical in appearance to simethicone) in a half glass of water immediately after consuming each dose of the Suprep. All of the bowel preparation solution and required water should be consumed at least 2 hours prior to colonoscopy.

Publications

(Includes publications given by the data provider as well as publications identified by ClinicalTrials.gov Identifier (NCT Number) in Medline.)Valiante F, Bellumat A, De Bona M, De Boni M. Bisacodyl plus split 2-L polyethylene glycol-citrate-simethicone improves quality of bowel preparation before screening colonoscopy. World J Gastroenterol. 2013 Sep 7;19(33):5493-9. doi: 10.3748/wjg.v19.i33.5493. (https://www.ncbi.nlm.nih.gov/pubmed/24023492)

Gentile M, De Rosa M, Cestaro G, Forestieri P. 2 L PEG plus ascorbic acid versus 4 L PEG plus simethicon for colonoscopy preparation: a randomized single-blind clinical trial. Surg Laparosc Endosc Percutan Tech. 2013 Jun;23(3):276-80. doi: 10.1097/SLE.0b013e31828e389d. (https://www.ncbi.nlm.nih.gov/pubmed/23751992)

Pontone S, Angelini R, Standoli M, Patrizi G, Culasso F, Pontone P, Redler A. Low-volume plus ascorbic acid vs high-volume plus simethicone bowel preparation before colonoscopy. World J Gastroenterol. 2011 Nov 14;17(42):4689-95. doi: 10.3748/wjg.v17.i42.4689. (https://www.ncbi.nlm.nih.gov/pubmed/22180711)

Jansen SV, Goedhard JG, Winkens B, van Deursen CT. Preparation before colonoscopy: a randomized controlled trial comparing different regimes. Eur J Gastroenterol Hepatol. 2011 Oct;23(10):897-902. doi: 10.1097/MEG.0b013e32834a3444. (https://www.ncbi.nlm.nih.gov/pubmed/21900786)

Park JJ, Lee SK, Jang JY, Kim HJ, Kim NH. The effectiveness of simethicone in improving visibility during colonoscopy. Hepatogastroenterology. 2009 Sep-Oct;56(94-95):1321-5. (https://www.ncbi.nlm.nih.gov/pubmed/19950784)

Tongprasert S, Sobhonslidsuk A, Rattanasiri S. Improving quality of colonoscopy by adding simethicone to sodium phosphate bowel preparation. World J Gastroenterol. 2009 Jun 28;15(24):3032-7. (https://www.ncbi.nlm.nih.gov/pubmed/19554657)

Sudduth RH, DeAngelis S, Sherman KE, McNally PR. The effectiveness of simethicone in improving visibility during colonoscopy when given with a sodium phosphate solution: a double-bind randomized study. Gastrointest Endosc. 1995 Nov;42(5):413-5. (https://www.ncbi.nlm.nih.gov/pubmed/8566629)

Lazzaroni M, Petrillo M, Desideri S, Bianchi Porro G. Efficacy and tolerability of polyethylene glycol-electrolyte lavage solution with and without simethicone in the preparation of patients with inflammatory bowel disease for colonoscopy. Aliment Pharmacol Ther. 1993 Dec;7(6):655-9. (https://www.ncbi.nlm.nih.gov/pubmed/8161673)

Shaver WA, Storms P, Peterson WL. Improvement of oral colonic lavage with supplemental simethicone. Dig Dis Sci. 1988 Feb;33(2):185-8. (https://www.ncbi.nlm.nih.gov/pubmed/3338367)

Wexner SD, Beck DE, Baron TH, Fanelli RD, Hyman N, Shen B, Wasco KE; American Society of Colon and Rectal Surgeons; American Society for Gastrointestinal Endoscopy; Society of American Gastrointestinal and Endoscopic Surgeons. A consensus document on bowel preparation before colonoscopy: prepared by a task force from the American Society of Colon and Rectal Surgeons (ASCRS), the American Society for Gastrointestinal Endoscopy (ASGE), and the Society of American Gastrointestinal and Endoscopic Surgeons (SAGES). Gastrointest Endosc. 2006 Jun;63(7):894-909. Erratum in: Gastrointest Endosc. 2006 Jul;64(1):154. (https://www.ncbi.nlm.nih.gov/pubmed/16733101)

Chiu HM, Lin JT, Wang HP, Lee YC, Wu MS. The impact of colon preparation timing on colonoscopic detection of colorectal neoplasms--a prospective endoscopist-blinded randomized trial. Am J Gastroenterol. 2006 Dec;101(12):2719-25. Epub 2006 Oct 6. (https://www.ncbi.nlm.nih.gov/pubmed/17026559)

McNally PR, Maydonovitch CL, Wong RK. The effect of simethicone on colonic visibility after night-prior colonic lavage. A double-blind randomized study. J Clin Gastroenterol. 1989 Dec;11(6):650-2. (https://www.ncbi.nlm.nih.gov/pubmed/2584664)

McNally PR, Maydonovitch CL, Wong RK. The effectiveness of simethicone in improving visibility during colonoscopy: a double-blind randomized study. Gastrointest Endosc. 1988 May-Jun;34(3):255-8. (https://www.ncbi.nlm.nih.gov/pubmed/3292345)

Wu L, Cao Y, Liao C, Huang J, Gao F. Systematic review and meta-analysis of randomized controlled trials of Simethicone for gastrointestinal endoscopic visibility. Scand J Gastroenterol. 2011 Feb;46(2):227-35. doi: 10.3109/00365521.2010.525714. Epub 2010 Oct 26. Review. (https://www.ncbi.nlm.nih.gov/pubmed/20977386)

Recruitment Information

Recruitment Status
Recruiting

Estimated Enrollment
800

Eligibility Criteria

Inclusion Criteria:

- Age greater than 18 years
- Outpatients who require elective colonoscopy for colorectal cancer screening at Iowa Endoscopy Center and at University of Florida Jacksonville

Exclusion Criteria:

- Allergy or hypersensitivity to any constituent of the lavage solution or to simethicone
- Presence of any contraindication to colonoscopy (i.e. uncontrolled congestive heart failure, New York Heart Association classification III-IV, history of myocardial infarction within 6 months, coagulopathy)
- Massive ascites
- Renal insufficiency
- Pregnancy
- History of colonic surgery
- History of anti-flatulence or laxative agent within one week
- Refusal/inability to give consent
- Patients undergoing colonoscopy for reasons other than colorectal cancer screening
- Mentally disabled
- Non-English-speaking patients

Sex/Gender
All

Ages
18 Years to N/A

Accepts Healthy Volunteers
Accepts Healthy Volunteers

Contacts
Tercio Lopes, MD   Limongister@gmail.com

Completion Date
July 2019

Primary Completion Date
July 2019

Basket Study of Entrectinib (RXDX-101) for the Treatment of Patients With Solid Tumors Harboring NTRK 1/2/3 (Trk A/B/C), ROS1, or ALK Gene Rearrangements (Fusions)

Study ID:
NCT02568267

Sponsor:
Ignyta, Inc.

Information provided by (Responsible Party):
Ignyta, Inc. (Ignyta, Inc.)

Tracking Information

First Submitted Date
October 2, 2015

Start Date
October 2015

Primary Completion Date
October 2019

Last Update Posted Date
February 12, 2018

Current Primary Outcome Measures

Objective Response Rate[Time Frame: Approximately 24 months]
Assessed by blinded independent central review (BICR) using RECIST v1.1

Current Secondary Outcome Measures

Duration of Response[Time Frame: Approximately 24 months]
Assessed by blinded independent central review (BICR) using RECIST v1.1

Time to Response[Time Frame: Approximately 24 months]
Assessed by blinded independent central review (BICR) using RECIST v1.1

Clinical Benefit Rate[Time Frame: Approximately 24 months]
Assessed by blinded independent central review (BICR) using RECIST v1.1

Intracranial Tumor Response[Time Frame: Approximately 24 months]
Assessed by blinded independent central review (BICR) using RANO or RANO-BM, as applicable

CNS Progression-free Survival[Time Frame: Approximately 24 months]
Assessed by blinded independent central review (BICR) using RANO or RANO-BM, as applicable

Progression-free Survival[Time Frame: Approximately 30 months]
Assessed by Kaplan-Meier method

Overall Survival[Time Frame: Approximately 36 months]
Assessed by Kaplan-Meier method

Descriptive Information

Offical Title

An Open-Label, Multicenter, Global Phase 2 Basket Study of Entrectinib for the Treatment of Patients With Locally Advanced or Metastatic Solid Tumors That Harbor NTRK1/2/3, ROS1, or ALK Gene Rearrangements

Brief Summary

This is an open-label, multicenter, global Phase 2 basket study of entrectinib (RXDX-101) for the treatment of patients with solid tumors that harbor an NTRK1/2/3, ROS1, or ALK gene fusion. Patients will be assigned to different baskets according to tumor type and gene fusion.

Study Type

Interventional

Study Phase

Phase 2

Condition

- Breast Cancer
- Cholangiocarcinoma
- Colorectal Cancer
- Head and Neck Neoplasms
- Lymphoma, Large-Cell, Anaplastic
- Melanoma
- Neuroendocrine Tumors
- Non-Small Cell Lung Cancer
- Ovarian Cancer
- Pancreatic Cancer
- Papillary Thyroid Cancer
- Primary Brain Tumors
- Renal Cell Carcinoma
- Sarcomas
- Salivary Gland Cancers
- Adult Solid Tumor

Intervention

Drug: Entrectinib

TrkA/B/C, ROS1, and ALK inhibitor

Other Names:
RXDX-101

Study Arms

Experimental: NTRK1/2/3-rearranged NSCLC
Oral entrectinib (RXDX-101)

Experimental: ROS1-rearranged NSCLC
Oral entrectinib (RXDX-101)

- Experimental: ALKor ROS1-rearranged NSCLC
with CNS-only progression previously treated with crizotinib

Oral entrectinib (RXDX-101)

Experimental: NTRK/1/2/3-rearranged mCRC
Oral entrectinib (RXDX-101)

Experimental: ROS1-rearranged mCRC
Oral entrectinib (RXDX-101)

Experimental: ALK-rearranged mCRC
Oral entrectinib (RXDX-101)

Experimental: NTRK1/2/3-rearranged other solid tumor
Oral entrectinib (RXDX-101)

Experimental: ROS1-rearranged other solid tumor
Oral entrectinib (RXDX-101)

Experimental: ALK-rearranged other solid tumor
Oral entrectinib (RXDX-101)

Recruitment Information

Recruitment Status

Recruiting

Estimated Enrollment

300

Completion Date

October 2020

Primary Completion Date

October 2019

Eligibility Criteria

Inclusion Criteria:

- Histologicallyor cytologically-confirmed diagnosis of locally advanced or metastatic solid tumor that harbors an NTRK1/2/3, ROS1, or ALK gene rearrangement
- Note: Patients diagnosed with anaplastic large cell lymphoma (ALCL) harboring a gene rearrangement of interest may be eligible provided they meet all other inclusion/exclusion criteria
- For patients enrolled via local molecular testing, an archival or fresh tumor tissue (unless medically contraindicated) is required to be submitted for independent central molecular testing at Ignyta's CLIA laboratory post-enrollment
- Measurable or evaluable disease
- Patients with CNS involvement, including leptomeningeal carcinomatosis, which is either asymptomatic or previously-treated and controlled, are allowed
- Prior anticancer therapy is allowed (excluding approved or investigational Trk, ROS1, or ALK inhibitors in patients who have tumors that harbor those respective gene rearrangements)
- Note: prior treatment with crizotinib is permitted only in ALKor ROS1-rearranged NSCLC patients presenting with CNS-only progression. Other ALK inhibitors are prohibited.
- At least 2 weeks or 5 half-lives, whichever is shorter, must have elapsed after prior chemotherapy or small molecule targeted therapy
- At least 4 weeks must have elapsed since completion of antibody-directed therapy
- Prior radiotherapy is allowed if more than 14 days have elapsed since the end of treatment
- Eastern Cooperative Oncology Group (ECOG) performance status ≤ 2 and minimum life expectancy of 4 weeks
- Adequate organ function as defined per protocol
- Ability to swallow entrectinib intact
- Other protocol specified criteria

Exclusion Criteria:

- Current participation in another therapeutic clinical trial
- Prior treatment with approved or investigational Trk, ROS1, or ALK inhibitors in patients who have tumors that harbor those respective gene rearrangements
- Note: prior treatment with crizotinib is permitted only in ALKor ROS1-rearranged NSCLC patients presenting with CNS-only progression. Other ALK inhibitors are prohibited.
- History of other previous cancer that would interfere with the determination of safety or efficacy
- Incomplete recovery from any surgery
- History of non-pharmacologically induced prolonged QTc interval
- History of additional risk factors for torsade de pointes
- Peripheral neuropathy Grade ≥ 2
- Known active infections
- Active gastrointestinal disease or other malabsorption syndromes
- Known interstitial lung disease, interstitial fibrosis, or history of tyrosine kinase inhibitor-induced pneumonitis
- Other protocol specified criteria

▩ **Sex/Gender**

All

▩ **Ages**

18 Years to N/A

▩ **Accepts Healthy Volunteers**

No

▩ **Contacts**

Ignyta Inc.   1-844-782-7875   STARTRKtrials@ignyta.com

Oxaliplatin Microdosing Assay in Predicting Exposure and Sensitivity to Oxaliplatin-Based Chemotherapy

Study ID:

NCT02569723

Sponsor:

University of California, Davis

Information provided by (Responsible Party):

University of California, Davis (University of California, Davis)

Tracking Information

▩ **First Submitted Date**

July 27, 2015

▩ **Start Date**

October 2015

▩ **Primary Completion Date**

December 2018

▩ **Last Update Posted Date**

January 9, 2018

▩ **Current Primary Outcome Measures**

Feasibility of 14C Oxaliplatin Microdose as a clinical assay to predict oxaliplatin exposure[Time Frame: 0-5 minutes predose, 5, 15, and 30 minutes, and at 1, 2, 4, 8, and 24 hours after carbon C 14 oxaliplatin microdose]

  Correlate area under curve from phase 0 microdosing with area under curve for therapeutic dose of oxaliplatin

▩ **Current Secondary Outcome Measures**

Duration of disease control (DDC) according to RECIST 1.1[Time Frame: Up to 2 years]

  Will characterize the repair of DNA adducts in PBMC, using descriptive statistics.

Incidence of adverse events according to the Common Terminology Criteria for Adverse Events version 4[Time Frame: Up to 2 years]

  Assess toxicity to both microdoses of carbon C 14 oxaliplatin. Toxicities potentially related to carbon C 14 oxaliplatin will be assessed from initiation of the study to at least 14 days after the administration of the FOLFOX-integrated microdose or until full recover of toxicity (whichever is longer). Safety will be assessed through summaries of adverse events and laboratory evaluations.

Response rate per Response Evaluation Criteria in Solid Tumors (RECIST) 1.1[Time Frame: Up to 2 years]

Will characterize the repair of DNA adducts in peripheral blood mononuclear cell (PBMC).

Descriptive Information

▦ Offical Title

Pilot Study of a Carbon 14 Oxaliplatin Microdosing Assay to Predict Exposure and Sensitivity to Oxaliplatin-Based Chemotherapy in Advanced Colorectal Cancer

▦ Brief Summary

This pilot clinical trial studies how well carbon C 14 oxaliplatin microdosing assay works in predicting exposure and sensitivity to oxaliplatin-based chemotherapy in patients with colorectal cancer that has spread to other places in the body and usually cannot be cured or controlled with treatment. Drugs used in chemotherapy, such as oxaliplatin, work in different ways to stop the growth of tumor cells, either by killing the cells, by stopping them from dividing, or by stopping them from spreading. Carbon C 14 is a radioactive form of carbon, exists in nature and in the body at a low level. Microdose carbon C 14 oxaliplatin diagnostic assay may help doctors understand how well patients respond to treatment and develop individualize oxaliplatin dosing in patients with colorectal cancer.

▦ Detailed Description

PRIMARY OBJECTIVES:

I. To evaluate the feasibility of [14C] (carbon C 14) oxaliplatin microdose as a clinical assay to predict oxaliplatin exposure.

SECONDARY OBJECTIVES:

I. To estimate the degree to which a [14C]oxaliplatin microdose predicts the observed pharmacokinetics of standard dose oxaliplatin.

II. To validate that intrapatient variation of exposure to a [14C]oxaliplatin microdose is less than 5%.

III. To detect the levels of oxaliplatin-deoxyribonucleic acid (DNA) adducts induced by oxaliplatin microdosing in peripheral blood mononuclear cells (PBMCs), and correlate the results with patient response and progression free survival on oxaliplatin-based chemotherapy.

IV. To develop preliminary safety data of [14C]oxaliplatin microdosing for future studies.

OUTLINE:

Patients receive carbon C 14 oxaliplatin microdose intravenously (IV) over 120 minutes. Beginning not more than 4 weeks after the initial carbon C 14 oxaliplatin microdose administration, patients receive FOLFOX comprised of leucovorin calcium IV, fluorouracil IV over 2 hours (over 46-48 hours via ambulatory infusion pump on days 1 and 2), and oxaliplatin (contain carbon C 14 microdose course I only) IV over 2 hours on day 1. Courses repeat every 14 days in the absence of disease progression or unacceptable toxicity.

After completion of study treatment, patients are followed up periodically.

▦ Study Type

Interventional

▦ Study Phase

N/A

▦ Condition

- Colon Adenocarcinoma

▦ Intervention

Drug: Carbon C 14 Oxaliplatin
 Intravenous infusion

Other Names:
 [14C] Oxaliplatin

Drug: Oxaliplatin

Intravenous infusion

Other Names:
 Eloxatin

▦ Study Arms

Experimental: carbon C 14 oxaliplatin and oxaliplatin

Patients receive carbon C 14 oxaliplatin microdose IV over 120 minutes. Beginning not more than 4 weeks after the initial carbon C 14 oxaliplatin microdose administration, patients receive FOLFOX6 comprised of leucovorin calcium IV, fluorouracil IV over 2 hours (over 46-48 hours via ambulatory infusion pump on days 1 and 2), and oxaliplatin (contain carbon C 14 microdose course I only) IV over 2 hours on day 1.

Recruitment Information

■ **Recruitment Status**

Recruiting

■ **Estimated Enrollment**

6

■ **Completion Date**

December 2020

■ **Primary Completion Date**

December 2018

■ **Eligibility Criteria**

Inclusion Criteria:

- Histologically or cytologically confirmed locally advanced or metastatic colon or rectal adenocarcinoma
- Intent to treat the patient with a leucovorin calcium, fluorouracil, and oxaliplatin (FOLFOX) chemotherapy regimen containing fluorouracil (5-FU), leucovorin, and oxaliplatin according to clinical standard practice; the intent should be to dose oxaliplatin at 85 mg/m^2 on an every 2 week basis
- Treatment with any additional Food and Drug Administration (FDA)-approved biologic agent (i.e. bevacizumab, cetuximab, or panitumumab) is allowed according to standard practice
- Prior radiation or surgery is allowed, but should be finished at least 2 weeks prior to study enrollment; if a participant has prior radiation therapy, at least one measurable lesion outside of the radiation field should be available for the evaluation of response to chemotherapy
- Any number of prior therapies other than oxaliplatin is allowed
- Zubrod performance status equal to or less than 2 (Karnofsky equal to or greater than 50%)
- Life expectancy of at least 3 months
- Absolute neutrophil count greater than or equal to 1,500/microL
- Platelets greater than or equal to 100,000/microL
- Total bilirubin less than 3 x institutional upper limit of normal (ULN)
- Aspartate aminotransferase (AST) (serum glutamic oxaloacetic transaminase) less than or equal to 5 x ULN
- Creatinine less than 1.5 x ULN
- Women of child bearing potential must not be pregnant; a pre-study pregnancy test must be negative
- Women of child-bearing potential must agree to use adequate contraception (hormonal or barrier method of birth control; abstinence) prior to study entry and for 30 days after study participation
- Men must agree to use adequate contraception (barrier method or abstinence) prior to study entry and for 30 days after study participation
- Ability to understand and willing to sign a written informed consent document

Exclusion Criteria:

- Prior treatment with oxaliplatin
- Patients must not receive concomitant radiation
- Uncontrolled intercurrent illness including, but not limited to, ongoing or active infection, symptomatic congestive heart failure, unstable angina pectoris, cardiac arrhythmia, or psychiatric illness/social situations that would limit compliance with study requirements
- Participants who are pregnant or nursing
- Participants who are allergic to any platinum agent
- Participants who have more than grade 1 peripheral neuropathy

■ **Sex/Gender**

All

■ **Ages**

18 Years to N/A

■ **Accepts Healthy Volunteers**

No

A Study of Toca 511, a Retroviral Replicating Vector, Combined With Toca FC in Patients With Solid Tumors or Lymphoma (Toca 6)

Study ID:

NCT02576665

Sponsor:

Tocagen Inc.

Information provided by (Responsible Party):

Tocagen Inc. (Tocagen Inc.)

Tracking Information

▦ **First Submitted Date**

October 12, 2015

▦ **Start Date**

July 2016

▦ **Primary Completion Date**

April 2019

▦ **Last Update Posted Date**

January 9, 2018

▦ **Current Primary Outcome Measures**

Changes from baseline in immune activity in tumor and peripheral blood[Time Frame: Baseline to Weeks 9-10]

Descriptive Information

▦ **Offical Title**

A Phase 1b Study of Toca 511, a Retroviral Replicating Vector, Combined With Toca FC in Patients With Solid Tumors or Lymphoma

▦ **Brief Summary**

The purpose of this trial is to evaluate changes in immune activity relative to baseline following treatment with Toca 511 and Toca FC in patients with solid tumors (including recurrent high grade glioma [rHGG]) or lymphoma. This is a multicenter, open-label study of Toca 511 and Toca FC. Patients with advanced solid tumors or lymphoma, for whom curative options are not available, will be enrolled into the study, subject to all entry criteria. Tumors must be accessible to biopsy and/or resection. Patients will be qualified based on the presence of specific molecular characteristics, documented by Foundation Medicine (or equivalent) genomic profile report, and specific tumor types.

Toca 511 will be administered by IV injection followed by (1) intratumoral injection following biopsy or (2) injection into the resection cavity wall following planned resection in the case of rHGG or brain metastases. Toca FC will be administered orally in cycles of therapy.

Patients not undergoing resection of brain tumors will undergo 2 biopsies to allow assessment of baseline and follow-up immune activity in the tumor. Changes in immune activity in peripheral blood will be measured in all patients.

▦ **Study Type**

Interventional

▦ **Study Phase**

Phase 1

▦ **Condition**

- Colorectal Cancer
- Triple Negative Breast Cancer
- Pancreatic Cancer
- Non-Small Cell Lung Cancer
- Head and Neck Cancer
- Ovarian Cancer
- Lymphoma
- Sarcoma
- Bladder Cancer
- Melanoma
- IDH1 Mutated Solid Tumors
- IDH1 Mutated or MGMT Methylated Recurrent HGG (Not Recruiting)

Intervention

Biological: Toca 511

Toca 511 consists of a purified retroviral replicating vector encoding a modified yeast cytosine deaminase (CD) gene. The CD gene converts the antifungal 5-fluorocytosine (5FC) to the anticancer drug 5-FU in cells that have been infected by the Toca 511 vector

Other Names:

vocimagene amiretrorepvec

RRV

retroviral replicating viral

Drug: Toca FC

Toca FC is an extended-release formulation of flucytosine. Toca FC is supplied as 500 mg white, oblong tablets with "TOCA FC" embossed on one side and "500" embossed on the other side

Other Names:

Flucytosine

5-FC

5-Fluorocytosine

Study Arms

Experimental: Toca 511/Toca FC

Toca 511: 14 mL intravenously daily for 3 days followed by up to 4 mL intratumorally or into resection cavity walls following biopsy or resection. Cutaneous melanoma patients may receive intralesional injections (up to 4 mL) daily for 5 days.

Toca FC: 220 mg/kg/day orally starting at Week 5-6. Cycles are 5to 7day courses of treatment every 4 to 6 weeks.

Recruitment Information

Recruitment Status

Recruiting

Estimated Enrollment

30

Completion Date

November 2019

Primary Completion Date

April 2019

Eligibility Criteria

Inclusion Criteria:

1. Patient has given written informed consent.

2. Patient is between 18 and 75 years of age, inclusive.

3. Patient has an advanced malignancy that has progressed or recurred following standard therapy for advanced disease, and for which no curative therapies are available.

4. Patient has histologically confirmed (1) colorectal cancer, triple negative breast cancer, pancreatic cancer, non-small cell lung cancer, head and neck cancer, ovarian cancer, lymphoma, sarcoma, bladder cancer, or melanoma with defects in one or more of the following genes: ABL2, ACVR1B, APC, ASXL1, ATM, ATR, BLM, BRCA1, BRCA2, CDK12, CDKN1A, CDKN1B, CDKN2A, CHD4, CYLD, DICER1, DNMT3A, ERBB3, EZH2, FGFR2, FLT3, GATA3, HGF, KDM6A, KDR, KEAP1, KIT, KMT2D, KRAS, MAGI2, MAP3K1, MED12, MET, MSH-2, MSH-6, MYC, NA, NF1, NF2, NOTCH1, NOTCH2, NRAS, NSD1, PIK3C2B, PIK3CA, PIK3CB, PIK3R1, PTCH1, PTPN11, RB1, RUNX1, SETD2, SMARCA4, SOX9, STAG2, TAF1, TBX3, TET2, TP53, XPO1; (2) documented IDH1 mutated solid tumor (other than glioma); or (3) documented IDH1 mutated or MGMT promoter methylation positive glioblastoma multiforme (GBM) or anaplastic astrocytoma. Note: Genetic abnormalities must be documented by Foundation Medicine (or equivalent) genomic profile report.

5. Patient has an estimated life expectancy of at least 6 months.

6. Patient has adequate organ function, as indicated by the following laboratory values

- Bone marrow: hemoglobin ≥ 10 g/dL, platelet count ≥ 100,000/mm3, absolute neutrophil count ≥ 1,500/ mm3, absolute lymphocyte count ≥ 500/ mm3.
- Liver: total bilirubin ≤ 1.5 x the upper limit of normal (ULN; unless known Gilbert's syndrome); alanine aminotransferase ≤ 2.5 x ULN (≤ 5.0 x ULN in patients with liver metastases).
- Kidney: estimated glomerular filtration rate (Cockcroft-Gault) ≥ 50 mL/min.

7. Women of childbearing potential (defined as not postmenopausal [ie, ≥ 12 months of non-therapy-induced amenorrhea] or not surgically sterile) must have a negative serum pregnancy test within 21 days prior to initiation of Toca 511, and be willing to use an effective means of contraception in addition to barrier methods (condoms).

8. Patient and partner are willing to use condoms for 12 months after receiving Toca 511 or until there is no evidence of the virus in his/her blood, whichever is longer.

9. Patients with solid tumors or lymphoma must have 1 or more tumors accessible to biopsy or resection, including biopsy allowing multiple cores from at least 1 lesion (fine needle aspiration is excluded), incisional or excisional biopsy, and/or resection. Note: Patients with resectable brain metastases must be undergoing planned resection. Patients with rHGG must be undergoing planned subtotal or gross total resection.

10. Patient has a tumor amenable to injection of Toca 511 (ie, ≥ 2 cm and not close to or invading major vessels).

11. Patient has an ECOG Performance Status score of 0 or 1 (solid tumors) or KPS score ≥ 70 (rHGG).

12. Patient has measurable disease by RECIST version 1.1 (solid tumors) or Lugano (lymphoma) criteria or evaluable or measureable disease by Macdonald criteria (rHGG).

13. Patients with GBM or anaplastic astrocytoma must be at first or second recurrence (including this recurrence) or have progressed following initial definitive multimodal therapy with surgery, temozolomide, and radiation (confirmed by diagnostic biopsy with local pathology review or contrast-enhanced magnetic resonance imaging [MRI]). If first recurrence is documented by MRI, an interval of at least 12 weeks after the end of prior radiation therapy is required, unless there is either histopathologic confirmation of recurrent tumor or new enhancement on MRI outside the radiotherapy treatment field.

Exclusion Criteria:

1. Patient has a history of other malignancy, unless the patient has been disease free for at least 5 years. Adequately treated basal cell carcinoma or squamous cell skin cancer is acceptable regardless of time, as well as localized prostate carcinoma or cervical carcinoma in situ, after curative treatment.

2. Patient has or had any active infection requiring antibiotic, antifungal, or antiviral therapy within the 2 weeks prior to administration of Toca 511.

3. Patient received chemotherapy within 2 weeks prior to initiation of treatment with Toca 511 (6 weeks for nitrosoureas).

4. Patient received investigational treatment within 2 weeks or immunotherapy or antibody therapy within 28 days prior to initiation of treatment with Toca 511, and/or has not recovered from toxicities associated with such treatment.

5. For patients with rHGG, the patient intends to undergo treatment with the Gliadel® wafer at the time of planned resection (ie, on-study surgery) or has received the Gliadel wafer < 30 days from the date of planned resection.

6. Patient has any bleeding diathesis, or must take anticoagulants or antiplatelet agents, including nonsteroidal anti inflammatory drugs, that cannot be stopped for biopsy or surgery.

7. Patient has severe pulmonary, cardiac, or other systemic disease, specifically:

- New York Heart Association > Class II congestive heart failure that is not controlled on standard therapy within 6 months prior to initiation of treatment with Toca 511.

- Uncontrolled or significant cardiovascular disease, clinically significant ventricular arrhythmia (such as ventricular tachycardia, ventricular fibrillation, or Torsades de pointes), clinically significant pulmonary disease (such as ≥ Grade 2 dyspnea, according to CTCAE 4.03).

- Any other disease, either metabolic or psychological, that as per Investigator assessment may affect the patient's compliance or place the patient at an increased risk of potential treatment complications.

8. Patient has a history of allergy or intolerance to flucytosine.

9. Patient has a condition that would prevent him or her from being able to swallow Toca FC tablets or absorb flucytosine.

10. Patient is human immunodeficiency virus seropositive.

11. Patient is breast feeding.

12. Patient has previously participated in the Toca 5 trial (Tg 511-15-01).

■ **Sex/Gender**

All

■ **Ages**

18 Years to 75 Years

■ **Accepts Healthy Volunteers**

No

■ **Contacts**

Jolene Shorr   (858) 412-8467   jshorr@tocagen.com
Mary Lovely   (858) 412-8473   mlovely@tocagen.com

Feasibility of the LUM Imaging System for Detection of Gastrointestinal Cancers

Study ID:

NCT02584244

Sponsor:

Lumicell, Inc.

Information provided by (Responsible Party):

Lumicell, Inc. (Lumicell, Inc.)

Tracking Information

■ **First Submitted Date**

October 16, 2015

■ **Start Date**

May 2016

■ **Primary Completion Date**

February 2018

■ **Last Update Posted Date**

December 7, 2017

■ **Current Primary Outcome Measures**

Determine optimal dose of LUM015 to be used according to tissue type based on optimal LUM015 activity in normal versus tumor tissue.[Time Frame: 1 day]

■ **Current Secondary Outcome Measures**

Assess toxicity in patients with gastrointestinal cancers by monitoring adverse events, including clinically significant abnormalities in CBC and serum chemistry tests from injection until first post-operative visit[Time Frame: 2 weeks]

Determine initial efficacy of LUM015 in labeling gastrointestinal cancers for molecular imaging by comparing imaging results with pathology.[Time Frame: 1 day]

Descriptive Information

■ **Offical Title**

Feasibility of the LUM Imaging System for Detection of Gastrointestinal Cancers

■ **Brief Summary**

The overall goal of this feasibility study is to assess the initial safety and efficacy of LUM015 in ex vivo far-red imaging of colorectal, pancreatic, and esophageal cancers (adenocarcinoma) using the LUM 2.6 Imaging Device.

■ **Detailed Description**

The overall goal of this feasibility study is to assess the initial safety and efficacy of a novel, intravenously administered cathepsin activatable imaging probe, LUM015, in ex vivo far-red imaging of colorectal, pancreatic, and esophageal cancers (adenocarcinoma) using the LUM 2.6 Imaging Device.

All subjects will have an established diagnosis of colorectal, pancreatic, or esophageal adenocarcinoma and are scheduled for resection of their primary tumors.

Patients will be seen by their surgeon in an office visit and undergo routine preoperative testing within four weeks of their planned surgery. During the pre-surgery visit a complete history and physical examination and standard of care pre-operative laboratory studies (including ECG) will be performed. On the day of their planned surgery, LUM015 will be administered by bolus intravenous injection 2-6 hours prior to surgery in the preoperative area. The patient will be monitored for adverse events until discharged from the hospital. Follow up of subjects will continue until their first post-operative visit.

Patients will undergo their planned surgical resection 2-6 hours after LUM015 is administered. All the surgical specimens (whether containing normal tissue or tumor tissue) will be sent to the pathology suite for imaging with the LUM 2.6 Imaging Device and routine diagnostic assessment. Imaged areas showing high fluorescence will be marked to guide pathology evaluation and determine whether the area contains tumor. Samples of imaged areas showing low fluorescence signal will also be evaluated by pathology to determine whether the area only contains normal tissue. After imaging, part of this tissue will be fresh frozen for correlative studies.

The patients are expected to be admitted to the hospital for the surgical procedure and remain in the hospital post-surgery as indicated and required by the surgeon per standard of care treatment. While in the hospital, the patient will be assessed for adverse events. Laboratory studies will also be performed during this time as a part of routine post-surgical care and to assess for any imaging agent related adverse events.

■ **Study Type**

Interventional

Study Phase

Phase 1/Phase 2

Condition

- Colorectal Cancer
- Pancreatic Cancer
- Esophageal Cancer

Intervention

Drug: LUM015

   Device: LUM 2.6 Imaging Device

Study Arms

Experimental: LUM Imaging System

   The first 3 patients will be injected at a dose of 0.5 mg/kg. If no or minimal activity is observed and no serious adverse events occur, the subsequent three patients will be injected with the second tier dose level of 1.0 mg/kg. If no or minimal activity is observed in in the second tier dosing group, and no serious adverse events occur, the following three patients will have the third tier dose of 1.5 mg/kg administered. An additional 12 patients will be recruited at the dose level that produces optimal LUM015 activity. Patients will undergo their planned surgical resection 2-6 hours after LUM015 injection. All surgical specimens will be sent to the pathology suite for imaging with the LUM 2.6 Imaging Device and routine diagnostic assessment.

Recruitment Information

Recruitment Status

Recruiting

Estimated Enrollment

21

Completion Date

March 2018

Primary Completion Date

February 2018

Eligibility Criteria

Inclusion Criteria:

1. Subjects must have histologically or cytologically confirmed esophageal, colorectal or pancreatic adenocarcinoma (inclusive of high grade dysplasia) on a biopsy prior to surgery and must be scheduled for surgical resection, inclusive of endoscopic mucosal resection, of the primary tumor. Subjects at any cancer stage will be enrolled.

2. Subjects may have previously received pre-operative radiation therapy.

3. Age of 18 years or older.

4. Subjects must be able and willing to follow study procedures and instructions.

5. Subjects must have received and signed an informed consent form.

6. Subjects must be sufficiently healthy to undergo surgery or an endoscopic procedure.

7. Subjects must have normal organ and marrow function as defined below:

- Leukocytes > 3,000/mcL
- Absolute neutrophil count > 1,500/mcL
- Platelets > 100,000/mcL
- total bilirubin within normal institutional limits (except in cases of malignant biliary obstruction)
- AST (SGOT)/ALT (SGPT) < 2.5 X institutional upper limit of normal
- Creatinine within normal institutional limits or creatinine clearance > 60 mL/min/1.73 m2 for subjects with creatinine levels above institutional normal.

8. Women of child-bearing potential must agree to use adequate contraception (hormonal or barrier method of birth control, abstinence) starting the day entering the study, and for 60 days after injection of the imaging agent. Should a woman become pregnant or suspect she is pregnant while participating in this study, she should inform her treating physician immediately.

9. Subjects with ECOG performance status of 0 or 1.

Exclusion Criteria:

1. Subjects who have taken an investigational drug within 30 days of enrollment.

2. Subjects with QTc interval > 480ms.

3. Subjects who have not recovered from adverse events due to pharmaceutical or diagnostic agents administered more than 4 weeks earlier.

4. Subjects with uncontrolled hypertension defined as persistent systolic blood pressure > 180 mm Hg, or diastolic blood pressure > 110 mm Hg; those subjects with known HTN should be under these values while under pharmaceutical therapy

5. History of anaphylactic reaction attributed to any contrast agent or drugs containing polyethylene glycol (PEG).

6. Pregnant women or lactating women

7. Subjects who are sexually active and not willing/able to use medically acceptable forms of contraception upon entering the study.

8. HIV-positive individuals on combination antiretroviral therapy.

9. Any subject for whom the investigator feels participation is not in the best interest of the subject.

10. Subjects previously treated with systemic therapies to treat cancer, such as neo-adjuvant chemotherapy or hormonal therapy.

Sex/Gender

All

Ages

18 Years to N/A

Accepts Healthy Volunteers

No

Contacts

Jorge Ferrer, Ph.D   617-571-0592   jmferrr@lumicell.com
Lori Gilmartin   lgilmartin@lumicell.com

A Study to Assess the Safety, Tolerability and Anti-tumour Activity of Ascending Doses of Selumetinib in Combination With MEDI4736 and Selumetinib in Combination With MEDI4736 and Tremelimumab in Patients With Advanced Solid Tumours

Study ID:

NCT02586987

Sponsor:

AstraZeneca

Information provided by (Responsible Party):

AstraZeneca (AstraZeneca)

Tracking Information

First Submitted Date

September 21, 2015

Primary Completion Date

October 5, 2018

Start Date

December 28, 2015

Last Update Posted Date

December 21, 2017

Current Primary Outcome Measures

Safety and tolerability of Selumetinib in combination with MEDI4736, and in combination with MEDI4736+ tremelimumab by assessment of Adverse Events[Time Frame: From screening until approximately 30 days after last dose of study drug at disease progression]

Safety and tolerability of Selumetinib in combination with MEDI4736, and in combination with MEDI4736+ tremelimumab by assessment of safety laboratory tests[Time Frame: From screening until approximately 30 days after last dose of study drug at disease progression]

Safety and tolerability of Selumetinib in combination with MEDI4736, and in combination with MEDI4736+ tremelimumab by assessment of blood pressure (BP)[Time Frame: From screening until approximately 30 days after last dose of study drug at disease progression]

Safety and tolerability of Selumetinib in combination with MEDI4736, and in combination with MEDI4736+ tremelimumab by assessment of Electrocardiogram (ECG)[Time Frame: From screening until approximately 30 days after last dose of study drug at disease progression]

Safety and tolerability of Selumetinib in combination with MEDI4736, and in combination with MEDI4736+ tremelimumab by assessment of physical examinations[Time Frame: From screening until approximately 30 days after last dose of study drug at disease progression]

Safety and tolerability of Selumetinib in combination with MEDI4736, and in combination with MEDI4736+ tremelimumab by assessment of Echocardiogram (ECHO)[Time Frame: From screening until approximately 30 days after last dose of study drug at disease progression]

Safety and tolerability of Selumetinib in combination with MEDI4736, and in combination with MEDI4736+ tremelimumab by assessment of pulse[Time Frame: From screening until approximately 30 days after last dose of study drug at disease progression]

Safety and tolerability of Selumetinib in combination with MEDI4736, and in combination with MEDI4736+ tremelimumab by assessment of body temperature[Time Frame: From screening until approximately 30 days after last dose of study drug at disease progression]

Safety and tolerability of Selumetinib in combination with MEDI4736, and in combination with MEDI4736+ tremelimumab by assessment of respiratory rate[Time Frame: From screening until approximately 30 days after last dose of study drug at disease progression]

Safety and tolerability of Selumetinib in combination with MEDI4736, and in combination with MEDI4736+ tremelimumab by assessment of Multigated Acquisition (MUGA)[Time Frame: From screening until approximately 30 days after last dose of study drug at disease progression]

Safety and tolerability of Selumetinib in combination with MEDI4736, and in combination with MEDI4736+ tremelimumab by assessment of Ophthalmic examination (best corrected visual acuity)[Time Frame: From screening until approximately 30 days after last dose of study drug at disease progression]

Safety and tolerability of Selumetinib in combination with MEDI4736, and in combination with MEDI4736+ tremelimumab by assessment of Ophthalmic examination (Intraocular pressure)[Time Frame: From screening until approximately 30 days after last dose of study drug at disease progression]

Safety and tolerability of Selumetinib in combination with MEDI4736, and in combination with MEDI4736+ tremelimumab by assessment of Ophthalmic examination (slit lamp fundoscopy)[Time Frame: From screening until approximately 30 days after last dose of study drug at disease progression]

Current Secondary Outcome Measures

Long-term tolerated dose and exposure predicted to result in biological activity (including but not limited to Response Evaluation Criteria in Solid Tumours (RECIST)[Time Frame: From screening until 30 days after last dose of study drug at disease progression, approximately 6 months however there is no maximum duration of treatment]

Objective response rate (ORR)[Time Frame: From screening until 30 days after last dose of study drug at disease progression, approximately 6 months however there is no maximum duration of treatment]

Change in tumour size[Time Frame: From screening until 30 days after last dose of study drug at disease progression, approximately 6 months however there is no maximum duration of treatment]

Best Objective Response (BoR)[Time Frame: From screening until 30 days after last dose of study drug at disease progression, approximately 6 months however there is no maximum duration of treatment]

Duration of Response (DoR)[Time Frame: From screening until 30 days after last dose of study drug at disease progression, approximately 6 months however there is no maximum duration of treatment]

Progression-free survival (PFS)[Time Frame: From screening until 30 days after last dose of study drug at disease progression, approximately 6 months however there is no maximum duration of treatment]

Overall survival (OS)[Time Frame: From screening until 30 days after last dose of study drug at disease progression, approximately 6 months however there is no maximum duration of treatment]

MEDI4736 and/or tremelimumab anti-drug antibody (ADA) level in Plasma[Time Frame: From screening until 30 days after last dose of study drug at disease progression, approximately 6 months however there is no maximum duration of treatment]

Descriptive Information

Offical Title

A Phase I, Open-Label, Multi-Centre Study to Assess the Safety, Tolerability and Preliminary Anti-tumour Activity of Ascending Doses of Selumetinib (AZD6244 Hyd-sulfate) in Combination With MEDI4736 and Selumetinib in Combination With MEDI4736 and Tremelimumab in Patients With Advanced Solid Tumours

Brief Summary

This is a Phase I, open-label, multi-centre, drug combination study of double and triple combination oral selumetinib (AZD6244 Hyd-sulfate) plus intravenous (IV) MEDI4736 and oral selumetinib plus IV MEDI4736 and IV tremelimumab in patients with advanced solid tumours.

Detailed Description

This is a Phase I, open-label, multi-centre, drug combination study of double and triple combination oral selumetinib (AZD6244 Hyd-sulfate) plus intravenous (IV) MEDI4736 and oral selumetinib plus IV MEDI4736 and IV tremelimumab in patients with advanced solid tumours refractory to standard therapy or for which no standard therapy exists. The safety, tolerability, and preliminary anti-tumour activity of ascending doses of Selumetinib (AZD6244 Hyd-sulfate) in Combination with MEDI4736 and Selumetinib in Combination with MEDI4736 and Tremelimumab will be investigated. Once safety and tolerability have been established for the relevant dose, expansion cohorts will commence in order to further evaluate safety, tolerability, and provide a preliminary evaluation of the mechanism of action and anti-tumour activity of the drug combination. Mandatory paired biopsy expansion cohorts will be tumour-type specific. Expansion cohorts will open independently for double and triple combination treatments.

Study Type

Interventional

Study Phase

Phase 1

Condition

- Lung Cancer
- Melanoma
- Head and Neck Carcinoma
- Gastroesophageal Cancer
- Breast Cancer
- Pancreatic Adenocarcinoma
- Colorectal Cancer
- Biliary Tract Cancer

Intervention

Drug: Selumetinib

Selumetinib oral

Drug: MEDI4736

MEDI4736 IV

Drug: Tremelimumab

Tremelimumab, IV

Study Arms

Experimental: Dose escalation: Selumetinib+MEDI4736

An oral formulation of selumetinib will be administered in combination with an IV dose of MEDI4736. 4 cohorts of double combination (Selumetinib+MEDI4736).

The decision to escalate to the next dose level/cohort will be made by the Safety Review Committee (SRC) following the completion of the dose limiting toxicity (DLT) assessment period for at least 3 evaluable patients in each cohort.

Experimental: Mandatory paired biopsy expansion cohort: Selumetinib+MEDI4736

One or more independent mandatory paired biopsy expansion cohorts for double combination treatment will start after safety and tolerability have been established for the relevant dose. It will be tumour-type specific for double combination, the tumor type will be determined from emerging data.

Experimental: Dose escalation: Selumetinib+MEDI4736+tremelimumab

An oral formulation of selumetinib will be administered in combination with an IV dose of MEDI4736 and an IV dose of tremelimumab.

For triple combination treatment, the starting dose of selumetinib (DL1) will be determined by the SRC based on emerging data from dose escalation cohorts of double combination treatment.

Experimental: Mandatory paired biopsy expansion cohort: triple combination

One or more independent mandatory paired biopsy expansion cohorts for triple combination treatment will start after safety and tolerability have been established for the relevant dose. It will be tumour-type specific for triple combination, the tumor type will be determined from emerging data.

Recruitment Information

Recruitment Status

Recruiting

Estimated Enrollment

60

Completion Date

October 5, 2018

Primary Completion Date

October 5, 2018

Eligibility Criteria

Inclusion Criteria:

1. Written informed consent and any locally-required authorization (eg, Health Insurance Portability and Accountability Act in the US, EU Data Privacy Directive in the EU) obtained from the patient prior to performing any protocol-related procedures, including pre-screening and screening evaluations

2. Age ≥18 years at time of study entry

3. Histological or cytological confirmation of locally advanced (stage IIIB) or metastatic (stage IV) solid tumours refractory to standard therapy or for which no standard therapy exists

4. World Health Organisation Eastern Cooperative Oncology Group (ECOG) performance status 0-1 with no deterioration over the previous 2 weeks and minimum life expectancy of 12 weeks

5. At least 1 lesion, not previously irradiated, that can be accurately measured at baseline as ≥10 mm in the longest diameter (except lymph nodes which must have short axis ≥15 mm) with computed tomography (CT) or magnetic resonance imaging (MRI) and which is suitable for accurate repeated assessment as per Response Evaluation Criteria in Solid Tumours (RECIST criteria v1.1)

6. Female patients and males with partners of childbearing potential should be using highly effective contraceptive measures. Females should not be breastfeeding and must have a negative pregnancy test prior to start of dosing if of childbearing potential or must have evidence of non-childbearing potential by fulfilling 1 of the criteria below at screening.

- Postmenopausal defined as aged more than 50 years and amenorrhoeic for at least 12 months following cessation of all exogenous hormonal treatments
- Women <50 years old would be considered postmenopausal if they have been amenorrheic for the past 12 months or more following cessation of exogenous hormonal treatments. The levels of luteinising hormone (LH) and follicle stimulating hormone (FSH) must also be in the postmenopausal range (as per the institution)
- Documentation of irreversible surgical sterilisation by hysterectomy and / or bilateral oophorectomy and/or bilateral salpingectomy but not tubal ligation

7. Male patients should be willing to use barrier contraception ie, condoms plus spermicide

8. Mandatory provision of tumour tissue sample available at study entry for exploratory biomarker research. Cytology samples for this exploratory biomarker research will not be acceptable

9. Patients must have mCRC and, if MSI status is known, non-high MSI status. MSI status will be evaluated based on previous results of local MSI testing, if available. Patients with known MSI-high status will be excluded; patients with MSS, MSI-low, or unknown MSI status may be enrolled

Exclusion Criteria:

Patients must not enter the study if any of the following exclusion criteria are fulfilled

1. Previous enrolment in the present study

2. Treatment with any of the following:

- Cytotoxic chemotherapy or other anticancer drugs within 28 days of the 1st dose of study treatment or any investigational agents within 5 half-lives of the product
- MEDI4736 or selumetinib in the present study (ie, dosing with MEDI4736 or selumetinib previously initiated in this study)
- Major surgical procedure, (excluding placement of vascular access) or significant traumatic injury within 4 weeks of the 1st dose of study treatment, or have an anticipated need for major surgery during the study
- Palliative radiotherapy with a wide field of radiation within 4 weeks or radiotherapy with a limited field of radiation for palliation within 2 weeks of the 1st dose of study treatment
- Prior exposure to immune-mediated therapy, including, but not limited to, other anti-CTLA4 (Cytotoxic T-lymphocyte antigen-4), anti-PD-1 (Programmed cell death 1), anti-PD-L1 (Programmed cell death ligand 1), or anti-PD-L2 (Programmed cell death ligand 2) antibodies, including therapeutic anticancer vaccines
- Receipt of live attenuated vaccine within 30 days prior to the first dose of IP
- Concurrent enrolment in another clinical study, unless it is an observational (non-interventional) clinical study or during the follow-up period of an interventional study

3. Any unresolved toxicity NCI CTCAE (National Cancer Institute Common Terminology Criteria for Adverse Events) Grade ≥2 from previous anticancer therapy with the exception of alopecia, vitiligo, and the laboratory values defined in the inclusion criteria

- Patients with Grade ≥2 neuropathy will be evaluated on a case-by-case basis and may be included after consultation with the medical monitor
- Patients with irreversible toxicity not reasonably expected to be exacerbated by treatment with selumetinib, MEDI4736 or tremelimumab may be included after consultation with the medical monitor

4. History of leptomeningeal carcinomatosis and brain metastases or spinal cord compression. Patients with suspected brain metastases at screening should have a CT / MRI of the brain prior to study entry

5. Active or prior documented autoimmune or inflammatory disorders (including inflammatory bowel disease [eg, colitis or Crohn's disease], diverticulitis [with the exception of diverticulosis], celiac disease, irritable bowel disease, or other serious GI (Gastrointestinal) chronic conditions associated with diarrhoea, systemic lupus erythematosus, Sarcoidosis syndrome, or Wegener syndrome [eg, granulomatosis with polyangiitis, Graves' disease; rheumatoid arthritis, hypophysitis, uveitis]) within the past 3 years prior to the start of treatment. The following are exceptions to this

criterion:

- Patients with vitiligo or alopecia
- Patients with hypothyroidism (eg, following Hashimoto syndrome) stable on hormone replacement or psoriasis not requiring systemic treatment

6. History of active primary immunodeficiency

7. **Current or prior use of immunosuppressive medication within 14 days before the 1st dose of MEDI4736. The following are exceptions to this criterion:**

- Intranasal, inhaled, topical steroids, or local steroid injections (eg, intra-articular injection)
- Systemic corticosteroids at physiologic doses not to exceed 10 mg/day of prednisone or its equivalent
- Steroids as premedication for hypersensitivity reactions (eg, CT scan premedication)

8. As judged by the investigator, any evidence of severe or uncontrolled systemic diseases, including uncontrolled hypertension, renal transplant, active bleeding diatheses, which in the investigator's opinion makes it undesirable for the patient to participate in the study or which would jeopardise compliance with the protocol or active infection including hepatitis B surface antigen (HBsAg), hepatitis C virus (HCV) antibody or human immunodeficiency virus (HIV) or known history of clinical diagnosis of tuberculosis

9. Screening for chronic conditions is not required

10. **Any of the following cardiac criteria:**

- Any factors that increase the risk of QT(ECG interval measured from the onset of the QRS complex to the end of the T wave) interval corrected for heart rate (QTc) prolongation or risk of arrhythmic events (eg, heart failure, hypokalaemia, congenital long QT syndrome, family history of long QT syndrome or unexplained sudden death under 40 years of age) or mean QTc >470 msec
- Uncontrolled hypertension (eg, BP ≥150/95 mmHg despite medical therapy)
- Acute coronary syndrome within 6 months prior to starting treatment
- Angina Canadian Cardiovascular Society Grade II-IV (despite medical therapy)
- Symptomatic heart failure (New York Heart Association II-IV)
- Prior or current cardiomyopathy
- Baseline LVEF (Left ventricular ejection fraction) <55% measured by echocardiography or MUGA. Appropriate correction to be used if a MUGA is performed.
- Atrial fibrillation with a ventricular rate >100 beats per minute at rest
- Severe valvular heart disease

11. **Any of the following ophthalmic criteria:**

- Current or past history of central serous retinopathy, detachment of retinal pigmented epithelium, or retinal vein occlusion
- Intraocular pressure (IOP) >21 mmHg
- Uncontrolled glaucoma (irrespective of IOP)

12. **Inadequate bone marrow reserve or organ function as demonstrated by any of the following laboratory values:**

- Absolute neutrophil count <1.5 x 109/L
- Platelet count <100 x 109/L
- Haemoglobin <90 g/L
- Alanine aminotransferase >2.5 x ULN (upper limit of normal) if no demonstrable liver metastases or >5 times ULN in the presence of liver metastases
- Aspartate aminotransferase >2.5 x ULN if no demonstrable liver metastases or >5 times ULN in the presence of liver metastases
- Serum bilirubin ≤1.5 x ULN. This will not apply to patients with confirmed Gilbert's syndrome (persistent or recurrent hyperbilirubinaemia [predominantly unconjugated bilirubin] in the absence of evidence of haemolysis or hepatic pathology), who will be allowed in consultation with their physician
- Creatinine clearance <50 mL/min (calculated by Cockcroft and Gault equation). Confirmation of creatinine clearance is only required when creatinine is >1.5 times ULN

13. Refractory nausea and vomiting, chronic GI diseases, inability to swallow the formulated product or previous significant bowel resection that would preclude adequate absorption of selumetinib

14. History of hypersensitivity to active or inactive excipients of MEDI4736 or selumetinib or drugs with a similar chemical structure or class to MEDI4736 or selumetinib

15. Judgment by the investigator that the patient should not participate in the study if the patient is unlikely to comply with study procedures, restrictions, and requirements

16. Involvement in the planning and conduct of the study (applies to both AZ staff or staff at the study site)

17. Previous allogeneic bone marrow transplant

18. Body weight <30 kg

■ **Sex/Gender**

All

Ages

18 Years to 99 Years

Accepts Healthy Volunteers

No

Contacts

AstraZeneca Clinical Study Information Center   1-877-240-9479   information.center@astrazeneca.com

Astrazeneca Cancer Study Locator Service   1-877-400-4656   Astrazeneca@emergingmed.com

L-Menthol Infusion as a Novel Technique During Colonoscopy

Study ID:

NCT02588248

Sponsor:

University Hospitals Cleveland Medical Center

Information provided by (Responsible Party):

University Hospitals Cleveland Medical Center (University Hospitals Cleveland Medical Center)

Tracking Information

First Submitted Date

October 6, 2015

Start Date

June 2016

Current Primary Outcome Measures

Adenoma Detection Rates[Time Frame: 2 weeks]
   Collected and recorded after pathology results are made available

Current Secondary Outcome Measures

Procedure time[Time Frame: immediate]
   Change in procedure time with compare to placebo

Advanced adenoma detection rates[Time Frame: 2 weeks]
   Collected and recorded after pathology results are made available

Cancer detection rates[Time Frame: 2 weeks]
   Collected and recorded after pathology results are made available

Patient comfort level recorded on post-procedure survey[Time Frame: 1 day]
   Pt reported comfort level recorded on post-procedure survey

Polyp Detection Rates[Time Frame: 2 weeks]
   Collected and recorded after pathology results are made available

Primary Completion Date

June 2017

Last Update Posted Date

November 30, 2016

Descriptive Information

Offical Title

L-Menthol Infusion as a Novel Technique During Colonoscopy: The MINT-C Study

Brief Summary

The primary objective of this double-blinded, prospective, randomized placebo-controlled study is to evaluate for change in endoscopic adenoma detection rates (ADR) with the use of peppermint oil solution vs placebo application during colonoscopy. The investigators hypothesize that ADR will be increased with the use of the peppermint oil solution and thus further reduce the risk of colon cancer by means of colonoscopy.

Detailed Description

Adult subjects who are undergoing colonoscopy for primary colorectal cancer screening or surveillance. The study will be carried out as a prospective, double-blinded, fully-masked randomized controlled trial. Prior to the trial entry, the participant's labs and medical record will be reviewed in the electronic records system. If the subject meets inclusion/exclusion criteria, he or she will be consented at bedside prior undergoing their scheduled procedure and receive standard care as otherwise. Experimental and placebo solution ingredients will be serially numbered and randomized in a 1:1 ratio using a variable block strategy and provided by the institutional investigational pharmacy. Research staff will draw up experimental or placebo solution in 4 syringes with a total of 20mL in each solution.

The solutions are identical in appearance and endoscopic delivery. To prevent olfactory detection of the peppermint oil solution an essential oil diffuser will be used in all endoscopy rooms using the same oil as in the experimental solution. Endoscopists will be instructed to deliver the contents of one syringe sprayed via the endoscope in the cecum and one in the sigmoid colon. The contents of the other two syringes are to be delivered at the discretion of the endoscopist. After the procedure, endoscopists and study participants will be surveyed to determine if blinding was effective and to assess patient comfort levels, respectively. The primary and secondary end points will be determined on an intention to treat basis.

Study Type

Interventional

Study Phase

Phase 3

Condition

- Colonic Polyps
- Colon Cancer

Intervention

Drug: Peppermint Oil
    Other Names:
    L-Menthol
    Other: Placebo

Study Arms

Experimental: Peppermint Oil
    1.6% Peppermint oil solution

Placebo Comparator: Placebo
    standard water solution

Recruitment Information

Recruitment Status

Recruiting

Estimated Enrollment

300

Completion Date

June 2017

Primary Completion Date

June 2017

Eligibility Criteria

Inclusion Criteria:

1. At least 50 years of age in Caucasians or 45 years of age in African-Americans.

2. Patients undergoing primary screening colonoscopy (either average risk or increased-risk) or surveillance colonoscopy after prior screening/surveillance colonoscopy.

3. Capable of understanding instructions, adhering to study schedules and requirements, and willing to provide informed consent.

Exclusion Criteria:

1. History of colectomy, partial or complete

2. Symptoms suggesting possible colorectal stenosis or cancer

3. Inflammatory bowel disease

4. Familial polyposis syndromes

5. History of, or current diagnosis of colorectal cancer

6. American Society of Anesthesia Physical Stats (ASA PS) score of IV or greater

7. Non-correctable coagulopathy

8. Currently receiving anti-thrombotic therapy, with an INR > 1.5

9. Poor prep, total BBPS score < 6, or any part of the colon < 2.

10. Patients with known allergy to peppermint oil or peppermint containing products.

11. Patients taking calcium channel blockers (Amlodipine, Nifedipine, Verapamil, Diltiazem, Dihydropyridine, Felodipine, etc).

■ **Sex/Gender**

All

■ **Ages**

45 Years to N/A

■ **Accepts Healthy Volunteers**

Accepts Healthy Volunteers

■ **Contacts**

Keyur P Parikh, MD   216-844-3217   keyur.parikh@uhhospitals.org

Peptide Vaccine in Advanced Pancreatic Ductal Adenocarcinoma or Colorectal Adenocarcinoma

Study ID:

NCT02600949

Sponsor:

M.D. Anderson Cancer Center

Information provided by (Responsible Party):

M.D. Anderson Cancer Center (M.D. Anderson Cancer Center)

Tracking Information

■ **First Submitted Date**

November 6, 2015

■ **Start Date**

May 2016

■ **Primary Completion Date**

May 2021

■ **Last Update Posted Date**

January 26, 2018

■ **Current Primary Outcome Measures**

Feasibility of Developing a Personalized Vaccine Within a Reasonable Timeframe for Participants with Metastatic Pancreatic Ductal Adenocarcinoma (PDA) and Colorectal Cancer (CRC)[Time Frame: 12 weeks]

Feasibility assessed by proportion of enrolled patients for whom a personalized vaccine is developed and ready to administer by the end of 12 weeks post-enrollment, and by proportion of enrolled patients who receive at least 1 dose of vaccine at any time post enrollment.

Toxicity of Personalized Vaccine in Participants with Metastatic Pancreatic Ductal Adenocarcinoma (PDA) and Colorectal Cancer (CRC)[Time Frame: 24 weeks]

Toxicity event defined as at least one grade 3 or 4 non-hematologic or grade 4 hematologic toxicity per CTCAE v4.0 that is deemed to be treatment-related. Toxicity endpoint defined as proportion of participants who experience at least one toxicity event within the first 24 weeks of the first dose of personalized vaccine.

■ **Current Secondary Outcome Measures**

Progression-Free Survival[Time Frame: 12 weeks]

Progression free complete response plus partial response plus stable disease (CR + PR + SD) defined based on response criteria according to RECIST 1.1 at 12 weeks post first vaccination (at second re-staging scan). Progression-free survival defined as time from first vaccination to evidence of progression on CT scan or death.

Descriptive Information

■ **Offical Title**

Pilot Study of the Feasibility and Safety of a Personalized Peptide Vaccine in Patients With Advanced Pancreatic Ductal Adenocarcinoma or Colorectal Adenocarcinoma

■ **Brief Summary**

The goal of this clinical research study is to learn if it is possible to make a vaccine for advanced pancreatic or colorectal cancer. In this study, you will receive the vaccine in combination with pembrolizumab. The safety of this vaccine in combination with pembrolizumab will also be studied.

This study will use your tumor cells (either from a fresh biopsy or from leftover tissue samples) and blood to help create a vaccine designed specifically for you based on what the study doctor and research staff can learn about the type of mutated proteins (a type of genetic change) in the tumor.

This is an investigational study. The study vaccine is not FDA approved or commercially available. It is currently being used for research purposes only. Pembrolizumab is FDA approved and commercially available for the treatment of melanoma, non-small cell lung cancer, and squamous cell head and neck cancer. It is considered investigational to use pembrolizumab to treat pancreatic or colorectal cancer.

The study doctor can explain how the vaccine is designed to work.

Up to 60 participants will be enrolled in this study. All will take part at MD Anderson.

Detailed Description

Tissue Collection:

Within 4 weeks after signing this informed consent document, as part of the screening tests:

°You will have leftover frozen tissue collected to create your vaccine, if available. If there is not enough frozen tissue available, then leftover tissue from a recent procedure performed as part of your standard of care will be collected. The study staff may ask you to take part in another MD Anderson clinical research study (PA15-0176) for collection of leftover tissue. The study doctor will discuss this with you and, if you decide to take part, you will sign a separate informed consent document.

After the tissue cells have been collected, your vaccine will be made.

The vaccine can also be made from blood cells. If you agree, you will be consented and enrolled under a separate protocol, PA14-0138, to have the leukapheresis procedure performed. Leukapheresis is a special type of blood draw procedure that separates the red blood cells, white blood cells, and other parts of your blood from each other. The consent form for this protocol will explain how the leukapheresis procedure is performed and its risks. The white blood cells collected from leukapheresis will be used in this study.

Baseline Tests:

You must receive at least 1 type of chemotherapy after you are enrolled in this study but before your first dose of vaccine. There is no limit to the number of types of chemotherapy you may receive. Your study doctor will decide when you will enter the treatment part of this study.

Within 28 days after your last dose of chemotherapy:

- You will have a physical exam.
- Blood (about 2 tablespoons) will be drawn for routine tests. The routine blood draw will include a pregnancy test if you can become pregnant.

Within 14 days before your first dose of vaccine, you will have an MRI or CT scan of the chest, abdomen, and pelvis.

Study Vaccine and Study Drug Administration:

About 28 days after your last dose of chemotherapy, you will receive the vaccine as an injection under the skin on Day 1 of Weeks 0, 1, 3, 4, 6 and then every 3 weeks until Week 30, then at Weeks 39 and 51.

Imiquimod cream will be applied over the injection site about 30 minutes after you receive the vaccine. This will be done each time you receive the vaccine.

You will also receive pembrolizumab by vein over about 30 minutes every 3 weeks until Week 51.

Study Visits:

On Day 1 of Weeks 0, 1, and 3:

- You will have a physical exam.
- Blood (about 6 tablespoons) will be drawn for routine tests and research tests for immune testing to test for genetic mutations.

On Day 1 of Week 4, blood (about 6 tablespoons) will be drawn for immune system testing and routine tests.

On Day 1 of Weeks 6, 9, 12, 15, and 18:

- You will have a physical exam.
- Blood (about 6 tablespoons) will be drawn for immune system testing and routine tests.
- You will have an MRI or CT scan of the chest, abdomen, and pelvis. You will not have these scans at Weeks 9 and 15.

On Day 1 of Weeks 16, 21, 24, 27, 33, 36, 42, 45, and 48:

- You will have a physical exam.
- Blood (about 2 tablespoons) will be drawn for routine tests.

On Day 1 of Weeks 30, 39, and 51:

- You will have a physical exam.
- Blood (about 6 tablespoons) will be drawn for immune system testing, tumor marker testing, and routine tests.
- You will have an MRI or CT scan of the chest, abdomen, and pelvis.

Length of Study:

You may receive the vaccine and pembrolizumab for up to 1 year.

You will no longer be able to receive the study vaccine if the disease gets worse, if intolerable side effects occur, or if you are unable to follow study directions.

Your participation on the study will be over after follow-up.

End-of-Study Visit:

About 8 weeks after your last study visit:

- You will have a physical exam.
- Blood (about 2 tablespoons) will be drawn for routine tests.

Follow-Up:

You will be called 2 times by the study staff in the 6 months after your last dose of vaccine and asked about any side effects you may have experienced since the end-of-study visit. Each call should last about 10 minutes.

If you left the study because you had side effects, you will be called by the study staff until that side effect has gone away or has become stable.

Study Type

Interventional

Study Phase

Phase 1

Condition

- Pancreatic Cancer
- Colorectal Cancer

Intervention

Biological: Peptide Vaccine

Vaccine given in a total volume of up to 1.0ml/shot consisting of a peptide cocktail injected subcutaneously into two to three separate sites of the subject's thighs for a total of up to 1.0ml per vaccination per cocktail. If subject is prescribed two cocktails then up to four to six sites on the subject's thighs may be used, provided that each vaccine cocktail is administered into different thighs. The total amount of peptide delivered will vary (range from approximately 200µg to 2.0mg) depending on how many peptides are identified and prescribed (range 1-5 per peptide cocktail, 2 total cocktails possible, maximum of 10 peptides).

Vaccinations given on Day 1 of Weeks 0, 1, 3, 4, 6 and then every 3 weeks until Week 30, then at Weeks 39 and 51.

Behavioral: Phone Call

Participant called 2 times by study staff in the 6 months after last dose of vaccine and asked about any side effects experienced since the end-of-study visit. Each call should take about 10 minutes.

Drug: Pembrolizumab

Pembrolizumab administered as a fixed dose of 200 mg infusion every three weeks over approximately 30 minutes until week 51.

Other Names:

Keytruda

MK-3475

SCH-900475

Study Arms

Experimental: Cohort A: Peptide Vaccine

Participants receive at least one line of chemotherapy prior to their first vaccination, as per treating physician.

Vaccine given on day 1, week 0, which will be at least 4 weeks after the end of their prior therapy.

Vaccine given in a total volume of up to 1.0ml/shot consisting of a peptide cocktail injected subcutaneously into two to three separate sites of the subject's thighs for a total of up to 1.0ml per vaccination per cocktail. If subject is prescribed two cocktails then up to four to six sites on the subject's thighs may be used, provided that each vaccine cocktail is administered into different thighs.

Participant called 2 times by study staff in the 6 months after last dose of vaccine and asked about any side effects experienced since the end-of-study visit.

Experimental: Cohort B: Peptide Vaccine + Pembrolizumab

Vaccine administered first followed by Pembrolizumab therapy.

Vaccine given in a total volume of up to 1.0ml/shot consisting of a peptide cocktail injected subcutaneously into two to three separate sites of the subject's thighs for a total of up to 1.0ml per vaccination per cocktail. If subject is prescribed two cocktails then up to four to six sites on the subject's thighs may be used, provided that each vaccine cocktail is administered into different thighs.

Pembrolizumab administered as a fixed dose of 200 mg infusion every three weeks over approximately 30 minutes until week 51.

Participant called 2 times by study staff in the 6 months after last dose of vaccine and asked about any side effects experienced since the end-of-study visit.

Recruitment Information

Recruitment Status

Recruiting

Estimated Enrollment

60

Completion Date

May 2022

Primary Completion Date

May 2021

Eligibility Criteria

Inclusion Criteria:

1. Patients must have metastatic Pancreatic Ductal Adenocarcinoma (PDA) or metastatic colorectal cancer (CRC) to be eligible. (PDA patients with an elevated tumor marker following a primary pancreatic surgery would be eligible).

2. Patients can have any lines (including zero) of prior therapy to sign consent prior to tissue harvest. Vaccination will not take place until at least one line of standard chemotherapy is given.

3. Patients must have adequate fresh or frozen tissue available. If tissue is needed, then subjects may have had it previously collected under protocol PA15-0176.

4. Age =/>18 years.

5. ECOG performance status <1 (Karnofsky >70%)

6. Life expectancy of greater than 6 months.

7. Patients must have normal organ and marrow function as defined below:: a) leukocytes =/>3,000/mcL; b) absolute neutrophil count =/>1,000/mcL; c) platelets =/>75,000/mcL; d)total bilirubin =/< 2.0 X institutional upper limit of normal; e) AST(SGOT)/ALT(SGPT) =/<2.5 X institutional upper limit of normal (except in gilberts disease where direct bilirubin will be used); f) calculated creatinine clearance =/>50 mL/min/1.73 m^2

8. Patients must demonstrate an ability to understand and the willingness to sign a written informed consent document.

9. The effects of a peptide based vaccine on the developing human fetus are unknown. For this reason, women of child-bearing potential and men must agree to use adequate The effects of a peptide based vaccine on the developing human fetus are unknown. For this reason, women of child-bearing potential and men must agree to use adequate contraception at study entry and for the duration of study participation. Should a woman become pregnant or suspect she is pregnant while participating in this study, she should inform her treating physician immediately. Birth control specifications: unless surgically sterile by bilateral tubal ligation or vasectomy of partner(s), sexually active participants must use birth control during and for >120 days after the study. Abstinence is also an acceptable form of birth control.

10. Inclusion criteria just prior to first vaccination (within 21 days) in addition to above inclusion criteria unless specified differently below : ECOG performance status =/<2 (Karnofsky =/>60%)

11. Inclusion criteria just prior to first vaccination (within 21 days): Life expectancy of greater than 4 months

12. Inclusion criteria just prior to first vaccination (within 21 days): Patients must have either measurable disease per RECIST v1.1 or evaluable disease defined as an elevated tumor biomarker (CA19-9, CEA or cfDNA mutation). Pancreatic cancer patients with an elevated tumor marker following a primary pancreatic surgery would be eligible

Exclusion Criteria:

1. Known history of testing positive for human immunodeficiency virus (HIV) or known acquired immunodeficiency syndrome (AIDS).HIV-positive patients on combination antiretroviral therapy are ineligible because of the potential for lack of efficacy of therapeutic cancer vaccine.

2. Patients with known brain metastases should be excluded from this clinical trial because of their poor prognosis and because they often develop progressive neurologic dysfunction that would confound the evaluation of neurologic and other adverse events.

3. Positive test for hepatitis B virus surface antigen (HBV sAg) or hepatitis C virus (ribonucleic acid or HCV antibody) indicating acute or chronic infection.

4. Subjects with active, known or suspected autoimmune disease. Subjects with vitiligo, type I diabetes mellitus, residual hypothyroidism due to autoimmune condition only requiring hormone replacement, psoriasis not requiring systemic treatment, or conditions not expected to recur in the absence of an external trigger are permitted to enroll.

5. Subjects with a condition requiring systemic treatment with either corticosteroids (> 10 mg daily prednisone equivalents) or other immunosuppressive medications. Inhaled or topical steroids and adrenal replacement doses > 10 mg daily prednisone equivalents are permitted in the absence of active autoimmune disease.

6. Uncontrolled concurrent illness including, but not limited to ongoing or active infection, symptomatic congestive heart failure, unstable angina pectoris, cardiac arrhythmia, or psychiatric illness/social situations that would limit compliance with study requirements.

7. Women of child bearing potential who are pregnant or breastfeeding. Women with a positive pregnancy test at enrollment or prior to administration of vaccine.

8. Has history of (non-infectious) pneumonitis that required steroids, evidence of interstitial lung disease or active, non-infectious pneumonitis

9. Known history of active TB (Bacillus Tuberculosis)

10. Hypersensitivity to pembrolizumab or any of its excipients.

11. Has a known additional malignancy that is progressing or requires active treatment.

12. Has a known history of Human Immunodeficiency Virus (HIV) (HIV 1/2 antibodies).

- 13. Exclusion criteria just prior to first vaccination (within 21 days) in addition to above exclusion criteria unless specified differently below: Patients who have had chemotherapy or radiotherapy within 2 weeks prior to entering the study or those who have not recovered to baseline from adverse events due to agents administered more than 2 weeks earlier (washout period).

- 14. Exclusion criteria just prior to first vaccination(within 21 days) in addition to above exclusion criteria unless specified differently below: Women of child bearing potential who are pregnant or breastfeeding. Women with a positive pregnancy test prior to administration of vaccine.

- 15. Exclusion criteria just prior to first vaccination (within 21 days) in addition to above exclusion criteria unless specified differently below: Uncontrolled concurrent illness including, but not limited to ongoing or active infection, symptomatic congestive heart failure, unstable angina pectoris, cardiac arrhythmia, or psychiatric illness/social situations that would limit compliance with study requirements.

- 16. Exclusion criteria just prior to first vaccination (within 21 days) in addition to above exclusion criteria unless specified differently below: Patients may not be receiving any other investigational agents.

- 17. Exclusion criteria just prior to first vaccination (within 21 days) in addition to above exclusion criteria unless specified differently below: Has received a live vaccine within 30 days of planned start of study therapy. Note: Seasonal influenza vaccines for injection are generally inactivated flu vaccines and are allowed; however intranasal influenza vaccines (e.g., Flu-Mist®) are live attenuated vaccines, and are not allowed.

Sex/Gender

All

Ages

18 Years to N/A

Accepts Healthy Volunteers

No

Contacts

Michael Overman, MD   713-792-2828

Tas-102 and Radioembolization With 90Y Resin Microspheres for Chemo-refractory Colorectal Liver Metastases

Study ID:

NCT02602327

Sponsor:

University of California, San Francisco

Information provided by (Responsible Party):

University of California, San Francisco (University of California, San Francisco)

Tracking Information

First Submitted Date

November 9, 2015

Start Date

October 2016

Current Primary Outcome Measures

Safety (adverse events)[Time Frame: 4 years]
    Safety (adverse events) of Tas-102 and 90Y radioembolization combination therapy.

Current Secondary Outcome Measures

Radiographic response[Time Frame: 4 years]

Primary Completion Date

September 2019

Last Update Posted Date

December 5, 2016

Radiographic overall response rate (measured in accordance to Response Evaluation Criteria in Solid Tumors [RECIST] version 1.1)

Progression-free survival (PFS)[Time Frame: 4 years]

Progression-free survival (PFS) following Tas-102 and 90Y radioembolization combination therapy (based on radiographic response).

Hepatic progression-free survival (HPFS)[Time Frame: 4 years]

Extrahepatic progression free survival (EHPFS)[Time Frame: 4 years]

Overall survival (OS)[Time Frame: 4 years]

Biomarker response[Time Frame: 4 years]

Proportion of patients with carcinoembryonic antigen (CEA) response with ≥ 50% decline from baseline (in patients with baseline level ≥ 3.2) post combination therapy with Tas-102 and 90Y radioembolization.

Descriptive Information

▦ Offical Title

Phase I Study of Tas-102 and Radioembolization With 90Y Resin Microspheres for Chemo-refractory Colorectal Liver Metastases

▦ Brief Summary

This is a phase I dose escalation study (3+3 design) with a dose expansion arm (12 patients) designed to evaluate safety of the combination of Tas-102 and radioembolization using Yttrium-90 (90Y) resin microspheres for patients with chemotherapy-refractory liver-dominant chemotherapy-refractory metastatic colorectal cancer (mCRC).

▦ Detailed Description

Randomized studies have demonstrated that Tas-102 has single agent activity against chemotherapy refractory colorectal cancer. A recent pre-clinical study has shown that Tas-102 may have activity as a radiation sensitizer in bladder cancer cell lines. Benefit of single agent Tas-102 against chemotherapy refractory colon cancer and the drug's promise a radiosensitizer make Tas-102 a potential candidate drug for testing in combination with radioembolization using Yttrium-90 resin microspheres in patients with liver-dominant chemotherapy-refractory mCRC. This is a phase I dose escalation study with a dose expansion arm designed to evaluate safety of the combination of Tas-102 and radioembolization using 90Y resin microspheres for patients with chemotherapy-refractory colon or rectal adenocarcinoma metastatic to the liver.

▦ Study Type

Interventional

▦ Study Phase

Phase 1

▦ Condition

- Colon Cancer
- Rectal Cancer
- Liver Metastases

▦ Intervention

Drug: Tas-102

Oral nucleoside antitumor agent consisting of α,α,α-trifluorothymidine (FTD) and 5-chloro-6-(2-iminopyrrolidin-1-yl) methyl-2,4 (1H,3H)-pyrimidinedione hydro chloride (TPI) at a molar ratio of 1:0.5.

Other Names:

Lonsurf

Device: SIR-Sphere

20-60mm resin microspheres containing Yttrium-90 (90Y, Y90) radioisotope

Other Names:

Yttrium-90 (Y90; 90Y) resin microspheres

▦ Study Arms

Experimental: Tas-102 and radioembolization

Combination therapy with Tas-102 and radioembolization using 90Y resin microspheres

Recruitment Information

Recruitment Status

Recruiting

Estimated Enrollment

24

Completion Date

September 2020

Primary Completion Date

September 2019

Eligibility Criteria

Inclusion Criteria:

1. Male or female, 18 years of age or older, and of any ethnic or racial group.

- 2. Diagnosis of unresectable metastatic colorectal adenocarcinoma with liver-dominant bilobar disease. Diagnosis may be made by histoor cyto-pathology, or by clinical and imaging criteria.

3. Disease progression or intolerance to at least two prior Food and Drug Administration-approved therapeutic regimens.

4. If extrahepatic disease is present, it must be asymptomatic.

5. If a primary tumor is in place, it must be asymptomatic.

6. Measurable target tumors using standard imaging techniques (RECIST v. 1.1 criteria).

7. Tumor replacement < 50% of total liver volume.

8. Current Eastern Cooperative Oncology Group (ECOG) performance status of 0 or 1 through screening to first treatment on study.

9. Completion of prior systemic therapy at least 14 days prior to enrollment.

10. Able to understand informed consent.

Exclusion Criteria:

1. At risk of hepatic or renal failure
- Serum creatinine > 1.5 mg/dl
- Serum bilirubin > 1.3 mg/ml
- Albumin < 2.0 g/dL
- Aspartate and/or alanine aminotransferase level > 5 times upper normal limit
- Any history of hepatic encephalopathy
- Cirrhosis or portal hypertension
- Clinically evident ascites (trace ascites on imaging is acceptable)

2. Contraindications to angiography and selective visceral catheterization
- Any bleeding diathesis or coagulopathy that is not correctable by usual therapy or hemostatic agents (e.g. closure device)
- Severe allergy or intolerance to contrast agents, narcotics, or sedatives that cannot be managed medically

3. Symptomatic lung disease

4. Prior therapy with Tas-102.

5. Contraindications to Tas-102
- Absolute neutrophil count < 1,500/μl
- Platelet count < 75,000/μl
- Allergy or intolerance to Tas-102

6. Unresolved toxicity of greater than or equal to National Cancer Institute Common Terminology Criteria for Adverse Events (NCI CTCAE) Grade 2 due to prior therapies.

7. Evidence of potential delivery of
- Greater than 30 Gy absorbed dose of radiation to the lungs during a single 90Y resin microsphere administration; or
- Cumulative delivery of radiation to the lungs > 50 Gy over multiple treatments.

8. Evidence of any detectable Tc-99m macro aggregated albumin flow to the stomach or duodenum, after application of established angiographic techniques to stop such flow.

9. Previous radiation therapy to the lungs and/or to the upper abdomen

10. Any prior arterial liver-directed therapy, including chemoembolization, bland embolization, and 90Y radioembolization

11. Any intervention for, or compromise of the ampulla of Vater

12. Active uncontrolled infection. Presence of latent or medication-controlled HIV and/or viral hepatitis is allowed.

13. Significant extrahepatic disease
- Symptomatic extrahepatic disease (including primary tumor, if unresected).
- Greater than 10 pulmonary nodules (each < 10 mm in diameter) or combined diameter of all pulmonary nodules > 80 mm.
- Peritoneal carcinomatosis

14. Life expectancy less than 3 months

15. Pregnant or lactating female

16. In the investigator's judgment, any co-morbid disease or condition that would place the patient at undue risk and preclude safe use of radioembolization or Tas-102.

■ **Sex/Gender**

All

■ **Ages**

18 Years to N/A

■ **Accepts Healthy Volunteers**

No

■ **Contacts**

Curt Johanson   (415) 353-2310   Curt.Johanson@ucsf.edu

Effectiveness of High Dose Vitamin D Supplementation in Stage III Colorectal Cancer

Study ID:

NCT02603757

Sponsor:

Legacy Health System

Information provided by (Responsible Party):

Legacy Health System (Legacy Health System)

Tracking Information

■ **First Submitted Date**

November 9, 2015

■ **Start Date**

March 2016

■ **Primary Completion Date**

December 2022

■ **Last Update Posted Date**

October 18, 2017

■ **Current Primary Outcome Measures**

Increase in serum Vitamin D3 level during chemotherapy in the active supplementation group compared to the control group.[Time Frame: 1 year]

■ **Current Secondary Outcome Measures**

Relapse-free survival (RFS)[Time Frame: 5 years]
   Overall survival (OS)[Time Frame: 5 years]

Descriptive Information

■ **Offical Title**

Prospective Pilot Study to Assess the Effectiveness of Vitamin D Supplementation for Patients Requiring Chemotherapy for Stage III Colorectal Cancer

■ **Brief Summary**

This is a pilot study to test whether there is an association between baseline Vitamin D levels, Vitamin D supplementation and survival in patients with stage III colon and stage II/III rectal cancer receiving chemotherapy. 70 patients with colon stage III or rectal stage II or III cancer that require chemotherapy will be screened and 60 patients will be enrolled. Patients will be randomized to standard dose (2000 IU daily) or high-dose (50,000 IU weekly) Vitamin D supplementation for 1 year after initiation of chemotherapy. Patients' Vitamin D levels will be checked throughout supplementation then followed for 5 years with occasional Vitamin D testing and surveying in order to collect information on recurrence and survival outcomes.

■ **Study Type**

Interventional

■ **Study Phase**

N/A

Condition

- Colon Cancer
- Rectal Cancer

Intervention

Dietary Supplement: cholecalciferol
    2,000 IU of Vitamin D3 daily and 50,000 IU Vitamin D3 daily

Other Names:
    Vitamin D3

Study Arms

Active Comparator: Group A
    Standard-dose of 2,000 IU Vitamin D3, daily

Experimental: Group B
    Higher-dose of 50,000 IU of Vitamin D3, weekly

Publications

(Includes publications given by the data provider as well as publications identified by ClinicalTrials.gov Identifier (NCT Number) in Medline.)Fiscella K, Winters P, Tancredi D, Hendren S, Franks P. Racial disparity in death from colorectal cancer: does vitamin D deficiency contribute? Cancer. 2011 Mar 1;117(5):1061-9. doi: 10.1002/cncr.25647. Epub 2010 Oct 13. (https://www.ncbi.nlm.nih.gov/pubmed/20945439)

Zgaga L, Theodoratou E, Farrington SM, Din FV, Ooi LY, Glodzik D, Johnston S, Tenesa A, Campbell H, Dunlop MG. Plasma vitamin D concentration influences survival outcome after a diagnosis of colorectal cancer. J Clin Oncol. 2014 Aug 10;32(23):2430-9. doi: 10.1200/JCO.2013.54.5947. Epub 2014 Jul 7. (https://www.ncbi.nlm.nih.gov/pubmed/25002714)

Ng K, Sargent DJ, Goldberg RM, Meyerhardt JA, Green EM, Pitot HC, Hollis BW, Pollak MN, Fuchs CS. Vitamin D status in patients with stage IV colorectal cancer: findings from Intergroup trial N9741. J Clin Oncol. 2011 Apr 20;29(12):1599-606. doi: 10.1200/JCO.2010.31.7255. Epub 2011 Mar 21. (https://www.ncbi.nlm.nih.gov/pubmed/21422438)

Brunner RL, Wactawski-Wende J, Caan BJ, Cochrane BB, Chlebowski RT, Gass ML, Jacobs ET, LaCroix AZ, Lane D, Larson J, Margolis KL, Millen AE, Sarto GE, Vitolins MZ, Wallace RB. The effect of calcium plus vitamin D on risk for invasive cancer: results of the Women's Health Initiative (WHI) calcium plus vitamin D randomized clinical trial. Nutr Cancer. 2011;63(6):827-41. doi: 10.1080/01635581.2011.594208. Epub 2011 Jul 20. (https://www.ncbi.nlm.nih.gov/pubmed/21774589)

Fakih MG, Andrews C, McMahon J, Muindi JR. A prospective clinical trial of cholecalciferol 2000 IU/day in colorectal cancer patients: evidence of a chemotherapy-response interaction. Anticancer Res. 2012 Apr;32(4):1333-8. (https://www.ncbi.nlm.nih.gov/pubmed/22493367)

Fedirko V, Bostick RM, Flanders WD, Long Q, Shaukat A, Rutherford RE, Daniel CR, Cohen V, Dash C. Effects of vitamin D and calcium supplementation on markers of apoptosis in normal colon mucosa: a randomized, double-blind, placebo-controlled clinical trial. Cancer Prev Res (Phila). 2009 Mar;2(3):213-23. doi: 10.1158/1940-6207.CAPR-08-0157. Epub 2009 Mar 3. (https://www.ncbi.nlm.nih.gov/pubmed/19258546)

Fernandez-Garcia NI, Palmer HG, Garcia M, Gonzalez-Martin A, del Rio M, Barettino D, Volpert O, Muñoz A, Jimenez B. 1alpha,25-Dihydroxyvitamin D3 regulates the expression of Id1 and Id2 genes and the angiogenic phenotype of human colon carcinoma cells. Oncogene. 2005 Sep 29;24(43):6533-44. (https://www.ncbi.nlm.nih.gov/pubmed/16007183)

Fedirko V, Bostick RM, Long Q, Flanders WD, McCullough ML, Sidelnikov E, Daniel CR, Rutherford RE, Shaukat A. Effects of supplemental vitamin D and calcium on oxidative DNA damage marker in normal colorectal mucosa: a randomized clinical trial. Cancer Epidemiol Biomarkers Prev. 2010 Jan;19(1):280-91. doi: 10.1158/1055-9965.EPI-09-0448. (https://www.ncbi.nlm.nih.gov/pubmed/20056649)

Bee CR, Sheerin DV, Wuest TK, Fitzpatrick DC. Serum vitamin D levels in orthopaedic trauma patients living in the northwestern United States. J Orthop Trauma. 2013 May;27(5):e103-6. doi: 10.1097/BOT.0b013e31825cf8fb. (https://www.ncbi.nlm.nih.gov/pubmed/22576645)

Morgan SL, Weinsier RL. Fundamentals of clinical nutrition, Mosby, St. Louis 1998. p.3

Recruitment Information

Recruitment Status

Recruiting

Estimated Enrollment

70

Eligibility Criteria

Inclusion Criteria:

- ≥ 18 years of age
- Willing to stop herbal medications as directed by physician

Completion Date

December 2022

Primary Completion Date

December 2022

- Willing to stop current supplemental Vitamin D (Multivitamin with Vitamin D component is acceptable)
- Willing to travel to Legacy Health/OHSU facility if necessary
- Agree to attend study visits outside of standard of care visits, if necessary
- Diagnosed with stage III colon or stage II/III rectal cancer that will receive neoadjuvant or adjuvant chemotherapy but have not yet started
- Baseline serum Vitamin D level below 52 ng/ml

Exclusion Criteria:

- ≤ 18 years of age
- Colon cancer stages I-II and IV or Rectal cancer stage I or IV
- Patients who do not undergo chemotherapy
- Patients with prior chemotherapy for this cancer
- No other prior malignancy except for adequately treated basal cell or squamous cell skin cancer, in situ cancer, or other cancer for which the patient has been disease-free for > 3 years
- Unable to comply with protocol
- Unable to provide written informed consent
- Unwilling or unable to stop oral supplemental Vitamin D
- Patients taking high-dose Vitamin D supplementation (50,000 IU weekly) prior to enrollment
- Patients with Vitamin D levels above 52 ng/ml at baseline testing
- Patients with hypercalcemia and/or any condition resulting in malabsorption
- Investigator does not believe study participation, for any reason, is in the best interest of the patient

Sex/Gender

All

Ages

18 Years to 99 Years

Accepts Healthy Volunteers

No

Contacts

Jennifer Stubbs, BS   503.413.7202   jstubbs@lhs.org

Local Ablative Strategies After Endovascular Radioembolization

Study ID:

NCT02611661

Sponsor:

Washington University School of Medicine

Information provided by (Responsible Party):

Washington University School of Medicine (Washington University School of Medicine)

Tracking Information

First Submitted Date

November 18, 2015

Start Date

January 19, 2016

Current Primary Outcome Measures

Primary Completion Date

February 28, 2019

Last Update Posted Date

December 18, 2017

Safety and tolerability of administering hepatic locoregional therapy following radioembolization as measured by occurrences of grade 3 or higher toxicities of interest[Time Frame: 30 days after completion of therapy (approximately 6 weeks)]

Strata 2, 3, and 4 only

The descriptions and grading scales found in the revised NCI Common Terminology Criteria for Adverse Events (CTCAE) version 4.0 will be utilized for all toxicity reporting.

▣ Current Secondary Outcome Measures

Late toxicity associated with radioembolization followed by dosimetry-guided subsequent hepatic locoregional therapy[Time Frame: Up to 6 months]

-The descriptions and grading scales found in the revised NCI Common Terminology Criteria for Adverse Events (CTCAE) version 4.0 will be utilized for all toxicity reporting.

Local recurrence rates associated with radioembolization followed by dosimetry-guided subsequent hepatic locoregional therapy[Time Frame: Up to 2 years]

Overall survival rates associated with radioembolization followed by dosimetry-guided subsequent hepatic locoregional therapy[Time Frame: Up to 2 years]

Response rates associated with radioembolization followed by dosimetry-guided subsequent hepatic locoregional therapy[Time Frame: Up to 6 months]

Complete Response (CR): Disappearance of all target lesions and non-target lesions. Normalization of tumor marker level.

Partial Response (PR): At least a 30% decrease in the sum of the diameters of target lesions, taking as reference the baseline sum diameters.

Progressive Disease (PD): At least a 20% increase in the sum of the diameters of target lesions, taking as reference the smallest sum on study (this includes the baseline sum if that is the smallest on study). In addition to the relative increase of 20%, the sum must also demonstrate an absolute increase of at least 5 mm. (Note: the appearance of one or more new lesions is also considered progressions).

Stable Disease (SD): Neither sufficient shrinkage to qualify for PR nor sufficient increase to qualify for PD, taking as reference the smallest sum diameters while on study.

Descriptive Information

▣ Offical Title

Local Ablative Strategies After Endovascular Radioembolization (LASER)

▣ Brief Summary

The rationale for this design is initial utilization of a standard-of-care therapy for mCRC (radioembolization) with a dose-calculation algorithm that has been verified as predictive for treatment response. Prediction of treatment failure will enable the proposed subsequent locoregional therapies which were selected based on safety profiles and feasibility. While the goal of this study is assessing feasibility and safety of this approach, the end goal of improving overall patient outcomes by improved hepatic tumor control.

▣ Detailed Description

As the median time to radiographic response ranges from 3-8 months in published data, utilization of post-treatment PET/MRI dosimetry offers a powerful mechanism for immediate (within 36 hours) prediction of lesions that are likely to fail radioembolization. This early prediction enables a window for subsequent locoregional therapy prior to re-initiation of systemic chemotherapy. The investigators propose to evaluate patients who are undergoing radioembolization for mCRC using PET/MRI derived dosimetry obtained within 36 hours of the radioembolization procedure. Patients with four tumors or fewer receiving an average dose (Davg) less than 30 Gy will be candidates for subsequent locoregional therapy (stereotactic body radiotherapy (SBRT) or microwave ablation). This strategy will ideally increase the therapeutic index of locoregional therapies, particularly in the patient population who has exhausted their options for systemic therapy.

- After radioembolization, patients will be divided into 5 strata as per the protocol schema. Patients who receive a Davg greater than 30 Gy in all hepatic lesions will be placed in Stratum 1 and will not undergo subsequent therapy. Patients with four or fewer lesions receiving a Davg less than 30 Gy will be placed in Strata 2, 3, or 4 based on distribution of the underdosed lesions. Stratum 2 will be comprised of patients with four or fewer underdosed lesions less than 3 cm which do not touch vasculature greater than 4 mm in size. Patients in this stratum will receive percutaneous microwave ablation to the underdosed lesions. Stratum 3 will be composed of patients with 4 or fewer underdosed lesions that are not amenable to microwave ablation by virtue of either size (greater than 3 cm) or proximity to hepatic vasculature greater than 4 mm in diameter. These patients will be treated with SBRT to the underdosed lesions. Patients with a combination of lesions some of which are amenable to microwave ablation and some of which are not (due to either size or proximity to vasculature) will be treated in Stratum 4 with a combined approach microwave ablation to all lesions which are amenable and SBRT to any remaining underdosed lesions. Finally, Stratum 5 will consist of patients with more than 4 underdosed lesions or with disease progression; these patients will be referred for further systemic therapy and are not candidates for further locoregional therapy on study.

▣ Study Type

Interventional

▣ Study Phase

Phase 1

▣ Condition

- Metastatic Colorectal Cancer

Intervention

Device: PET/MRI

   Radiation: Percutaneous ablation

   Radiation: Stereotactic body radiotherapy

   Other Names:

   SBRT

Study Arms

Other: Stratum 1: Observe

   PET/MRI within 36 hours of standard of care hepatic radioembolization received off study

   No further treatment just observation

Experimental: Stratum 2: Percutaneous ablation

   PET/MRI within 36 hours of standard of care hepatic radioembolization received off study

   Percutaneous ablation can be radiofrequency ablation (RFA), microwave ablation (MWA), cryoablation, and irreversible electroporation

Experimental: Stratum 3: SBRT

   PET/MRI within 36 hours of standard of care hepatic radioembolization received off study

   The planned SBRT dose will be 30 Gy in 5 fractions of 6 Gy each. It is recommended that each fraction be separated by a minimum of 12 hours and a maximum of 8 days.

Experimental: Stratum 4: SBRT + Percutaneous Ablation

   PET/MRI within 36 hours of standard of care hepatic radioembolization received off study

   Percutaneous ablation can be radiofrequency ablation (RFA), microwave ablation (MWA), cryoablation, and irreversible electroporation

   The planned SBRT dose will be 30 Gy in 5 fractions of 6 Gy each. It is recommended that each fraction be separated by a minimum of 12 hours and a maximum of 8 days.

No Intervention: Stratum 5: Referral for systemic therapy

   PET/MRI within 36 hours of standard of care hepatic radioembolization received off study

   Referred for further systemic therapy and are not candidates for further locoregional therapy on study.

Recruitment Information

Recruitment Status

Recruiting

Estimated Enrollment

40

Completion Date

July 31, 2019

Primary Completion Date

February 28, 2019

Eligibility Criteria

Inclusion Criteria:

- Diagnosis of colorectal carcinoma with intrahepatic metastases; limited extrahepatic metastasis is allowed as long as the overall metastatic burden is hepatic dominant.
- Local surgical resection is not possible due to tumor or patient factors.
- Prior locoregional therapy is allowed if completed at least 2 weeks prior to enrollment.
- Prior chemotherapy is allowed if stopped/completed at least 2 weeks prior to enrollment.
- At least 18 years old.
- ECOG performance status ≤ 1.
- Scheduled to undergo radioembolization for treatment of intrahepatic metastases.
- Able to understand and willing to sign an IRB-approved written informed consent document.

Exclusion Criteria:

- Child-Pugh score 8 or greater.
- ALT or AST ≥ 6 x ULN.
- Prior history of abdominal irradiation. Patients who have received prior pelvic radiation for colorectal cancer are eligible; however, prior radiation treatment plans must be reviewed prior to enrollment.
- Presence of any contraindications to MRI scanning.

- GFR < 30 ml/min/1.73m2 (if receiving contrast for MRI).
- Currently on dialysis (if receiving contrast for MRI).
- Prior allergic reaction to gadolinium-based contrast agents (if receiving contrast for MRI).
- Pregnant or nursing. Women of childbearing potential must have a negative pregnancy test within 14 days of study entry.
- Uncontrolled intercurrent illness including, but not limited to, ongoing or active infection, symptomatic congestive heart failure, unstable angina pectoris, cardiac arrhythmia, or psychiatric illness/social situations that would limit compliance with study requirements.

Sex/Gender

All

Ages

18 Years to N/A

Accepts Healthy Volunteers

No

Contacts

Parag Parikh, M.D.   314-362-9703   parikh@wustl.edu

A Trial of mFOLFIRI With MEK162 in Patients With Advanced KRAS Positive Metastatic Colorectal Cancers

Study ID:

NCT02613650

Sponsor:

University of Utah

Information provided by (Responsible Party):

University of Utah (University of Utah)

Tracking Information

First Submitted Date

November 12, 2015

Start Date

May 12, 2016

Current Primary Outcome Measures

Incidence of dose limiting toxicities (DLTs) of combination MEK162 and mFOLFIRI[Time Frame: Patient safety will be evaluated throughout the treatment period (treatment with MEK162 and mFOLFIRI which is expected to last 6-10 months for each patient)]

Primary Completion Date

January 2020

Last Update Posted Date

February 17, 2017

Descriptive Information

Offical Title

A Phase 1b Trial of a Combination of mFOLFIRI With MEK162 in Patients With Advanced KRAS Positive Metastatic Colorectal Cancers

Brief Summary

This is a Phase 1b, open label, dose-finding study to determine the Maximum Tolerated Dose (MTD) of MEK162 in combination with mFOLFIRI, and to evaluate the response rate, clinical benefit rate and additional safety parameters of the treatment combination

Study Type

Interventional

Study Phase

Phase 1

- **Condition**
  - Advanced KRAS Positive Metastatic Colorectal Cancer
- **Intervention**

  Drug: MEK162 and mFOLFIRI

  MEK162 in combination with mFOLFIRI in a 14 day cycle

  MEK162 will be given single agent 6 day lead in and then will be given in combination with mFOLFIRI

  mFOLFIRI Administered Day 1 of each cycle Irinotecan 180mg/m2 iv over 90 minutes on day 1 5-fluoruracil 1200mg/m2 continuous infusion for 48 hours (2400mg/m2 in 48 hours)

  Followed by MEK162 Taken twice daily orally on Days 1-12 of each cycle

  Level -1: mFOLFIRI at 80% + MEK162 30 mg twice daily 1 week on and 1 week off Level 1: mFOLFIRI + MEK162 30 mg twice daily Level 2: mFOLFIRI + MEK162 45 mg twice daily

  Other Names:

  Binimetinib

- **Study Arms**

  Experimental: MEK162 and mFOLFIRI, all patients

Recruitment Information

- **Recruitment Status**

  Recruiting

- **Estimated Enrollment**

  30

- **Completion Date**

  January 2020

- **Primary Completion Date**

  January 2020

- **Eligibility Criteria**

  Inclusion Criteria:

  - Age > 18 years old
  - Patients with histologically confirmed KRAS positive metastatic colorectal cancer.
  - Patients must have progressed during or after first-line treatment for metastatic disease with oxaliplatin and fluoropyrimidines based chemotherapy (with failure within six months) or not be a candidate for oxaliplatin (i.e. neuropathy).
  - ECOG Performance Status 0-1
  - Able to provide informed consent and willing to sign an approved consent form that conforms to federal and institutional guidelines.
  - Women of childbearing potential must have a negative blood pregnancy test at the screening visit
  - Adequate bone marrow, organ function and laboratory parameters as defined by the protocol
  - Adequate cardiac function as defined by the protocol
  - Must have recovered from adverse effects of any prior surgery, radiotherapy or other antineoplastic therapy. Alopecia and CTCAE grade 1 peripheral neuropathy is acceptable
  - Willingness and ability to comply with all study procedures and able to take oral medications

  Dose Expansion Phase Additional Inclusion Criteria

  - Patients must be willing and able to undergo biopsy according to the institute's own guidelines and requirements for such procedures
  - Patients must have measurable disease as defined by RECIST v1.1 (at least one lesion ≥ 10mm in at least one dimension when assessed by CT or MRI, or a cutaneous lesion with clearly defined margins that measures ≥ 10 mm in at least one dimension)
  - Patients must be irinotecan refractory. Patients must have progressed on prior irinotecan therapy but must be able to tolerate standard irinotecan doses.

  Exclusion Criteria:

  - UGT1A1

  28 homozygous patients

  - Previous treatment with any MEK inhibitor
  - Treatment with systemic antineoplastic therapy (including unconjugated therapeutic antibodies and toxin immunoconjugates) or any investigational therapy within 4 weeks (<6 weeks for nitrosurea or mitomycin-C, antibodies except for trastuzumab) or within 5-half lives of the investigational therapy prior to starting study treatment, whichever is longer
  - Patient received radiotherapy within 2 weeks prior to the first dose of study treatment except localized radiation therapy for symptomatic bone metastasis.
  - Have had a diagnosis of another malignancy, unless the patient has been disease-free for at least 3 years following the

completion of curative intent therapy, with the following exceptions:

- Patients with treated non-melanoma skin cancer, in situ carcinoma, or cervical intraepithelial neoplasia, regardless of the disease-free duration, are eligible for this study if definitive treatment for the condition has been completed.
- Patients with organ-confined prostate cancer with no evidence of recurrent or progressive disease based on prostate-specific antigen (PSA) values are also eligible for this study if hormonal therapy has been initiated or a radical prostatectomy has been performed.
- History or current evidence of retinal vein occlusion (RVO) or current risk factors for RVO (e.g. uncontrolled glaucoma or ocular hypertension, history of hyperviscosity or hypercoagulability syndromes.
- Personal history of Gilbert's syndrome.
- Uncontrolled arterial hypertension defined by blood pressure >140 (systolic) or100 (diastolic) mmHg at rest (average 3 consecutive readings at least 5 minutes apart) despite appropriate medical therapy.
- Impaired cardiovascular function or clinically significant cardiovascular diseases, including any of the following:
- History of acute coronary syndromes (including myocardial infarction, unstable angina, coronary artery bypass grafting, coronary angioplasty, or stenting) <6 months prior to screening,
- Symptomatic chronic heart failure; evidence of clinically significant cardiac arrhythmias and/or conduction abnormalities < 6 months prior to screening except atrial fibrillation and paroxysmal supraventricular tachycardia.
- Known positive serology for HIV, active Hepatitis B, and/or active Hepatitis C infection (Note: if not suspected, testing is not required at baseline).
- Patients who have neuromuscular disorders that are associated with elevated CK (e.g., inflammatory myopathies, muscular dystrophy, amyotrophic lateral sclerosis, spinal muscular atrophy).
- Patients who are planning on embarking on a new strenuous exercise regimen after first dose of study treatment. Muscular activities, such as strenuous exercise, that can result in significant increases in plasma CK levels should be avoided while on MEK162 treatment.
- Impairment of gastrointestinal function or gastrointestinal disease (e.g., ulcerative disease, uncontrolled nausea, vomiting, diarrhea, malabsorption syndrome, or small bowel resection that under the judgment of the PI may impair absorption of study drugs).
- Any other condition that would, in the Investigator's judgment, contraindicate the patient's participation in the clinical study due to safety concerns or compliance with clinical study procedures, e.g., infection/inflammation, intestinal obstruction, unable to swallow medication.(patients may not receive drug through a feeding tube), social/ psychological issues, etc.
- Patients who have undergone major surgery ≤ 3 weeks prior to starting study drug or who have not recovered from side effects of such procedure.
- Pregnant or nursing (lactating) women, where pregnancy is defined as the state of a female after conception and until the termination of gestation, confirmed by a positive hCG laboratory test.
- Women of child-bearing potential, defined as all women physiologically capable of becoming pregnant, unless they are using highly effective methods of contraception throughout the study and for 15 days after study drug discontinuation.
- Sexually active males unless they use a condom during intercourse while taking the drug and for 15 days after stopping treatment and should not father a child in this period. A condom is required to be used also by vasectomized men in order to prevent delivery of the drug via seminal fluid.
- Medical, psychiatric, cognitive or other conditions that may compromise the patient's ability to understand the patient information, give informed consent, comply with the study protocol or complete the study.

■ Sex/Gender

All

■ Ages

18 Years to N/A

■ Accepts Healthy Volunteers

No

■ Contacts

Adam Blair   801-213-5759   adam.blair@hci.utah.edu

Accelerated Enhanced RECOVERy Following Minimally Invasive Colorectal Cancer Surgery (RecoverMI)

Study ID:

NCT02613728

Sponsor:

M.D. Anderson Cancer Center

Information provided by (Responsible Party):

M.D. Anderson Cancer Center (M.D. Anderson Cancer Center)

Tracking Information

■ **First Submitted Date**

November 23, 2015

■ **Start Date**

May 13, 2016

■ **Current Primary Outcome Measures**

Cumulative Hospital Length of Stay (LOS)[Time Frame: 30 days post transplant]

■ **Current Secondary Outcome Measures**

Failure Rate (FR) in the RecoverMI Arm[Time Frame: 30 days]
   Patient Satisfaction[Time Frame: 30 days]

■ **Primary Completion Date**

May 2019

■ **Last Update Posted Date**

September 25, 2017

Descriptive Information

■ **Offical Title**

Accelerated Enhanced RECOVERy Following Minimally Invasive Colorectal Cancer Surgery (RecoverMI)

■ **Brief Summary**

The goal of this clinical research study is to learn if RecoverMI care can help to shorten the time that patients are in the hospital after surgery and if it can help them recover sooner.

RecoverMI includes the following parts:

- Preoperative Education
- Early oral intake
- Early mobilization
- Telemedicine

■ **Detailed Description**

Study Groups:

If you are found to be eligible to take part in this study, you will be randomly assigned (as in the flip of a coin) to 1 of 2 study groups. This is done because no one knows if one group is the same, better, or worse than the other group.

- If you are assigned to Group 1, you will receive standard enhanced care after your surgery.
- If you are assigned to Group 2, you will receive routine care after surgery, but you will also receive accelerated recovery, early discharge, and Telemedicine. Participants will be loaned an iPad to use for video-conferencing and text messaging in this study.

This is an investigational study. The study doctor can explain how RecoverMI is designed to work.

Up to 32 participants will be enrolled in this study. All will take part at MD Anderson.

■ **Study Type**

Interventional

■ **Study Phase**

N/A

■ **Condition**

- Colorectal Cancer

■ **Intervention**

Behavioral: Accelerated Recovery Plan
   Behavioral: Early Discharge
   Other: Telemedicine
   Behavioral: Standard Enhanced Care

■ **Study Arms**

Active Comparator: Standard of Care Arm
   Standard enhanced care following minimally invasive colorectal cancer surgery

Experimental: Intervention (RecoverMI) Arm

Routine care with Accelerated Recovery Plan, Early Discharge, and Telemedicine following minimally invasive colorectal cancer surgery

Recruitment Information

■ **Recruitment Status**

Recruiting

■ **Estimated Enrollment**

32

■ **Eligibility Criteria**

Inclusion Criteria:

1. Patient has histologically proven colorectal cancer or polyp(s) that is planned to be treated by surgical resection performed with curative intent.

2. Patient is >/= 18 years and younger than 80 years.

3. Elective minimally invasive operation.

4. No planned ostomy creation at time of enrollment.

5. Serum creatinine <1.5 measured within 30 days of surgery.

6. Ability to speak, read, and understand English.

Exclusion Criteria:

1. Strong, self-reported history of postoperative nausea and vomiting.

2. History of congestive heart failure. Systolic heart failure defined as Ejection Fraction (EF) </= 40%), or diastolic heart failure defined as EF >40% PLUS systemic manifestation of heart failure.

■ **Sex/Gender**

All

■ **Ages**

18 Years to 79 Years

■ **Accepts Healthy Volunteers**

No

■ **Contacts**

George Chang, MD, MS   713-563-1875

■ **Completion Date**

May 2019

■ **Primary Completion Date**

May 2019

A ProspectiveTrial Comparing THUNDERBEAT to the Ligasure Energy Device During Laparoscopic Colon Surgery

Study ID:

NCT02628093

Sponsor:

Weill Medical College of Cornell University

Information provided by (Responsible Party):

Weill Medical College of Cornell University (Weill Medical College of Cornell University)

Tracking Information

■ **First Submitted Date**

December 4, 2015

■ **Start Date**

February 17, 2016

■ **Current Primary Outcome Measures**

Overall time for dissection of the soft tissues[Time Frame: up to 5 weeks]

■ **Primary Completion Date**

May 2018

■ **Last Update Posted Date**

July 12, 2017

from the start of colon mobilization to specimen removal from the abdominal cavity

Current Secondary Outcome Measures

dissection time for each stage of the surgery[Time Frame: up to 5 weeks]

Descriptive Information

Offical Title

A Randomized Controlled Trial Comparing THUNDERBEAT to the Ligasure Energy Device During Laparoscopic Colon Surgery

Brief Summary

- Prospective randomized controlled study, at Colon and Rectal Surgery, WMC/NYPH. Subjects undergoing Laparoscopic Left Colectomy will be randomized into 1 of 2 groups based on the instrument used for tissue dissection and vessel ligation: Group 1 THUNDERBEAT Group 2
- Ligasure Population

Detailed Description

- Prospective randomized controlled study, at Colon and Rectal Surgery, WMC/NYPH. Subjects undergoing Laparoscopic Left Colectomy will be randomized into 1 of 2 groups based on the instrument used for tissue dissection and vessel ligation: Group 1 THUNDERBEAT Group 2
- Ligasure Population: 60 subjects, with colon neoplasm or diverticulitis will be invited in the study after surgery is deemed necessary Study Procedures: This project will consist only of prospective data collection. No interventions will be done for research purpose. Data will be collected prospectively on: -Patients (before, during and after surgery) -The THUNDERBEAT and LigaSure instruments Data will be collected on data collection sheets and entered in a password protected database Primary Outcomes/DefinitionsOverall time for dissection of the soft tissues necessary for specimen removal during colon resection, measured in minutes, from the start of colon mobilization to specimen removal from the abdominal cavity.

Study Type

Interventional

Study Phase

N/A

Condition

- Colon Cancer

Intervention

Device: THUNDERBEAT

Tissue dissection and vessels ligation

Device: LIGASURE

Tissue dissection and vessels ligation

Study Arms

Other: THUNDERBEAT

THUNDERBEAT energy device (Olympus) will be used for dissection of tissue and ligation of vessels

Other: LIGASURE

LIGASURE energy device will be used for dissection of tissue and ligation of vessels

Recruitment Information

Recruitment Status

Recruiting

Completion Date

July 2018

Estimated Enrollment

60

Primary Completion Date

May 2018

Eligibility Criteria

Inclusion Criteria:

- Patients that will be undergoing a Left Laparoscopic Colon Resection
- Older than 18 years old
- ASA 1 to 3

- Elective surgeries
- Patients who willingly provide informed consent

Exclusion Criteria:
- Morbidly obese patients (BMI >35)
- Patients with acute diverticulitis
- Patients with multiple previous abdominal surgeries
- Patients on anticoagulants
- Patients who can not, tolerate a major surgery
- Patients for whom electrosurgery is contraindicated
- Patients who are pregnant
- Patient with IBDs

Sex/Gender

All

Ages

18 Years to N/A

Accepts Healthy Volunteers

No

Contacts

Koiana Trencheva, M.S.   646-962-2342   kivanova@med.cornell.edu

Safety Study of MGD009 in B7-H3-expressing Tumors

Study ID:

NCT02628535

Sponsor:

MacroGenics

Information provided by (Responsible Party):

MacroGenics (MacroGenics)

Tracking Information

First Submitted Date

November 20, 2015

Primary Completion Date

December 2018

Start Date

September 2015

Last Update Posted Date

October 5, 2017

Current Primary Outcome Measures

Number of participants with adverse events[Time Frame: 28 days after last dose of study drug]
adverse events, serious adverse events

Current Secondary Outcome Measures

Peak plasma concentration[Time Frame: 8 days]
PK of MGD009

Number of participants that develop anti-drug antibodies[Time Frame: first dose through 28 days after last dose of study drug]
Proportion of patients who develop anti-MGD0009 antibodies, immunogenicity

Change in tumor volume[Time Frame: Weeks 6, 15, 24, 33, 42, 51, 60, 69, 78, 87, 96, 105]
Anti-tumor activity of MGD006 using both conventional RECIST 1.1 and immune-related RECIST criteria.

Descriptive Information

Offical Title

Phase 1, First-in-Human, Open Label, Dose Escalation Study of MGD009, A Humanized B7-H3 x CD3 Dual-Affinity Re-Targeting (DART) Protein in Patients With Unresectable or Metastatic B7-H3-Expressing Neoplasms

Brief Summary

The purpose of this study is to evaluate the safety of MGD009 when given to patients with B7-H3-expressing tumors. The study will also evaluate what is the highest dose of MGD009 that can be given safely. Assessments will be done to see how the drug acts in the body (pharmacokinetics (PK), pharmacodynamics (PD) and to evaluate potential anti-tumor activity of MGD009.

Detailed Description

This study is a Phase 1 open-label, dose escalation, cohort expansion, and efficacy follow-up study of MGD009 administered intravenously (IV) on an every-other-week schedule for up to one year (14 cycles).

The dose escalation phase is designed to characterize the safety and tolerability of MGD009 and to define the maximum tolerated or maximum administered dose (MTD/MAD). This phase will enroll patients with mesothelioma, bladder cancer, melanoma, squamous cell carcinoma of the head and neck (SCCHN), non-small cell lung cancer (NSCLC), clear cell renal cell carcinoma (ccRCC), ovarian cancer, thyroid cancer, triple-negative breast cancer (TNBC), pancreatic cancer, colon cancer, soft tissue sarcoma, or prostate cancer.

- In the cohort expansion phase, 6 cohorts of 16 patients each will be enrolled to further evaluate the safety and potential efficacy of MGD009 administered at the MTD/MAD dose in patients with mesothelioma, bladder cancer, melanoma, SCCHN, NSCLC, or other specific tumors that express high levels of B7-H3. Preand on-study biopsies are required for melanoma patients in the cohort expansion phase.

The survival follow-up phase consists of the 2-year period after the final dose of study drug.

All tumor evaluations will be carried out by both Response Evaluation Criteria in Solid Tumors (RECIST) and immune-related response criteria (irRC).

Study Type

Interventional

Study Phase

Phase 1

Condition

- Mesothelioma
- Bladder Cancer
- Melanoma
- Squamous Cell Carcinoma of the Head and Neck
- Non Small Cell Lung Cancer
- Clear Cell Renal Cell Carcinoma
- Ovarian Cancer
- Thyroid Cancer
- Breast Cancer
- Pancreatic Cancer
- Prostate Cancer
- Colon Cancer
- Soft Tissue Sarcoma

Intervention

Biological: MGD009
    B7-H3 x CD3 DART protein

Study Arms

Experimental: MGD009
    Humanized B7-H3 x CD3 Dual-Affinity Re-Targeting (DART®) Protein

Recruitment Information

Recruitment Status

Recruiting

Estimated Enrollment

114

Eligibility Criteria

Inclusion Criteria:

- Histologically and/or cytologically proven unresectable locally advanced or metastatic tumors that express B7-H3 on the membrane or vasculature. The requirement for previous systemic therapy may be waived if a person was intolerant of standard

Completion Date

December 2020

Primary Completion Date

December 2018

front-line therapy
- **Dose escalation phase prior systemic treatment requirements:**
- mesothelioma, pancreatic cancer: 1-3 prior treatments
- urothelial, SCHNN, prostate, soft tissue sarcoma, prostate cancer, TNBC, ccRCC, NSCLC: 1-5 prior treatments
- ovarian cancer: 2-4 prior treatments
- colon cancer: 2-4 prior treatments
- melanoma: at least 1 prior treatment (including immunotherapy).
- Patients with prior immune checkpoint inhibitors must have related toxicities reduced to Grade 0, 1, or baseline
- Measurable disease per RECIST 1.1 criteria
- Easter Cooperative Oncology Group (ECOG) performance status 0 or 1
- Acceptable laboratory parameters and adequate organ reserve.

Exclusion Criteria:

- Patients with central nervous system (CNS) involvement must have been treated, be asymptomatic, do not exhibit progression of CNS metastases on MRI or CT within 28 days, and do not have concurrent leptomeningeal disease or cord compression.
- Clinically significant pulmonary compromise (e.g. require supplemental oxygen)
- History of autoimmune disease with certain exceptions such as vitiligo, resolved childhood atopic dermatitis, psoriasis not requiring systemic therapy within the past 2 years, patients with history of Grave's disease that are now euthyroid clinically and by lab testing
- History of clinically-significant cardiovascular disease
- History of clinically-significant gastrointestinal (GI) disease; GI perforation within 1 year; GI bleeding or acute pancreatitis within 3 months; or diverticulitis within 4 weeks of first study drug administration
- Active viral, bacterial, or systemic fungal infection requiring parenteral treatment within 7 days of first study drug administration
- Known history of hepatitis B or C infection or known positive test for hepatitis B surface antigen or core antigen, or hepatitis C polymerase chain reaction (PCR)
- Known positive testing for human immunodeficiency virus or history of acquired immune deficiency syndrome
- History of allogeneic bone marrow, stem cell, or solid organ transplant
- Treatment with systemic cancer therapy or investigational therapy within 4 weeks of first study drug administration; radiation within 2 weeks; corticosteroids (greater than or equal to 10 mg prednisone or equivalent per day) or other immune suppressive drugs within 2 weeks of first study drug administration
- Trauma or major surgery within 4 weeks of first study drug administration
- Known hypersensitivity to recombinant proteins, polysorbate 80, or any excipient contained in the drug or vehicle formulation for MGD009

Sex/Gender

All

Ages

18 Years to N/A

Accepts Healthy Volunteers

No

Contacts

Bing Nie   240-552-8084   nieb@macrogenics.com

Phase I Study of Enadenotucirev and PD-1 Inhibitor in Subjects With Metastatic or Advanced Epithelial Tumors

Study ID:

NCT02636036

Sponsor:

PsiOxus Therapeutics Ltd

Information provided by (Responsible Party):

PsiOxus Therapeutics Ltd (PsiOxus Therapeutics Ltd)

Tracking Information

First Submitted Date

November 20, 2015

Start Date

January 2016

Current Primary Outcome Measures

Maximum Tolerated and/or Maximum Feasible Dose[Time Frame: 12 months]

Maximum tolerated dose (MTD) / maximum feasible dose (MFD) of enadenotucirev administered IV in combination with nivolumab.

Current Secondary Outcome Measures

to assess the blood levels of enadenotucirev following combination treatment[Time Frame: 12 months]

Enadenotucirev blood level samples will be taken on each enadenotucirev dosing day, pre-dose on pembrolizumab dosing day and at the end of study treatment visit. Measurements of enadenotucirev will be in vp/ml

To examine the anti-tumor activity of combination treatment with enadenotucirev and nivolumab[Time Frame: 12 months]

Overall response rate according to RECIST Version 1.1

To examine the anti-tumor activity of combination treatment with enadenotucirev and nivolumab[Time Frame: 12 months]

Overall response rate according to irRECIST Version 1.1

Primary Completion Date

March 2019

Last Update Posted Date

February 16, 2017

Descriptive Information

Offical Title

A Phase I Multicenter, Open Label Study of Enadenotucirev Combined With PD-1 Inhibitor in Subjects With Metastatic or Advanced Epithelial Tumors

Brief Summary

This is a Phase I multicenter, open label, nonrandomized study of enadenotucirev administered in combination with nivolumab in subjects with metastatic or advanced epithelial tumors (with focus on CRC, UCC, SCCHN and salivary gland cancer) not responding to standard therapy.

Study Type

Interventional

Study Phase

Phase 1

Condition

- Colorectal Cancer
- Bladder Carcinoma
- Squamous Cell Carcinoma of the Head and Neck
- Salivary Gland Cancer

Intervention

Biological: enadenotucirev
Biological: nivolumab

Study Arms

Experimental: enadenotucirev and nivolumab

Recruitment Information

Recruitment Status

Recruiting

Estimated Enrollment

30

Eligibility Criteria

Inclusion Criteria:

Completion Date

June 2019

Primary Completion Date

March 2019

- Adult males or females aged 18 years or over
- Diagnosis of metastatic or advanced CRC, UCC, SCCHN, salivary gland cancer or NSCLC with tumor accessible for biopsy
- Dose expansion only: Subjects must have at least one measurable site of disease according to Response Evaluation Criteria in Solid Tumors (RECIST) criteria; this lesion must be outside a previously irradiated area
- **Disease status:**
- Dose escalation phase only: Subject not responding to standard therapy or for whom no standard treatment exists
- **Dose expansion phase: Subject not responding to standard therapy or for whom no standard treatment exists with:**
- CRC No more than four different prior lines of systemic therapy for advanced disease
- UCC and SCCHN and salivary gland cancer No more than three different prior treatment regimens in the advanced/metastatic setting with a maximum of two chemotherapy-containing regimens
- NSCLC Prior treatment regimens must include a platinum-based therapy
- Eastern Cooperative Oncology Group (ECOG) performance status 0 or 1
- Predicted life expectancy of 3 months or more
- Ability to comply with study procedures in the Investigator's opinion
- Recovered to Grade 1 from the effects (excluding alopecia) of any prior therapy for their malignancies
- **Adequate renal function:**
- Creatinine ≤1.5 mg/dL or calculated creatinine clearance using the Cockcroft-Gault formula ≥60 mL/min or measured creatinine clearance
- Proteinuria: dipstick ≤2+
- **Adequate hepatic function:**
- Serum bilirubin <1.5 mg/dL (except subjects with Gilbert's syndrome who may have total bilirubin <3.0 mg/mL)
- Aspartate aminotransferase and alanine aminotransferase ≤3 x upper limit of normal (ULN)
- Albumin ≥3 g/dL
- Lipase: 1.5 x ULN. Subjects with lipase >1.5 x ULN may enrol if there are neither clinical or radiographic signs of pancreatitis
- Amylase: 1.5 x ULN. Subjects with amylase >1.5 x ULN may enrol if there are neither clinical or radiographic signs of pancreatitis
- **Adequate bone marrow function:**
- Absolute neutrophil count ≥1.5 x 109/L
- Platelets ≥100 x 109/L
- Hemoglobin ≥90 g/L
- Adequate coagulation tests: international normalized ratio ≤1.5
- Normal thyroid and pituitary functions
- For females of childbearing potential (defined as <2 years after last menstruation or not surgically sterile), a negative serum pregnancy test must be documented in the 14 days before the first dose of study treatment For females who are not postmenopausal (24 months of amenorrhea) or surgically sterile (absence of ovaries and/or uterus): agreement to use two adequate methods of contraception, during the study treatment period and for at least 6 months after the last dose of study treatment For males: agreement to use a barrier method of contraception during the study treatment period and for at least 6 months after the last dose of study treatment
- Subjects must provide written informed consent to participate
- Willing to consent to tumor biopsies during the study

Exclusion Criteria:

- Pregnant or breastfeeding females
- Known history or evidence of significant immunodeficiency due to underlying illness (e.g. human immunodeficiency virus [HIV]/acquired immunodeficiency syndrome [AIDS]) and/or medication (e.g. systemic corticosteroids or other immunosuppressive medications, including cyclosporine, azathioprine, interferons in the 4 weeks before the first dose of study treatment). Subjects with a condition requiring systemic treatment with either corticosteroids (>10 mg daily prednisolone equivalent) or other immunosuppressive medications within 14 days of the first dose of study treatment. Inhaled or topical steroids and adrenal replacement steroid doses are permitted in the absence of autoimmune disease
- Splenectomy
- Prior allogeneic or autologous bone marrow or organ transplantation
- Subjects with active, known or suspected auto-immune disease or a syndrome that requires systemic or immunosuppressive agents; subjects with vitiligo, type I diabetes mellitus, residual hypothyroidism due to autoimmune disease only requiring hormone replacement, psoriasis not requiring systemic treatment or conditions not expected to recur in the absence of an external trigger are permitted to enrol
- History of idiopathic pulmonary fibrosis, drug induced pneumonitis, evidence of active pneumonia or pneumonitis on computed tomography scan
- Active infections requiring antibiotics, physician monitoring or recurrent fevers >100.4°F (38.0°C) associated with a clinical diagnosis of active infection
- Active viral disease or positive test for hepatitis B virus using hepatitis B surface antigen test or positive test for hepatitis C

virus (HCV) using HCV ribonucleic acid or HCV antibody test indicating acute or chronic infection. Positive test for HIV or AIDS; testing is not required in the absence of history

- Use of the following antiviral agents: ribavirin, adefovir, lamivudine or cidofovir within 7 days prior to the first dose of study treatment; or pegylated interferon in the 14 days before the first dose of study treatment
- Prior treatment with PD-1 and programmed death ligand (PD-L)1 inhibitors
- Administration of an investigational drug in the 28 days before the first dose of study treatment
- Major surgery or treatment with any chemotherapy, radiation therapy, biologics for cancer or investigational therapy in the 28 days before the first dose of study treatment (subjects with prior cytotoxic or investigational products <3 weeks prior to study treatment might be eligible after discussion between the Investigator and Medical Monitor, if toxicities from the prior treatment have been resolved to NCI CTCAE Grade 1). All toxicities attributed to prior anti-cancer therapy other than alopecia and fatigue must have resolved to Grade 1 or baseline before the first dose of study treatment. Subjects with toxicities attributed to prior anti-cancer therapy which are not expected to resolve and result in long lasting sequelae, such as neuropathy after platinum based therapy, are permitted to enrol
- Other prior malignancy active within the previous 3 years except for local or organ confined early stage cancer that has been definitively treated with curative intent, does not require ongoing treatment, has no evidence of residual disease and has a negligible risk of recurrence and is therefore unlikely to interfere with the primary and secondary endpoints of the study, including response rate and safety
- Symptomatic brain metastases or any leptomeningeal metastasis that is symptomatic and/or requires treatment. Subjects with brain metastases are eligible if these have been locally treated (surgery, radiotherapy). There must also be no requirement for immunosuppressive doses of systemic corticosteroids (>10 mg/day prednisone equivalent) for at least 2 weeks before the first dose of study treatment
- Any serious or uncontrolled medical disorder that, in the opinion of the Investigator or the Medical Monitor, may increase the risk associated with study participation or study treatment administration, impair the ability of the subject to receive protocol therapy or interfere with the interpretation of study results
- Known allergy to enadenotucirev, nivolumab or their excipients
- Any other medical or psychological condition that would preclude participation in the study or compromise ability to give informed consent
- Dependence on continuous supplemental oxygen use

Sex/Gender

All

Ages

18 Years to N/A

Accepts Healthy Volunteers

No

Contacts

PsiOxus Therapeutics   enquiries@psioxus.com

Pembrolizumab Combined With Itacitinib (INCB039110) and/or Pembrolizumab Combined With INCB050465 in Advanced Solid Tumors

Study ID:
NCT02646748

Sponsor:
Incyte Corporation

Information provided by (Responsible Party):
Incyte Corporation (Incyte Corporation)

Tracking Information

First Submitted Date
January 4, 2016

Start Date
January 2016

Primary Completion Date
June 2019

Last Update Posted Date
December 19, 2017

Current Primary Outcome Measures

Evaluation of safety and tolerability as measured by the frequency, duration, and severity of adverse events[Time Frame: Duration of study treatment and up to 120 days after the last dose of study drug]

Current Secondary Outcome Measures

Objective Response Rate (ORR) as determined by radiographic disease assessments per immune-related Response Evaluation Criteria In Solid Tumors (irRECIST) v1.1 criteria[Time Frame: Every 9 weeks for the first year on study]

Progression Free Survival (PFS) as measured by the duration from the date of first dose until the earliest date of disease progression or death as measured by immune-related Response Evaluation Criteria In Solid Tumors (irRECIST) v1.1[Time Frame: Every 9 weeks for the first year on study]

Duration of response (DOR) as measured from the time of the earliest response complete response (CR) or partial response (PR) until disease progression per irRECIST v1.1[Time Frame: Every 9 weeks for the first year on study]

Descriptive Information

Offical Title

A Platform Study Exploring the Safety, Tolerability, Effect on the Tumor Microenvironment, and Efficacy of Pembrolizumab + INCB Combinations in Advanced Solid Tumors

Brief Summary

This is an open-label, multicenter, Phase 1b platform study in subjects with advanced or metastatic solid tumors (Part 1a) and subjects with selected solid tumors (Part 1b and Part 2). Two treatment groups (Group A and Group B) will be evaluated

Part 1a utilizes a 3+3 design to evaluate pembrolizumab and INCB combinations in advanced solid tumors. Group A will evaluate a JAK inhibitor with JAK1 selectivity itacitinib (INCB039110) in combination with pembrolizumab (MK-3475) and Group B will evaluate a PI3K-delta inhibitor (INCB050465) in combination with pembrolizumab to determine the maximum tolerated dose (MTD) or PAD and recommend a dose for the Part 1b safety expansion with each combination.

Once the recommended dose has been identified in Part 1a, subjects with select solid tumor types will be enrolled into safety expansion cohorts based upon prior treatment history with a PD-1 pathway-targeted agent (Part 1b) for each combination.

Part 2 utilizes a Simon 2-Stage design to evaluate INCB050465 in combination with pembrolizumab in patients with small cell lung cancer (SCLC) and a 1 stage design to evaluate the combination in patients with non-small cell lung cancer (NSCLC) and urothelial cancer (UC).

Detailed Description

This is an open-label, Phase 1b, 3 Part (Part 1a, Part 1b, and Part 2), multi-center study.

Part 1a utilizes a 3+3 design to evaluate pembrolizumab and INCB combinations in advanced solid tumors. Group A will evaluate a JAK inhibitor with JAK1 selectivity itacitinib (INCB039110) in combination with pembrolizumab (MK-3475) and Group B will evaluate a PI3K-delta inhibitor (INCB050465) in combination with pembrolizumab to determine the maximum tolerated dose (MTD) or PAD and recommend a dose for the Part 1b safety expansion with each combination.

Once the recommended dose has been identified in Part 1a, subjects with endometrial cancer, gastric cancer, melanoma, microsatellite unstable (MSI) colorectal cancer or other MMR-deficient tumors, non-small cell lung cancer, renal cell carcinoma, head and neck squamous cell carcinoma, triple negative breast cancer, pancreatic ductal carcinoma, or transitional cell carcinoma of the genitourinary tract will be enrolled into safety expansion cohorts based upon prior treatment history with a PD-1 pathway-targeted agent (Part 1b) for each combination.

Part 2 utilizes a Simon 2-Stage design to evaluate INCB050465 in combination with pembrolizumab in patients with small cell lung cancer (SCLC) and a 1 stage design to evaluate the combination in patients with non-small cell lung cancer (NSCLC) and urothelial cancer (UC).

Study Type

Interventional

Study Phase

Phase 1

Condition

- Advanced Solid Tumors
- Endometrial Cancer
- Melanoma
- CRC (Colorectal Cancer)
- MMR-deficient Tumors
- RCC (Renal Cell Carinoma)
- SCCHN (Head and Neck Squamous Cell Carcinoma)
- Breast Cancer
- Pancreatic Ductal Adenocarcinoma

- Small Cell Lung Cancer
- NSCLC (Non-small Cell Lung Cancer)
- UC (Urothelial Cancer)

Intervention

Drug: Pembrolizumab

Pembrolizumab 200 mg IV Q3W.

Drug: itacitinib

Itacitinib tablets administered orally once daily.

Other Names:

INCB039110

Drug: INCB050465

INCB050465 tablets administered orally once daily.

Study Arms

Experimental: pembrolizumab + itacitinib

Part 1a Group A will utilize an open-label 3+3 dose-escalation design based on observing each dose level for a period of 21 days.

Part 1b Group A-1 and Group A-2 will evaluate the MTD or PAD of itacitinib in combination with pembrolizumab in subjects with select solid tumors.

Experimental: pembrolizumab + INCB050465

Part 1a Group B will utilize an open-label 3+3 dose-escalation design based on observing each dose level for a period of 21 days.

Part 1b Group B-1 and Group B-2 will evaluate the MTD or PAD of INCB050465 in combination with pembrolizumab in subjects with select solid tumors.

Part 2 will evaluate the combination of INCB050465 in combination with pembrolizumab in subjects with small cell lung cancer, non-small lung cancer and urothelial cancer.

Recruitment Information

Recruitment Status

Recruiting

Estimated Enrollment

237

Completion Date

August 2019

Primary Completion Date

June 2019

Eligibility Criteria

Inclusion Criteria:

- Male or female, age 18 years or older.
- Willingness to provide written informed consent for the study.
- Has a core or excisional baseline tumor biopsy specimen available or willingness to undergo a pre study treatment tumor biopsy to obtain the specimen.
- Eastern Cooperative Oncology Group (ECOG) performance status of 0 to 1.
- Presence of measureable disease based on RECIST v1.1
- For Part 1a: Subjects with histologically or cytologically confirmed advanced or metastatic solid tumors that have failed prior standard therapy (including subject refusal or intolerance).
- For Part 1b: Subjects with histologically or cytologically confirmed advanced or metastatic endometrial cancer, gastric cancer, melanoma, microsatellite unstable (MSI) colorectal cancer or other MMR-deficient tumors, non-small cell lung cancer, renal cell carcinoma, head and neck squamous cell carcinoma, triple negative breast cancer, pancreatic ductal carcinoma, or transitional cell carcinoma of the genitourinary tract that have had disease progression after available therapies for advanced or metastatic disease that are known to confer clinical benefit, been intolerant to treatment, or refused standard treatment.
- For Part 1b: Must have documented confirmed disease progression on a prior PD-1 pathway targeted agent or must be PD-1 pathway-targeted treatment naïve.

For Part 2

For subjects with SCLC:

Subjects with histologically or cytologically confirmed advanced or metastatic SCLC. Must not have had previous treatment with antibodies that modulate T-cell function or checkpoint pathways. Must have disease progression on or after platinum-based chemotherapy or must be intolerant to or refuse standard treatment. Must not have received more than 2 lines of prior therapy.

For subjects with NSCLC:

Subjects with a histologically or cytologically confirmed diagnosis of Stage IIIB, Stage IV, or recurrent NSCLC. Have not received more than 1 prior systemic therapy for metastatic NSCLC. No prior therapy with checkpoint inhibitors (anti-PD-1/PD-L1 or anti-CTLA-4). Have confirmation that EGFR or ALK-directed therapy is not indicated as primary therapy (documentation of absence of tumor activating EGFR mutations AND ALK gene rearrangements treatable with a tyrosine kinase inhibitor (TKI) OR presence of a KRAS mutation). If participant's tumor is known to have a predominantly squamous histology, molecular testing for EGFR mutation and ALK translocation will not be required as this is not part of current diagnostic guidelines. Have measurable disease based on RECIST 1.1.

For subjects with UC:

Subjects with a histologically or cytologically confirmed diagnosis of advanced/unresectable (inoperable) or metastatic urothelial cancer of the renal pelvis, ureter, bladder, or urethra. Have had 1 prior treatment of systemic chemotherapy containing a platinum agent or is considered ineligible to receive cisplatin-based combination therapy. No prior therapy with checkpoint inhibitors (anti-PD-1/PD-L1 or anti-CTLA-4). Have measurable disease based on RECIST 1.1.

Exclusion Criteria:

- Laboratory parameters not within the protocol-defined range.
- Receipt of anticancer medications or investigational drugs within a defined interval before the first administration of study drug.
- Received an immune-suppressive based treatment for any reason within 14 days prior to the first dose of study treatment.
- Has not recovered from toxic effect of prior therapy to < Grade 1.
- Active or inactive autoimmune process.
- Has received a live vaccine within 30 days of planned start of study therapy.
- Active infection requiring systemic therapy.

■ **Sex/Gender**

All

■ **Ages**

18 Years to N/A

■ **Accepts Healthy Volunteers**

No

■ **Contacts**

Incyte Corporation Call Center   1.855.463.3463

Study of the Safety, Tolerability and Efficacy of KPT-8602 in Patients With Relapsed/Refractory Cancer Indications

Study ID:

NCT02649790

Sponsor:

Karyopharm Therapeutics Inc

Information provided by (Responsible Party):

Karyopharm Therapeutics Inc (Karyopharm Therapeutics Inc)

Tracking Information

■ **First Submitted Date**

January 6, 2016

■ **Start Date**

January 2016

■ **Primary Completion Date**

June 2018

■ **Last Update Posted Date**

January 25, 2018

■ **Current Primary Outcome Measures**

- Evaluate dose limiting toxicities of KPT-8602[Time Frame: From first dose through Cycle 128 days]

Descriptive Information

■ **Offical Title**

A Phase 1/2 Open-Label Study of the Safety, Tolerability and Efficacy of the Selective Inhibitor of Nuclear Export (SINE) Compound KPT-8602 in Patients With Relapsed/Refractory Cancer Indications

■ **Brief Summary**

This is a first-in-human, multi-center, open-label clinical study with separate dose escalation (Phase 1) and expansion (Phase 2) stages to assess preliminary safety, tolerability, and efficacy of the second generation oral XPO1 inhibitor KPT-8602 in patients with relapsed/refractory multiple myeloma (MM), colorectal cancer (CRC), metastatic castration resistant prostate cancer (mCRPC), and higher risk myelodysplastic syndrome (MDS).

Dose escalation and dose expansion may be included for all parts of the study as determined by ongoing study results.

■ **Study Type**

Interventional

■ **Study Phase**

Phase 1/Phase 2

■ **Condition**

- Multiple Myeloma (MM)
- Colorectal Cancer (CRC)
- Metastatic Castration Resistant Prostate Cancer (mCRPC)
- Higher Risk Myelodysplastic Syndrome (MDS)

■ **Intervention**

Drug: KPT-8602

■ **Study Arms**

Experimental: KPT-8602

> Multiple myeloma 5-60mg monotherapy, 20mg KPT-8602 + low dose dexamethasone, 30mg KPT-8602 + low dose dexamethasone
>
> starting dose for CRC,mCRPC, MDS is 20 mg KPT-8602

Recruitment Information

■ **Recruitment Status**

Recruiting

■ **Estimated Enrollment**

103

■ **Completion Date**

December 2018

■ **Primary Completion Date**

June 2018

■ **Eligibility Criteria**

INCLUSION CRITERIA

1. Written informed consent obtained prior to any screening procedures and in accordance with federal, local, and institutional guidelines.

2. Age ≥ 18 years.

3. Adequate hepatic function:

a. total bilirubin ≤ 2 times the upper limit of normal (ULN) (except patients with Gilbert's syndrome [hereditary indirect hyperbilirubinemia] who must have a total bilirubin of ≤ 3 times ULN), b. aspartate aminotransferase (AST) and alanine aminotransferase (ALT) ≤ 2.5 times ULN (except patients with known liver involvement of their tumor who must have their AST and ALT ≤ 5.0 times ULN).

4. Adequate renal function: estimated creatinine clearance of ≥ 30 mL/min, calculated using the formula of Cockcroft and Gault (140-Age) • Mass (kg)/(72 • creatinine mg/dL); multiply by 0.85 if female.

5. Contraception:

1. RRMM, CRC, and higher risk MDS patients: Female patients of child-bearing potential must agree to use dual methods of contraception (including one highly effective and one effective method of contraception) and have a negative serum pregnancy test at Screening, and male patients must use an effective barrier method of contraception if sexually active with a female of child-bearing potential. For both male and female patients, effective methods of contraception must be used throughout the study and for 3 months following the last dose.

2. RR mCRPC patients: Patients must use an effective barrier method of contraception if sexually active with a female of child-bearing potential. Effective methods of contraception must be used throughout the study and for 3 months following the last dose.

INDICATION-SPECIFIC INCLUSION CRITERIA

Relapsed/Refractory Multiple Myeloma (Parts A1, A2, and B):

6. Symptomatic, histologically confirmed MM and evidence of disease progression, based on IMWG guidelines.

7. Patients must have measurable disease as defined by at least one of the following:

- Serum M-protein ≥ 0.5 g/dL by serum protein electrophoresis (SPEP) or for immunoglobulin (Ig) A myeloma, by quantitative IgA. If SPEP is felt to be unreliable for routine M-protein measurement (e.g., for patients with IgA MM), then quantitative Ig levels by nephelometry; or

- Urinary M-protein excretion at least 200 mg/24 hours; or

- Serum free light chain (FLC) whereby the involved light chain measures ≥10 mg/dL and with an abnormal ratio.

8. Previously treated with ≥ 3 prior regimens (lines of therapy) that included at least one of each of the following: an immunomodulatory drug, a proteasome inhibitor, and a steroid.

9. MM refractory to the patient's most recent anti-MM regimen.

10. Patients receiving hematopoietic growth factor support including erythropoietin, darbepoetin, granulocyte-colony stimulating factor, granulocyte macrophage-colony stimulating factor, and platelet stimulators can continue to do so, but must be transfusion independent for at least one (1) week prior to Cycle 1 Day 1 (C1D1) in the study.

11. Adequate hematopoietic function: total white blood cell (WBC) count ≥ 1500/mm3, absolute neutrophil count (ANC) ≥ 800/mm3, hemoglobin (Hb) ≥ 8.0 g/dL, and platelet count ≥ 75,000/mm3.

12. Eastern Cooperative Oncology Group (ECOG) performance status of ≤ 1.

13. Life expectancy of ≥ 4 months.

Relapsed/Refractory Colorectal Cancer (Part C):

14. Histological or cytological documentation of adenocarcinoma of the colon or rectum.

15. Measurable disease by RECIST v1.1.

16. Metastatic disease not suitable for upfront curative-intent surgery.

17. Patients with site-defined KRAS status (wild-type or mutant) from a fresh or archival tumor biopsy prior to enrollment.

1. All patients must be willing to have fresh biopsies to obtain tumor tissue for biomarker analysis.

18. Documented evidence of progressive disease according to RECIST v1.1.

19. Prior treatment (with completion of a course of therapy, or to disease progression or intolerability) with each of the following:

1. Fluoropyrimidine-, oxaliplatin-, irinotecan-based chemotherapies (e.g., FOLFOX and FOLFIRI)

2. An anti-EGFR therapy, if KRAS wild-type

3. Prior third line treatment with regorafenib or TAS-102; will be assessed on an individual basis

• Note: The requirement for prior third line regorafenib will be assessed on an individual basis by the Investigator in consultation with the Karyopharm Medical Monitor

4. Radiation and surgery are not considered as prior anticancer regimens

20. Patients should not be transfusion dependent.

21. Adequate hematopoietic function: ANC ≥ 1000/mm3, hemoglobin (Hb) ≥ 9.0 g/dL, and platelet count ≥ 100,000/mm3.

22. Eastern Cooperative Oncology Group (ECOG) performance status of ≤ 1.

23. Life expectancy of ≥ 4 months.

Relapsed/Refractory Metastatic Castration Resistant Prostate Cancer (Parts D and E):

24. Histologically confirmed adenocarcinoma of the prostate with archival tumor tissue available for molecular analyses. If the patient does not have a prior histological diagnosis, then a fresh biopsy at screening may be used for this purpose.

a. Optional: All patients will be asked to have fresh biopsies to obtain tumor tissue for biomarker analysis.

25. Surgically or medically castrated, with testosterone levels of <50 ng/dL (<2.0 nM). If the patient is being treated with luteinizing hormone-releasing hormone (LHRH) agonists (patient who have not undergone orchiectomy), and patients must have shown to progress on this per inclusion criterion 26.

26. Documented mCRPC progression as assessed by the Investigator with one of the following:

1. Prostate specific antigen (PSA) progression defined by a minimum of 3 rising PSA levels (at approximately Day -30 and approximately Day -45) with an interval of >1 week between each determination. The PSA values at the Screening visit should be >2 µg/L (>2 ng/mL); patients on systemic glucocorticoids for control of symptoms must have documented PSA progression by Prostate Cancer Working Group 3 (PCWG3) while on systemic glucocorticoids prior to commencing C1D1 of treatment.

2. Radiographic progression of soft tissue disease by modified RECIST criteria 1.1 or of bone metastasis with 2 or more documented new bone lesions on a bone scan with or without PSA progression.

27. Initial response (per modified PCWG3 Guidelines) to second generation anti-hormonal therapy (examples: abiraterone, enzalutamide, TAK 700), but later relapsed. Disease relapse would be defined as progressive disease at the time of entry per inclusion criterion 26.

28. Zero to 2 previous taxane-based chemotherapy regimens. If docetaxel chemotherapy is used more than once, this will be considered as one regimen. Patients may have had prior exposure to cabazitaxel treatment. Patients may be taxane naïve.

29. At least 2 weeks from completion of any radiotherapy including a single fraction of radiotherapy for the purposes of palliation (confined to one field) is permitted.

30. Patients should not be transfusion dependent.

31. Albumin >2.5 g/dL.

32. Adequate hematopoietic function: ANC ≥ 1000/mm3, hemoglobin (Hb) ≥ 9.0 g/dL, and platelet count ≥ 100,000/mm3.

33. Part E only: Patients currently receiving treatment with abiraterone and appropriate to continue in the opinion of the Investigator. Patients must also have been on and continue on a stable dose of corticosteroids (prednisone or dexamethasone) for 30 days prior to C1D1.

34. Eastern Cooperative Oncology Group (ECOG) performance status of ≤ 1.

35. Life expectancy of ≥ 4 months.

Higher Risk Myelodysplastic Syndrome (Part F):

36. Documented diagnosis of MDS with 5-19% myeloblasts, (MDS-EB-2 by the 2016 WHO classification).

- The marrow histopathology must be documented by recent bone marrow biopsy

- Patients should be intermediate-2 or high-risk MDS by International Prognostic Scoring System (IPSS)

37. Patients believed to be IPSS high risk, without clearly meeting IPSS categories above should be discussed with the Medical Monitor prior to enrolling. This includes patients with unusual cytogenetic patterns, or those who would normally be high risk by International Prognostic Scoring System-Revised (IPSS-R).

38. Documented evidence of progressive disease as defined by the 2006 International Working Group (IWG) Response Criteria for MDS. This includes hypomethylating agent failures (HMA).

39. HMA refractory patients including:

1. ≥2 cycles of azacitidine and/or decitabine or experimental agents (such as SGI-110 or ASTX727 or similar) with clear progressive disease (PD) (no count recovery with ≥50% increase in bone marrow blasts)

OR

2. ≥4 cycles of azacitidine and/or decitabine (or other hypomethylating therapy) with lack of improvement (no CR/CRi/PR/HI).

40. Patients receiving a stable dose of erythropoiesis-stimulating agent (ESA) for at least 1 month at the time of study entry may continue to receive ESA, but changes in dosing of ESA or new start of ESA in less than 30 days are not permitted.

41. Eastern Cooperative Oncology Group (ECOG) performance status of ≤ 2.

EXCLUSION CRITERIA

Patients in All Parts of the Study:

1. Female patients who are pregnant or lactating.

2. Major surgery within 4 weeks before C1D1.

3. Impaired cardiac function or clinically significant cardiac diseases, including any of the following:

1. Unstable angina or acute myocardial infarction ≤ 3 months prior to C1D1;

2. Clinically significant heart disease (e.g., symptomatic congestive heart failure [e.g., >NYHA Class 2]; uncontrolled arrhythmia, or hypertension; history of labile hypertension or poor compliance with an antihypertensive regimen).

4. Uncontrolled active severe systemic infection requiring parenteral antibiotics, antivirals, or antifungals within one week prior to C1D1.

5. Patients with known symptomatic brain metastasis are not suitable for enrollment. Patients with asymptomatic, stable, treated brain metastases are eligible for study entry.

6. Patients with a known history of human immunodeficiency virus (HIV); HIV testing is not required as part of this study.

7. Known, active hepatitis A, B, or C infection; or known to be positive for HCV RNA or HBsAg (HBV surface antigen).

8. Prior malignancies:

1. Patients in All Parts of the Study: Patients with adequately resected basal or squamous cell carcinoma of the skin, or adequately resected carcinoma in situ (i.e. cervix) may enroll irrespective of the time of diagnosis.

2. Patients with Relapsed/refractory MM, CRC, and mCRPC only: Prior malignancies which may interfere with the interpretation of the study. Cancer treated with curative intent < 5 years previously will not be allowed unless approved by the Sponsor. Cancer treated with curative intent > 5 years previously and without evidence of recurrence will be allowed.

3. Patients with Higher Risk MDS only: Concomitant malignancies or previous malignancies with less than a 1-year disease free interval at the time of enrollment.

9. Patients with active central nervous system (CNS) malignancy. Patients who have only had prophylactic intrathecal or intravenous chemotherapy against CNS disease are eligible.

10. Patients with gastrointestinal tract disease (or uncontrolled vomiting or diarrhea) that could interfere with the absorption of KPT-8602.

11. Serious psychiatric or medical conditions that, in the opinion of the Investigator, could interfere with treatment, compliance, or the ability to give consent.

12. Patients unwilling to comply with the protocol including required biopsies and sample collections required to measure disease.

INDICATION-SPECIFIC EXCLUSION CRITERIA

Relapsed/Refractory Multiple Myeloma (Parts A1, A2, and B):

13. Time since the last prior therapy for treatment of RRMM:

1. Radiation, chemotherapy, immunotherapy or any other anticancer therapy, including investigational anticancer therapy ≤ 2 weeks prior to C1D1.

2. Palliative steroids for disease related symptoms are allowed up to 3 days prior to C1D1.

3. Patients must have recovered or stabilized (≤ Grade 1 or to their baseline) from toxicities related to their previous treatment except for alopecia.

14. Patients with active graft versus host disease after allogeneic stem cell transplantation. At least 3 months must have elapsed since completion of allogeneic stem cell transplantation 15. Grade > 2 peripheral neuropathy or Grade 2 peripheral neuropathy with pain within 2 weeks prior to C1D1.

Relapsed/Refractory Colorectal Cancer (Part C):

16. Radiotherapy, chemotherapy, or any other anticancer therapy, including investigational anticancer therapy, within 2 weeks prior to Screening. Patients must have recovered from clinically significant toxicities. The site of irradiation should have evidence of progressive disease (new lesions or increase in lesion size) if this is the only site of disease.

17. Patients who have been treated with their most recent chemotherapy or investigational drugs ≤21 days or 5 half-lives (whichever is longer) prior to the first dose of study treatment, and/or have any acute toxicities due to prior chemotherapy and/or radiotherapy that have not resolved to a NCI-CTCAE v4.03 Grade 0 or Grade 1 with the exception of chemotherapy induced alopecia and Grade 2 peripheral neuropathy.

Relapsed/Refractory Metastatic Castration Resistant Prostate Cancer (Parts D and E):

17. Patients who have been treated with their most recent chemotherapy or investigational drugs ≤21 days or 5 half-lives (whichever is longer) prior to the first dose of study treatment, and/or have any acute toxicities due to prior chemotherapy and/or radiotherapy that have not resolved to a NCI-CTCAE v4.03 Grade 0 or Grade 1 with the exception of chemotherapy induced alopecia and Grade 2 peripheral neuropathy.

18. Initiating bisphosphonate therapy or adjusting bisphosphonate dose/regimen within 30 days prior to C1D1. Patients on a stable bisphosphonate or denosumab regimen are eligible and may continue.

Higher risk Myelodysplastic Syndrome (Part F):

19. IPSS low or intermediate-1 risk MDS. 20. Evidence of transformation to AML by World Health Organization (WHO) (≥20% blasts in bone marrow or peripheral blood).

21. Patients receiving granulocyte-colony stimulating factor (G-CSF) or granulocyte macrophage-colony stimulating factor (GM-CSF) within the 3 weeks prior to C1D1.

- **Sex/Gender**

  All

- **Ages**

  18 Years to N/A

- **Accepts Healthy Volunteers**

  No

- **Contacts**

  Michael Kauffman, M.D., Ph.D.   mkauffman@karyopharm.com
  Sharon Shacham, PhD

Phase 1/1b Study to Evaluate the Safety and Tolerability of CPI-444 Alone and in Combination With Atezolizumab in Advanced Cancers

Study ID:

NCT02655822

Sponsor:

Corvus Pharmaceuticals, Inc.

Information provided by (Responsible Party):

Corvus Pharmaceuticals, Inc. (Corvus Pharmaceuticals, Inc.)

Tracking Information

- **First Submitted Date**

  January 8, 2016

- **Start Date**

  January 2016

■ **Current Primary Outcome Measures**

Incidence of dose-limiting toxicities (DLTs) of CPI-444 as a single agent and in combination with atezolizumab[Time Frame: 28 days following first administration of CPI-444]

Objective response rate per RECIST v1.1 criteria of CPI-444 as a single agent and in combination with atezolizumab[Time Frame: From start of treatment to end of treatment, up to 36 months]

Incidence of treatment-emergent adverse events, as assessed by NCI CTCAE v.4.03, of CPI-444 as a single agent and in combination with atezolizumab[Time Frame: Continuously, up to 36 months]

Mean and median Area under the curve (AUC) of CPI-444[Time Frame: Day 14 of Cycle 1]

Mean and median Maximum concentration (Cmax) of CPI-444[Time Frame: Day 14 of Cycle 1]

Identify the MDL (maximum dose level) of single agent CPI-444[Time Frame: From start of treatment to end of treatment, up to 36 months.]

Descriptive Information

■ **Offical Title**

A Phase 1/1b, Open-Label, Multicenter, Repeat-Dose, Dose-Selection Study of CPI-444 as Single Agent and in Combination With Atezolizumab in Patients With Selected Incurable Cancers

■ **Brief Summary**

This is a phase 1/1b open-label, multicenter, dose-selection study of CPI-444, an oral small molecule targeting the adenosine-A2A receptor on T-lymphocytes and other cells of the immune system. This trial will study the safety, tolerability, and anti-tumor activity of CPI-444 as a single agent and in combination with atezolizumab, a PD-L1 inhibitor against various solid tumors. CPI-444 blocks adenosine from binding to the A2A receptor. Adenosine suppresses the anti-tumor activity of T cells and other immune cells.

■ **Detailed Description**

This is a phase 1/1b open-label, multicenter, dose-selection study of CPI-444, an oral small molecule targeting the adenosine-A2A receptor on T-lymphocytes and other cells of the immune system. This trial will study the safety, tolerability, and anti-tumor activity of CPI-444 as a single agent and in combination with atezolizumab, an intravenous PD-L1 inhibitor. CPI-444 blocks adenosine from binding to the A2A receptor. Adenosine suppresses the anti-tumor activity of T cells and other immune cells.

■ **Study Type**

Interventional

■ **Study Phase**

Phase 1

■ **Condition**

- Non-Small Cell Lung Cancer
- Malignant Melanoma
- Renal Cell Cancer
- Triple Negative Breast Cancer
- Colorectal Cancer
- Bladder Cancer
- Metastatic Castration Resistant Prostate Cancer

■ **Intervention**

Drug: CPI-444

100 mg orally twice daily for the first 14 days of each 28-day cycle.

Drug: CPI-444

100 mg orally twice daily for 28 days of each 28-day cycle.

Drug: CPI-444

200 mg orally once daily for the first 14 days of each 28-day cycle.

Drug: CPI-444 + atezolizumab

CPI-444 orally in combination with atezolizumab intravenously.

Drug: CPI-444

Start with150mg orally twice daily for 28-day cycles; then, increase increments by 100mg/day for 6 dose levels.

■ **Study Arms**

Experimental: Cohort 1
CPI-444

Experimental: Cohort 2
CPI-444

Experimental: Cohort 3
CPI-444

Experimental: Cohort 4
CPI-444 + atezolizumab

Experimental: Cohort 5
CPI-444

Recruitment Information

■ **Recruitment Status**

Recruiting

■ **Estimated Enrollment**

534

■ **Eligibility Criteria**

Inclusion Criteria

1. Eastern Cooperative Oncology Group (ECOG) Performance Status 0-1.

2. Documented incurable cancer with one of the following histologies: non-small cell lung cancer, malignant melanoma, renal cell cancer, triple negative breast cancer, colorectal cancer with microsatellite instability (MSI), bladder cancer, and metastatic castration resistant prostate cancer.

3. At least 1 measurable lesion per Response Evaluation Criteria in Solid Tumors (RECIST 1.1).

4. At least 1 but not more than 5 prior systemic therapies for advanced/recurrent or progressing disease.

Exclusion Criteria

1. History of severe hypersensitivity reaction to monoclonal antibodies.

2. Any active autoimmune disease or a documented history of serious autoimmune disease within the past 5 years requiring immunosuppressive therapy.

3. History of idiopathic pulmonary fibrosis, organizing pneumonia, drug-induced pneumonitis, idiopathic pneumonitis, or clinical symptoms of active pneumonitis.

4. The use of any investigational medication or device in the 30 days prior to screening and throughout the study is prohibited.

5. If a patient is currently receiving denosumab, this must be discontinued prior to enrollment. Substitution with biphosphonates are acceptable.

■ **Completion Date**

December 2018

■ **Primary Completion Date**

June 2018

■ **Sex/Gender**

All

■ **Ages**

18 Years to N/A

■ **Accepts Healthy Volunteers**

No

PF-06671008 Dose Escalation Study in Advanced Solid Tumors

Study ID:

NCT02659631

Sponsor:

Pfizer

Information provided by (Responsible Party):

Pfizer (Pfizer)

Tracking Information

■ **First Submitted Date**

January 15, 2016

■ **Start Date**

April 28, 2016

■ **Primary Completion Date**

March 27, 2021

■ **Last Update Posted Date**

February 1, 2018

■ **Current Primary Outcome Measures**

Number of participants with Dose-Limiting Toxicities (DLT) [Part 1][Time Frame: Baseline through Day 21]

> First cycle DLTs in order to determine the maximum tolerated dose

Number of participants with objective response[Time Frame: Baseline, every 6 weeks until disease progression or unacceptable toxicity up to 24 months]

> Objective response as determined by RECIST v1.1

■ **Current Secondary Outcome Measures**

Maximum Observed Plasma Concentration (Cmax)[Time Frame: C1D1 0, 1, 2, 4, 8, 24 hrs post, D4, D8 0, 1, 2, 4, 8, 24 hrs post, D11, D15 0, 1 or 2 hrs post, C2D1 0, 1 or 2, 4, 24 hrs post, D4, D8 and D15 0, 1 or 2 hrs post, 0, 1 or 2 hrs post on D1, 8 and 15 of subsequent cycles, and up to 24 months]

> Time to Reach Maximum Observed Plasma Concentration (Tmax)[Time Frame: C1D1 0, 1, 2, 4, 8, 24 hrs post, D4, D8 0, 1, 2, 4, 8, 24 hrs post, D11, D15 0, 1 or 2 hrs post, C2D1 0, 1 or 2, 4, 24 hrs post, D4, D8 and D15 0, 1 or 2 hrs post, 0, 1 or 2 hrs post on D1, 8 and 15 of subsequent cycles, and up to 24 months]

> Plasma Decay Half-Life (t1/2)[Time Frame: C1D1 0, 1, 2, 4, 8, 24 hrs post, D4, D8 0, 1, 2, 4, 8, 24 hrs post, D11, D15 0, 1 or 2 hrs post, C2D1 0, 1 or 2, 4, 24 hrs post, D4, D8 and D15 0, 1 or 2 hrs post, 0, 1 or 2 hrs post on D1, 8 and 15 of subsequent cycles, and up to 24 months]

> Area Under the Curve from Time Zero to End of Dosing Interval (AUCtacu)[Time Frame: C1D1 0, 1, 2, 4, 8, 24 hrs post, D4, D8 0, 1, 2, 4, 8, 24 hrs post, D11, D15 0, 1 or 2 hrs post, C2D1 0, 1 or 2, 4, 24 hrs post, D4, D8 and D15 0, 1 or 2 hrs post, 0, 1 or 2 hrs post on D1, 8 and 15 of subsequent cycles, and up to 24 months]

> Area Under the Curve from time zero to infinity (AUCinf)[Time Frame: C1D1 0, 1, 2, 4, 8, 24 hrs post, D4, D8 0, 1, 2, 4, 8, 24 hrs post, D11, D15 0, 1 or 2 hrs post, C2D1 0, 1 or 2, 4, 24 hrs post, D4, D8 and D15 0, 1 or 2 hrs post, 0, 1 or 2 hrs post on D1, 8 and 15 of subsequent cycles, and up to 24 months]

> Systemic Clearance[Time Frame: C1D1 0, 1, 2, 4, 8, 24 hrs post, D4, D8 0, 1, 2, 4, 8, 24 hrs post, D11, D15 0, 1 or 2 hrs post, C2D1 0, 1 or 2, 4, 24 hrs post, D4, D8 and D15 0, 1 or 2 hrs post, 0, 1 or 2 hrs post on D1, 8 and 15 of subsequent cycles, and up to 24 months]

> Number of participants with objective response (Part 1)[Time Frame: Baseline and every 6 weeks for the first 6 months, then every 12 weeks until disease progression, unacceptable toxicity, or up to 24 months]

> Response rate by RECIST v1.1

Number of participants with PFS (Part 2)[Time Frame: Baseline and every 6 weeks for the first 6 months, then every 12 weeks until disease progression or unacceptable toxicity, or up to 24 months]

> Number of participants with OS (Part 2)[Time Frame: Baseline and every 6 weeks until disease progression or unacceptable toxicity, or up to 24 months]

Descriptive Information

■ **Offical Title**

A Phase 1 Dose Escalation Study Evaluating The Safety And Tolerability Of Pf-06671008 In Patients With Advanced Solid Tumors

■ **Brief Summary**

The study will evaluate the safety, pharmacokinetics and pharmacodynamics of increasing doses of PF-06671008 in patients with advanced solid tumors with the potential to have P-cadherin expression. The study will then expand to look at the selected dose in patients with P-cadherin expressing TNBC, CRC or NSCLC.

■ **Study Type**

Interventional

■ **Study Phase**

Phase 1

- ▓ **Condition**
  - Neoplasms
- ▓ **Intervention**

  Drug: PF-06671008

  Dose Escalation Phase Part 1

  Drug: PF-06671008

  Dose Expansion Phase Part 2
- ▓ **Study Arms**

  Experimental: PF-06671008

Recruitment Information

- ▓ **Recruitment Status**

  Recruiting
- ▓ **Estimated Enrollment**

  110
- ▓ **Eligibility Criteria**

  Key Inclusion Criteria
  - Diagnosis of tumor type with the potential to have P-cadherin expression that is resistant to standard therapy or for which no standard therapy is available
  - Performance status of 0 or 1
  - Adequate bone marrow, kidney and liver function

  Key Exclusion Criteria
  - Known CNS disease including, but not limited to, metastases
  - Current or history of seizure disorder
  - History of or active autoimmune disorders
  - Active bacterial, fungal or viral infection
  - Major surgery, anti-cancer therapy, or radiation therapy within 4 weeks of study treatment
  - Requirement for systemic immune suppressive medication
  - Grade 2 or greater peripheral neuropathy
- ▓ **Sex/Gender**

  All
- ▓ **Ages**

  18 Years to N/A
- ▓ **Accepts Healthy Volunteers**

  No
- ▓ **Contacts**

  Pfizer CT.gov Call Center   1-800-718-1021   ClinicalTrials.gov   Inquiries@pfizer.com

- ▓ **Completion Date**

  March 27, 2021
- ▓ **Primary Completion Date**

  March 27, 2021

A Study of Niclosamide in Patients With Resectable Colon Cancer

Study ID:

NCT02687009

Sponsor:

Michael Morse, MD

Information provided by (Responsible Party):

Duke University (Michael Morse, MD)

Tracking Information

First Submitted Date

February 10, 2016

Start Date

April 17, 2017

Primary Completion Date

July 2020

Last Update Posted Date

April 20, 2017

Current Primary Outcome Measures

Dose limiting toxicity[Time Frame: 5 DAYS]

> The NCI Common Toxicity Criteria version 4.0 will be used to grade adverse events to determine dose limiting toxicity for safety measure

Dose limiting toxicity[Time Frame: 30 DAYS]

> he NCI Common Toxicity Criteria version 4.0 will be used to grade adverse events to determine dose limiting toxicity for safety measure

Current Secondary Outcome Measures

Niclosamide blood levels[Time Frame: 1 DAY]

> Niclosamide blood levels[Time Frame: 2 days]

> Niclosamide blood levels[Time Frame: 8 days]

Descriptive Information

Offical Title

A Phase I Study of Niclosamide in Patients With Resectable Colon Cancer

Brief Summary

This study evaluates the safety of Niclosamide in patients with colon cancer that are undergoing primary resection of their tumor. This is a phase I study with three dosage levels to determine the maximum tolerated dose (MTD).

Detailed Description

Niclosamide is a drug traditionally used in parasitic infections that has recently been shown to regulated the Wnt signaling pathway in cells at the level of the Frizzled receptor.

The Wnt pathway is critical for embryogenesis, differentiation of progenitor cells, and supports proliferation of neoplastic tissue. In cancer, activation of the Wnt pathway leads to increased transcription of genes important for growth, proliferation, differentiation, apoptosis, genetic stability, migration, and angiogenesis. The Wnt pathway has particular importance in colorectal cancer.

The purpose of this study is to obtain safety data along with pharmacokinetic data and information on the changes in the WNT pathway signalling following niclosamide administration in humans. This phase I study will support future studies in patients with more advanced cancer and other cancers with dysregulation of the Wnt pathway.

Study Type

Interventional

Study Phase

Phase 1

Condition

- Colon Cancer

Intervention

Drug: Niclosamide

> Niclosamide will be taken orally in the morning of each day from day 1-7 prior to surgery for resection of primary tumor. Niclosamide tablets must be chewed well prior to swallowing.

Other Names:

> Yomensan

Study Arms

Experimental: Niclosamide

Publications

(Includes publications given by the data provider as well as publications identified by ClinicalTrials.gov Identifier (NCT Number) in Medline.)Osada T, Chen M, Yang XY, Spasojevic I, Vandeusen JB, Hsu D, Clary BM, Clay TM, Chen W, Morse MA, Lyerly

HK. Antihelminth compound niclosamide downregulates Wnt signaling and elicits antitumor responses in tumors with activating APC mutations. Cancer Res. 2011 Jun 15;71(12):4172-82. doi: 10.1158/0008-5472.CAN-10-3978. Epub 2011 Apr 29. (https://www.ncbi.nlm.nih.gov/pubmed/21531761)

Recruitment Information

Recruitment Status

Recruiting

Estimated Enrollment

18

Completion Date

July 2022

Primary Completion Date

July 2020

Eligibility Criteria

Inclusion Criteria:

- Histologically confirmed diagnosis of colon adenocarcinoma with a plan to undergo surgical resection no sooner than 7 days from the projected date of study drug initiation. Patients with rectal cancer not receiving pre-operative chemoradiotherapy are also eligible.
- Karnofsky performance status greater than or equal to 70%
- Age ≥ 18 years.
- Adequate hematologic function, with ANC > 1500/microliter, hemoglobin ≥ 9 g/dL (may transfuse or use erythropoietin to achieve this level), platelets ≥ 100,000/microliter; INR <1.5, PTT <1.5X ULN
- Adequate renal and hepatic function, with serum creatinine < 1.5 mg/dL, bilirubin < 1.5 mg/dL (except for Gilbert's syndrome which will allow bilirubin ≤ 2.0 mg/dL), ALT and AST ≤ 2.5 x upper limit of normal.
- Ability to understand and provide signed informed consent that fulfills Institutional Review Board's guidelines.
- Ability to return to Duke University Medical Center for adequate follow-up, as required by this protocol.

Exclusion Criteria:

- Patients with concurrent cytotoxic chemotherapy or radiation therapy are excluded
- Known active brain or leptomeningeal metastases (defined as symptomatic metastases) or continued requirement for glucocorticoids for brain or leptomeningeal metastases. Treated, asymptomatic metastases are permitted provided the patient has been off steroids for at least 1 month prior to day 1 of study drug.
- Patients with serious intercurrent chronic or acute illness, such as cardiac disease (NYHA class III or IV), hepatic disease, or other illness considered by the Principal Investigator as unwarranted high risk for investigational drug treatment.
- Patients with a medical or psychological impediment to probable compliance with the protocol should be excluded.
- Concurrent (or within the last 5 years) second malignancy other than non melanoma skin cancer, cervical carcinoma in situ, controlled superficial bladder cancer, or other carcinoma in situ that has been treated.
- Presence of a known active acute or chronic infection including: a urinary tract infection, HIV or viral hepatitis.
- Patients with prior use of niclosamide or allergies to niclosamide will be excluded from the protocol.
- Concomitant use of strong CYP3A4, CYP 1A2, or CYP2C9 substrates (See http://medicine.iupui.edu/clinpharm/ddis/main-table).
- Pregnant and nursing women should be excluded from the protocol since this research may have unknown and harmful effects on an unborn child or on young children. If the patient is sexually active, the patient must agree to use a medically acceptable form of birth control while receiving treatment and for a period of 12 months following the last dose of niclosamide. It is not known whether the treatment used in this study could affect the sperm and could potentially harm a child that may be fathered while on this study.
- Patients with complete bowel obstruction or who are at high risk for GI perforation or severe hemorrhage. Patients with inflammatory bowel disease.

Sex/Gender

All

Ages

18 Years to 99 Years

Accepts Healthy Volunteers

No

Contacts

Michael A Morse, MD   919-684-5705   michael.morse@dm.duke.edu
Wanda Honeycutt, RN BSN CCRP   919-668-1861   wanda.honeycutt@dm.duke.edu

Study of Safety and Efficacy of Ribociclib and Trametinib in Patients With Metastatic or Advanced Solid Tumors

Study ID:

NCT02703571

Sponsor:

Novartis Pharmaceuticals

Information provided by (Responsible Party):

Novartis (Novartis Pharmaceuticals)

Tracking Information

▓ **First Submitted Date**

March 4, 2016

▓ **Start Date**

June 29, 2016

▓ **Primary Completion Date**

December 15, 2018

▓ **Last Update Posted Date**

February 12, 2018

▓ **Current Primary Outcome Measures**

Incidence of dose limiting toxicities (DLTs)[Time Frame: 21-day cycle one of treatment]

Phase I part:

The primary variable is the incidence of DLTs during the first 21 days of therapy. Estimation of the MTD of the combination treatment will be based upon the estimation of the probability of DLT during the first 21 days of therapy for patients in the DDS.

Objective Response Rate (ORR)[Time Frame: Until progression of disease up to 1 year]

Phase II part:

The primary variable used to evaluate the efficacy of the ribociclib and trametinib combination is the ORR, defined as the proportion of patients with a best overall confirmed CR or PR, as assessed per RECIST 1.1 by investigator assessment.

▓ **Current Secondary Outcome Measures**

Duration of response (DOR)[Time Frame: Until progression of disease up to 1 year]

Among patients with a confirmed response (PR or CR) per RECIST 1.1, DOR is defined as the time from first documented response (PR or CR) to the date of first documented disease progression or death due to any cause. The distribution function of DOR will be estimated using the Kaplan-Meier method. The median DOR along with 95% CI will be presented by treatment arm.

Time to response[Time Frame: Until progression of disease up to 1 year]

Time to overall response of CR or PR (TTR) is defined as the time from start of study drug to first documented response (CR or PR, which must be confirmed subsequently) for patients with a confirmed CR or PR. TTR will be summarized by treatment arm, using descriptive statistics.

Disease control rate[Time Frame: Until progression of disease up to 1 year]

Disease control rate (DCR) is defined as the proportion of patients with best overall response of CR, PR, or SD per RECIST 1.1. DCR will be estimated and the binomial exact 95% CI will be provided by arm.

Progression disease rate[Time Frame: Until progression of disease up to 1 year]

Progression disease rate defined as the proportion of patients with a progression disease as assessed per RECIST 1.1 by investigator assessment.

Progression free survival[Time Frame: Until progression of disease up to 1 year]

Progression-free survival (PFS) is defined as the time from the date of the first dose of study drug to the date of first documented disease progression per RECIST 1.1 or death due to any cause.

overall survival[Time Frame: Until death up to 1 year]

Overall survival (OS) is defined as the time from the date of first dose of study drug to the date of death due to any cause.

Descriptive Information

▓ **Offical Title**

A Phase I/II Study of Safety and Efficacy of Ribociclib (LEE011) in Combination With Trametinib (TMT212) in Patients With Metastatic or Advanced Solid Tumors

Brief Summary

Phase Ib dose escalation in advanced solid tumors to identify dose for Phase II dose expansion in advanced or metastatic pancreatic cancer and KRAS-mutant colorectal cancer. Open-label, nonrandomized.

Study Type

Interventional

Study Phase

Phase 1/Phase 2

Condition

- Solid Tumors
- Pancreatic Cancer
- Colorectal Cancer

Intervention

Drug: ribociclib

Other Names:

LEE011

Drug: Trametinib

Other Names:

TMT212

Study Arms

Experimental: Advanced or metastatic pancreatic cancer

Patients in the Phase II portion of the study who have advanced or metastatic pancreatic cancer

Experimental: KRAS-mutant colorectal cancer

Patients in the Phase II portion of the study who have KRAS-mutant colorectal cancer

Recruitment Information

Recruitment Status

Recruiting

Estimated Enrollment

124

Completion Date

May 2, 2019

Primary Completion Date

December 15, 2018

Eligibility Criteria

Inclusion Criteria (All):

- Written informed consent must
- Patient has histologically and/or cytologically confirmed malignancies:

Phase I:

- Patients with advanced or metastatic solid tumors who have failed at least one prior line of systemic antineoplastic therapy in the advanced setting without a standard of care treatment option available;

Phase II:

- Advanced or metastatic pancreatic adenocarcinoma who have failed at least one prior systemic antineoplastic therapies in the advanced setting
- Advanced or metastatic KRAS-mutant CRC who have failed at least two prior systemic antineoplastic therapies in the advanced setting without a standard of care treatment option available. Testing for KRAS mutation in patients with CRC using locally approved diagnostic kit will be used for eligibility.
- Phase II only: patient must have measurable disease
- Patient has an ECOG performance status 0 or 1.
- Patient has adequate bone marrow and organ function
- Patient must have specified laboratory values within normal limits or corrected to within normal limits with supplements before the first dose of study medication on Cycle 1 Day 1:
- Standard 12-lead ECG values defined

Exclusion Criteria:

Phase II only:

- Patient has received prior treatment with a MEK inhibitor or a CDK4/6 inhibitor.

Phase I and Phase II:

- Patient with a known hypersensitivity to the study drugs or any of the excipients of ribociclib or trametinib.
- Patient is concurrently using other anti-cancer therapy.
- Patient has received radiotherapy ≤ 4 weeks or limited field radiation for palliation ≤ 2 weeks prior to Cycle 1 Day 1
- Patient has received local therapy to liver ≤ 3 months of C1D1
- History of liver disease as follow:
- Cirrhosis
- Autoimmune hepatitis
- Portal hypertension
- Drug induced liver steatosis
- Prior systemic anti-cancer treatment within 28 days prior to Cycle 1 Day 1
- Prior therapy with anthracyclines at cumulative doses of 450 mg/ m2 or more for doxorubicin or 900 mg/m2 or more for epirubicin.
- Patient is currently receiving warfarin or other coumadin derived anti-coagulant
- Patient has a history of deep venin thrombosis or pulmonary embolism within 6 months of screening.
- Patient has a concurrent malignancy or malignancy within 3 years prior to Cycle 1 Day 1, with the exception of adequately treated basal or squamous cell carcinoma or curatively resected cervical cancer.
- Patients with central nervous system (CNS) involvement
- Patient has impairment of GI function or GI disease that may significantly alter the absorption of the study drugs
- History of interstitial lung disease or pneumonitis.
- Clinically significant, uncontrolled heart disease and/or cardiac repolarization abnormality
- Patient is currently receiving any strong inducers or inhibitors of CYP3A4/5 and/or Substances that have a narrow therapeutic window and are predominantly metabolized through CYP3A4/5 and cannot be discontinued 7 days prior to Cycle 1 Day 1:
- Patient is currently receiving or has received systemic corticosteroids ≤ 2 weeks prior to starting study drug, or who have not fully recovered from side effects of such treatment.
- History of retinal vein occlusion (RVO)

Other protocol-defined inclusion/exclusion criteria may apply.

■ **Sex/Gender**

All

■ **Ages**

18 Years to N/A

■ **Accepts Healthy Volunteers**

No

■ **Contacts**

Novartis Pharmaceuticals   1-888-669-6682   novartis.email@novartis.com
Novartis Pharmaceuticals   +41613241111   novartis.email@novartis.com

Open-Label Safety and Tolerability Study of INCB057643 in Subjects With Advanced Malignancies

Study ID:

NCT02711137

Sponsor:

Incyte Corporation

Information provided by (Responsible Party):

Incyte Corporation (Incyte Corporation)

Tracking Information

First Submitted Date

March 9, 2016

Start Date

May 2016

Primary Completion Date

November 2021

Last Update Posted Date

November 30, 2017

Current Primary Outcome Measures

Safety and tolerability of INCB057643 as monotherapy and in combination with standard of care (SOC) agents in patients with advanced malignancies; assessed by clinical laboratory assessments, physical examinations, 12 lead ECGs, and adverse events (AEs)[Time Frame: From screening through at least 30 days after end of treatment, up to approximately 24 months]

Current Secondary Outcome Measures

Pharmacokinetics of INCB057643 as monotherapy in the fasted state and in the fed state (food effect; Part 2 only) and when administered in combination with Standard of Care (SOC) agents in the fasted state assessed by plasma and urine concentrations[Time Frame: Protocol-defined timepoints in treatment Cycle 1 and 2, up to approximately 1 month.]

Measurement of cellular myc protein concentrations before and after administration of INCB057643 when administered as monotherapy[Time Frame: PD in plasma at pre-dose and 0.5, 1, 2, 4, 6 and 8 hours postdose, up to approximately 1 month.]

Identify cell populations and changes in cell populations, including, but not limited to, markers for tumor cell or immune cell populations before and after administration of INCB057643 when administered as monotherapy[Time Frame: Sparse correlative whole blood and plasma up to approximately 24 months.]

Efficacy of INCB057643 when administered as monotherapy and in combination with SOC agents based on the investigator assessment of response using criteria appropriate for each disease in subjects with advanced malignancies criteria[Time Frame: Efficacy measures from screening through end of treatment and follow-up (every 9 weeks), up to approximately 24 months]

Measurement of biomarkers that may predict pharmacologic activity or response to INCB57643 when administered as monotherapy and in combination with SOC agents criteria[Time Frame: Efficacy measures from screening through end of treatment and follow-up (every 9 weeks), up to approximately 24 months]

Efficacy assessed by progression-free survival (PFS) or event-free survival (EFS) per disease-specific response criteria[Time Frame: Efficacy measures from screening through end of treatment and follow-up (every 9 weeks), up to approximately 24 months]

Efficacy assessed by duration of response (DOR) per disease-specific response criteria[Time Frame: Efficacy measures from screening through end of treatment and follow-up (every 9 weeks), up to approximately 24 months]

Efficacy assessed by overall survival (OS) per disease-specific response criteria[Time Frame: Efficacy measures from screening through end of treatment and follow-up (every 9 weeks), up to approximately 24 months]

Subjects' self-reported myelofibrosis (MF)-related symptom burden assessment in subjects with MF after administration of INCB057643 in combination with ruxolitinib.[Time Frame: Protocol-defined time points up to approximately 24 months.]

Descriptive Information

Offical Title

A Phase 1/2, Open-Label, Dose-Escalation/Dose-Expansion, Safety and Tolerability Study of INCB057643 in Subjects With Advanced Malignancies

Brief Summary

The purpose of the Study is to select a dose and assess the safety and tolerability of INCB057643 as a monotherapy (Part 1 and Part 2) and in combination with standard-of-care (SOC) agents (Part 3 and Part 4) for subjects with advanced malignancies.

Part 1 will determine the maximum tolerated dose of INCB057643 and/or a tolerated dose that demonstrates sufficient pharmacologic activity. Part 2 will further evaluate the safety, preliminary efficacy, PK, and PD of the dose(s) selected in Part 1 in select tumor types including solid tumors, lymphomas and other hematologic malignancies. Part 3 will determine the tolerated dose of INCB057643 in combination with select SOC agents; and assess the safety and tolerability of the combination therapy in select advanced solid tumors and hematologic malignancies. Part 4 will further evaluate the safety, preliminary efficacy, PK, and PD of the selected dose combination from Part 3 in 4 specific advanced solid tumor and hematologic malignancies.

Study Type

Interventional

Study Phase

Phase 1/Phase 2

Condition

- Solid Tumors and Hematologic Malignancy

Intervention

Drug: INCB057643

Initial cohort dose of INCB057643 at the protocol-specified starting dose (Part 1), with subsequent dose escalations based on protocol-specific criteria. The recommended treatment group-specific dose(s) will be taken forward into expansion cohorts (Part 2).

Drug: INCB057643

Initial cohort dose of INCB057643 at the protocol-specified starting dose (Part 3), with subsequent dose escalations based on protocol-specific criteria. The recommended treatment group-specific dose(s) will be taken forward into expansion cohorts (Part 4).

Drug: Gemcitabine

Standard of Care (SOC) agents

Drug: Paclitaxel

Standard of Care (SOC) agents

Drug: Rucaparib

Standard of Care (SOC) agents

Drug: Abiraterone

Standard of Care (SOC) agents

Drug: Ruxolitinib

Standard of Care (SOC) agents

Drug: Azacitidine

Standard of Care (SOC) agents

Study Arms

Experimental: INCB057643

Experimental: INCB057643 + Standard of Care (SOC) agents

Recruitment Information

Recruitment Status

Recruiting

Estimated Enrollment

420

Completion Date

December 2021

Primary Completion Date

November 2021

Eligibility Criteria

Inclusion Criteria:

- Histologically or cytologically confirmed diagnosis of relapsed or refractory advanced or metastatic malignancies:
- Part 1: solid tumors or lymphomas, or hematologic malignancies
- Part 2: histologically confirmed disease in specific tumor types
- Part 3: advanced solid tumor or hematologic malignancy
- Part 4: select advanced solid tumor or hematologic malignancy
- For Part 1 and 2, subjects must have progressed following at least 1 line of prior therapy and there is no further established therapy that is known to provide clinical benefit (including subjects who are intolerant to the established therapy)
- For Parts 3 and 4, subjects must have progressed following at least 1 line of prior therapy, and the treatment with the select SOC agent is relevant for the specific disease cohort.
- Life expectancy > 12 weeks, for MF subjects in Parts 3 and 4, life expectancy > 24 weeks
- Eastern Cooperative Oncology Group (ECOG) performance status
- Parts 1 and 3: 0 or 1
- Parts 2 and 4: 0, 1, or 2
- Willingness to avoid pregnancy or fathering children

Exclusion Criteria:

- Inadequate bone marrow function per protocol-specified hemoglobin, platelet count, and absolute neutrophil count
- Inadequate organ function per protocol-specified total bilirubin, AST and ALT, creatinine clearance and alkaline phosphatase.
- Receipt of anticancer medications or investigational drugs within protocol-specified intervals
- Unless approved by the medical monitor, may not have received an allogeneic hematopoietic stem cell transplant within 6

months before treatment, or have active graft-versus-host-disease following allogeneic transplant

- Unless approved by the medical monitor, may not have received autologous hematopoietic stem cell transplant within 3 months before treatment
- Any unresolved toxicity ≥ Grade 2 (except stable Grade 2 peripheral neuropathy or alopecia) from previous anticancer therapy
- Radiotherapy within the 2 weeks before initiation of treatment. Palliative radiation treatment to nonindex or bone lesions performed less than 2 weeks before treatment initiation may be considered with medical monitor approval
- Currently active and uncontrolled infectious disease requiring systemic antibiotic, antifungal, or antiviral treatment
- Untreated brain or central nervous system (CNS) metastases or brain/CNS metastases that have progressed
- History or presence of abnormal electrocardiogram (ECG) that, in the investigator's opinion, is clinically meaningful
- Type 1 diabetes or uncontrolled Type 2 diabetes
- HbA1c of ≥ 8% (all subjects will have HbA1c test at screening)
- Any sign of clinically significant bleeding
- Coagulation panel within protocol-specified parameters

Sex/Gender

All

Ages

18 Years to N/A

Accepts Healthy Volunteers

No

Contacts

Incyte Corporation Call Center   1.855.463.3463

Cetuximab and Pembrolizumab in Treating Patients With Colorectal Cancer That is Metastatic or Cannot Be Removed by Surgery

Study ID:

NCT02713373

Sponsor:

Roswell Park Cancer Institute

Information provided by (Responsible Party):

Roswell Park Cancer Institute (Roswell Park Cancer Institute)

Tracking Information

First Submitted Date

March 11, 2016

Primary Completion Date

January 13, 2019

Start Date

August 5, 2016

Last Update Posted Date

February 7, 2018

Current Primary Outcome Measures

Incidence of adverse events, categorized and graded according to National Cancer Institute (NCI) Common Terminology Criteria for Adverse Events version 4.0 (CTCAE v4.0)[Time Frame: Up to 30 days after last dose of study drug]

The frequency of toxicities will be tabulated by maximum grade by preferred term within a patient across all cycles.

Progression free survival (PFS), evaluated according to Response Evaluation Criteria In Solid Tumors (RECIST) 1.1[Time Frame: At 6 months]

Will be tabulated and will be compared to the null values using exact tests. Distributions of PFS will be estimated using the Kaplan-Meier method.

Tumor response rate, evaluated according to RECIST 1.1[Time Frame: Up to 2 years]

Will be tabulated and will be compared to the null values using exact tests.

Objective tumor response using immune-related RECIST[Time Frame: Up to 2 years]
Will be tabulated.

Overall survival (OS)[Time Frame: Up to death, withdrawal of consent, or the end of the study, whichever occurs first, assessed up to 2 years]
Distributions of OS will be estimated using the Kaplan-Meier method.

Progression Free Survival (PFS)[Time Frame: At 6 months]
PFS will be tested using an exact binomial test. Distributions of PFS will be estimated using the Kaplan-Meier method.

Descriptive Information

■ Offical Title

A Phase Ib/II Study of Cetuximab and Pembrolizumab in Metastatic Colorectal Cancer

■ Brief Summary

This phase I/II trial studies the side effects and best dose of cetuximab when given together with pembrolizumab in treating patients with colorectal cancer that has spread from the primary site (place where it started) to other places in the body (metastatic) or that cannot be removed by surgery. Monoclonal antibodies, such as cetixumab and pembrolizumab, may block tumor growth in different ways by targeting certain cells.

■ Detailed Description

PRIMARY OBJECTIVES:

I. To estimate the objective response rate of patients with metastatic colorectal cancer treated with pembrolizumab and cetuximab.

II. To estimate the 6-month progression free survival (PFS) rate of patients with metastatic colorectal cancer treated with pembrolizumab and cetuximab.

III. To examine the adverse event profile of combining pembrolizumab and cetuximab.

SECONDARY OBJECTIVES:

I. To examine the PFS of patients with metastatic colorectal cancer treated with pembrolizumab and cetuximab.

II. To determine the objective response rate by immune-related response criteria (irRC) of patients with metastatic colorectal cancer.

III. To examine the overall survival of patients with metastatic colorectal cancer treated with pembrolizumab and cetuximab.

EXPLORATORY OBJECTIVES:

I. Identify tumor and peripheral blood biomarkers of response and/or resistance to the study treatment.

OUTLINE:

Patients receive cetuximab intravenously (IV) over 120 minutes on day 1, 8, and 15 (as monotherapy for cycle 1 only) and pembrolizumab IV over 30 minutes on day 1. Treatment repeats every 3 weeks for 24 months in the absence of disease progression or unacceptable toxicity. Patients may continue pembrolizumab treatment for up to 1 year if they experience disease progression.

After completion of the study treatment, patients are followed up every 3 months for up to 2 years.

■ Study Type

Interventional

■ Study Phase

Phase 1/Phase 2

■ Condition

- Recurrent Colorectal Carcinoma
- Stage IVA Colorectal Cancer
- Stage IVB Colorectal Cancer

■ Intervention

Biological: Cetuximab
Given IV

Other Names:

Chimeric Anti-Epidermal Growth Factor Receptor (EGFR) Monoclonal Antibody

Chimeric MoAb C225

Chimeric Monoclonal Antibody C225

Erbitux

IMC-C225

Other: Laboratory Biomarker Analysis

Correlative studies

Biological: Pembrolizumab

Given IV

Other Names:

Keytruda

Lambrolizumab

MK-3475

SCH 900475

Study Arms

Experimental: Arm I (cetuximab and pembrolizumab)

Patients receive cetuximab IV over 120 minutes on day 1 (days 1, 7, and 14 of course 1 only) and pembrolizumab IV over 30 minutes on day 1. Treatment repeats every 3 weeks for 24 months in the absence of disease progression or unacceptable toxicity. Patients may continue pembrolizumab treatment for up to 1 year if they experience disease progression.

Recruitment Information

Recruitment Status

Recruiting

Estimated Enrollment

42

Completion Date

January 13, 2020

Primary Completion Date

January 13, 2019

Eligibility Criteria

Inclusion Criteria:

- Have a pathologically confirmed diagnosis of colorectal cancer, which is metastatic or otherwise unresectable
- Have received at least 1 prior systemic therapy in the metastatic or unresectable disease setting; patients who have recurred within six months of adjuvant chemotherapy are not required to have received an additional line of chemotherapy
- Retrovirus-associated deoxyribonucleic acid (DNA) sequence (RAS) wild-type; v-Ki-ras2 Kirsten rat sarcoma viral oncogene homolog (KRAS) testing must be completed, with full KRAS and neuroblastoma RAS viral (v-ras) oncogene homolog (NRAS) testing strongly advised; the presence of known mutations in KRAS or NRAS is exclusionary; primary tumor or metastatic tumor may be tested; (note: in the case of multiple genomic evaluations with conflicting results e.g. KRAS mutant in one sample, but wild-type in another the patient may be included as RAS wild-type, if clinically justified, after review with the principal investigator [PI])
- Naive to anti-EGFR therapy (cetuximab or panitumumab)
- Have an Eastern Cooperative Oncology Group (ECOG) performance status =< 2
- Have measurable disease per Response Evaluation Criteria in Solid Tumors (RECIST) 1.1 criteria present
- Be willing to provide tissue from a newly obtained core or excisional biopsy of a tumor lesion; newly-obtained is defined as a specimen obtained up to 30 days prior to initiation of treatment on day 1; subjects for whom newly-obtained samples cannot be provided (e.g. inaccessible or subject safety concern) may submit an archived specimen only upon agreement from the principal investigator
- Hemoglobin >= 8 g/dL (performed within 14 days of treatment initiation)
- Absolute neutrophil count >= 1000/mm3 (performed within 14 days of treatment initiation)
- Platelet count >= 100,000/mm3 (performed within 14 days of treatment initiation)
- Serum creatinine =< 2 upper limit of normal (ULN) or, >= 15 mL/min for participants with creatinine levels > 2 ULN (performed within 14 days of treatment initiation)
- Aspartate aminotransferase (AST) (serum glutamic oxaloacetic transaminase [SGOT]) and alanine aminotransferase (ALT) (serum glutamate pyruvate transaminase [SGPT]) =< 2.5 ULN or, =< 5 ULN for participants with liver metastases (performed within 14 days of treatment initiation)
- Female participants of childbearing potential are to have a negative serum pregnancy test
- Female participants of child-bearing potential must agree to use an acceptable method of birth control, be surgically sterile, or abstain from heterosexual activity for the course of the study through 120 days after the last dose of study medication; participants of childbearing potential are those who have not been surgically sterilized or have not been free from menses for > 1 year; should a woman become pregnant or suspect she is pregnant while she or her partner is participating in this study, she should inform her treating physician immediately

- Male participants must agree to use an adequate method of contraception starting with the first dose of study therapy through 120 days after the last dose of study therapy
- Participant or legal representative must understand the investigational nature of this study and sign an Independent Ethics Committee/Institutional Review Board approved written informed consent form prior to receiving any study related procedure

Exclusion Criteria:

- Participants who have had chemotherapy, targeted therapies, radiotherapy, or used an investigational device within 2 weeks prior to the first dose of treatment or those who have not recovered from adverse events (i.e., =< grade 1 or at baseline) due to agents administered more than 2 weeks earlier; note: participants with =< grade 2 neuropathy are an exception to this criterion and may qualify for the study
- Has a diagnosis of immunodeficiency or is receiving systemic steroid therapy or any other form of immunosuppressive therapy within 7 days prior to the first dose of trial treatment
- Has a known history of active TB (Bacillus Tuberculosis)
- Hypersensitivity to pembrolizumab or any of its excipients
- Has a known additional malignancy that requires active treatment; exceptions include basal cell carcinoma of the skin or squamous cell carcinoma of the skin that has undergone potentially curative therapy or in situ cervical cancer
- Has known active central nervous system (CNS) metastases and/or carcinomatous meningitis; participants with previously treated brain metastases may participate provided they are stable (without evidence of progression by imaging for at least four weeks prior to the first dose of trial treatment and any neurologic symptoms have returned to baseline), have no evidence of new or enlarging brain metastases, and are not using steroids for at least 7 days prior to trial treatment; this exception does not include carcinomatous meningitis which is excluded regardless of clinical stability
- Has active autoimmune disease that has required systemic treatment in the past 2 years (i.e. with use of disease modifying agents, corticosteroids or immunosuppressive drugs); replacement therapy (e.g., thyroxine, insulin, or physiologic corticosteroid replacement therapy for adrenal or pituitary insufficiency) is not considered a form of systemic treatment
- Has known history of, or any evidence of active, non-infectious pneumonitis
- Uncontrolled clinically significant intercurrent illness including, but not limited to, ongoing or active infection, symptomatic congestive heart failure, unstable angina pectoris, unstable cardiac arrhythmia, or psychiatric illness, substance abuse disorders or social situations that would limit compliance with study requirements
- Is pregnant or breastfeeding, or expecting to conceive or father children within the projected duration of the trial, starting with the pre-screening or screening visit through 120 days after the last dose of trial treatment
- Has a known history of human immunodeficiency virus (HIV or HIV 1/2 antibodies); testing not required
- Has known active hepatitis B (e.g., hepatitis B surface antigen [HBsAg] reactive) or hepatitis C (e.g., hepatitis C virus [HCV] ribonucleic acid [RNA] [qualitative] is detected); testing not required
- Has received a live vaccine within 30 days of planned start of study therapy (note: seasonal influenza vaccines for injection are generally inactivated flu vaccines and are allowed; however intranasal influenza vaccines (e.g., Flu-Mist®) are live attenuated vaccines, and shingles are not allowed)
- Received an investigational agent within 30 days prior to starting study treatment
- Has a history or current evidence of any condition, therapy, or laboratory abnormality that might confound the results of the trial, interfere with the subject's participation for the full duration of the trial, or is not in the best interest of the subject to participate, in the opinion of the treating investigator
- Unwilling or unable to follow protocol requirements

Sex/Gender

All

Ages

18 Years to N/A

Accepts Healthy Volunteers

No

Safety and Efficacy Study of AMG 820 and Pembrolizumab Combination in Select Advanced Solid Tumor Cancer

Study ID:

NCT02713529

Sponsor:

Amgen

Information provided by (Responsible Party):

Amgen (Amgen)

Tracking Information

First Submitted Date

March 3, 2016

Start Date

April 14, 2016

Primary Completion Date

March 18, 2019

Last Update Posted Date

December 2, 2017

Current Primary Outcome Measures

Number of participants with treatment related adverse events as assessed by CTCAE version 4.0[Time Frame: 12 months]

Objective response rate of tumors using irRECIST criteria for total measureable tumor burden[Time Frame: 12 months]

Analyze CT/MRI scans using a modified criteria (irRECIST) adapting the immune-related response criteria to conventional RECIST 1.1 (irRECIST accounts for index and measureable lesions in total tumor burden).

Number of participants with treatment emergent adverse events as assessed by CTCAE version 4.0[Time Frame: 12 months]

Current Secondary Outcome Measures

Objective response rate of tumors using RECIST 1.1 criteria for total measurable tumor burden[Time Frame: 12 months]

Analyze CT/MRI scans using defined criteria for bidimensional measurements of index lesions.

Maximum observed concentration [Cmax] of AMG820[Time Frame: 12 months]

Analyze serum concentration of AMG 820 after intravenous infusion administration of AMG 820 in combination with pembrolizumab.

CD4, CD8, and CD68 cell numbers in pre-treatment tumor biopsy tissue[Time Frame: 12 months]

Minimum observed concentration [Cmin] of AMG 820[Time Frame: 12 months]

Analyze serum concentration of AMG 820 after intravenous infusion administration of AMG 820 in combination with pembrolizumab.

Area Under the Curve [AUC] of AMG820[Time Frame: 12 months]

Analyze serum concentration of AMG 820 after intravenous infusion administration of AMG 820 in combination with pembrolizumab.

Descriptive Information

Offical Title

A Phase1b/2 Study Assessing Safety and Anti-tumor Activity of AMG 820 in Combination With Pembrolizumab in Select Advanced Solid Tumors

Brief Summary

A multi-center Phase 1b/2 study testing the combination of AMG 820 and pembrolizumab in subjects with select advanced solid tumors.

Detailed Description

Phase 1b is AMG 820 dose determining and aimed at assessing the safety and tolerability of the selected starting dose of AMG 820 in combination with pembrolizumab. Phase 2 of the study will further evaluate safety and tolerability and additionally test whether AMG 820 can enhance the anti-tumor activity observed historically with pembrolizumab alone and/or overcome lack of response to pembrolizumab monotherapy in subjects with select solid tumors.

Study Type

Interventional

Study Phase

Phase 1/Phase 2

Condition

- Pancreatic Cancer
- Colorectal Cancer
- Non-Small Cell Lung Cancer

Intervention

Biological: AMG820 and pembrolizumab

Treatment with AMG820 and pembrolizumab

Study Arms

Experimental: AMG820 and pembrolizumab
    Treatment with AMG820 and pembrolizumab

Recruitment Information

Recruitment Status

Recruiting

Estimated Enrollment

197

Completion Date

April 19, 2019

Primary Completion Date

March 18, 2019

Eligibility Criteria

Inclusion Criteria:

- Pathologically documented, advanced colorectal, pancreatic or non-small cell lung cancer that is refractory to standard treatment, or the subjects have been intolerant to or refuse standard treatment.
- Measurable disease per RECIST 1.1 guidelines.
- Eastern Cooperative Oncology Group (ECOG) performance status of 0 1
- Adequate hematologic, renal, and hepatic function determined by laboratory blood and urine tests.
- Availability of recent tumor tissue with 3 months prior to enrollment, when feasible.

Exclusion Criteria:

- Has known active central nervous system metastases
- History of other malignancy with the past 2 years with some exceptions
- Evidence of active non-infectious pneumonitis/interstitial lung disease
- Evidence of other active autoimmune disease that has required prolonged systemic treatment in past 2 years.
- Evidence of clinically significant immunosuppression such as organ or stem cell transplantation, any severe congenital or acquired cellular and/or humoral immune deficiency, concurrent opportunistic infection.
- Receiving systemic immunostimulatory agents within 6 weeks or 5 half-lives, whichever is shorter, prior to first dose of study treatment (except ant PD-1/PD-L1 treatment if recruited into Group 4a or 4b).
- Evidence of active infection within 2 weeks prior to first dose of study treatment.
- Prior chemotherapy, radiotherapy, biological cancer therapy or major surgery within 28 days prior to enrollment
- Currently participating or has participated in a study (treatment period only) of an investigational agent or used an investigational device within 28 days of enrollment
- Received live vaccine within 28 days prior to enrollment
- Adverse event due to cancer therapy administered more than 28 days prior to enrollment that has not recovered to CTCAE grade 1 or better.
- Positive for human immunodeficiency virus (HIV), Hepatitis B or C
- Women planning to become pregnant or who are lactating/breastfeeding while on study through 4 months after receiving the last dose of study drug.

Sex/Gender

All

Ages

18 Years to N/A

Accepts Healthy Volunteers

No

Contacts

Amgen Call Center   866-572-6436   medinfo@amgen.com

Curcumin in Combination With 5FU for Colon Cancer

Study ID:

NCT02724202

Sponsor:

Baylor Research Institute

Information provided by (Responsible Party):

Baylor Research Institute (Baylor Research Institute)

Tracking Information

First Submitted Date

March 16, 2016

Start Date

March 2016

Primary Completion Date

March 2018

Last Update Posted Date

April 1, 2016

Current Primary Outcome Measures

Determine the safety using curcumin in patients with metastatic colon cancer; where toxicities will be graded according to the NCI Common Terminology Criteria for Adverse Events (CTCAE) Version 4.0.[Time Frame: 12 weeks]

Events will be recorded from the time of informed consent signature through the 30 days following the last study treatment.

Current Secondary Outcome Measures

Overall Response[Time Frame: 12 months]

Recorded from the start of the treatment until disease progression/recurrence. The patient's best response assignment will depend on the finding of target and non-target disease and will also take into consideration the appearance of new lesions.

Evidence of altered biomarker status (circulating DNA methylation status, miRNA profile) at 8 weeks post-treatment according to RECIST version 1.1 and survival criteria.[Time Frame: Baseline, Week 2, Week 8]

Blood will be collected at baseline, after completing one cycle of curcumin treatment (2 weeks), and after completing three 2 week-cycles of 5FU (6 weeks) for inflammatory and epigenetic chemoresponsive biomarker profiling.

Duration of response[Time Frame: 12 months]

Duration of progression free survival[Time Frame: 12 months]

Duration of overall survival[Time Frame: 12 months]

Duration of Quality of Life[Time Frame: Baseline, 12 months]

All subjects will complete the quality of life survey at Baseline, 5FU treatment visits and follow-up visits.

Descriptive Information

Offical Title

A Pilot, Feasibility Study of Curcumin in Combination With 5FU for Patients With 5FU-Resistant Metastatic Colon Cancer

Brief Summary

The purpose of this study is to test the safety and find the response rate of combining the dietary supplement, curcumin, with the standard of care, FDA-approved chemotherapy drug 5-fluorouracil (5FU, Adracil) and see what effects (good and bad) that the combined treatments have on colon cancer.

Detailed Description

Confirm clinical safety and identify clinical response rate of combination treatment with curcumin and 5FU in chemorefractory CRC patients. To determine whether curcumin administration induces systemic alterations in inflammatory and epigenetic biomarkers in patients with chemoresistant metastatic colorectal cancer (CRC). To correlate altered biomarker findings with clinical response according to RECIST V1.1 and survival criteria.

Study Type

Interventional

Study Phase

Early Phase 1

Condition

- Metastatic Colon Cancer

Intervention

Drug: Curcumin

Curcumin is supplied as soft-gel capsule. It is a micronized rhizome extract containing phospholipids and 500mg of pure curcuminoids (95% curcumin, 5% desmethoxycurcumin) suspended in turmeric essential oil.

Other Names:

BCM-95

Drug: 5-flurorouracil

Fluorouracil is an anti-cancer (antineoplastic or cytotoxic) chemotherapy drug. Fluorouracil is classified as an antimetabolite.

Other Names:

5FU

Adracil

Study Arms

Experimental: Open Label

All subjects will receive induction oral curcumin 500 mg twice per day for 2 weeks. Patients will continue on curcumin at same dose for an additional 6 weeks while being treated with 3 cycles of 5FU.

Recruitment Information

Recruitment Status

Recruiting

Estimated Enrollment

14

Completion Date

March 2018

Primary Completion Date

March 2018

Eligibility Criteria

Inclusion Criteria:

- Male or female 18 years or older, at the time of signing the informed consent.
- Capable of giving written informed consent, which includes compliance with the requirements and restrictions listed in the consent form.
- Histologically or cytologically confirmed diagnosis of metastatic colorectal cancer that is not response to standard 5FU based therapies.
- Performance Status (PS) score of 0 to 2 according to the Eastern Cooperative Oncology Group (ECOG) scale.
- Able to swallow and retain oral medication.
- A female subject is eligible to participate if she is of:
- Non-childbearing potential defined as pre-menopausal females with a documented tubal ligation or hysterectomy; or postmenopausal defined as 12 months of spontaneous amenorrhea (in questionable cases a blood sample with simultaneous follicle stimulating hormone (FSH) >40 mili-internation unit (MIU)/ml and estradiol <40 pg/ml (140pmol/L) is confirmatory
- Child-bearing potential and agrees to use a contraception method of abstinence, intrauterine device (IUD), barrier methods or birth control pills prior to the start of dosing to sufficiently minimize the risk of pregnancy at that point and until three months after the last dose of the study medication.
- Male subjects must agree to use a method of contraception. This criterion must be followed from the time of the first dose of study medication until three months after the last dose of study medication.
- Adequate organ system function defined as follows:

System Laboratory Values Hematologic Absolute neutrophil count (ANC) ≥ 1.5 x 10^9/L Hemoglobin ≥ 9.5 g/dL Platelets ≥ 75 x 10^9/L For subjects not on warfarin-based anticoagulants: Prothrombin time/International normalized ratio (PT/INR) and partial thromboplastin time (PTT) ≤ 1.1x upper limit of normal (ULN) INR (subjects on warfarin-based anticoagulant): 2-3 x ULN Hepatic Total bilirubin ≤ 1.5x ULN (isolated bilirubin > 1.5x ULN is acceptable if bilirubin is fractionated and direct bilirubin < 35%) Aspartate aminotransferase (AST) and alanine transaminase (ALT) 1 ≤ 1.5x ULN Albumin ≥ 2.5 g/dL Renal Creatinine ≤ ULN; or Calculated creatinine clearance2 ≥ 50 mL/min; or Metabolic Fasting Serum Glucose < 250 mg/dL Cardiac Left Ventricular Ejection fraction (LVEF) ≥ lower limit of normal (LLN) by echocardiogram (ECHO) Blood pressure Systolic < 160 mm Hg and Diastolic < 100 mm Hg.

1. If liver metastases are present, AST and ALT ≤ 2.5x ULN is permitted

2. As calculated by Cockroft-Gault formula.

Exclusion Criteria:

- Chemotherapy, radiotherapy, immunotherapy, or other anti-cancer therapy including investigational drugs within 28 days or 5 half-lives, whichever is shorter prior to the first dose of any one of the investigational drugs described in this study.
- Unresolved toxicity by National Cancer Institute (NCI) Common Terminology Criteria for Adverse Events, Version 4.0 (NCI-CTCAE V4) of > Grade 1 from previous anti-cancer therapy.
- Presence of active GI disease or other condition that could affect gastrointestinal absorption (malabsorption syndrome) or predispose a subject to GI ulceration.
- Evidence of mucosal or internal bleeding
- Any major surgery within the last four weeks
- Uncontrolled diabetes mellitus
- Any malignancy related to human immunodeficiency virus (HIV), known history of HIV, history of known Hepatitis B virus (HBV) surface antigen positivity (subjects with documented laboratory evidence of HBV clearance may be enrolled) or positive

Hepatitis C virus (HCV) antibody.

- Known active infection requiring parenteral or oral anti-infective treatment.
- **Subjects with brain metastases are excluded if their brain metastases are:**
- Symptomatic
- Treated (surgery, radiation therapy) but not clinically and radiographically stable one month after therapy (as assessed by at least 2 distinct contrast enhanced MRI or CT scans over at least a one month period), or
- Asymptomatic and untreated but > 1 cm in the longest dimension
- History or evidence of current clinically significant uncontrolled arrhythmias.
- Subjects with controlled atrial fibrillation for >1 month prior to study Day 1 are eligible.
- History of acute coronary syndromes (including unstable angina), myocardial infarction, coronary angioplasty, or stenting or bypass grafting within six months of screening.
- Class II, III, or IV heart failure as defined by the New York Heart Association (NYHA) functional classification system.
- Any serious or unstable pre-existing medical, psychiatric, or other condition (including lab abnormalities) that could interfere with subject's safety or providing informed consent.
- Known immediate or delayed hypersensitivity to any of the components of the study treatment(s).
- Evidence of severe or uncontrolled systemic diseases (unstable or uncompensated respiratory, hepatic, renal, or cardiac disease, including unstable hypertension).
- Pregnant or lactating females.

Sex/Gender

All

Ages

18 Years to N/A

Accepts Healthy Volunteers

No

Contacts

Grace Townsend   214-818-8382   Grace.Townsend@BSWhealth.org

S1415CD, Trial Assessing CSF Prescribing Effectiveness and Risk (TrACER)

Study ID:
NCT02728596

Sponsor:
Southwest Oncology Group

Information provided by (Responsible Party):
Southwest Oncology Group (Southwest Oncology Group)

Tracking Information

First Submitted Date
March 30, 2016

Primary Completion Date
April 2020

Start Date
October 2016

Last Update Posted Date
January 4, 2018

Current Primary Outcome Measures

Change in FN-related HRQL (patient report) assessed using the Functional Assessment of Cancer Therapy -Febrile Neutropenia (FACT-N)[Time Frame: Baseline to up to 14 days]

A linear mixed effects model will be fit to assess the effect of the intervention on HRQL. Component-level characteristics, patient-level clinical and demographic variables will be adjusted.

Change in patient knowledge of PP-CSF benefits (patient report)[Time Frame: Baseline to up to 14 days (1 course)]

Linear mixed effects model with a time variable and an interaction between randomized group and time will be used to analyze change in the patient knowledge score. Random effects will be used to accommodate both the correlation among measures from the same patient as well as the correlation among patients from the same component. Component-level characteristics, patient-level clinical and demographic variables will be adjusted.

Change in patient knowledge of PP-CSF indications (patient report)[Time Frame: Baseline to up to 14 days]

Linear mixed effects model with a time variable and an interaction between randomized group and time will be used to analyze change in the patient knowledge score. Random effects will be used to accommodate both the correlation among measures from the same patient as well as the correlation among patients from the same component. Component-level characteristics, patient-level clinical and demographic variables will be adjusted.

Change in patient knowledge of PP-CSF out-of-pocket costs (patient report)[Time Frame: Baseline to up to 6 months]

Linear mixed effects model with a time variable and an interaction between randomized group and time will be used to analyze change in the patient knowledge score. Random effects will be used to accommodate both the correlation among measures from the same patient as well as the correlation among patients from the same component. Component-level characteristics, patient-level clinical and demographic variables will be adjusted.

Change in patient knowledge of PP-CSF risks (patient report)[Time Frame: Baseline to up to 14 days (1 course)]

Linear mixed effects model with a time variable and an interaction between randomized group and time will be used to analyze change in the patient knowledge score. Random effects will be used to accommodate both the correlation among measures from the same patient as well as the correlation among patients from the same component. Component-level characteristics, patient-level clinical and demographic variables will be adjusted.

Incidence of febrile neutropenia (clinical) graded according to the National Cancer Institute (NCI) Common Toxicity Criteria version 4.0[Time Frame: Within 14 days after the completion of first course of therapy]

Incidence of febrile neutropenia (clinical) graded according to the NCI Common Toxicity Criteria version 4.0[Time Frame: Within 6 months]

Overall survival (clinical)[Time Frame: Time from date of registration to date of death due to any cause, assessed up to 12 months]

A Cox proportional hazards model will be used to model survival. Component-level characteristics, patient-level clinical and demographic variables will be adjusted. A separate analysis of cause-specific survival to address FN-related deaths will also be conducted.

Patient adherence to PP-CSF prescription (clinical and patient report)[Time Frame: Within 14 days after the completion of first course of therapy]

For the home and clinic settings, separate mixed effects logistic models will be used to assess the effect of the intervention on adherence to PP-CSF orders, treating adherence after the start of the study. Component-level characteristics, patient-level clinical and demographic variables will be adjusted.

Prophylactic and FN-related antibiotic use (clinical)[Time Frame: Within 30 days of therapy]

Prophylactic and FN-related antibiotic use will be measured as total number of antibiotic agents used and duration of antibiotic use. A linear mixed effects model will be fit to assess the effect of the intervention on duration of antibiotics use with number of days. Mixed effects Poisson models will be used to assess the effect of the intervention on total number of antibiotics agents used. Three separate models will be fit, with the following outcomes: (i) the number of times antibiotics were used as prophylaxis, (ii) the number of times antibiotics were used as treatment for FN, and (iii) t

Proportion completing initial systemic therapy regimen: a) at planned duration and b) at planned dose intensity (clinical)[Time Frame: Up to 12 months]

Two separate mixed effects logistic models will be used to assess the effect of the intervention on completion of the initial systemic therapy regimen (i) at planned duration and (ii) at planned dose intensity. Component-level characteristics, patient-level clinical and demographic variables will be adjusted.

Rate of CSF prescribing as primary prophylaxis (clinical)[Time Frame: Time from initiation of granulocyte CSFs during the first cycle of myelosuppressive systemic therapy, given 24 to 72 hours after cessation of systemic therapy, assessed up to 12 months]

PP-CSF use is observed and reported. Separate mixed effects logistic models will be fit to assess the effect of the intervention on PP-CSF use.

Rate of FN-related emergency department (ED) visits and hospitalizations (clinical)[Time Frame: At 6 months]

A mixed effects Poisson model will be used to assess the effect of the intervention on FN-related ED visits and hospitalizations. Robust variance estimation will be used to relax the strong assumptions about the variance made by Poisson regression. If a large number of zero counts is observed, then zero-inflated Poisson regression will be used.

Descriptive Information

▦ Offical Title

- A Pragmatic Trial to Evaluate a Guideline-Based Colony Stimulating Factor Standing Order Intervention and to Determine the Effectiveness of Colony Stimulating Factor Use as a Prophylaxis for Patients Receiving Chemotherapy With Intermediate Risk for Febrile Neutropenia Trial Assessing CSF Prescribing Effectiveness and Risk (TrACER)

▦ Brief Summary

This randomized clinical trial studies prophylactic colony stimulating factor management in patients with breast, colorectal or non-small cell lung cancer receiving chemotherapy and with risk of developing febrile neutropenia. Patients receiving chemotherapy may develop febrile neutropenia. Febrile neutropenia is a condition that involves fever and a low number of neutrophils (a type of white blood cell) in the blood. Febrile neutropenia increases the risk of infection. Colony stimulating factors are medications sometimes given to patients receiving chemotherapy to prevent febrile neutropenia. Colony stimulating factors are given to patients based on guidelines. Some clinics have an automated system that helps doctors decide when to prescribe them when there is a high risk of developing febrile neutropenia. Gathering information about the use of an automated system to prescribe prophylactic colony stimulating factor may help doctors use colony stimulating factor when it is needed.

Detailed Description

PRIMARY OBJECTIVES:

I. To compare the use of primary prophylactic colony stimulating factor (PP-CSF) according to recommended clinical practice guidelines among patients registered at intervention components versus usual care components.

II. To compare the rate of febrile neutropenia (FN) among patients registered at intervention components versus usual care components.

III. To compare the rate of FN among intermediate risk patients registered at intervention components by component treatment assignment (administer PP-CSF to intermediate risk patients versus not).

SECONDARY OBJECTIVES:

I. To compare the rate of FN among low-risk patients registered at intervention components versus usual care components.

II. To compare the FN-related health-related quality of life (HRQOL) among low-risk patients registered at intervention components versus usual care components.

III. To compare patient adherence to PP-CSF prescribing among patients registered at intervention components versus usual care components.

IV. To compare patient knowledge of the indications for, efficacy of, and side effects associated with PP-CSF between the initiation and conclusion of the first cycle of myelosuppressive systemic therapy among patients registered at intervention components versus usual care components.

V. To compare the proportion of patients completing the initial systemic therapy regimen at planned duration and at planned dose intensity among patients registered at intervention components versus usual care components.

VI. To compare antibiotic use both as prophylaxis and as treatment for FN among patients registered at intervention components versus usual care components.

VII. To compare the rate of FN-related emergency department visits and hospitalizations among intermediate risk patients registered to Intervention components by component treatment assignment (administer PP-CSF to intermediate risk patients versus not).

VIII. To compare the FN-related health-related quality of life (HRQOL) among intermediate risk patients registered to intervention components by component treatment assignment (administer PP-CSF to intermediate risk patients versus not).

IX. To compare overall survival among intermediate risk patients registered to intervention components by component treatment assignment (administer PP-CSF to intermediate risk patients versus not).

TERTIARY OBJECTIVES:

I. To characterize and descriptively report the differences among cohort components and the intervention and usual care components.

II. To evaluate the time to invasive recurrence in non-metastatic patients by component treatment assignment

OUTLINE: Patients are randomized to 1 of 4 clinic groups.

CLINIC GROUP 1 (CLINIC WITH AUTOMATED SYSTEM): Patients with a high risk of developing FN receive CSF based on the automated system recommendations. The automated system suggests that CSFs not be used for drugs that have a low risk of FN.

CLINIC GROUP 2 (CLINIC WITH NO AUTOMATED SYSTEM): Patients receive CSF based on clinical practice guidelines.

CLINIC GROUP 3 (CLINIC WITH AUTOMATED SYSTEM): Patients with a high or moderate risk of developing FN receive CSF based on the automated system recommendations. The automated system suggests that CSFs not be used for drugs that have a low risk of FN.

CLINIC GROUP 4 (CLINIC WITH AUTOMATED SYSTEM): Patients with a high risk of developing FN receive CSF based on the automated system recommendations. The automated system suggests that CSF not be used for drugs that have a moderate risk of FN.

After completion of study treatment, patients are followed up for 12 months.

Study Type

Interventional

Study Phase

N/A

Condition

- Febrile Neutropenia
- Stage 0 Breast Cancer
- Stage 0 Colorectal Cancer

- Stage 0 Non-Small Cell Lung Cancer
- Stage I Colorectal Cancer
- Stage IA Breast Cancer
- Stage IA Non-Small Cell Lung Carcinoma
- Stage IB Breast Cancer
- Stage IB Non-Small Cell Lung Carcinoma
- Stage IIA Breast Cancer
- Stage IIA Colorectal Cancer
- Stage IIA Non-Small Cell Lung Carcinoma
- Stage IIB Breast Cancer
- Stage IIB Colorectal Cancer
- Stage IIB Non-Small Cell Lung Carcinoma
- Stage IIC Colorectal Cancer
- Stage IIIA Breast Cancer
- Stage IIIA Colorectal Cancer
- Stage IIIA Non-Small Cell Lung Cancer
- Stage IIIB Breast Cancer
- Stage IIIB Colorectal Cancer
- Stage IIIB Non-Small Cell Lung Cancer
- Stage IIIC Breast Cancer
- Stage IIIC Colorectal Cancer
- Stage IV Breast Cancer
- Stage IV Non-Small Cell Lung Cancer
- Stage IVA Colorectal Cancer
- Stage IVB Colorectal Cancer

Intervention

Other: Preventive Intervention

Receive PP-CSF

Other Names:

PREVENTATIVE

Prevention

Prevention Measures

Prophylaxis

PRYLX

Other: Quality-of-Life Assessment

Ancillary studies

Other Names:

Quality of Life Assessment

Other: Questionnaire Administration

Ancillary studies

Study Arms

Experimental: Clinic group 1 (clinic with automated system)

Patients with a high risk of developing FN receive CSF based on the automated system recommendations. The automated system suggests that CSFs not be used for drugs that have a low risk of FN.

Experimental: Clinic group 2 (clinic with no automated system)

Patients receive CSF based on clinical practice guidelines.

Experimental: Clinic group 3 (clinic with automated system)

Patients with a high or moderate risk of developing FN receive CSF based on the automated system recommendations. The automated system suggests that CSFs not be used for drugs that have a low risk of FN.

Active Comparator: Clinic group 4 (clinic with automated system)

Patients with a high risk of developing FN receive CSF based on the automated system recommendations. The automated system suggests that CSF not be used for drugs that have a moderate risk of FN.

Recruitment Information

■ **Recruitment Status**

Recruiting

■ **Estimated Enrollment**

3960

■ **Completion Date**

April 2020

■ **Primary Completion Date**

April 2020

■ **Eligibility Criteria**

Inclusion Criteria:

- Patients must have a current diagnosis of breast cancer, non-small cell lung cancer, or colorectal cancer; cancer may be metastatic or non-metastatic
- Patients must be planning to receive one of the study-allowed regimens as their initial treatment for their current diagnosis
- Patients must be registered prior to their first cycle of systemic therapy (chemotherapy, immunotherapy, biologic therapy, or combination regimens) for this diagnosis; if patient has had any prior systemic therapy for another malignancy, patient must not have had any systemic therapy in the 180 days just prior to registration
- Patients must not have any known contraindication to CSFs prior to registration, including prior hypersensitivity to Escherichia coli-derived proteins, filgrastim, pegfilgrastim, or tbo-filgrastim
- Patients must be able to understand and provide information for the patient-completed study forms in either English or Spanish
- Patients may have had a prior malignancy
- Patients must not be participating or plan to participate in other clinical trials that involve investigational systemic cancer treatments or investigational uses of CSF
- Patients must be informed of the investigational nature of this study and must sign and give written informed consent in accordance with institutional and federal guidelines
- As a part of the Oncology Patient Enrollment Network (OPEN) registration process the treating institution's identity is provided in order to ensure that the current (within 365 days) date of institutional review board approval for this study has been entered in the system

■ **Sex/Gender**

All

■ **Ages**

18 Years to N/A

■ **Accepts Healthy Volunteers**

No

■ **Contacts**

Kimberly F. Kaberle   210-614-8808   kkaberle@swog.org
Dana Sparks, MAT   210-614-8808   dsparks@swog.org

Trial of Liver Resection Versus No Surgery in Patients With Liver and Unresectable Pulmonary Metastases From Colorectal Cancer (Liver Resection With Unresectable Lung Nodules From Colorectal Adenocarcinoma LUNA)

Study ID:

NCT02738606

Sponsor:

M.D. Anderson Cancer Center

Information provided by (Responsible Party):

M.D. Anderson Cancer Center (M.D. Anderson Cancer Center)

Tracking Information

■ **First Submitted Date**

April 12, 2016

■ **Start Date**

May 25, 2016

■ **Current Primary Outcome Measures**

Overall Survival[Time Frame: 3 years]

Overall survival time defined as the time period from the date of randomization to the date of death or the date of last follow-up if the patients are alive at the time of last follow-up.

■ **Primary Completion Date**

May 1, 2020

■ **Last Update Posted Date**

August 22, 2017

Descriptive Information

■ **Offical Title**

Randomized Controlled Phase II Trial of Liver Resection Versus No Surgery in Patients With Liver and Unresectable Pulmonary Metastases From Colorectal Cancer

■ **Brief Summary**

The goal of this clinical research study is to compare the effect of having liver resection with standard of care chemotherapy to having standard of care chemotherapy alone in patients whose colorectal cancer has spread to their liver and lungs.

■ **Detailed Description**

Study Groups:

If you are found to be eligible to take part in this study, you will be randomly assigned (as in the flip of a coin) to 1 of 2 study groups. This is done because no one knows if one study group is better, the same, or worse than the other group. You will have an equal chance to be assigned to either group.

- If you are assigned to Group 1, you will have liver resection surgery, followed by standard of care chemotherapy. The chemotherapy you receive will depend on what the doctor thinks is in your best interest.
- If you are assigned to Group 2, you will receive standard of care chemotherapy that your doctor thinks is in your best interest.

You will sign a separate consent form explaining how the standard of care chemotherapy works, the chemotherapy schedule, and its risks.

Group 1:

If you are in Group 1, you will have standard of care liver resection surgery. A portion of the liver that is affected by the tumor will be removed either with many small incisions or one large incision. An ultrasound device will be used to help the doctor see the affected area. The study doctor will explain this procedure in more detail and you will sign a separate consent form explaining the standard of care surgery and its risks.

Study Visits:

Both groups will have study visits every 3-6 months while on study. The following tests and procedures will be performed:

- You will have a physical exam.
- You will have a chest x-ray or CT scan to check status of disease.
- You will have an abdominal and pelvic CT scan, PET/CT scan, or an MRI scan to check the status of the disease.
- Blood (about 3 tablespoons) will be drawn for routine tests.
- Blood (about 2 teaspoons) will be drawn for biomarker testing.
- You will complete the quality of life survey you completed during screening.

Length of Study:

You will be on study for up to 3 years. You will be taken off study if the disease gets worse or intolerable side effects occur.

This is an investigational study. Liver resection surgery for patients with colorectal cancer that is able to be resected can be done with standard techniques using FDA-approved devices. Liver resection surgery for patients with colorectal cancer that can only be partially resected is considered investigational.

Up to 80 participants will take part in this study. All will be enrolled at MD Anderson.

■ **Study Type**

Interventional

■ **Study Phase**

Phase 2

Condition
- Colorectal Cancer
- Other Diseases of Intestines

Intervention

Procedure: Liver Resection Surgery

Participants undergo standard of care liver resection surgery.

Drug: Chemotherapy

Standard of care chemotherapy decided by participant's physician.

Behavioral: Survey

Quality of life survey completed at baseline and every 3-6 months at follow up.

Other Names:

Questionnaire

Study Arms

Experimental: Liver Resection Surgery + Chemotherapy Group

Participants have liver resection surgery, followed by standard of care. Standard of care chemotherapy decided by participant's physician.

Quality of life survey completed at baseline and every 3-6 months at follow up.

Active Comparator: Chemotherapy Group

Standard of care chemotherapy decided by participant's physician.

Quality of life survey completed at baseline and every 3-6 months at follow up.

Recruitment Information

Recruitment Status

Recruiting

Estimated Enrollment

80

Completion Date

May 1, 2020

Primary Completion Date

May 1, 2020

Eligibility Criteria

Inclusion Criteria:

1. Patients with synchronous or metachronous diagnosis of resectable liver metastases by computed tomography (CT) or magnetic resonance imaging (MRI) of the abdomen: a) Patients requiring percutaneous or intraoperative ablation of liver metastases < 2 cm in size are eligible. b) Patients who underwent prior liver resection or ablation for colorectal liver metastases are eligible.

2. Patients previously treated with systemic chemotherapy and/or biologic agents for colorectal cancer are eligible.

3. The primary tumor in the colon or rectum may be intact or resected.

4. Low-volume lung metastases are defined as solid pulmonary nodules < 2 cm with non-spiculated contours, no benign-appearing calcifications, and </= 14 in number, diagnosed by computed tomography of the chest or positron emission tomography (PET).

5. Lung metastases will be unresectable due to anatomic location, distribution, or patients' comorbidities, as determined by review of imaging by a faculty member in the Department of Thoracic & Cardiovascular Surgery.

6. Patients 18 years of age and older.

7. Patients must sign a study-specific consent form.

8. Patients will undergo CT imaging of the chest, abdomen, and pelvis to evaluate lung and liver metastases within 30 days of registration. For patients who cannot tolerate CT contrast or have hepatic steatosis that reduces the sensitivity of CT, MRI of the liver will be performed.

Exclusion Criteria:

1. Radiographic evidence of disease other than liver and lungs, with the exception of mediastinal lymph nodes < 2 cm and hepatoduodenal ligament lymphadenopathy, diagnosed by computed tomography, magnetic resonance imaging, or positron emission tomography.

2. Inadequate liver function, as evidenced by serum bilirubin >/= 2 mg/dL, international normalized ratio (INR) >/= 1.7, and/or platelet count < 50,000/microL.

3. Eastern Cooperative Oncology Group (ECOG) performance status of 3-4.

4. Patient refusal to participate in randomization.

5. Pregnant women are excluded from this study.

6. Planned stereotactic body radiation therapy (SBRT) for the pulmonary metastases.

Sex/Gender

All

Ages

18 Years to N/A

Accepts Healthy Volunteers

No

Contacts

Yun Shin Chun, MD   713-563-9682

A Phase 1 Clinical Study of AZD4635 and Durvalumab in Patients With Advanced Solid Malignancies

Study ID:

NCT02740985

Sponsor:

AstraZeneca

Information provided by (Responsible Party):

AstraZeneca (AstraZeneca)

Tracking Information

First Submitted Date

February 29, 2016

Start Date

June 17, 2016

Primary Completion Date

August 13, 2019

Last Update Posted Date

January 17, 2018

Current Primary Outcome Measures

The incidence of Dose-Limiting Toxicities (DLTs) in patients receiving AZD4635 monotherapy orally.[Time Frame: 3 weeks (One Cycle)]

A Bayesian Logistic Regression Model (BLRM) based approach will be used to identify the set of AZD4635 doses where the incidence of DLTs is no larger than 33%. It is planned that 24 to 36 patients in total will be included in the dose-escalation part of Phase Ia. In each cohort, up to 3 patients will be initially assessed. Dose escalation to the next higher dose level for the next cohort group of 3 patients will occur if all 3 patients in the initial cohort complete the first 3 weeks of dosing without a DLT. Following the first DLT, the BLRM model will be run and the output made available to the safety review committee (SRC) to guide further dosing decisions. Each dose cohort will include a maximum of 6 patients.

The incidence of Dose-Limiting Toxicities (DLTs) in patients receiving AZD4635 orally in combination with intravenous durvalumab.[Time Frame: 4 weeks (One Cycle)]

A Bayesian Logistic Regression Model (BLRM) based approach will be used to identify the set of AZD4635 doses where the incidence of DLTs is no larger than 33%. It is planned that 24 to 36 patients in total will be included in the dose-escalation part of Phase Ia. In each cohort, up to 3 patients will be initially assessed. Dose escalation to the next higher dose level for the next cohort group of 3 patients will occur if all 3 patients in the initial cohort complete the first 3 weeks of dosing without a DLT. Following the first DLT, the BLRM model will be run and the output made available to the safety review committee (SRC) to guide further dosing decisions. Each dose cohort will include a maximum of 6 patients.

Current Secondary Outcome Measures

The plasma concentration of AZD4635 after administration in the monotherapy portion of the study[Time Frame: Predose and 0.5, 1, 2, 3, 4, 6, 8, 10, and 24 hr post dose on Days 1 and 15 in Cycles 0 and 1. Also 48, 72, and 96 hr post-dose in Cycle 0 and predose in Cycle 2 and alternating cycles thereafter.]

Plasma concentration of AZD4635 will be determined by inspection of the concentration-time profile. The date and time of collection of each sample will be recorded.

The concentration of AZD4635 and metabolites in urine[Time Frame: A predose sample of urine will be collected. Quantitative collection of all urine will done in the following post-dose intervals: 0-4 hours, 4-8 hours, and 8-24 hours.]

The amount of AZD4635 (and metabolites) in urine will be determined in all patients. Pooled collections of urine 0 to 4 hours post dose, 4 to 8 hours post dose, and 8 to 24 hours post dose. Patients will collect all urine at home and bring the 8 to 24 hour pooled collection to the clinic. The total volume of each pooled sample will be recorded after which a 10 mL aliquot will be taken for analysis.

The plasma concentration of AZD4635 when given in combination with durvalumab[Time Frame: Predose and 0.5, 1, 2, 3, 4, 6, 8, and 24 hr post dose on Day 1 in Cycles 0, 2, and 4. Also 48, 72, and 96 hr post-dose in Cycle 0 and predose in Cycles 1, 3, 5, and 7.]

Plasma concentration of AZD4635 will be determined by inspection of the concentration-time profile. The date and time of collection of each sample will be recorded.

The concentration of durvalumab and anti-drug antibody in plasma when given in combination with AZD4635[Time Frame: Preinfusion and end of infusion on Day 1 of Cycles 2 and 5. Preinfusion of Day 1 of Cycles 3 and 8 and 90-days after the last dose of durvalumab.]

Plasma concentration of durvalumab and anti-drug antibody will be determined by inspection of the concentration-time profile. The date and time of collection of each sample will be recorded.

The effect of AZD4635 on QTc interval[Time Frame: In screening and on Days 1 and 15 in Cycle 1, Day 1 of each cycle therafter, and at the end of treatment and at each progression-free follow-up visit.]

Twelve-lead ECGs will be obtained after the patient has been resting semi-supine for at least 10 minutes. For each time point 3 ECG recordings should be taken at about 2to 5 minute intervals.

Tumour Response[Time Frame: Tumour response will be assessed 6 weeks after the start of treatment and then every 8 weeks thereafter up to 1 year.]

Categorization of objective tumour response assessment will be based on the RECIST Version 1.1 guidelines for response (CR (complete response), PR (partial response), SD (stable disease), and PD (progressive disease).

For patients who only have non-measurable disease at baseline, categorization of objective tumour response assessment will be based on the RECIST Version 1.1 guideline for response for non-target lesions (NTLs): CR, PD, and Non CR/Non PD.

Descriptive Information

Offical Title

A Phase I, Open-Label, Multicenter Study to Assess Safety, Tolerability, Pharmacokinetics, and Preliminary Anti-Tumor Activity of Ascending Doses of AZD4635 Both as Monotherapy and in Combination With Durvalumab in Patients With Advanced Solid Malignancies.

Brief Summary

This is a Phase I, open-label, multicenter study of continuous oral dosing of AZD4635 administered as a single agent and then in combination with a PD-L1 antibody, durvalumab. The study design allows an escalation of dose with intensive safety monitoring to ensure the safety of the patients. The primary objective of the study is to determine the maximum tolerated dose of AZD4635 in combination with durvalumab.

Detailed Description

The study will be conducted in two segments. The first segment of the study (Phase 1a) will be a dose escalation design in order to determine the Maximum Tolerated Dose (MTD) of AZD4635 given as monotherapy and in combination with durvalumab. The MTD will be determined by assessing adverse events and the incidence of abnormal laboratory measures. Once the maximum tolerated monotherapy dose of AZD4635 has been determined, combination dosing with durvalumab will start in a new cohort of patients at one dose level lower than the highest tolerated dose of AZD4635 monotherapy. The combination therapy cohorts in Phase 1a will also have a 2-week monotherapy lead-in after which patients who tolerate monotherapy AZD4635 will then continue twice daily dosing of AZD4635 in combination with durvalumab (anti programmed-death ligand 1 [PD-L1]) at the fixed dose of 1.5 grams IV every 4 weeks.

When the maximum-tolerated dose in the combination setting is determined, additional patients with advanced solid malignancies will be enrolled to a dose expansion portion to explore further the safety, tolerability, pharmacokinetics (PK), and biological activity at the selected doses. Approximately 24 to 36 patients with advanced solid malignancies will be treated in Phase 1a. When the maximum-tolerated dose in the combination setting is determined, additional patients with advanced solid malignancies will be enrolled to a dose expansion portion to explore further the safety, tolerability, pharmacokinetics (PK), and biological activity at the selected doses. Approximately 24 to 36 patients with advanced solid malignancies will be treated in Phase 1a. If the MTD for either AZD4635 monotherapy or the AZD4635/durvalumab combination is not reached dose expansion may take place at dose levels of AZD4635 and durvalumab other than MTD.

The second segment of the study (Phase 1b) will consist of an additional expansion cohorts in tumour types where there is a rationale for potential efficacy of the study treatment. The additional dose expansion cohorts will use doses that do not exceed the highest tolerated dose determined during the dose escalation segment of the study in patients with:

- Post-immunotherapy non-small cell lung cancer (NSCLC) (AZD4635 monotherapy or AZD4635 in combination with durvalumab).
- Other post-immunotherapy solid tumours (AZD 4635 monotherapy).
- Immune checkpoint-naïve metastatic castrate-resistant prostate carcinoma (mCRPC) (AZD4635 monotherapy or AZD4635 in combination with durvalumab).
- Immune checkpoint-naïve colorectal carcinoma (CRC) (AZD4635 monotherapy).
- Other immune checkpoint-naïve solid tumours (AZD4635 monotherapy).

- ▨ **Study Type**

  Interventional

- ▨ **Study Phase**

  Phase 1

- ▨ **Condition**

  - Advanced Solid Malignancies
  - Non-Small Cell Lung Cancer (NSCLC)
  - Metastatic Castrate-Resistant Prostate Carcinoma (mCRPC)
  - Colorectal Carcinoma (CRC)

- ▨ **Intervention**

  Drug: AZD4635

  AZD4635 will be administered orally as a nanosuspension on a continuous schedule. The drug product will be constituted extemporaneously as an oral suspension by the patient immediately prior to dosing.

  Drug: Durvalumab

  Durvalumab will be administered by intravenous infusion once every 4 weeks. Durvalumab should be reconstituted using aseptic techniques with sterile water for injection. The reconstituted solution will be diluted with 0.9% (w/v) saline prior to IV infusion.

  Other Names:

  MEDI4736

- ▨ **Study Arms**

  Experimental: AZD4635 Monotherapy

  AZD4635 monotherapy will be given twice daily in a dose escalation scheme in Part 1a. Patients will receive a single dose of AZD4635 on Day 1 and will have blood samples collected to assess pharmacokinetics over 24 hours. On Day 2, twice daily dosing will commence and continue daily. Other dosing schedules (e.g., once daily, three times daily) may be investigated during the study on the basis of emerging safety, PK, and exploratory mechanism of action (MOA) data. During monotherapy dosing, a cycle will be 3 weeks. The Safety Review Committee (SRC) will determine whether dose escalation should occur based on safety assessments in the first cycle supported by a Bayesian Logistic Regression Model (BLRM) approach.

  In Phase 1b additional expansion cohorts will be investigated based on the activity observed in the Phase 1a monotherapy dose escalation cohorts as well as monotherapy responses seen in other A2aR inhibitor studies.

  Experimental: AZD4635 + Durvalumab Combination

  In the combination therapy cohorts AZD4635 will be given as monotherapy during a 2-week lead-in. After the 2-week lead-in durvalumab will be given by IV infusion on Day 1 of each 4-week cycle. Other dosing schedules (e.g., once daily, three times daily) may be investigated during the study on the basis of emerging safety, PK, and exploratory mechanism of action (MOA) data. During combination therapy dosing, a cycle will be 4 weeks. The Safety Review Committee (SRC) will determine whether dose escalation should occur based on safety assessments in the first cycle supported by a Bayesian Logistic Regression Model (BLRM) approach.

  In Phase 1b additional expansion cohorts receiving combination therapy with AZD4635 and durvalumab will be investigated in patients with non small-cell lung cancer or metastatic castrate-resistant prostate cancer.

Recruitment Information

- ▨ **Recruitment Status**

  Recruiting

- ▨ **Estimated Enrollment**

  156

- ▨ **Eligibility Criteria**

  Inclusion Criteria

  1. Age ≥ 18.

  2. Availability of an archival tumor tissue sample. If archival tumour tissue is not available, then tissue from a fresh biopsy can be used.

  3. Patients in the Phase 1a dose escalation combination cohorts must have at least 1 tumour lesion amenable to biopsy and must be medically fit and willing to undergo a biopsy during screening and, unless clinically contraindicated, after 2 weeks on monotherapy.

  4. Phase 1a: histological or cytological confirmation of a solid, malignant tumor (excluding CNS tumors), that is refractory to standard therapies or for which no standard therapies exist.

- ▨ **Completion Date**

  August 13, 2019

- ▨ **Primary Completion Date**

  August 13, 2019

5. Eastern Cooperative Oncology Group (ECOG) performance 0-1.

6. Normotensive or well controlled blood pressure (BP) (<140/90).

7. Females should be using adequate contraceptive measures from the time of screening until 3 months after study discontinuation, should not be breast feeding and must have negative pregnancy test prior to the start of dosing.

8. Male patients should be willing to use barrier contraception for the duration of the study and for 3 months after treatment discontinuation.

9. To participate in Phase 1b patients must have disease that is suitable for repeated measurements, either:

- at least one lesion that can be accurately assessed at baseline by computed tomography (TC), magnetic resonance imaging (MRI) or X-ray, that is suitable for repeated measurement.
- for patients with mCRC patients must have measurable PSA above normal limits per local ranges.

10. A minimum of 10 patients with mCRPC, CRC and 'other' tumors will be required to have a site of disease that is safely accessible for biopsy (paired) upon enrollment. Accessible lesions are defined as those which are biopsiable (at screening) and amenable to repeat biopsy (after 2 weeks of monotherapy), unless clinically contraindicated. In the case that the second sample is not taken, the patient will remain in the study and there will be no penalty or loss of benefit to the patient and they will not be excluded from other aspects of the study.

The tumor-specific cohorts will be closely monitored to ensure the desired number of biopsiable patients are enrolled. The requirement for biopsies must be made clear to each patient at the time of initial approach by the Investigator.

11. For post immunotherapy patients with NSCLC all of the following apply:

- Patients must have advanced or metastatic NSCLC with histological or cytological confirmation. Patients with known EGFR-activating mutations or ALK rearrangements are excluded.
- Patient must have previously received one (but no more) line of previous therapy with an anti-PD-1/PD-L1 mAb therapy either alone or in combination and have either progressed or responded and then stopped responding.

12. For other post immunotherapy patients all of the following must apply:

- Patients must have an immune checkpoint resistant malignancy (for example, RCC, head and neck carcinoma or MSI high cancers which have approved settings for anti-PD1 treatment), confirmed histologically or cytologically.
- Patients must have previously received at least one line (and not more than 2 lines) of previous therapy with an anti-PD-1/PD-L1 mAb therapy, either alone or in combination, and have either progressed or responded and then stopped responding.

13. For immune checkpoint naïve CRPC patients all of the following must apply:

- Patients must have metastatic prostate cancer with histological or cytological confirmation.
- Patients must be castrate-resistant (i.e., developed progression of metastases following surgical castration or during medical androgen ablation therapy). Patients receiving medical castration therapy with gonadotropin-releasing hormone analogues should continue this treatment during this study. Patients must have immune checkpoint naïve histologically/cytologically confirmed advanced or metastatic CRC.
- Patients must have previously received and progressed on standard-of-care therapy(ies).

14. For other immune checkpoint naïve patients all of the following must apply:

- histologically/cytologically confirmed advanced solid tumor type that has received and progressed on standard-of-care therapy(ies).

Exclusion Criteria

1. Treatment with any of the following:

1. nitrosourea or mitomycin C within 6 weeks of the first dose

2. any investigational agents or drugs from a previous clinical study within 28 days

3. any investigational medicinal product or other systemic anticancer treatment within 4 weeks or within 8 weeks after immunotherapy or other long half-life antibody therapy

4. Rx or non-Rx drugs or other products known to be sensitive BCRP or OAT1 substrates or to be potent inhibitors/inducers of CYP1A2, which cannot be discontinued 2 weeks prior to Day 1 of dosing and withheld throughout the study until 2 weeks after the last dose of AZD4635.

5. herbal preparations/medications are not allowed throughout the study, including but not limited to St. John's Wort, kava, ephedra (ma huang), gingko biloba, dehydroepiandrosterone, yohimbe, saw palmetto, and ginseng.

6. Concomitant therapy with another A1R antagonist that would increase the risk of seizure (e.g., theophylline, aminophylline).

7. Ongoing treatment with Coumadin.

8. Ongoing corticosteroid use.

2. Major surgery within 4 weeks of the first dose of study treatment

3. Radiotherapy with a wide field of radiation within 4 weeks or radiotherapy with a limited field of radiation for palliation within 2 weeks of the first dose of study treatment.

4. With the exception of alopecia, any unresolved toxicities from prior therapy greater than CTCAE Grade 1 at the time of starting study treatment.

5. History of seizures, central nervous system tumors or CNS metastasis, prior traumatic brain injury, prior stroke, or other predisposing risk of seizure. Due to the incidence of silent CNS metastases in patients with advanced NSCLC, such patients must undergo mandatory screening with brain MRI or CT scan to determine eligibility.

6. Significant mental illness in the 4-week period preceding drug administration.

7. Evidence of severe or uncontrolled systemic disease, including uncontrolled hypertension, active bleeding diatheses, or active infection.

8. Any of the following cardiac criteria: mean resting corrected QT interval (QTcF) >470 msec obtained from 3 ECGs; clinically important abnormalities in rhythm, conduction, or morphology of resting ECGs, e.g., complete left bundle branch block, third degree heart block; any factors that increase the risk of QTc prolongation or risk of arrhythmic events; ejection fraction <55% or the lower limit of normal of the institutional standard.

9. Inadequate bone marrow reserve or organ function as demonstrated by any of the following laboratory values: Absolute neutrophil count < 1.5 x 10 (exp9)/L; Platelet count < 100 x 10 (exp9)/L; Hemoglobin <90 g/L; ALT and/or AST >2.5 times the upper limit of normal (ULN) if no demonstrable liver metastases or >5 times ULN in the presence of liver metastases; Total bilirubin >1.5 times ULN; Creatinine >1.5 times ULN concurrent with creatinine clearance <50 mL/min

10. Refractory nausea and vomiting, chronic gastrointestinal diseases, or previous significant bowel resection that would preclude adequate absorption of AZD4635.

11. Organ transplant that requires the use of immunosuppressive treatment.

12. Active or prior documented autoimmune or inflammatory disorders within the past 3 years prior to the start of treatment.

13. Patients with prior ≥ Grade 3, serious, or life threatening immune-mediated reactions following prior anti-PD-1 or other immune-oncology therapies

14. History of hypersensitivity to AZD4635 or drugs with a similar chemical structure or class to AZD4635.

15. Patients with a known microsatellite instability (MSI) high biomarker based on local laboratory assessment are excluded from Phase 1b post immunotherapy cohort enrollment.

Sex/Gender

All

Ages

18 Years to 130 Years

Accepts Healthy Volunteers

No

Contacts

AstraZeneca Clinical Study Information Center   1-877-240-9479   information.center@astrazeneca.com
AstraZeneca Cancer Study Location Service   1-877-400-4656   AstraZeneca@emergingmed.com

A Study of Napabucasin (BBI-608) in Combination With FOLFIRI in Adult Patients With Previously Treated Metastatic Colorectal Cancer

Study ID:

NCT02753127

Sponsor:

Boston Biomedical, Inc

Information provided by (Responsible Party):

Boston Biomedical, Inc (Boston Biomedical, Inc)

Tracking Information

First Submitted Date

April 25, 2016

Start Date

June 2016

Primary Completion Date

June 2020

Last Update Posted Date

December 14, 2017

Current Primary Outcome Measures

Overall Survival[Time Frame: 36 months]

To assess the effect of napabucasin plus biweekly FOLFIRI versus biweekly FOLFIRI on the Overall Survival of patients with previously treated metastatic colorectal cancer.

Current Secondary Outcome Measures

Progression Free Survival[Time Frame: 36 months]

Defined as the time from randomization to the first objective documentation of disease progression or death due to any cause.

Objective Response Rate[Time Frame: 36 months]

Defined as the proportion of patients with a documented complete response or partial response (CR + PR) based on RECIST 1.1.

Disease Control Rate[Time Frame: 36 months]

Defined as the proportion of patients with a documented complete response, partial response, and stable disease (CR + PR + SD) based on RECIST 1.1.

Number of Patients with Adverse Events[Time Frame: 36 months]

All patients who have received at least one dose of napabucasin will be included in the safety analysis according to the National Cancer Institute Common Toxicity Criteria for Adverse Events (NCI CTCAE) version 4.0. The incidence of adverse events will be summarized by type of adverse event and severity.

Quality of Life (QoL)[Time Frame: 36 months]

QoL will be measured using the European Organization for Research and Treatment of Cancer Quality of Life questionnaire (EORTC-QLQ-C30) in patients with pretreated metastatic CRC treated with napabucasin plus biweekly FOLFIRI versus biweekly FOLFIRI.

Descriptive Information

Offical Title

A Phase III Study of BBI-608 in Combination With 5-Fluorouracil, Leucovorin, Irinotecan (FOLFIRI) in Adult Patients With Previously Treated Metastatic Colorectal Cancer (CRC).

Brief Summary

This is an international multi-center, prospective, open-label, randomized phase 3 trial of the cancer stem cell pathway inhibitor napabucasin plus standard bi-weekly FOLFIRI versus standard bi-weekly FOLFIRI in patients with previously treated metastatic colorectal cancer (CRC).

Study Type

Interventional

Study Phase

Phase 3

Condition

- Colorectal Cancer

Intervention

Drug: Napabucasin

Napabucasin 240 mg will be administered orally, twice daily, with doses separated by approximately 12 hours (480 mg total daily dose).

Other Names:

BBI-608

BBI608

BB608

Drug: Fluorouracil

Other Names:

5-FU

Carac

Efudex

Fluoroplex

Adrucil

Drug: Leucovorin

Other Names:

Folinic Acid

Drug: Irinotecan

Other Names:

Camptosar

Drug: Bevacizumab

Other Names:

Avastin

Study Arms

Experimental: Napabucasin plus FOLFIRI

Addition of bevacizumab to the FOLFIRI regimen will be permissible. FOLFIRI chemotherapy infusion will start at least 2 hours following the first daily dose of napabucasin and will be administered every 2 weeks. Irinotecan/leucovorin infusion will follow bevacizumab infusion in selected patients to receive standard dose of bevacizumab (5 mg/kg). Irinotecan 180 mg/m^2 together with leucovorin 400 mg/m^2 will be administered intravenously, over approximately 90 minutes and 2 hours, respectively, starting on Day 1 of Cycle 1, following bevacizumab infusion or at least 2 hours following the first daily dose of napabucasin if bevacizumab is not administered. 5-FU 400 mg/m^2 bolus will be administered intravenously immediately following irinotecan/leucovorin infusion, followed by 5-FU 1200 mg/m^2/day (total 2400 mg/m^2) continuous infusion. This regimen will be repeated on Day 1 of every 14 day cycle.

Active Comparator: FOLFIRI

Addition of bevacizumab to the FOLFIRI regimen will be permissible. FOLFIRI chemotherapy infusion will be administered every 2 weeks. Irinotecan/leucovorin infusion will follow bevacizumab infusion in selected patients to receive standard dose of bevacizumab (5 mg/kg). Irinotecan 180 mg/m^2 together with leucovorin 400 mg/m^2 will be administered intravenously, over approximately 90 minutes and 2 hours, respectively, starting on Day 1 of Cycle 1, following bevacizumab infusion. 5-FU 400 mg/m^2 bolus will be administered intravenously immediately following irinotecan/leucovorin infusion, followed by 5-FU 1200 mg/m^2/day (total 2400 mg/m^2) continuous infusion. This regimen will be repeated on Day 1 of every 14 day cycle.

Recruitment Information

Recruitment Status

Recruiting

Estimated Enrollment

1250

Completion Date

N/A

Primary Completion Date

June 2020

Eligibility Criteria

Inclusion Criteria:

1. Written, signed consent for trial participation must be obtained from the patient appropriately in accordance with applicable ICH guidelines and local and regulatory requirements prior to the performance of any study specific procedure.

2. Must have histologically confirmed advanced CRC that is metastatic.

3. Must have failed treatment with one regimen containing a fluoropyrimidine, oxaliplatin with or without bevacizumab for metastatic disease. All patients must have received a minimum of 6 weeks of the first-line regimen that included bevacizumab (if applicable), oxaliplatin and a fluoropyrimidine in the same cycle. Treatment failure is defined as radiologic progression during or < 6 months after the last dose of first-line therapy.

4. FOLFIRI therapy is appropriate for the patient and is recommended by the Investigator.

5. Imaging investigations including CT/MRI of chest/abdomen/pelvis or other scans as necessary to document all sites of disease performed within 21 days prior to randomization. Patients with either measurable disease or non-measurable evaluable disease are eligible.

6. Must have an Eastern Cooperative Oncology Group (ECOG) Performance Status of 0 or 1.

7. Must be ≥ 18 years of age.

8. For male or female patient of child producing potential: Must agree to use contraception or take measures to avoid pregnancy during the study and for 180 days for female and male patients, of the final FOLFIRI dose. Patients who receive single agent napabucasin without FOLFIRI must agree to use contraception or take measures to avoid pregnancy during the study and for 30 days for female patients and 90 days for male patients, of the final napabucasin dose.

9. Women of child bearing potential (WOCBP) must have a negative serum or urine pregnancy test within 5 days prior to randomization. The minimum sensitivity of the pregnancy test must be 25 IU/L or equivalent units of HCG.

10. Must have alanine transaminase (ALT) ≤ 3 × institutional upper limit of normal (ULN) [≤ 5 × ULN in presence of liver metastases] within 14 days prior to randomization.

11. Must have hemoglobin (Hgb) ≥ 9.0 g/dL within 14 days prior to randomization. Must not have required transfusion of red blood cells within 1 week of baseline Hgb assessment.

12. Must have total bilirubin ≤ 1.5 × institutional ULN [≤ 2.0 x ULN in presence of liver metastases] within 14 days prior to randomization.

13. Must have creatinine ≤ 1.5 × institutional ULN or Creatinine Clearance > 50 ml/min (as calculated by the Cockcroft-Gault equation) within 14 days prior to randomization.

14. Must have absolute neutrophil count ≥ 1.5 x 10^9/L within 14 days prior to randomization.

15. Must have platelet count ≥ 100 x 10^9/L within 14 days prior to randomization. Must not have required transfusion of platelets within 1 week of baseline platelet assessment.

16. Patient must have adequate nutritional status with Body Mass Index (BMI) > 18 kg/m^2 and body weight of > 40 kg with serum albumin > 3 g/dL.

17. Other baseline laboratory evaluations, listed in Section 6.0, must be done within 14 days prior to randomization.

18. Patient must consent to provision of, and Investigator(s) must confirm access to and agree to submit a representative formalin fixed paraffin block of tumor tissue in order that the specific correlative marker assays may be conducted. Submission of the tissue does not have to occur prior to randomization. Where local center regulations prohibit submission of blocks of tumor tissue, two 2 mm cores of tumor from the block and 10-30 unstained slides of whole sections of representative tumor tissue are preferred. Where two 2 mm cores of tumor from the block are unavailable, 10-30 unstained slides of whole sections of representative tumor tissue alone are acceptable. Where no previously resected or biopsied tumor tissue exists or is available, on the approval of the Sponsor/designated CRO, the patient may still be considered eligible for the study.

19. Patient must consent to provision of a sample of blood in order that the specific correlative marker assays may be conducted.

20. Patients must be accessible for treatment and follow-up. Patients registered on this trial must receive protocol treatment and be followed at the participating center. This implies there must be reasonable geographical limits placed on patients being considered for this trial. Investigators must ensure that the patients randomized on this trial will be available for complete documentation of the treatment, response assessment, adverse events, and follow-up.

21. Protocol treatment is to begin within 2 calendar days of patient randomization.

22. The patient is not receiving therapy in a concurrent clinical study and the patient agrees not to participate in other interventional clinical studies during their participation in this trial while on study treatment. Patients participating in surveys or observational studies are eligible to participate in this study.

Exclusion Criteria:

1. Anti-cancer chemotherapy or biologic therapy if administered prior to the first planned dose of study medication (napabucasin or FOLFIRI) within period of time equivalent to the usual cycle length of the regimen. An exception is made for oral fluoropyrimidines (e.g. capecitabine, S-1), where a minimum of 10 days since last dose must be observed prior to the first planned dose of study medication. Standard dose of bevacizumab (5 mg/kg) may be administered prior to FOLFIRI infusion, per Investigator decision, for as long as permanent decision to include or exclude bevacizumab is made prior to patient randomization. Radiotherapy, immunotherapy (including immunotherapy administered for non-malignant diseaseneoplastic treatment purposes), or investigational agents within four weeks of first planned dose of study medication, with the exception of a single dose of radiation up to 8 Gy (equal to 800 RAD) with palliative intent for pain control up to 14 days before randomization.

2. More than one prior chemotherapy regimen administered in the metastatic setting.

3. Major surgery within 4 weeks prior to randomization.

4. Patients with any known brain or leptomeningeal metastases are excluded, even if treated.

5. Women who are pregnant or breastfeeding. Women should not breastfeed while taking study treatment and for 4 weeks after the last dose of napabucasin or while undergoing treatment with FOLFIRI and for 180 days after the last dose of FOLFIRI.

6. Gastrointestinal disorder(s) which, in the opinion of the Qualified/Principal Investigator, would significantly impede the absorption of an oral agent (e.g. intestinal occlusion, active Crohn's disease, ulcerative colitis, extensive gastric and small intestine resection).

7. Unable or unwilling to swallow napabucasin capsules daily.

8. Prior treatment with napabucasin.

9. Uncontrolled intercurrent illness including, but not limited to, ongoing or active infection, clinically significant non-healing or healing wounds, symptomatic congestive heart failure, unstable angina pectoris, clinically significant cardiac arrhythmia, significant pulmonary disease (shortness of breath at rest or mild exertion), uncontrolled infection or psychiatric illness/social situations that would limit compliance with study requirements.

10. Known hypersensitivity to 5-fluorouracil/leucovorin

11. Known dihydropyrimidine dehydrogenase (DPD) deficiency

12. Known hypersensitivity to irinotecan

13. Chronic inflammatory bowel disease (Crohn's disease or ulcerative colitis)

14. Patients receiving treatment with St. John's wort or Phenytoin.

15. Patients who plan to receive yellow fever vaccine during the course of the study treatment.

16. Abnormal glucuronidation of bilirubin, known Gilbert's syndrome

17. Patients with QTc interval > 470 milliseconds

18. For patients to be treated with a regimen containing bevacizumab:

- History of cardiac disease: congestive heart failure (CHF) > New York Heart Association (NYHA) Class II; active coronary artery disease, myocardial infarction within 6 months prior to study entry; unevaluated new onset angina within 3 months or unstable angina (angina symptoms at rest) or cardiac arrhythmias requiring anti-arrhythmic therapy (beta blockers or digoxin are permitted).

- Current uncontrolled hypertension (systolic blood pressure [BP] > 150 mmHg or diastolic pressure > 90 mmHg despite optimal medical management) as well as prior history of hypertensive crisis or hypertensive encephalopathy.

- History of arterial thrombotic or embolic events (within 6 months prior to study entry)
- Significant vascular disease (e.g., aortic aneurysm, aortic dissection, symptomatic peripheral vascular disease)
- Evidence of bleeding diathesis or clinically significant coagulopathy
- Major surgical procedure (including open biopsy, significant traumatic injury, etc.) within 28 days, or anticipation of the need for major surgical procedure during the course of the study as well as minor surgical procedure (excluding placement of a vascular access device or bone marrow biopsy) within 7 days prior to study enrollment
- Proteinuria at screening as demonstrated by urinalysis with proteinuria ≥ 2+ (patients discovered to have ≥2+ proteinuria on dipstick urinalysis at baseline should undergo a 24 hour urine collection and must demonstrate ≤ 1g of protein in 24 hours to be eligible).
- History of abdominal fistula, gastrointestinal perforation, peptic ulcer, or intra-abdominal abscess within 6 months
- Ongoing serious, non-healing wound, ulcer, or bone fracture
- Known hypersensitivity to any component of bevacizumab
- History of reversible posterior leukoencephalopathy syndrome (RPLS)
- History of hypersensitivity to Chinese hamster ovary (CHO) cells or other human or humanized recombinant antibodies.

19. Patients with a history of other malignancies except: adequately treated non-melanoma skin cancer, curatively treated in-situ cancer of the cervix, or other solid tumors curatively treated with no evidence of disease for > 3 years.

20. Any active disease condition which would render the protocol treatment dangerous or impair the ability of the patient to receive protocol therapy.

21. Any condition (e.g. psychological, geographical, etc.) that does not permit compliance with the protocol.

Sex/Gender

All

Ages

18 Years to N/A

Accepts Healthy Volunteers

No

Contacts

Boston Biomedical   617-674-6800

Evaluation the Efficacy of Colon Capsule Endoscopy (CCE) Versus Computed Tomographic Colonography (CTC) in the Identification of Colonic Polyps in a Screening Population.

Study ID:

NCT02754661

Sponsor:

Medtronic MITG

Information provided by (Responsible Party):

- Medtronic MITG (Medtronic MITG)

Tracking Information

First Submitted Date

April 25, 2016

Start Date

September 2016

Primary Completion Date

November 2017

Last Update Posted Date

January 26, 2018

Current Primary Outcome Measures

Diagnostic yield (proportion of subjects shown to have an actionable lesion, defined as any polyp or mass lesion ≥6 mm) by CCE as compared to CTC. Diagnostic yield of CCE/CTC will be calculated in relation to the confirmatory Optical colonoscopy results[Time Frame: 5-6 weeks from randomized procedure]

■ Current Secondary Outcome Measures

Accuracy measures of CCE versus CTC in the detection of polyps ≥6 mm will be assessed in relation to the confirmatory OC results on a "per subject" basis: Negative predictive value (NPV), Positive predictive value (PPV); Sensitivity; Specificity[Time Frame: 5-6 weeks from randomized procedure]

Descriptive Information

■ Offical Title

Multicenter, Prospective, Randomized Study Comparing the Diagnostic Yield of Colon Capsule Endoscopy Versus Computed Tomographic Colonography in a Screening Population

■ Brief Summary

The primary objective of this multicenter, prospective, randomized study is to assess the diagnostic yield of CCE versus CTC in a screening population.

■ Detailed Description

This is a multicenter, prospective, randomized study to evaluate the efficacy of CCE versus CTC in the identification of colonic polyps in a screening population.

- Subjects will be enrolled at up to 20 clinical sites in the United States. Subjects who meet the eligibility criteria will be screened by the gastroenterology site for study participation at a baseline visit which will also include a blood test for renal function (eGFR), and will be evaluated on the randomized procedure day (CCE versus CTC) and again on the day of both the blinded and unblinded OC procedures. Telephone follow-ups will be conducted 5 9 days after the CCE/CTC procedure and 5 9 days after the unblinded OC procedure to assess subject well-being and capture any AEs, regardless of relationship to the CCE, CTC, or OC procedures.

All CCE RAPID® videos and CTC images will be evaluated by local and central readers. All study analyses will be based on central reader results for both CCE and CTC. Two sets of central readers will be utilized, one set for reading of the CCE RAPID® videos and one set for reading the CTC studies. Both groups of readers will be experts in the reading process for their respective procedures. Readers will provide a report of their findings to the sponsor within 2 weeks of capsule ingestion or CTC procedure in order to allow subjects to return within 5 weeks capsule ingestion or CTC procedure to undergo confirmatory OC. The first OC procedure will be performed with the clinician blinded to the CCE or CTC results. Immediately following this blinded procedure, the clinician will review the CCE or CTC results report provided by the sponsor from the central readers, and a second unblinded OC procedure will be performed if there are discrepancies between the CCE/CTC findings and OC.

Colonoscopy must not be performed by the same person who conducts the local CCE reading, or anyone who has reviewed CCE/CTC results for that subject.

Bowel preparation regimens for all three procedure types will be standardized across sites.

■ Study Type

Interventional

■ Study Phase

N/A

■ Condition

- Colorectal Cancer Screening

■ Intervention

Device: COLON Capsule endoscopy

Device: Computed Tomographic Colonography

■ Study Arms

Experimental: COLON Capsule endoscopy

Subjects will be instructed to follow a detailed dietary and colon preparation regimen prior to and during the CCE procedure day. With the exception of Gastrografin, all colon preparation products will be standard colon cleansing products approved by the FDA.

Between 45 and 75 minutes after the final PEG ingestion, the subject will swallow the PillCam COLON Capsule with a cup of water.

If necessary, capsule position will be monitored to ensure adequate booster administration. Subjects will keep a timed diary of key preparation steps and bowel activity, including capsule excretion. Subjects will be allowed to leave the unit 10 hours after capsule ingestion if the capsule is not yet excreted. Subjects leaving before excretion will be instructed to disconnect the recorder at excretion or 12 hours after capsule ingestion (whichever comes first).

Active Comparator: Computed Tomographic Colonography

Subjects will be instructed to follow a detailed dietary and colon preparation regimen prior to and during the Computed Tomographic Colonography (CTC) procedure day.

The CTC procedure and study interpretation will be conducted in accordance with the ACR-SAR-SCBT-MR Practice

Parameter for the Performance of CT Colonography in Adults. Colon insufflation will be performed with the subject in the lateral decubitus or supine position.With the subject in the supine position, a CT scout image will be taken to confirm adequate colon distention. If adequate bowel distention is not achieved, additional air will be insufflated into the colon. After scanning the subject in the supine position, the subject will be placed in the prone position, and additional CO_2 will be administered. Subsequently, CT will be performed with the subject in the prone position. If a prone position is not possible for the subject, a left lateral decubitus position is preferred for optimal gas and fluid redistribution.

Recruitment Information

Recruitment Status

Recruiting

Estimated Enrollment

320

Completion Date

April 2018

Primary Completion Date

November 2017

Eligibility Criteria

Inclusion Criteria:

1. Subject is between 50 and 75 years of age.

2. Subject is classified as average risk per the American Gastroenterological Association Guidelines on Colorectal Cancer Screening: Individuals without a personal or family history of CRC or adenomas, inflammatory bowel disease, or high-risk genetic syndromes.

3. Subject is willing and able to participate in the study procedures and to understand and sign the informed consent.

Exclusion Criteria:

1. Subject with history of colorectal cancer or adenoma (including those identified by computed tomography [CT], optical colonoscopy, sigmoidoscopy, etc.).

2. Subject with history of negative colonoscopy within 10 years, as these subjects would be defined as not requiring screening in this timeframe. For subjects with alternative screening methods, refer to applicable guidelines.

3. Subject with currently suspected or diagnosed with hematochezia, melena, iron deficiency with or without anemia, or any other rectal bleeding, including positive fecal occult blood test of any variety.

4. Subject with any current condition believed to have an increased risk of capsule retention such as suspected or known bowel obstruction, stricture, or fistula.

5. Subject with current dysphagia or any swallowing disorder.

6. Subject with current serious medical conditions that would increase the risk associated with CCE, CTC, or colonoscopy that are so severe that screening would have no benefit.

7. Subject with a cardiac pacemaker or other implanted electromedical device.

8. Subject expected to undergo MRI examination within 7 days after ingestion of the capsule.

9. Subject with clinical evidence of renal disease, including clinically significant laboratory abnormalities of renal function within the past 6 months, or at any time in the past if not tested within the last 6 months, defined as creatinine, blood urea nitrogen (BUN), and/or glomerular filtration rate (GFR) outside of the local laboratory reference range.

10. Subject with a diagnosis of gastroparesis or small bowel or large bowel dysmotility.

11. Subject with allergies or known contraindication to the medications or preparation agents used in the procedure as described in the relevant instructions for use.

12. Subject has an estimated life expectancy of less than 6 months.

13. Subject is considered to be part of a vulnerable population (e.g. prisoners or those without sufficient mental capacity).

14. Subject is pregnant, suspected pregnant, or is actively breast-feeding. Females of child-bearing potential will be required to provide either a urine pregnancy test or serum pregnancy test as part of the participant's standard of care regardless of their participation in the study (except for subjects who are surgically sterile or are post-menopausal for at least two years).

15. Subject has participated in an investigational drug or device research study within 30 days of enrollment that may interfere with the subject's safety or ability to participate in this study.

Sex/Gender

All

Ages

50 Years to 75 Years

Accepts Healthy Volunteers

Accepts Healthy Volunteers

Contacts

Liron Bar Yaakov   972-526060466   liron.bar-yaakov@covidien.com

Tremelimumab (Anti-CTLA-4) Plus Durvalumab (MEDI4736) (Anti-PD-L1) in the Treatment of Resectable Colorectal Cancer Liver Metastases

Study ID:
NCT02754856

Sponsor:
M.D. Anderson Cancer Center

Information provided by (Responsible Party):
M.D. Anderson Cancer Center (M.D. Anderson Cancer Center)

Tracking Information

▦ **First Submitted Date**

April 26, 2016

▦ **Start Date**

July 28, 2016

▦ **Primary Completion Date**

July 2021

▦ **Last Update Posted Date**

September 13, 2017

▦ **Current Primary Outcome Measures**

Feasibility of Tremelimumab plus MEDI4736 with FOLFOX and Bevacizumab in Candidates for Resection of Colorectal Cancer Liver Metastases[Time Frame: 15 weeks]

> Feasibility assessed by whether or not the patient successfully goes to surgery following the planned treatments, scans, and biopsy. Combination regimen considered feasible if at least 80% of patients successfully undergo surgery. It will be infeasible if fewer than 60% of patients can undergo surgery.

▦ **Current Secondary Outcome Measures**

Relapse-free survival (RFS) of Tremelimumab plus MEDI4736 with FOLFOX and Bevacizumab in Candidates for Resection of Colorectal Cancer Liver Metastases[Time Frame: 56 weeks]

> Relapse-free survival (RFS) assessed from the date of study entry until relapse or death from any cause.

Descriptive Information

▦ **Offical Title**

Pilot Study Assessing the Safety and Tolerability of the Neoadjuvant Use of Tremelimumab (Anti-CTLA-4) Plus Durvalumab (MEDI4736) (Anti-PD-L1) in the Treatment of Resectable Colorectal Cancer Liver Metastases

▦ **Brief Summary**

The goal of this clinical research study is to learn if tremelimumab in combination with MEDI4736 can help to control colorectal cancer that has spread to the liver. The safety of these drugs will also be studied.

This is an investigational study. MEDI4736 and tremelimumab are not FDA approved or commercially available. They are currently being used for research purposes only.

The study doctor can explain how the study drugs are designed to work.

Up to 35 participants will take part in this study. All will be enrolled at MD Anderson.

▦ **Detailed Description**

Study Drug Administration:

If you are found to be eligible to take part in this study, you will receive tremelimumab by vein over about 1 hour and MEDI4736 by vein over about 4 hours during Week 11. After Week 11, you will receive MEDI4736 alone by vein over about 1 hour during Weeks 21, 25, 29, and 33.

Between Weeks 15 and 17, you will have your already scheduled liver surgery. This means you will receive tremelimumab before your surgery and MEDI4736 after your surgery.

Study Visits:

During Week 1:

- You will have a physical exam.
- Blood (about 6 tablespoons) will be drawn for routine tests and for testing related to your immune system.
- If you can become pregnant, part of the above routine blood sample will be used for a pregnancy test. Urine may also be collected for this test.

During Week 4 :

- You will have a physical exam.
- Blood (about 6 teaspoons) will be drawn for routine tests and for testing related to your immune system.
- You will have a CT scan.
- If you can become pregnant, part of the above routine blood sample will be used for a pregnancy test. Urine may also be collected for this test.

Between Weeks 4 and 8:

- You will have a physical exam.
- Blood (about 4 tablespoons) will be drawn for tests related to the immune system.
- You will have liver surgery as part of your standard care. You will sign a separate consent form for this procedure.

After your liver surgery

Between 0-2 weeks after your liver surgery:

- You will also have a physical exam.
- Blood (about 7 tablespoons) will be drawn for routine tests, to check the status of the disease, and for tests related to your immune system.

During Week 1:

- You will have a physical exam.
- Blood (about 4 teaspoons) will be drawn for routine tests.
- If you can become pregnant, part of the above routine blood sample will be used for a pregnancy test. Urine may also be collected for this test.

During Weeks 5 and 9:

- You will have a physical exam.
- Blood (about 4 teaspoons) will be drawn for routine tests.

During Week 13 and every 14 weeks after that until 2 years:

- You will have a physical exam.
- Blood (about 8 teaspoons) will be drawn for routine tests and to check the status of the disease.
- You will have a CT scan or MRI.

At Week 17, instead of coming into the clinic, the study staff may call you to ask how you are doing. If you are called, it should last about 5-10 minutes.

Length of Study:

You may receive tremelimumab and MEDI4736 for 1 week and MEDI4736 alone for up to an additional 4 weeks. You will no longer be able to take the study drugs if the disease gets worse, if intolerable side effects occur, or if you are unable to follow study directions.

Your participation on this study will be over after follow-up.

Follow-Up:

If you stop treatment for any reason, you will be asked to come to the hospital so your study doctor may check your health and follow up any ongoing side effects or discomfort until they get better.

If the disease has gotten better or remained the same, your doctor will continue to check on the status of the disease as part of your standard of care, which may include imaging scans and/or blood draws for routine tests.

The study staff will call you 2 times every year starting about 2 years after surgery to ask you how you are doing. These calls should last about 5-10 minutes.

Follow-up will continue for 5 years or until you withdraw from the study, whichever happens first.

Study Type

Interventional

Study Phase

Phase 1

Condition

- Colorectal Cancer
- Liver Metastases

Intervention

Drug: Tremelimumab

Tremelimumab 75 mg by vein as a flat dose during Week 11.

Drug: MEDI4736

MEDI4736 1500 mg by vein as a flat dose during Week 11. After Week 11, participant receives MEDI4736 alone by vein during Weeks 21, 25, 29, and 33.

Other Names:

Durvalumab

Procedure: Liver Resection

Participant undergoes scheduled liver resection between Weeks 15 and 17.

Study Arms

Experimental: Tremelimumab + MEDI4736

Participants receive Tremelimumab by vein over about 1 hour and MEDI4736 by vein over about 4 hours during Week 11. After Week 11, participants receives MEDI4736 alone by vein over about 1 hour during Weeks 21, 25, 29, and 33.

Between Weeks 15 and 17, participant undergoes scheduled liver surgery.

Recruitment Information

Recruitment Status

Recruiting

Estimated Enrollment

35

Completion Date

July 2021

Primary Completion Date

July 2021

Eligibility Criteria

Inclusion Criteria:

1. Patients must have histologically or cytologically confirmed colorectal cancer with liver metastases deemed resectable by a general or liver surgeon (resectability may involve the use of ablative techniques to some but not all liver metastases). Those patients with known disease outside of the liver are not eligible (except for patients with primary lesions in place that are planned for resection or nonspecific lung metastases <1cm).

2. Patients must have measurable disease, defined as at least one lesion that can be accurately measured in at least one dimension (longest diameter to be recorded) as =/>10 mm with spiral CT scan.

3. All lines of prior therapy accepted. Subjects with prior hepatic or extra-hepatic resections of metastatic disease will be included.

4. Age =/>18 years. Because no dosing or adverse event data are currently available on the use of tremelimumab in combination with durvalumab in patients <18 years of age, children are excluded from this study.

5. Life expectancy of greater than 6 months.

6. ECOG performance status =/<1 (Karnofsky =/>70%).

7. Patients must have normal organ and marrow function as defined: a) leukocytes =/>3,000/mcL; b) absolute neutrophil count =/>1,500/mcL; c) platelets =/>100,000/mcL; d) total bilirubin < 1.5 X institutional normal limits (subjects with known Gilbert syndrome are eligible with total bilirubin < 3.0 mg/dL); e) AST(SGOT)/ALT(SGPT) =/< 3 X institutional upper limit of normal; f) creatinine within normal institutional limits OR g) creatinine clearance =/>60 mL/min/1.73 m^2 for patients with creatinine levels above institutional normal.

8. Known or ordered molecular testing for MSI, BRAF, and KRAS status.

9. Evidence of post-menopausal status or negative urinary or serum pregnancy test for female pre-menopausal patients. Women will be considered post-menopausal if they have been amenorrheic for 12 months without an alternative medical cause. The following age-specific requirements apply: Women <50 years of age would be considered post-menopausal if they have been amenorrheic for 12 months or more following cessation of exogenous hormonal treatments and if they have luteinizing hormone and follicle-stimulating hormone levels in the post-menopausal range for the institution or underwent surgical sterilization (bilateral oophorectomy or hysterectomy).

10. Continuation from criteria above: Women >/= 50 years of age would be considered post-menopausal if they have been amenorrheic for 12 months or more following cessation of all exogenous hormonal treatments, had radiation-induced menopause with last menses >1 year ago, had chemotherapy-induced menopause with last menses >1 year ago, or underwent surgical sterilization (bilateral oophorectomy, bilateral salpingectomy or hysterectomy).

11. Ability to understand and the willingness to sign a written informed consent document.

12. Weight >30kg (required for flat dose-based administration of study agents)

Exclusion Criteria:

1. Prior chemotherapy < 2 weeks prior to study drug treatment and treatment related adverse events that have not recovered to baseline or grade 1 (alopecia excluded). Prior radiation therapy <4weeks prior to study drug treatment.

2. Patients may not be receiving any other investigational agents.

3. Active or prior documented autoimmune or inflammatory disorders (including inflammatory bowel disease [eg, colitis or Crohn's disease], diverticulitis [with the exception of diverticulosis], systemic lupus erythematosus, Sarcoidosis syndrome, or Wegener syndrome [granulomatosis with polyangiitis, Graves' disease, rheumatoid arthritis, hypophysitis, uveitis, etc.]). The following are exceptions to this criterion: a) Patients with vitiligo or alopecia; b) Patients with hypothyroidism (eg, following Hashimoto syndrome) stable on hormone replacement; c) Any chronic skin condition that does not require systemic therapy; d) Patients without active disease in the last 5 years may be included but only after consultation with the study physician; d) Patients with celiac disease controlled by diet alone.

4. Subjects with a condition requiring systemic treatment with either corticosteroids (>10mg daily prednisone equivalents) or other immunosuppressive medications within 14 days of study drug administration. Inhaled or topical steroids and adrenal replacement doses > 10mg daily prednisone equivalents are permitted in the absence of active autoimmune disease.

5. Prior exposure to T cell checkpoint inhibitor therapies, including durvalumab and tremelimumab.

6. Uncontrolled intercurrent illness including, but not limited to, ongoing or active infection, interstitial lung disease, symptomatic congestive heart failure, unstable angina pectoris, cardiac arrhythmia, or psychiatric illness/social situations that would limit compliance with study requirements.

7. Known allergy or hypersensitivity to any of the study drugs or any of the study drug excipients.

8. History of active primary immunodeficiency

9. Women who are pregnant, which includes women with a positive pregnancy test at enrollment or prior to the administration of study medication, or breastfeeding are not allowed on study.

10. Receipt of a live vaccine within 30 days of study entry.

11. Any unresolved toxicity NCI CTCAE Grade >/=2 from previous anticancer therapy with the exception of alopecia, vitiligo, and the laboratory values defined in the inclusion criteria: a) Patients with Grade >/=2 neuropathy will be evaluated on a case-by-case basis after consultation with the Study Physician; b) Patients with irreversible toxicity not reasonably expected to be exacerbated by treatment with durvalumab or tremelimumab may be included only after consultation with the Study Physician.

12. Any concurrent chemotherapy, biologic, or hormonal therapy for cancer treatment. Concurrent use of hormonal therapy for non-cancer-related conditions (e.g., hormone replacement therapy) is acceptable.

13. Major surgical procedure within 28 days prior to the first dose of IP. Note: Local surgery of isolated lesions for palliative intent is acceptable.

14. History of allogenic organ transplantation.

15. Known active infection including tuberculosis (clinical evaluation that includes clinical history, physical examination and radiographic findings, and TB testing in line with local practice), hepatitis B (known positive HBV surface antigen (HBsAg) result), hepatitis C, or human immunodeficiency virus (positive HIV 1/2 antibodies). Patients with a past or resolved HBV infection (defined as the presence of hepatitis B core antibody [anti-HBc] and absence of HBsAg) are eligible. Patients positive for hepatitis C (HCV) antibody are eligible only if polymerase chain reaction is negative for HCV RNA.

16. Female patients who are pregnant or breastfeeding or male or female patients of reproductive potential who are not willing to employ effective birth control from screening to 90 days after the last dose of durvalumab monotherapy or180 days after the last dose of durvalumab + tremelimumab combination therapy.

Sex/Gender

All

Ages

18 Years to N/A

Accepts Healthy Volunteers

No

Contacts

Michael Overman, MD   713-792-2828

A Study of LY3039478 in Participants With Advanced or Metastatic Solid Tumors

Study ID:

NCT02784795

Sponsor:

Eli Lilly and Company

Information provided by (Responsible Party):

Eli Lilly and Company (Eli Lilly and Company)

Tracking Information

First Submitted Date

May 25, 2016

Start Date

November 4, 2016

Primary Completion Date

April 2018

Last Update Posted Date

January 8, 2018

▧ Current Primary Outcome Measures

Maximum Tolerated Dose (MTD) of LY3039478[Time Frame: Cycle 1 (up to 28 Days)]

▧ Current Secondary Outcome Measures

Pharmacokinetics (PK): Area Under the Plasma Concentration Time Curve (AUC) of LY3039478 in Combination with Taladegib, LY3023414, Abemaciclib, Cisplatin/Gemcitabine, and Gemcitabine/Carboplatin[Time Frame: Predose Cycle 1 Day 1 through Predose Cycle 2 Day 1 (up to 28 Day Cycles)]

PK: AUC of Taladegib and its Active Metabolite LSN3185556, in Combination with LY3039478[Time Frame: Predose Cycle 1 Day 1 through Predose Cycle 2 Day 1 (up to 28 Day Cycles)]

PK: AUC of LY3023414 in Combination with LY3039478[Time Frame: Predose Cycle 1 Day 1 through Predose Cycle 2 Day 1 (up to 28 Day Cycles)]

PK: AUC of Abemaciclib and its Major Active Metabolites LSN2839567 and LSN3106726, in Combination with LY3039478[Time Frame: Predose Cycle 1 Day 1 through Predose Cycle 2 Day 1 (up to 28 Day Cycles)]

Duration of Response (DoR)[Time Frame: Date of Complete Response (CR) or Partial Response (PR) to Date of Objective Disease Progression (Estimated up to 12 Months)]

Progression Free Survival (PFS)[Time Frame: Baseline to Objective Disease Progression or Death (Estimated up to 12 Months)]

Descriptive Information

▧ Offical Title

A Phase 1b Study of LY3039478 in Combination With Other Anticancer Agents in Patients With Advanced or Metastatic Solid Tumors

▧ Brief Summary

The main purpose of this study is to evaluate the safety of the study drug known as LY3039478 in combination with other anticancer agents in participants with advanced or metastatic solid tumors.

▧ Study Type

Interventional

▧ Study Phase

Phase 1

▧ Condition

- Solid Tumor
- Breast Cancer
- Colon Cancer
- Cholangiocarcinoma
- Soft Tissue Sarcoma

▧ Intervention

Drug: LY3039478

  Administered orally

  Drug: Taladegib

  Administered orally

Other Names:

  LY2940680

  Drug: Abemaciclib

  Administered orally

Other Names:

  LY2835219

  Drug: Cisplatin

  Administered IV

  Drug: Gemcitabine

  Administered IV

  Drug: Carboplatin

Administered IV

Drug: LY3023414

Administered orally

Study Arms

Experimental: LY3039478 + Taladegib

LY3039478 given orally 3 times per week (TIW) in combination with taladegib given orally daily on a 28 day cycle. A single dose of taladegib will also be given on day 1 during a 3-day lead-in period.

Experimental: LY3039478 + LY3023414

LY3039478 given orally TIW in combination with LY3023414 given orally every 12 hours on a 28-day cycle. A single dose of LY3023414 will also be given on day 1 during a 3-day lead-in period.

Experimental: LY3039478 + Abemaciclib

LY3039478 given orally TIW in combination with abemaciclib given orally every 12 hours on a 28-day cycle. A single dose of abemaciclib will also be given on day 1 during a 3-day lead-in period.

Experimental: LY3039478 + Cisplatin/Gemcitabine

LY3039478 given orally TIW in combination with cisplatin and gemcitabine given as intravenous (IV) infusions on days 1 and 8 of a 21 day cycle.

Experimental: LY3039478 + Gemcitabine/Carboplatin

LY3039478 given orally TIW in combination with gemcitabine and carboplatin given as IV infusions on days 1 and 8 of a 21 day cycle.

Recruitment Information

Recruitment Status

Recruiting

Estimated Enrollment

163

Completion Date

September 2018

Primary Completion Date

April 2018

Eligibility Criteria

Inclusion Criteria:

- For all parts: The participant must be, in the judgment of the investigator, an appropriate candidate for experimental therapy after available standard therapies have failed to provide clinical benefit for their advanced or metastatic cancer.
- For dose escalation for all combinations: The participant must have histological or cytological evidence of cancer, either a solid tumor or a lymphoma, which is advanced or metastatic.
- For Part A dose confirmation: All participants must have histological evidence of advanced or metastatic soft tissue sarcoma or breast cancer. Breast cancer participants must have prescreened mutations, amplification, or gene/protein expression alterations related to Notch pathway.
- For Part B dose confirmation: All participants must have histological evidence of advanced or metastatic colon cancer or soft tissue sarcoma. Colon cancer participants must have prescreened mutations, amplification, or gene/protein expression alterations related to Notch pathway.
- For Part C dose confirmation: All participants must have histological evidence of advanced or metastatic breast cancer and prescreened mutations, amplification, or gene/protein expression alterations related to Notch pathway.
- For Part D dose confirmation: All participants must have histological evidence of cholangiocarcinoma and prescreened mutations, amplification, or gene/protein expression alterations related to Notch pathway. Participants must not have received >1 line of prior systemic therapy for metastatic or resectable disease (that is, participants may have received adjuvant gemcitabine and then later gemcitabine/cisplatin for recurrent metastatic disease).
- For Part E dose confirmation: All participants must have histological evidence of locally advanced or metastatic triple negative breast cancer (TNBC) and prescreened mutations, amplification, or gene/protein expression alterations related to Notch pathway. Participants must not have received >2 lines of systemic treatment for advanced or metastatic TNBC.
- Have adequate organ function.
- Have a performance status of ≤1 on the Eastern Cooperative Oncology Group (ECOG) scale.
- Have discontinued all previous therapies for cancer.

Exclusion Criteria:

- Have current acute leukemia.
- Have current or recent (within 3 months of study drug administration) gastrointestinal disease with chronic or intermittent diarrhea, or disorders that increase the risk of diarrhea, such as inflammatory bowel disease.

Sex/Gender

All

A Phase 1 Study of TSR-022, an Anti-TIM-3 Monoclonal Antibody, in Patients With Advanced Solid Tumors

Study ID:

NCT02817633

Sponsor:

Tesaro, Inc.

Information provided by (Responsible Party):

Tesaro, Inc. (Tesaro, Inc.)

Tracking Information

■ **First Submitted Date**

June 22, 2016

■ **Start Date**

July 2016

■ **Primary Completion Date**

December 2019

■ **Last Update Posted Date**

October 10, 2017

■ **Current Primary Outcome Measures**

- Safety and tolerability of TSR-022 using Common Terminology Criteria for Adverse Events (CTCAE v.4.03) in patients with advanced solid tumors[Time Frame: Part 1 Dose Escalation Approximately 2 years]

  Anti-tumor activity of TSR-022 in patients with solid tumors, in terms of objective response rate (ORR) as assessed by the Investigators using Response Evaluation Criteria in Solid Tumors (RECIST) v. 1.1[Time Frame: Part 2 Expansion Approximately 2 years]

  Recommended Phase 2 dose (RP2D) and schedule as monotherapy and in combination with an anti-PD-1 antibody[Time Frame: Part 1 and Part 2 Approximately 4 years]

■ **Current Secondary Outcome Measures**

- Safety and tolerability of TSR-022 using CTCAE v.4.03[Time Frame: Part 2 Approximately 2 years]

  Incidence of treatment-emergent AEs (TEAEs), SAEs, immune-related AEs (irAEs), TEAEs leading to death, and AEs leading to discontinuation occurring while patients are on treatment or up to 90 days after the last dose of study drug as assessed by CTCAE v4.03

- Overall Response Rate (ORR) by RECIST v. 1.1 (Part 1)[Time Frame: Part 1 and Part 2 Approximately 4 years]

  ORR by immune-related RECIST (irRECIST)[Time Frame: Part 1 and Part 2 Approximately 4 years]

  Duration of response (DOR) by RECIST v 1.1[Time Frame: Part 1 and Part 2 Approximately 4 years]

  Disease control rate (DCR) by RECIST v 1.1 and by irRECIST[Time Frame: Part 1 and Part 2 Approximately 4 years]

  Progression-free survival (PFS) by RECIST v 1.1 and by irRECIST[Time Frame: Part 1 and Part 2 Approximately 4 years]

  Overall survival (OS)[Time Frame: Part 1 and Part 2 Approximately 4 years]

  PK Parameter: AUC, 0-last assessment[Time Frame: Part 1 and Part 2 Approximately 4 years]

  PK Parameter: AUC, 0 to infinity[Time Frame: Part 1 and Part 2 Approximately 4 years]

  PK Parameter: AUC at steady state[Time Frame: Part 1 and Part 2 Approximately 4 years]

  PK Parameter: Minimum Concentration (Cmin)[Time Frame: Part 1 and Part 2 Approximately 4 years]

  PK Parameter: Maximum Concentration (Cmax)[Time Frame: Part 1 and Part 2 Approximately 4 years]

- PK Parameter: Clearance (CL)[Time Frame: Part 1 and Part 2 Approximately 4 years]
- PK Parameter: Cmin at steady state (Cmin,ss)[Time Frame: Part 1 and Part 2 Approximately 4 years]

- PK Parameter: Cmax at steady state (Cmax, ss)[Time Frame: Part 1 and Part 2 Approximately 4 years]
- PK Parameter: Volume of Distribution (Vz)[Time Frame: Part 1 and Part 2 Approximately 4 years]
- PK Parameter: terminal half-life (t1/2)[Time Frame: Part 1 and Part 2 Approximately 4 years]
- Pharmacodynamic profile as assessed by receptor occupancy[Time Frame: Part 1 and 2 Approximately 4 years]

Immunogenicity as assessed by the presence of anti-drug antibodies[Time Frame: Part 1 and 2 -Approximately 4 years]

Descriptive Information

▩ Offical Title

A Phase 1 Dose Escalation and Cohort Expansion Study of TSR-022, an Anti-TIM-3 Monoclonal Antibody, in Patients With Advanced Solid Tumors

▩ Brief Summary

This is a multicenter, open-label, first-in-human Phase 1 study evaluating the anti-TIM-3 (T cell immunoglobulin and mucin containing protein-3) antibody TSR-022, as a monotherapy and in combination with an anti-PD-1 antibody, in patients with advanced solid tumors who have limited available treatment options. The study will be conducted in 2 parts: dose escalation and cohort expansion.

▩ Study Type

Interventional

▩ Study Phase

Phase 1

▩ Condition

- Advanced or Metastatic Solid Tumors

▩ Intervention

Drug: TSR-022

    TSR-022 is a humanized monoclonal IgG4 antibody

    Drug: anti-PD-1 antibody

▩ Study Arms

- Experimental: Part 1Dose Escalation

    1a: Dose escalation TSR-022 alone

    1b: Dose escalation TSR-022 in combination with an anti-PD-1 antibody

    1c: TSR-022 dose in combination with an anti-PD-1 antibody

- Experimental: Part 2Expansion Cohorts

    Part 2 of the study will further explore the safety and clinical activity of TSR-022 as monotherapy and in combination with anti-PD-1 antibody in patients with select tumor types

Recruitment Information

▩ Recruitment Status

Recruiting

▩ Estimated Enrollment

627

▩ Completion Date

June 2020

▩ Primary Completion Date

December 2019

▩ Eligibility Criteria

Partial Inclusion Criteria:

- Patient with advanced or metastatic solid tumor and has disease progression or treatment intolerance after treatment with available therapies
- Agreement to biopsies before and during treatment, depending on study part
- Female patients must have a negative serum pregnancy test or be of non-childbearing potential.
- Required that female patients of childbearing potential use two methods of contraception with their partner
- Eastern Cooperative Oncology Group (ECOG) performance status of ≤ 1 and adequate organ function

Partial Exclusion Criteria:

- Received prior therapy with an anti-CTLA-4, anti-PD-1, anti-PD1-ligand-1 (anti-PD-L1), or anti-PD-1 ligand-2 (anti-PD-L2) agent within 8 weeks prior to initiation of study treatment depending on study part

- Known uncontrolled central nervous system (CNS) metastases and/or carcinomatous meningitis or known malignancy that progressed or required active treatment within the last 2 years
- Pregnant, breastfeeding, or expecting to conceive children within projected duration of study
- History of human immunodeficiency virus (HIV), interstitial lung disease, active Hepatitis B or Hepatitis C, or ≥Grade 3 immune-related AE with prior immunotherapy
- Autoimmune disease that required systemic treatment
- Not recovered from radiation and chemotherapy-induced AEs
- Participated in another investigational study (drug or device) within 4 weeks of first dose
- Received prior anticancer therapy within 21 days of first dose
- Not recovered from AEs and/or complications from major surgery prior to first dose
- Received a vaccine within 7 days of first dose

Sex/Gender

All

Ages

18 Years to N/A

Accepts Healthy Volunteers

No

Contacts

Clinical Trial Management Group   ClinicalTrialsTSR022@tesarobio.com

Trial of Intraperitoneal (IP) Oxaliplatin in Combination With Intravenous FOLFIRI

Study ID:

NCT02833753

Sponsor:

University of Massachusetts, Worcester

Information provided by (Responsible Party):

University of Massachusetts, Worcester (University of Massachusetts, Worcester)

Tracking Information

First Submitted Date

July 12, 2016

Start Date

July 2016

Current Primary Outcome Measures

Primary Completion Date

July 2019

Last Update Posted Date

July 24, 2017

Define the maximum tolerated dose (MTD) of intraperitoneal (IP) oxaliplatin given with systemic FOLFIRI in patients with peritoneal carcinomatosis (PC) of colorectal or appendiceal origin[Time Frame: 8 weeks]

Descriptive Information

Offical Title

Phase I Trial of Intraperitoneal Oxaliplatin in Combination With Intravenous FOLFIRI (5-fluorouracil, Leucovorin and Irinotecan) for Peritoneal Carcinomatosis From Colorectal and Appendiceal Cancer

Brief Summary

This is a Phase I dose escalation study to determine how much chemotherapy can be safely administered into the abdomen while experiencing the fewest possible side effects.

Detailed Description

There are two common combinations of chemotherapy drugs used to treat cancer of the colon, rectum, or appendix that has spread to the abdomen. One uses 5-fluorouracil (also called 5-FU), leucovorin and oxaliplatin, and is called FOLFOX. The other uses 5-FU, leucovorin, and irinotecan, and is called FOLFIRI. The Food and Drug Administration (FDA) has approved each of these combinations as treatment for colon or rectal cancer. Each is given through the veins.

FOLFOX and FOLFIRI do not work well for tumors growing in the abdominal cavity. The investigators are trying to determine if giving chemotherapy called oxaliplatin directly into the abdominal cavity will have a greater effect on the cancer.

The FDA has approved oxaliplatin to be given to people through their veins to treat advanced colorectal cancer. Giving oxaliplatin directly into the abdomen in this study is experimental and is not approved by the FDA. This study will give the standard chemotherapy FOLFIRI through the veins and oxaliplatin directly into the abdomen. This is the first time intraperitoneal oxaliplatin is being given in combination with FOLFIRI.

Study Type

Interventional

Study Phase

Phase 1

Condition

- Colorectal Cancer
- Appendix Cancer
- Peritoneal Carcinomatosis

Intervention

Drug: Oxaliplatin

Intraperitoneal oxaliplatin will be given along with standard chemotherapy FOLFIRI.

Level 1: Oxaliplatin 25mg/m2 IP every 2 weeks on day #1 of chemotherapy Level 2: Oxaliplatin 55mg/m2 IP every 2 weeks on day #1 of chemotherapy Level 3: Oxaliplatin 85mg/m2 IP every 2 weeks on day #1 of chemotherapy

Study Arms

Experimental: Dose Escalation

Single arm dose finding for intraperitoneal Oxaliplatin. All patients will receive experimental treatment.

The first cohort of 3 patients will receive dose level 1. The second cohort of 3 patients will receive dose level 2. The Third cohort of 3 patients with receive dose level 3.

Publications

(Includes publications given by the data provider as well as publications identified by ClinicalTrials.gov Identifier (NCT Number) in Medline.)Falcone A, Ricci S, Brunetti I, Pfanner E, Allegrini G, Barbara C, Crinò L, Benedetti G, Evangelista W, Fanchini L, Cortesi E, Picone V, Vitello S, Chiara S, Granetto C, Porcile G, Fioretto L, Orlandini C, Andreuccetti M, Masi G; Gruppo Oncologico Nord Ovest. Phase III trial of infusional fluorouracil, leucovorin, oxaliplatin, and irinotecan (FOLFOXIRI) compared with infusional fluorouracil, leucovorin, and irinotecan (FOLFIRI) as first-line treatment for metastatic colorectal cancer: the Gruppo Oncologico Nord Ovest. J Clin Oncol. 2007 May 1;25(13):1670-6. (https://www.ncbi.nlm.nih.gov/pubmed/17470860)

Loupakis F, Cremolini C, Masi G, Lonardi S, Zagonel V, Salvatore L, Cortesi E, Tomasello G, Ronzoni M, Spadi R, Zaniboni A, Tonini G, Buonadonna A, Amoroso D, Chiara S, Carlomagno C, Boni C, Allegrini G, Boni L, Falcone A. Initial therapy with FOLFOXIRI and bevacizumab for metastatic colorectal cancer. N Engl J Med. 2014 Oct 23;371(17):1609-18. doi: 10.1056/NEJMoa1403108. (https://www.ncbi.nlm.nih.gov/pubmed/25337750)

Franko J, Shi Q, Goldman CD, Pockaj BA, Nelson GD, Goldberg RM, Pitot HC, Grothey A, Alberts SR, Sargent DJ. Treatment of colorectal peritoneal carcinomatosis with systemic chemotherapy: a pooled analysis of north central cancer treatment group phase III trials N9741 and N9841. J Clin Oncol. 2012 Jan 20;30(3):263-7. doi: 10.1200/JCO.2011.37.1039. Epub 2011 Dec 12. (https://www.ncbi.nlm.nih.gov/pubmed/22162570)

Elias D, Lefevre JH, Chevalier J, Brouquet A, Marchal F, Classe JM, Ferron G, Guilloit JM, Meeus P, Goéré D, Bonastre J. Complete cytoreductive surgery plus intraperitoneal chemohyperthermia with oxaliplatin for peritoneal carcinomatosis of colorectal origin. J Clin Oncol. 2009 Feb 10;27(5):681-5. doi: 10.1200/JCO.2008.19.7160. Epub 2008 Dec 22. (https://www.ncbi.nlm.nih.gov/pubmed/19103728)

Sadeghi B, Arvieux C, Glehen O, Beaujard AC, Rivoire M, Baulieux J, Fontaumard E, Brachet A, Caillot JL, Faure JL, Porcheron J, Peix JL, François Y, Vignal J, Gilly FN. Peritoneal carcinomatosis from non-gynecologic malignancies: results of the EVOCAPE 1 multicentric prospective study. Cancer. 2000 Jan 15;88(2):358-63. (https://www.ncbi.nlm.nih.gov/pubmed/10640968)

Armstrong DK, Bundy B, Wenzel L, Huang HQ, Baergen R, Lele S, Copeland LJ, Walker JL, Burger RA; Gynecologic Oncology Group. Intraperitoneal cisplatin and paclitaxel in ovarian cancer. N Engl J Med. 2006 Jan 5;354(1):34-43. (https://www.ncbi.nlm.nih.gov/pubmed/16394300)

Fajardo AD, Tan B, Reddy R, Fleshman J. Delayed repeated intraperitoneal chemotherapy after cytoreductive surgery for colorectal and appendiceal carcinomatosis. Dis Colon Rectum. 2012 Oct;55(10):1044-52. doi: 10.1097/DCR.0b013e318265ad42. (https://www.ncbi.nlm.nih.gov/pubmed/22965403)

Elias D, Bonnay M, Puizillou JM, Antoun S, Demirdjian S, El OA, Pignon JP, Drouard-Troalen L, Ouellet JF, Ducreux M. Heated intra-operative intraperitoneal oxaliplatin after complete resection of peritoneal carcinomatosis: pharmacokinetics and tissue distribution. Ann Oncol. 2002 Feb;13(2):267-72. (https://www.ncbi.nlm.nih.gov/pubmed/11886004)

Elias D, Matsuhisa T, Sideris L, Liberale G, Drouard-Troalen L, Raynard B, Pocard M, Puizillou JM, Billard V, Bourget

P, Ducreux M. Heated intra-operative intraperitoneal oxaliplatin plus irinotecan after complete resection of peritoneal carcinomatosis: pharmacokinetics, tissue distribution and tolerance. Ann Oncol. 2004 Oct;15(10):1558-65. (https://www.ncbi.nlm.nih.gov/pubmed/15367418)

Gervais MK, Dubé P, McConnell Y, Drolet P, Mitchell A, Sideris L. Cytoreductive surgery plus hyperthermic intraperitoneal chemotherapy with oxaliplatin for peritoneal carcinomatosis arising from colorectal cancer. J Surg Oncol. 2013 Dec;108(7):438-43. doi: 10.1002/jso.23431. Epub 2013 Sep 9. (https://www.ncbi.nlm.nih.gov/pubmed/24018983)

Ceelen W, De Somer F, Van Nieuwenhove Y, Vande Putte D, Pattyn P. Effect of perfusion temperature on glucose and electrolyte transport during hyperthermic intraperitoneal chemoperfusion (HIPEC) with oxaliplatin. Eur J Surg Oncol. 2013 Jul;39(7):754-9. doi: 10.1016/j.ejso.2012.07.120. Epub 2012 Aug 9. (https://www.ncbi.nlm.nih.gov/pubmed/22878060)

Mehta AM, Van den Hoven JM, Rosing H, Hillebrand MJ, Nuijen B, Huitema AD, Beijnen JH, Verwaal VJ. Stability of oxaliplatin in chloride-containing carrier solutions used in hyperthermic intraperitoneal chemotherapy. Int J Pharm. 2015 Feb 1;479(1):23-7. doi: 10.1016/j.ijpharm.2014.12.025. Epub 2014 Dec 20. (https://www.ncbi.nlm.nih.gov/pubmed/25535649)

Fuchs CS, Marshall J, Mitchell E, Wierzbicki R, Ganju V, Jeffery M, Schulz J, Richards D, Soufi-Mahjoubi R, Wang B, Barrueco J. Randomized, controlled trial of irinotecan plus infusional, bolus, or oral fluoropyrimidines in first-line treatment of metastatic colorectal cancer: results from the BICC-C Study. J Clin Oncol. 2007 Oct 20;25(30):4779-86. (https://www.ncbi.nlm.nih.gov/pubmed/17947725)

Teefey P, Bou Zgheib N, Apte SM, Gonzalez-Bosquet J, Judson PL, Roberts WS, Lancaster JM, Wenham RM. Factors associated with improved toxicity and tolerability of intraperitoneal chemotherapy in advanced-stage epithelial ovarian cancers. Am J Obstet Gynecol. 2013 Jun;208(6):501.e1-7. doi: 10.1016/j.ajog.2013.03.012. Epub 2013 Mar 15. (https://www.ncbi.nlm.nih.gov/pubmed/23507546)

Eisenhauer EA, Therasse P, Bogaerts J, Schwartz LH, Sargent D, Ford R, Dancey J, Arbuck S, Gwyther S, Mooney M, Rubinstein L, Shankar L, Dodd L, Kaplan R, Lacombe D, Verweij J. New response evaluation criteria in solid tumours: revised RECIST guideline (version 1.1). Eur J Cancer. 2009 Jan;45(2):228-47. doi: 10.1016/j.ejca.2008.10.026. (https://www.ncbi.nlm.nih.gov/pubmed/19097774)

Recruitment Information

▧ Recruitment Status

Recruiting

▧ Estimated Enrollment

16

▧ Completion Date

July 2019

▧ Primary Completion Date

July 2019

▧ Eligibility Criteria

Inclusion Criteria:

- The patient must be 18 years of age or older and capable of providing informed consent indicating awareness of the investigational nature of this trial, in keeping with institutional policy
- Patients must be willing to return for follow-up
- The patient must consent to participate in the trial and must have signed an approved informed consent form conforming to institutional policy
- The patient must have histopathologically or cytologically confirmed colon, rectal or appendiceal adenocarcinoma with synchronous or metachronous peritoneal dissemination of disease.(Stage IV peritoneal based disease only)
- The patient must have active measurable disease by either abdominal computerized axial tomography (CT)/ Magnetic resonance imaging (MRI) or laparoscopy.

At the time of enrollment, the patient must have: (within 14 days of enrollment)

- Absolute neutrophil count (ANC) > 1200/mm3 and platelet count > 140,000/mm3
- An international normalized ratio (INR) ≤ 1.5 (patients who are therapeutically anticoagulated for non-related medical conditions such as atrial fibrillation and whose antithrombotic treatment can be withheld for operation will be eligible)
- Adequate hepatic function must be met as evidenced by total serum bilirubin ≤ 1.5 mg/dl (patients with total bilirubin >1.5 mg/dL eligible only with Gilbert's syndrome); alkaline phosphatase < 2.5 times the upper limit of normal; and, aspartate aminotransferase (AST) less than 1.5 times upper limit of normal [alkaline phosphatase and AST cannot both exceed the upper limit of normal]
- Serum renal functional parameters, blood urea nitrogen (BUN) and creatinine are within normal limits (estimated glomerular filtration rate (eGFR) >50)
- Prior to enrollment the patient must have had a complete history and physical examination, electrocardiogram, within three months of enrollment
- Satisfactory cardiopulmonary function (as determined by Physician)
- Patients can have received prior systemic chemotherapy, radiation or surgery
- Patients must be able to undergo placement of an intraperitoneal (IP) catheter and a Port-A Cath, if not already present
- Patients must have an Eastern Cooperative Oncology Group (ECOG) performance status of 2 or less
- Women of reproductive age and men who are sexually active must be willing to practice effective contraception
- Patients will be allowed to have secondary malignancies as long as they do not require active concomitant treatment

- **Sex/Gender**

  All

- **Ages**

  18 Years to 99 Years

- **Accepts Healthy Volunteers**

  No

- **Contacts**

  Bradley Switzer, MD   774-442-3716   bradley.switzer@umassmemorial.org

  Laura Lambert, MD   508-334-5274   laura.lambert@umassmemorial.org

Pembrolizumab + Poly-ICLC in MRP Colon Cancer

Study ID:

NCT02834052

Sponsor:

Asha Nayak

Information provided by (Responsible Party):

Augusta University (Asha Nayak)

Tracking Information

- **First Submitted Date**

  June 15, 2016

- **Start Date**

  January 10, 2018

- **Primary Completion Date**

  January 2020

- **Last Update Posted Date**

  January 12, 2018

- **Current Primary Outcome Measures**

  Phase 1: Determine the maximum tolerated dose of poly-ICLC that can be combined with pembrolizumab[Time Frame: 12 months]

  > A minimum of 3 participants will be treated at dose level 1 (1mg).

  > If 0 out of 3 participants experience dose limiting toxicities (DLT), then dose escalation will proceed to dose level 2 (2mg).

  > If 1 out of 3 participants experience DLT, a cohort of additional 3 participants will be assigned to the same dose level (1mg).

  > If 2 or more participants of 3 (or 6) experience DLT at dose level 1, then enrollment of participants will be stopped.

  Phase 1 and 2: Determine the response rate of metastatic MRP colon cancer (that has progressed following two lines of therapy in the metastatic setting) to the combination of pembrolizumab and poly-ICLC[Time Frame: From baseline to disease progression (Expected 12-24 months)]

  > Response rate will be determined using RECIST 1.1 criteria, calculated as the number of participants with complete response (CR) or partial response (PR)

- **Current Secondary Outcome Measures**

  Determine the adverse event profile and dose limiting toxicities of the combination of pembrolizumab and poly-ICLC[Time Frame: 12 months]

  > The adverse event profile will be presented by dose level of the combination treatment for the phase I portion

  Determine the progression free survival rate of recurrent metastatic MRP colon cancer to the combination of pembrolizumab and poly-ICLC[Time Frame: From baseline to disease progression (up to 24 months)]

  > The progression free survival rate for the combination of pembrolizumab and poly-ICLC administered at the Recommended Phase 2 Dose (RP2D) will be estimated, including the correspondent 95% confidence interval.

  Determine the 20-week progression free survival rate of recurrent metastatic MRP colon cancer to the combination of pembrolizumab and poly-ICLC[Time Frame: 20 weeks]

  > The 20-week progression free survival rate for the combination of pembrolizumab and poly-ICLC administered at the Recommended Phase 2 Dose (RP2D) will be estimated along with the correspondent 95% confidence interval.

  Determine the overall survival rate for recurrent metastatic MRP colon cancer response to the combination of pembrolizumab and poly-ICLC[Time Frame: From baseline to disease progression (up to 24 months)]

The overall survival rate of response to the combination of pembrolizumab and poly-ICLC administered at the Recommended Phase 2 Dose (RP2D) will be estimated along with the correspondent 95% confidence interval.

Determine the duration of response of recurrent metastatic MRP colon cancer to the combination of pembrolizumab and poly-ICLC[Time Frame: From baseline to disease progression (up to 24 months)]

The duration of response to the combination of pembrolizumab and poly-ICLC administered at the Recommended Phase 2 Dose (RP2D) will be estimated along with the correspondent 95% confidence interval.

Descriptive Information

▣ Offical Title

A Phase I/II Trial of Pembrolizumab (MK-3475) and Poly-ICLC in Patients With Metastatic Mismatch Repair-proficient (MRP) Colon Cancer

▣ Brief Summary

The main purpose of this study is to determine the dose of poly-ICLC that is safe and tolerable when it is combined with pembrolizumab in patients with colon cancer. This study will also evaluate how the combination of pembrolizumab and poly-ICLC activates the immune system in the patient's blood and inside the tumor; how it affects the size and number of tumor(s) in each patient; and how effective the combination is in patients with colon cancer that is unlikely to respond to pembrolizumab alone.

▣ Detailed Description

Mismatch repair genes normally serve to fix the small glitches that occur when DNA is copied as cells divide. In 1993, researchers discovered that mutations in human mismatch repair genes play a key role in the development of certain forms of colorectal cancer; individuals who are deficient in these mismatch repair genes are at high risk for colorectal cancer. Accumulating evidence has shown that immunotherapy may be most effective against these cancers.

Programmed cell death protein 1, also known as PD-1, functions as an immune checkpoint, down-regulating the immune system by preventing the activation of T-cells, which in turn reduces autoimmunity and promotes self-tolerance. A new class of immunotherapy drugs that block PD-1, the PD-1 inhibitors, activate the immune system to attack tumors and are therefore used with varying success to treat some types of cancer.

Current clinical trials are showing that patients whose tumors are mismatch repair deficient are more likely to respond to immune-boosting anti-PD-1 drugs—such as pembrolizumab—than those with tumors proficient in mismatch repair. The idea is that the greater the number of DNA glitches in a tumor cell, the more abnormal proteins it will produce—and the more abnormal proteins that are generated, the greater the odds that the body's immune cells will regard the tumor cells as "foreign" and target them for destruction. Thus far, PD-1 inhibitors have shown great promise for mismatch repair deficient cancer patients, but not for mismatch repair proficient (MRP) cancer patients.

In this clinical trial, the investigators hypothesize that treating MRP colon cancer patients with immunostimulating agent poly-ICLC will generate an inflammatory response, increasing epitope recognition and development of tumor reactive T-cells at the tumor site. However, interferon alpha and gamma produced by the poly-ICLC will increase PD-L1 expression and limit new T-cell development. Thus, PD1 blockade will increase the effectiveness of treatment with pembrolizumab.

▣ Study Type

Interventional

▣ Study Phase

Phase 1/Phase 2

▣ Condition

- Metastatic Colon Cancer
- Solid Tumor

▣ Intervention

Drug: pembrolizumab

200mg pembrolizumab will be given intravenously on Day 1 of each 3-week cycle

Other Names:

MK-3475

Keytruda

Drug: Poly-ICLC

The maximum tolerated dose of Poly ICLC will be given twice weekly, in each 3-week cycle:

Week 1, Days 1 and 4

Week 2, Days 8 and 11

Week 3, Days 15 and 18

Other Names:

polyinosinic-polycytidylic acid-polylysine-carboxymethylcellulose

Hiltonol

Study Arms

Experimental: Phase 1

This "Run In" phase is aimed to determine if poly-ICLC can be safely combined with standard dosages of pembrolizumab:

i. Pembrolizumab will be administered 200 mg intravenously (IV) every 3 weeks (q3w)

ii. Poly-ICLC will be administered intramuscularly (IM) twice weekly at one of two dose levels: 1 mg or 2 mg

Each dose level will enroll 3-6 participants, up to 12 participants total, depending on the occurrence of dose limiting toxicities (DLT) at each dosing level.

Participants may receive treatment for 1 year (~17 cycles).

Experimental: Phase 2

In Phase 2, all participants will receive the standard pembrolizumab dose (200 mg IV q3w) in addition to the maximum tolerated dose of poly-ICLC (either 1 mg or 2 mg), as determined by the Phase 1 arm.

Up to 30 participants will be treated in Phase 2. Participants may receive treatment for 1 year (~17 cycles).

Recruitment Information

Recruitment Status

Recruiting

Estimated Enrollment

42

Completion Date

January 2021

Primary Completion Date

January 2020

Eligibility Criteria

- Diagnosis/Condition for Entry into the Trial Phase 1 Presence of histologically confirmed malignancy that has progressed following at least one therapy and able to be visualized on imaging. Measurable disease is not required. Patients with known targetable mutations must have progressive disease on the appropriated targeted drug therapy.
- Phase 2 Presence of MRP colon cancer that has progressed following at least two lines of therapy. Ten patients will be included who have disease that can be biopsied preand post-therapy.

Inclusion Criteria:

- Be willing and able to provide written informed consent for the trial
- Have measurable disease based on RECIST 1.1 (Phase 2)
- Be willing to provide tissue from a newly obtained core or excisional biopsy of a tumor lesion
- Have a performance status of 0 or 1 on the ECOG Performance Scale
- Have adequate organ function, according to screening labs performed within 10 days of treatment initiation
- Subjects of childbearing potential must be willing to use an adequate method of contraception for the course of the study through 120 days after the last dose of study medication

Exclusion Criteria:

- Currently participating/previously participated in a therapeutic study and received study therapy or used an investigational device within 4 weeks of the first dose of treatment
- Has a diagnosis of immunodeficiency or is receiving systemic steroid therapy or any other form of immunosuppressive therapy within 7 days prior to the first dose of trial treatment
- Has a known history of active TB (Bacillus Tuberculosis)
- Hypersensitivity to pembrolizumab or any of its excipients
- Has a known additional malignancy that is progressing or requires active treatment. Exceptions include basal cell carcinoma of the skin or squamous cell carcinoma of the skin that has undergone potentially curative therapy or in situ cervical cancer
- Has received prior therapy with an anti-PD-1, anti-PD-L1, or anti-PD-L2 agent
- Has a known history of Human Immunodeficiency Virus (HIV) (HIV 1/2 antibodies), active Hepatitis B (e.g., HBsAg reactive) or Hepatitis C (e.g., HCV RNA [qualitative] is detected).
- Has known active central nervous system (CNS) metastases and/or carcinomatous meningitis.
- Has active autoimmune disease that has required systemic treatment in the past 2 years

Sex/Gender

All

Ages

18 Years to N/A

Accepts Healthy Volunteers

No

Contacts

Lisa Marshall, MSN, RN, CNL, CCRC   706-721-5095   lmarshall@augusta.edu

Carrie McAteer, BA, CCRC   706-721-1409   mmcateer@augusta.edu

PI Pembro in Combination With Stereotactic Body Radiotherapy for Liver Metastatic Colorectal Cancer

Study ID:

NCT02837263

Sponsor:

University of Wisconsin, Madison

Information provided by (Responsible Party):

University of Wisconsin, Madison (University of Wisconsin, Madison)

Tracking Information

First Submitted Date

July 15, 2016

Start Date

August 2016

Primary Completion Date

March 2018

Last Update Posted Date

August 29, 2017

Current Primary Outcome Measures

Recurrence rate at 1 year[Time Frame: 1 year]

Determine the recurrence rate at 1 year following clearance of metastatic disease in the setting of treatment with SBRT and pembrolizumab

Current Secondary Outcome Measures

Time to recurrence estimated using the Kaplan-Meier method[Time Frame: 1 year]

The 95% confidence of the median time to recurrence will be calculated using the Brookmeyer-Crowley method

Disease-free survival estimated using the Kaplan-Meier method[Time Frame: 1 year]

The 95% confidence of the median time to disease free survival calculated using the Brookmeyer-Crowley method.

Overall survival estimated using the Kaplan-Meier method[Time Frame: 1 year]

The 95% confidence of the median time to overall survival calculated using the Brookmeyer-Crowley method.

Descriptive Information

Offical Title

Pembrolizumab in Combination With Stereotactic Body Radiotherapy for Liver Metastatic Colorectal Cancer

Brief Summary

The purpose of this research study is:

- To find out how safe the study drug, pembrolizumab, is when combined with stereotactic body radiotherapy (SBRT) to the liver.
- To see how well subjects can tolerate treatment with pembrolizumab and SBRT.
- To find out how often colorectal cancer comes back 1 year after surgically removing all known disease and being treated with SBRT and pembrolizumab.

Detailed Description

This is a phase 1b feasibility study to evaluate the use of PD-1 blockade in combination with ablative radiotherapy for the treatment of metastatic colorectal cancer (CRC). This study will examine the sequential combination of stereotactic body radiotherapy (SBRT) and pembrolizumab for patients for whom the goal is eradicating all known sites of disease. It is very likely that for many patients the SBRT therapy will be completed following other modalities including operative resection or ablation.

Study Type

Interventional

Study Phase

Phase 1

Condition

- Colorectal Cancer
- Colorectal Adenocarcinoma
- Stage IVA Colorectal Cancer
- Stage IVB Colorectal Cancer
- Metastatic Carcinoma in the Liver

Intervention

Radiation: Stereotactic body radiotherapy (SBRT)

SBRT treatment will consist of 40-60 Gy delivered in five fractions prescribed to the planning target volume (PVT). Image guidance with MRI, megavoltage CT or cone beam CT scans would be required.

SBRT will be initiated on Day 0. This should be initiated within 4 weeks of signing informed consent. An additional 2 weeks will be allowed if necessary due to SBRT treatment planning.

Other Names:

Stereotactic Body Radiation Therapy

Drug: Pembrolizumab

Pembrolizumab is a potent and highly selective humanized monoclonal antibody (mAb) of the IgG4/kappa isotype designed to directly block the interaction between PD-1 and its ligands, PD-L1 and PD-L2. KeytrudaTM (pembrolizumab) has recently been approved in the United Stated for the treatment of patients with unresectable or metastatic melanoma and disease progression following ipilumumab and, if BRAF V600 mutation positive, a BRAF inhibitor.

Other Names:

Pembro

Keytruda

Study Arms

Experimental: SBRT + Pembrolizumab

Subjects will receive stereotactic body radiotherapy (SBRT) within 4 weeks of enrollment. Following SBRT, subjects will receive one cycle of pre-operative pembrolizumab given as an IV over approximately 30 minutes. Surgical management to remove all known sites of metastatic disease should occur 2 weeks post pembrolizumab treatment. Approximately 4-8 weeks after surgery subjects will being the second phase of pembrolizumab treatment. They will receive this treatment every 3 weeks (cycle) for 8 more cycles after surgery. Prior to the 5th cycle of pembrolizumab subjects will also have tumor imaging (CT or MRI).

Recruitment Information

Recruitment Status

Recruiting

Estimated Enrollment

15

Eligibility Criteria

Inclusion Criteria:

- Willing and able to provide written informed consent/assent for the trial
- Have a diagnosis of histologically confirmed metastatic colorectal cancer to the liver (no other sites of metastatic disease)

Histologic confirmation of a colorectal primary tumor is acceptable if accompanied by radiographic evidence of metastatic disease

- Tumor must be mismatch repair (MMR) proficient as determined by microsatellite instability or immunohistochemistry for for MMR proteins
- Microsatellite instability testing must be MSI-stable or MSI-low
- Or IHC for MMR proteins must demonstrate intact MMR proteins

Completion Date

December 2020

Primary Completion Date

March 2018

- Participant must be candidate for SBRT to at least one intrahepatic lesion. There is no limit on the number of intrahepatic lesions the patient may have
- Participant must be a surgical candidate with therapeutic goal of eradicating all known disease with one additional surgery
- Prior resection of extra-hepatic metastatic disease allowed if completed more than 12 months previous to study enrollment and now new extra-hepatic disease has been found
- Have measurable disease based on RECIST 1.1
- Fresh or archived colorectal cancer tissue, preferably from a hepatic metastatic site. Archival tissue is acceptable for enrolled into this study. Participants who have no archival tissue available do not need to undergo a new biopsy solely for the purpose of this study
- Participants must have received at least one prior line or chemotherapy including an irinotecan or oxaliplatin-fluoropyrimidine-based systemic treatment for colorectal cancer
- Have performance status of 0 or 1 on the ECOG Performance Scale
- Demonstrate an adequate organ function as defined in Table 1. These labs should be repeated if not completed within 10 days of SBRT treatment initiation
- Female participants of childbearing potential should have a negative urine or serum pregnancy test within 10 days of initiating SBRT. If the urine test is positive or cannot be confirmed as negative, a serum pregnancy test will be required
- Female participants of childbearing potential should be willing to use 2 methods of birth control or be surgically sterile, or abstain from heterosexual activity for the course of the study through 120 days after the last dose of study medication (Reference Section 5.7.2). Participants of childbearing potential are those who have not been surgically sterilized or have not been free from menses for >1 year
- Male participant should agree to use an adequate method of contraception starting with the first dose of study therapy through 120 days after the last dose of study therapy

Exclusion Criteria:

- Current participation and receiving study therapy or previous participation in a study of an investigational agent and received study therapy or used an investigational device within 4 weeks of the initiation of SBRT
- Prior anti-cancer monoclonal antibody (mAb) within 4 weeks prior to study Day 1 (first day of SBRT treatment) or who has not recovered (i.e. < Grade 1 or at baseline) from adverse events due to agents administered more than 4 weeks earlier
- Prior chemotherapy, targeted small molecule therapy, or radiation therapy within 2 weeks prior to study Day 1 or who has not recovered (i.e. < Grade 1 or at baseline) from adverse events due to a previously administered agent. Prior radiotherapy to the liver is not allowed
- Participants with < Grade 2 neuropathy are an exception to this criterion and may qualify for the study
- If the participant received major surgery, they must have recovered adequately from the toxicity and/or complications from the intervention prior to starting therapy
- Participant has a diagnosis of immunodeficiency or is receiving systemic steroid therapy or any other form of immunosuppressive therapy within 7 days prior to the initiation of SBRT
- Participant has a known history of active TB (Bacillus Tuberculosis)
- Hypersensitivity to pembrolizumab or any of its excipients
- Participant has had a prior anti-cancer monoclonal antibody (mAb) within 4 weeks prior to study Day 1 (first day or SBRT treatment) or who has not recovered (i.e., ≤ Grade 1 or at baseline) from adverse events due to agents administered more than 4 weeks earlier
- Participant has had prior chemotherapy, targeted small molecule therapy, or radiation therapy within 2 weeks prior to study Day 1 or who has not recovered (i.e., ≤ Grade 1 or at baseline) from adverse events due to a previously administered agent. Prior radiotherapy to the liver is not allowed. (Notes: Participants with ≤ Grade 2 neuropathy are an exception to this criterion and may qualify for the study. If participant received major surgery, they must have recovered adequately from the toxicity and/or complications from the intervention prior to starting therapy.)
- Participant has a known additional malignancy that is progressing or requires active treatment. Exceptions include basal cell carcinoma of the skin or squamous cell carcinoma of the skin that has undergone potentially curative therapy or in situ cervical cancer.
- Participant has known active central nervous system (CNS) metastases and/or carcinomatous meningitis. Participants with previously resected brain metastases may participate provided it has been at least 6 months and no CNS progression has been identified.
- Participant has active autoimmune disease that has required systemic treatment in the past 2 years (i.e. with use of disease modifying agents, corticosteroids or immunosuppressive drugs). Replacement therapy (eg., thyroxine, insulin, or physiologic corticosteroid replacement therapy for adrenal or pituitary insufficiency, etc.) is not considered a form of systemic treatment.
- Participant has known history of, or any evidence of active, non-infectious pneumonitis.
- Participant has an active infection requiring systemic therapy.
- Participant has a history or current evidence of any condition, therapy, or laboratory abnormality that might confound the results of the trial, interfere with the participant's participation for the full duration of the trial, or is not in the best interest of the participant to participate, in the opinion of the treating investigator.
- Participant has known psychiatric or substance abuse disorders that would interfere with cooperation with the requirements of the trial.
- Participant is pregnant or breastfeeding, or expecting to conceive or father children within the projected duration of the trial,

starting with the pre-screening or screening visit through 120 days after the last dose of trial treatment.

- Participant has received prior therapy with an anti-PD-1, anti-PD-L1, or anti-PD-L2 agent.
- Participant has a known history of Human Immunodeficiency Virus (HIV) (HIV 1/2 antibodies).
- Participant has known active Hepatitis B (e.g., HBsAg reactive) or Hepatitis C (e.g., HCV RNA [qualitative or quantitative] is detected).
- Participant has received a live vaccine within 30 days of planned start of study therapy.

▦ Sex/Gender

All

▦ Ages

18 Years to N/A

▦ Accepts Healthy Volunteers

No

▦ Contacts

Cancer Connect   800-622-8922   cancerconnect@uwcarbone.wisc.edu

TAS-OX for Refractory Metastatic Colon Cancer

Study ID:

NCT02848079

Sponsor:

Yale University

Information provided by (Responsible Party):

Yale University (Yale University)

Tracking Information

▦ **First Submitted Date**

July 21, 2016

▦ **Start Date**

August 2016

▦ **Primary Completion Date**

July 2019

▦ **Last Update Posted Date**

July 26, 2017

▦ **Current Primary Outcome Measures**

Overall Response Rate measured by Response Evaluation Criteria In Solid Tumor (RECIST) 1.1 criteria[Time Frame: up to 30 days following discontinuation of treatment]

▦ **Current Secondary Outcome Measures**

Progression Free Survival assessed according to RECIST criteria version 1.1.[Time Frame: from the date of start of treatment to the date of first documented progression or any cause of death assessed up to 12 months.]

Overall Survival assessed by time to death from start of study[Time Frame: from the date of start of treatment to the date of any cause of death assessed up to 24 months.]

safety and tolerability assessed with Common Terminology Criteria for Adverse Events (CTCAE)[Time Frame: assessed from start of treatment up to discontinuation of treatment or up to 12 months.]

Descriptive Information

▦ **Offical Title**

TAS-102 and Oxaliplatin (TAS-OX) for Refractory Metastatic Colon Cancer

▦ **Brief Summary**

This study will examine the safety and effectiveness of oxaliplatin in combination with TAS-102 (TAS-OX) for treatment of patients with metastatic colorectal cancer whose cancer has progressed or recurred after FOLFOX chemotherapy.

▦ **Detailed Description**

TAS-102 is an oral agent, which consists of a combination of a novel antimetabolite 5-trifluorothymidine (FTD) and a thymidine phosphorylase inhibitor (TPI) that prevents degradation of FTD. It has demonstrated activity in chemorefractory metastatic colorectal cancer (mCRC) patients. In the Japanese randomized phase II trial, TAS-102 improved medial overall survival when compared to placebo (9.0 vs.6.6 months, Hazard Ratio (HR) 0.56) in patients with mCRC refractory to 5-fluorouracil (5-FU), irinotecan and oxaliplatin. Subsequently, a randomized phase III study conducted in 13 countries (RECOURSE trial) confirmed this benefit on overall survival when compared to placebo (7.1 months vs. 5.3 months, HR 0.68) in patients with refractory metastatic colorectal cancer (CRC) 5.

Oxaliplatin is a third generation platinum compound, which is active when used together with 5-FU in the treatment of mCRC (FOLFOX). FOLFOX chemotherapy, which is frequently combined with anti-angiogenic agent Bevacizumab, is widely accepted as the preferred first-line regimen in the treatment of this disease in the US. Oxaliplatin is also frequently reintroduced in more advanced settings. Reintroduction is seen after progression on maintenance therapy, after resolution of previous treatment limiting neuropathy, after disease recurrence post adjuvant treatment or post metastasectomy. In the control arm of a randomized study of FOLFOX4 or FOLFOX7 with oxaliplatin in a stop-and-go fashion in advanced colorectal cancer (OPTIMOX1 study), oxaliplatin was reintroduced in 27% of patients. Although patients derive clinical benefit when oxaliplatin is reintroduced, the response rates are not as robust as during initial exposures. Decreased efficacy may be at least in part due to prolonged exposure and resultant resistance to 5-FU, which is a backbone in maintenance and in oxaliplatin containing regimens. Hence, the investigators propose exploring the safety and efficacy of oxaliplatin in combination with an alternative anti-metabolite TAS-102 (TAS-OX).

TAS-102 has demonstrated activity in 5-FU refractory mCRC, so the investigators hypothesize that TAS-OX may serve as an alternative drug combination for patients who have progressed or recurred after FOLFOX, and who are candidates for additional oxaliplatin therapy.

This is a 2-part clinical trial with TAS-102 in combination with oxaliplatin. The first part will be a dose-finding run-in phase and will enroll 3-18 patients. The second part, the focus of this study, will be a single arm cohort , which will further evaluate the safety, as well as efficacy, of TAS-OX in the treatment of mCRC. The subjects in part 2 will be treated with the drug doses determined in Part 1 of the trial. Up to 50 patients will be enrolled in part 2. Anticipated enrollment may be as high as 68 patients. Maximum potential enrollment is listed under anticipated enrollment, below.

Study Type

Interventional

Study Phase

Phase 1/Phase 2

Condition

- Colorectal Neoplasms

Intervention

Drug: combined TAS-102 and TAS-OX

Combination treatment with TAS-102 and oxaliplatin. TAS-102 is an oral medication; oxaliplatin (TAS-OX) is given by infusion.

Study Arms

Experimental: combined TAS-102 and oxaliplatin
Combination treatment with TAS-102 and oxaliplatin

Recruitment Information

Recruitment Status

Recruiting

Estimated Enrollment

68

Completion Date

December 2020

Primary Completion Date

July 2019

Eligibility Criteria

Inclusion Criteria:

1. Histologically confirmed stage IV colon cancer (American Joint Commission on Cancer (AJCC) 7th edition) that has progressed after at least 2 lines of standard therapy that included 5-FU, irinotecan and oxaliplatin. Patients who could not tolerate standard agents because of unacceptable, but reversible, toxicity necessitating their discontinuation will be allowed to participate.

2. Patients who had received adjuvant chemotherapy and had recurrence during or within 6 months of completion of the adjuvant chemotherapy will be allowed to count the adjuvant therapy as one chemotherapy regimen.

3. Progression of disease must be documented on the most recent scan.

4. Presence of measurable disease (not required for Phase 1 portion of the trial).

5. Retrovirus-associated DNA sequences (RAS) mutation and mismatch repair (MMR) status must be determined (or tissue availability for testing if not already determined)

6. Age 18 years or older.

7. Eastern Cooperative Oncology Group (ECOG) performance status 0-1.

8. Life expectancy of at least 3 months.

9. Patient with adequate organ function:

1. Absolute neutrophil count (ANC) ≥ 1.5 x 109/L

2. Hemoglobin ≥ 9 g/dL

3. Platelets (PLT) ≥ 75 x 109/L

4. Aspartate aminotransferase (AST)/Alanine aminotransferase (ALT) ≤ 5 x Upper limit of normal (ULN)

5. Total serum bilirubin of ≤1.5 mg/dL (except for Grade 1 hyperbilirubinemia due solely to a medical diagnosis of Gilbert's syndrome).

6. Albumin ≥ 2.5 g/dL

7. Serum creatinine ≤ 1.5 x institutional ULN (Cockcroft and Gault formula)

10. Adequate contraception if applicable.

11. Women who are nursing must discontinue nursing prior to enrollment in the program.

12. Ability to take oral medication (i.e. no feeding tube).

13. Patient able and willing to comply with study procedures as per protocol.

14. Patient able to understand and willing to sign and date the written voluntary informed consent form (ICF) at screening visit prior to any protocol-specific procedures.

Exclusion Criteria:

1. Patients who have previously received TAS-102.

2. Grade 2 or higher peripheral neuropathy.

3. Symptomatic Central nervous system (CNS) metastases requiring treatment.

4. Other active malignancy within the last 3 years (except for non-melanoma skin cancer or a non-invasive/in situ cancer).

5. Pregnancy or breast feeding.

6. Current therapy with other investigational agents.

7. Active infection with body temperature ≥38°C due to infection.

8. Major surgery within prior 4 weeks (the surgical incision should be fully healed prior to drug administration).

9. Any anticancer therapy within prior 3 weeks of first dose of study drug.

10. History of allergic reactions attributed to compounds of similar chemical or biologic composition to TAS-102.

11. Current therapy with other investigational agents or participation in another clinical study or any investigational agent received within prior 4 weeks.

12. Grade 3 or higher hypersensitivity reaction to oxaliplatin, or grade 1-2 hypersensitivity reaction to oxaliplatin not controlled with pre-medication.

13. Unresolved toxicity of greater than or equal to Common Terminology Criteria for Adverse Events (CTCAE) Grade 2 attributed to any prior therapies (excluding anemia, alopecia, skin pigmentation, and platinum-induced neurotoxicity).

14. Extended field radiation within prior 4 weeks of first dose of study drug or limited field radiation within prior 2 weeks of first dose of study drug.

15. Psychological, familial, or sociological condition potentially hampering compliance with the study protocol and follow-up schedule.

16. Involvement in the planning and/or conduct of the study.

17. Previous enrollment in the present study.

- Sex/Gender

All

- Ages

18 Years to N/A

- Accepts Healthy Volunteers

No

- Contacts

Kamil Sadowski   kamil.sadowski@yale.edu

Stephanie Brogan   203 737 4156   stephanie.brogan@yale.edu

CAR-T Hepatic Artery Infusions for CEA-Expressing Liver Metastases

Study ID:

NCT02850536

Sponsor:

Roger Williams Medical Center

Information provided by (Responsible Party):

Roger Williams Medical Center (Roger Williams Medical Center)

Tracking Information

▦ **First Submitted Date**

July 14, 2016

▦ **Start Date**

February 1, 2017

▦ **Primary Completion Date**

December 2017

▦ **Last Update Posted Date**

February 3, 2017

▦ **Current Primary Outcome Measures**

Safety of CAR-T cell hepatic artery infusions delivered using the Surefire Infusion System (SIS) as Measured by Number of Participants with Adverse Events[Time Frame: 10 weeks]

> To determine the safety and regimen limiting toxicity (RLT) of anti-CEA CAR-T hepatic artery infusions (HAI) via the Surefire Infusion System (SIS) for CEA-expressing liver metastases

▦ **Current Secondary Outcome Measures**

Radiographic treatment response by MRI[Time Frame: 10 weeks]

> Changes in tumor size

Radiographic treatment response by PET[Time Frame: 10 weeks]

> Changes in tumor metabolic activity

CAR-T detection in liver tumors[Time Frame: 10 weeks]

> Quantification of CAR-T cells in liver tumor core biopsies

CAR-T detection in normal liver tissue[Time Frame: 10 weeks]

> Quantification of CAR-T cells in normal liver core biopsies

CAR-T detection in extrahepatic sites[Time Frame: 10 weeks]

> Quantification of CAR-T in blood samples

Serum Cytokine Levels[Time Frame: 10 weeks]

> Measurement of cytokines as indicators of immune response

CEA level[Time Frame: 10 weeks]

> Measurement of serum tumor marker (ng/ml)

Tumor biopsy[Time Frame: 10 weeks]

> Assessment of tumor necrosis and fibrosis

Descriptive Information

▦ **Offical Title**

Phase Ib Trial of CAR-T Hepatic Artery Infusions Delivered With the Surefire Infusion System (SIS) for CEA-Expressing Liver Metastases

▦ **Brief Summary**

This is an open label, fixed dose, phase Ib trial of anti-CEA CAR-T cell infusions delivered via the hepatic artery using the Surefire Infusion System (SIS) for patients with CEA-expressing liver metastases.

▦ **Detailed Description**

Patients undergo leukapheresis from which peripheral blood mononuclear cells are purified. T cells are activated and then re-engineered to express chimeric antigen receptors (CARs) specific for CEA. Cells are expanded in culture and returned to the patient by percutaneous hepatic artery infusion at specific cell doses. Prior to the first dose, each patient will undergo diagnostic angiography to verify suitable arterial anatomy. Three anti-CEA CAR-T doses per patient are planned at 1-week intervals. Low dose interleukin-2 will be given via an ambulatory infusion pump for 4 weeks. Normal liver and tumor biopsies will be obtained at the time of the initial diagnostic angiogram and during the final session following the 3rd CAR-T infusion.

Study Type

Interventional

Study Phase

Phase 1

Condition

- Liver Metastases

Intervention

Biological: anti-CEA CAR-T cells
  Gene modified patient T cells

Other Names:
  Designer T cells

Study Arms

Experimental: anti-CEA CAR-T cells
  Three infusions of gene-modified anti-CEA T cells over the course of 3 weeks into the hepatic artery via a percutaneous approach along with low dose IL-2.

Recruitment Information

Recruitment Status

Recruiting

Estimated Enrollment

5

Completion Date

December 2017

Primary Completion Date

December 2017

Eligibility Criteria

Inclusion Criteria:

- Patient with histologically confirmed diagnosis of CEA+ adenocarcinoma and liver metastases. Patient must have either histologic confirmation of the liver metastases or histologic documentation of the primary tumor and definitive radiologic evidence of liver involvement. Measurable disease is required with lesions of > 1.0 cm by CT. Soluble CEA is not acceptable as the sole measure of disease. Limited extrahepatic disease is acceptable if confined to the lungs or peritoneal cavity.
- Tumor must be CEA-expressing as demonstrated by elevated serum CEA levels (≥10ng/ml) or immunohistochemistry on a biopsy specimen. Archived tissue is acceptable for determination of CEA expression.
- Patient must be at least 18 years of age.
- Patient able to understand and sign informed consent.
- Patient with a life expectancy of greater than four months.
- Patient failed at least one line of standard systemic chemotherapy and has unresectable disease.
- Patient with performance status of 0 to 1 (ECOG).
- Patient with adequate organ function as defined in protocol.
- Acceptable hepatic vascular anatomy as determined by CT, MR, or conventional angiography. A nuclear medicine study will be performed to document the absence of a significant hepatic-pulmonary shunt (<20%).

Exclusion Criteria:

- Female patients of childbearing age will be tested for pregnancy. Pregnant patients will be excluded from the study. Males who are actively seeking to have children will be made aware of the unknown risks of this study protocol on human sperm and the need to practice birth control.
- Patients with serious or unstable renal, hepatic, pulmonary, cardiovascular, endocrine, rheumatologic, or allergic disease based on history, physical exam and laboratory tests will be excluded, as outlined in section 5.2.8.
- Patients with active clinical disease caused by CMV, hepatitis B or C, HIV or tuberculosis will be excluded from the study.
- Patients who have had cytotoxic and/or radiation therapy within 4 weeks prior to entry into the trial or 4 weeks prior to infusion will be excluded. Patients with other concurrent malignancies will be excluded.
- Patients requiring systemic steroids will be excluded.
- Patients with unsuitable hepatic vascular anatomy will be excluded from the study.
- Patients with extrahepatic metastatic disease beyond the lungs or abdominal/ retroperitoneal lymph nodes.
- Patients with >50% liver replacement at time of treatment will be excluded.
- Previous external beam radiotherapy to the liver.

- Portal vein thrombosis.

Sex/Gender

All

Ages

18 Years to N/A

Accepts Healthy Volunteers

Accepts Healthy Volunteers

Contacts

Ashley Moody, RN   401-456-2268   ALarkin@chartercare.org

Tracey MacDermott   303-724-2757   Tracey.MacDermott@ucdenver.edu

A Study of LY3214996 Administered Alone or in Combination With Other Agents in Participants With Advanced/Metastatic Cancer

Study ID:

NCT02857270

Sponsor:

Eli Lilly and Company

Information provided by (Responsible Party):

Eli Lilly and Company (Eli Lilly and Company)

Tracking Information

First Submitted Date

August 3, 2016

Start Date

September 2016

Primary Completion Date

April 2019

Last Update Posted Date

February 8, 2018

Current Primary Outcome Measures

Number of Participants with LY3214996 Dose Limiting Toxicities (DLTs)[Time Frame: Cycle 1 (21 Days)]

Current Secondary Outcome Measures

Pharmacokinetics (PK): Area Under the Concentration-Time Curve (AUC) of LY3214996 Administered as Monotherapy and when Administered in Combination with Nab-Paclitaxel Plus Gemcitabine, and Abemaciclib[Time Frame: Cycle 1 Day 1 through Cycle 2 Day 1 (up to 28 Day Cycles)]

PK: AUC of Gemcitabine when Administered with LY3214996[Time Frame: Cycle 1 Day 1 through Cycle 1 Day 15 (28 Day Cycles)]

PK: AUC of Nab-Paclitaxel when Administered with LY3214996[Time Frame: Cycle 1 Day 1 through Cycle 1 Day 15 (28 Day Cycles)]

PK: AUC of Abemaciclib and its Metabolites when Administered with LY3214996[Time Frame: Cycle 1 Day 1 through Cycle 2 Day 1 (up to 22 Day Cycles)]

PK: AUC of Midazolam and its 1'-Hydroxymidazolam Metabolite when Administered Alone and in Combination with LY3214996[Time Frame: Cycle 1 Day 1 through Cycle 1 Day 16 (21 Day Cycles)]

Objective Response Rate (ORR): Percentage of Participants With a Complete (CR) or Partial Response (PR)[Time Frame: Baseline to Measured Progressive Disease or Start of New Anti-Cancer Therapy (Estimated up to 6 Months)]

Duration of Response (DoR)[Time Frame: Date of Complete Response (CR) or Partial Response (PR) to Date of Objective Disease Progression or Death Due to Any Cause (Estimated up to 12 Months)]

Time to First Response (TTR)[Time Frame: Baseline to Date of CR or PR (Estimated up to 6 Months)]

Progression Free Survival (PFS)[Time Frame: Baseline to Progressive Disease or Death of Any Cause (Estimated up to 12 Months)]

Descriptive Information

▦ Offical Title

A Phase 1 Study of an ERK1/2 Inhibitor (LY3214996) Administered Alone or in Combination With Other Agents in Advanced Cancer

▦ Brief Summary

The purpose of this study is to determine the safety of an extracellular signal regulated kinase (ERK1/2) inhibitor LY3214996 administered alone or in combination with other agents in participants with advanced cancer.

▦ Study Type

Interventional

▦ Study Phase

Phase 1

▦ Condition

- Advanced Cancer
- Metastatic Melanoma
- Metastatic Non-small Cell Lung Cancer
- Metastatic Pancreatic Ductal Adenocarcinoma
- Colorectal Cancer

▦ Intervention

Drug: LY3214996

   Administered orally

   Drug: Midazolam

   Administered orally

Drug: Abemaciclib

   Administered orally

Other Names:

   LY2835219

Drug: Nab-paclitaxel

   Administered IV

Drug: Gemcitabine

   Administered IV

▦ Study Arms

Experimental: LY3214996 Dose Escalation

   LY3214996 given orally once a day (or twice a day) for 21 days.

Experimental: LY3214996 + Midazolam

   (Preliminary Drug-Drug Interactions [DDI])

   LY3214996 given orally (dose timing will be determined) and midazolam given orally on cycle 1 day 1 and cycle 1 day 16 (21 day cycles except cycle 1 only = 22 days).

Experimental: LY3214996 Monotherapy

   LY3214996 given orally (dose timing will be determined) during each 21 day cycle.

Experimental: LY3214996 + Abemaciclib

   Dose Escalation and ExpansionLY3214996 given orally (dose timing will be determined) and abemaciclib given orally (single dose given during lead in period) twice a day every 12 hours during 21 day cycle.

Experimental: LY3214996 + Nab-Paclitaxel + Gemcitabine

   Dose Escalation and ExpansionLY3214996 given orally (dose timing will be determined) and nab-paclitaxel given intravenously (IV) on day 1, 8, and 15 and gemcitabine IV on day 1, 8, and 15 during each 28 day cycle.

Recruitment Information

Recruitment Status

Recruiting

Estimated Enrollment

136

Completion Date

September 2019

Primary Completion Date

April 2019

Eligibility Criteria

Inclusion Criteria:

- Have advanced or metastatic cancer (solid tumors) and be an appropriate candidate for experimental therapy.
- Part B2: Have advanced/metastatic cancer carrying activating mitogen-activated protein kinase (MAPK) pathway alteration
- Part B3: Have metastatic melanoma carrying BRAF mutation, refractory/relapsed after treatment with Raf and/or MEK inhibitors
- Part B4: Have metastatic melanoma carrying NRAS mutation
- Part C: Have advanced unresectable cancer (dose escalation) and advanced/unresectable/metastatic NSCLC carrying BRAF or RAS mutation and colorectal cancer carrying RAS mutation (dose expansion)
- Part D: Have metastatic pancreatic ductal adenocarcinoma (dose escalation and dose expansion)
- Have discontinued previous treatments for cancer and have resolution, except where otherwise stated in the inclusion criteria, of all clinically significant toxic effects of prior chemotherapy, surgery, or radiotherapy to Grade ≤1 by National Cancer Institute (NCI) Common Terminology Criteria for Adverse Events (CTCAE), Version 4.0.
- Have adequate organ function.
- Have a performance status of 0 to 1 on the Eastern Cooperative Oncology Group (ECOG) scale.

Exclusion Criteria:

- Have serious preexisting medical conditions.
- Have a known human immunodeficiency virus (HIV) infection or known activated/reactivated hepatitis A, B, or C.
- Have symptomatic central nervous system malignancy or metastasis.
- Have current hematologic malignancies, acute or chronic leukemia.
- Have a second primary malignancy that in the judgment of the investigator or Lilly may affect the interpretation of results.
- Have prior malignancies. Participants with carcinoma in situ of any origin and participants with prior malignancies who are in remission and whose likelihood of recurrence is very low, as judged by the Lilly clinical research physician, are eligible for this study.
- Have a mean QT interval corrected for heart rate (QTc) of ≥470 milliseconds on screening electrocardiogram (ECG) as calculated using the Bazett's formula at several consecutive days of assessment.
- Have participated, within the last 28 days in a clinical trial involving an investigational product or are currently enrolled in a clinical trial involving an investigational product or any other type of medical research judged not to be scientifically or medically compatible with this study.
- Have previously completed or withdrawn from this study or any other study investigating an ERK1/2 inhibitor.
- If female, is pregnant, breastfeeding, or planning to become pregnant.
- Have history or findings of central or branch retinal artery or venous occlusion with significant vision loss or other retinal diseases that cause current visual impairment or would likely cause visual impairment over the time period of the study.
- Currently using concomitant medications that are strong inhibitors or inducers of CYP3A4.

Sex/Gender

All

Ages

18 Years to N/A

Accepts Healthy Volunteers

No

Contacts

There may be multiple sites in this clinical trial. 1-877-CTLILLY (1-877-285-4559) or   1-317-615-4559

Continuous 24h Intravenous Infusion of Mithramycin, an Inhibitor of Cancer Stem Cell Signaling, in People With Primary Thoracic Malignancies or Carcinomas, Sarcomas or Germ Cell Neoplasms With Pleuropulmonary Metastases

Study ID:

NCT02859415

Sponsor:

National Cancer Institute (NCI)

Information provided by (Responsible Party):

National Institutes of Health Clinical Center (CC) (National Cancer Institute (NCI))

Tracking Information

▦ **First Submitted Date**

August 6, 2016

▦ **Start Date**

August 6, 2016

▦ **Primary Completion Date**

August 3, 2028

▦ **Last Update Posted Date**

January 10, 2018

▦ **Current Primary Outcome Measures**

Maximum tolerated dose[Time Frame: at the end of first 14 day cycle at each dose level]

> The number of patients experiencing DLT.Toxicity information recorded will include the type, severity, time of onset, time of resolution, and the probable association with the study regimen. Tables will be constructed to summarize the observed incidence by severity and type of toxicity.

Overall response rate[Time Frame: every 8 weeks until at disease progression]

> Response rates will be calculated as the percent of patients whose best response is a CR or PR.

Descriptive Information

▦ **Offical Title**

Phase I/II Evaluation of Continuous 24h Intravenous Infusion of Mithramycin, an Inhibitor of Cancer Stem Cell Signaling, in Patients With Primary Thoracic Malignancies or Carcinomas, Sarcomas or Germ Cell Neoplasms With Pleuropulmonary Metastases

▦ **Brief Summary**

Background:

Mithramycin is a new cancer drug. In another study, people with chest cancer took the drug 6 hours a day for 7 straight days. Many of them had liver damage as a side effect. It was discovered that only people with certain genes got this side effect. Researchers want to test mithramycin in people who do not have those certain genes.

<TAB>

Objectives:

To find the highest safe dose of mithramycin that can be given to people with chest cancer who have certain genes over 24 hours instead of spread out over a longer period of time. To see if mithramycin given as a 24-hour infusion shrinks tumors.

Eligibility:

People ages 18 and older who have chest cancer that is not shrinking with known therapies, and whose genes will limit the chance of liver damage from mithramycin

Design:

Participants will be screened with:

Medical history

Physical exam

Blood and urine tests

Lung and heart function tests

X-rays or scans of their tumor

Liver ultrasound

Tumor biopsy

Participants will be admitted to the hospital overnight. A small plastic tube (catheter) will be inserted in the arm or chest. They will get mithramycin through the catheter over about 24 hours.

If they do not have bad side effects or their cancer does not worsen, they can repeat the treatment every 14 days.

Participants will have multiple visits for each treatment cycle. These include repeats of certain screening tests.

After stopping treatment, participants will have weekly visits until they recover from any side effects.

▪ Detailed Description

Background:

Increasing evidence indicates that activation of stem cell gene expression is a common mechanism by which environmental carcinogens mediate initiation and progression of thoracic malignancies. Similar mechanisms appear to contribute to extra-thoracic malignancies that metastasize to the chest. Utilization of pharmacologic agents, which target gene regulatory networks mediating stemness may be novel strategies for treatment of these neoplasms. Recent studies performed in the Thoracic Epigenetics Laboratory, TGIB/NCI, demonstrate that under exposure conditions potentially achievable in clinical settings, mithramycin diminishes stem cell gene expression and markedly inhibits growth of lung and esophageal cancer and malignant pleural mesothelioma (MPM) cells in vitro and in vivo. These findings add to other recent preclinical studies demonstrating impressive anti-tumor activity of mithramycin in epithelial malignancies and sarcomas that frequently metastasize to the thorax.

Primary Objectives:

- Phase I component: To determine pharmacokinetics, toxicities, and maximum tolerated dose (MTD) of mithramycin administered as a continuous 24hr infusion in patients with primary thoracic malignancies or carcinomas, sarcomas or germ cell tumors metastatic to the chest.
- Phase II component: To determine objective response rates (CR+PR) of mithramycin administered as 24h intravenous infusions in patients with primary thoracic malignancies or carcinomas, sarcomas or germ cell tumors metastatic to the chest.

Eligibility:

- Patients with histologically or cytologically proven primary malignancies involving lungs, esophagus, thymus, pleura, chest wall or mediastinum, or extra-thoracic malignancies metastatic to the chest.
- Patients with germline SNPs in ABCB4 and ABCB11 that are associated with resistance to mithramycin-induced hepatotoxicity.
- Patients must have had or refused first-line standard therapy for their malignancies.
- Patients must be 18 years or older with an ECOG performance status of 0-2, without evidence of unstable or decompensated myocardial disease. Patients must have adequate pulmonary reserve evidenced by FEV1 and DLCO equal to or greater than 30% predicted; pCO2 less than 55 mm Hg and pO(2) greater than or equal to 60 mm Hg on room air ABG.
- Patients must have a platelet count greater than or equal to 100,000, an ANC equal to or greater than 1500 without transfusion or cytokine support, a normal PT, and adequate hepatic function as evidenced by a total bilirubin of <1.5 times upper limits of normal. Serum creatinine within normal institutional limits or creatinine clearance greater than or equal to 60 mL/min/1.73 m(2) for patients with creatinine levels above institutional normal

Design:

- Single arm Phase I dose escalation to define pharmacokinetics, toxicities and MTD.
- Patient cohorts will receive 24h infusions of mithramycin targeting total doses currently administered during 7 daily six hour infusions at 30-50mcg/kg.
- The 24 h infusions will be administered every 14 days (1 cycle). Four cycles will constitute one course of therapy.
- Pharmacokinetics and toxicity assessment to define MTD will be assessed during cycle 1 of the first course of therapy.
- Due to uncertainties regarding potential cumulative toxicities, no intra-patient dose escalation will be allowed.
- Once MTD has been defined, patients will be stratified into two cohorts (primary thoracic malignancy vs neoplasm of non-thoracic origin metastatic to the chest) to determine clinical response rates at the MTD, using a Simon Optimal Two Stage Design for Phase II Clinical Trials targeting an objective response rate (RECIST) of 30%.
- Following each course of therapy, patients will undergo restaging studies. Patients exhibiting objective response to therapy or stable disease by RECIST criteria will be offered an additional course of therapy.
- Patients exhibiting disease progression will be removed from study.
- Biopsies of index lesions will be obtained at baseline and on day 4 of the first and if feasible second cycle of therapy for analysis of pharmacodynamic endpoints. An additional biopsy may be requested in patient exhibiting objective responses following one course of therapy.

▪ Study Type

Interventional

▪ Study Phase

Phase 1/Phase 2

▪ Condition

- Esophageal Neoplasms
- Lung Neoplasms

- Mesothelioma
- Thymus Neoplasms
- Neoplasms, Germ Cell and Embryonal

▦ Intervention

Drug: Mithramycin

Phase 1: 24 hour intravenous infusion of mithramycin given once every 14 days at escalating doses; Phase 2: 24 hour intravenous infusion of mithramycin given once every 14 days at MTD established in phase 1

▦ Study Arms

Experimental: 1

phase 1 dose escalation cohort

Experimental: 2

phase 2 primary thoracic malignancies cohort

Recruitment Information

▦ **Recruitment Status**

Recruiting

▦ **Estimated Enrollment**

100

▦ **Completion Date**

August 3, 2028

▦ **Primary Completion Date**

August 3, 2028

▦ **Eligibility Criteria**

- **INCLUSION CRITERIA:**
- Diagnosis: Patients with measurable inoperable, histologically confirmed non-small cell lung cancer (NSCLC), small cell lung cancer (SCLC), esophageal carcinoma, thymic epithelial neoplasms, germ cell tumors, malignant pleural mesotheliomas or chest wall sarcomas, as well as patients with gastric, colorectal, pancreas or renal cancers, germ cell tumors and sarcomas metastatic to thorax are eligible.
- Histologic confirmation of disease in the Laboratory of Pathology, CCR, NCI, NIH.
- Germline ABCB4 (CC) and ABCB11 (GG or GC) genotypes determined by pharmacogenomics analysis of peripheral blood mononuclear cells.
- Disease amenable to biopsy via percutaneous approach or other minimally invasive procedures such as thoracoscopy, bronchoscopy, laparoscopy, or GI endoscopy
- Age greater than or equal to18
- ECOG status 0-2
- Patients must have had, or refused first-line standard chemotherapy for their inoperable malignancies.
- Patients must have had no chemotherapy, biologic therapy, or radiation therapy for their malignancy for at least 30 days prior to treatment. Patients may have received localized radiation therapy to non-target lesions provided that the radiotherapy is completed 14 days prior to commencing therapy, and the patient has recovered from any toxicity. At least 3 half-lives must have elapsed since monoclonal antibody treatment. At least six weeks must have elapsed between mitomycin C or nitrosourea treatment.
- **Patients must have adequate organ and marrow function as defined below:**

1. Hematologic and Coagulation Parameters:
- Peripheral ANC greater than or equal to 1500/mm(3)
- Platelets greater than or equal to 100,000/ mm(3) (transfusion independent)
- Hemoglobin greater than or equal to 8 g/dL (PRBC transfusions permitted)
- PT/PTT within normal limits (11.6 15.2 / 25.3 37.3 sec)

2. Hepatic Function
- Bilirubin (total) < 1.5 times upper limit of normal (ULN)
- ALT (SGPT) less than or equal to 3.0 times ULN
- Albumin > 2 g/dL

3. Renal Function
- Creatinine within normal institutional limits or creatinine clearance greater than or equal to 60 mL/min/1.73 m(2) for patients with creatinine levels above institutional normal.
- Normal ionized calcium, magnesium and phosphorus (can be on oral supplementation)
- Cardiac Function: Left ventricular ejection fraction (EF) >40% by echocardiogram, MUGA, or cardiac MR.
- Ability of subject to understand, and be willing to sign informed consent
- Female and male patients (and when relevant their partners) must be willing to practice birth control (including abstinence)

during and for two months after treatment if female of childbearing potential or male having sexual contact with a female of childbearing potential.

- Patients must be willing to undergo 2 tumor biopsies

EXCLUSION CRITERIA:

- Clinically significant systemic illness (e.g. serious active infections or significant cardiac, pulmonary, hepatic or other organ dysfunction), that in the judgment of the PI would compromise the patient s ability to tolerate protocol therapy or significantly increase the risk of complications
- Patients with cerebral metastases
- **Patients with any of the following pulmonary function abnormalities will be excluded:**

FEV, < 30% predicted; DLCO, < 30% predicted (post-bronchodilator); pO2 < 60 mm Hg or pCO2 greater than or equal to 55 mm Hg on room air arterial blood gas.

- Patients with evidence of active bleeding, intratumoral hemorrhage or history of bleeding diatheses, unless specifically occurring as an isolated incident during reversible chemotherapy-induced thrombocytopenia
- Patients on therapeutic anticoagulation Note: prophylactic anticoagulation (i.e. intralumenal heparin) for venous or arterial access devices is allowed.
- **Patients who are concurrently receiving or requiring any of the following agents, which may increase the risk for mithramycin related toxicities, such as hemorrhage:**
- Thrombolytic agents
- Aspirin or salicylate-containing products, which may increase risk of hemorrhage
- Dextran
- Dipyridamole
- Sulfinpyrazone
- Valproic acid
- Clopidogrel
- Lactating or pregnant females (due to risk to fetus or newborn, and lack of testing for excretion in breast milk).
- Patients with history of HIV, HBV or HCV due to potentially increased risk of mithramycin toxicity in this population.
- Hypersensitivity to mithramycin
- Patients who in the opinion of the investigator may not be able to comply with the safety monitoring requirements of the study.

▦ **Sex/Gender**

All

▦ **Ages**

18 Years to 100 Years

▦ **Accepts Healthy Volunteers**

No

▦ **Contacts**

Tricia Kunst, R.N.   (240) 760-6234   kunstt@mail.nih.gov

CB-839 + Capecitabine in Solid Tumors and Fluoropyrimidine Resistant PIK3CA Mutant Colorectal Cancer

Study ID:

NCT02861300

Sponsor:

Case Comprehensive Cancer Center

Information provided by (Responsible Party):

Case Comprehensive Cancer Center (Case Comprehensive Cancer Center)

Tracking Information

▦ **First Submitted Date**

August 5, 2016

▦ **Start Date**

August 31, 2016

Primary Completion Date

July 2018

Last Update Posted Date

January 31, 2018

Current Primary Outcome Measures

PHASE 1: Recommended dose for phase II study[Time Frame: At least 21 days of treatment]

The Phase I study has been designed to define the recommended phase II dose of CB-839 and capecitabine. A traditional 3+3 dose escalation design will be adopted. Nine to twenty-four patients are expected to be enrolled, depending on the number of dose escalations and assuming that a total of 6 patients will be treated at the final recommended phase II dose level. Patients who complete the first 21 day treatment cycle of CB-839 and capecitabine chemotherapy will be included in the analysis.

PHASE 2: Number of patients with response to treatment[Time Frame: Up to 18 months after beginning treatment]

In the phase II component of this study, the primary endpoint is response rate. Response rate will be determined using RECIST criteria.

RECIST response categories: Progressive disease (PD): >=20% increase in sum of longest diameter (LD) of target lesion(s), taking as reference smallest sum LD recorded since treatment started. Complete response (CR): disappearance of all target lesions. Partial response (PR): >=30% decrease in sum of LD of target lesion(s), taking as reference baseline sum LD. Stable disease (SD): neither sufficient shrinkage to qualify as PR nor sufficient increase to qualify as PD.

Current Secondary Outcome Measures

PHASE 1: proportion of patient who respond to treatment[Time Frame: At least 21 days of treatment]

Response rate will be determined using RECIST criteria.

RECIST response categories: Progressive disease (PD): >=20% increase in sum of longest diameter (LD) of target lesion(s), taking as reference smallest sum LD recorded since treatment started. Complete response (CR): disappearance of all target lesions. Partial response (PR): >=30% decrease in sum of LD of target lesion(s), taking as reference baseline sum LD. Stable disease (SD): neither sufficient shrinkage to qualify as PR nor sufficient increase to qualify as PD.

Descriptive Information

Offical Title

Phase I/II Study of CB-839 and Capecitabine in Patients With Advanced Solid Tumors and Fluoropyrimidine Resistant PIK3CA Mutant Colorectal Cancer

Brief Summary

This study has two portions. The main goal of the Phase I portion of this research study is to see what doses of CB-839 and capecitabine can safely be given to patients without having too many side effects. Other purposes of this research study will be to determine what side effects are seen with this combination of medicines. The Phase II portion of the study will test how many patients show shrinkage in their tumor with this combination of medicines and what changes occur inside the cancer cells and blood cells after treatment.

Detailed Description

Phase I Primary Objective:

To determine the safety, tolerability and recommended phase II dose (RP2D) of combination CB-839 and capecitabine chemotherapy in patients with advanced solid tumors for whom there are no remaining treatment options or for whom capecitabine is an acceptable therapy.

Phase II Primary Objective:

To determine the response rate of combination CB-839 and capecitabine chemotherapy in patients with metastatic PIK3CA mutant colorectal cancers who are refractory to fluoropyrimidine therapy.

Phase I Secondary Objectives:

To determine the dose-limiting toxicities and maximum tolerated dose of combination therapy with CB-839 and capecitabine in patients with advanced solid tumors for whom there are no remaining treatment options or for whom single agent capecitabine is an acceptable therapy.

To determine the antitumor response as assessed by RECIST criteria of combination therapy with CB-839 and capecitabine in patients with advanced solid tumors for whom there are no remaining treatment options or for whom single agent capecitabine is an acceptable therapy.

Phase II Secondary Objectives:

To determine the progression free survival following treatment with CB-839 and capecitabine chemotherapy in patients with metastatic PIK3CA mutant colorectal cancer and are refractory to fluoropyrimidine therapy.

To determine the overall survival following treatment with CB-839 and capecitabine chemotherapy in patients who have metastatic PIK3CA mutant colorectal cancer and are refractory to fluoropyrimidine therapy.

Study Type

Interventional

Study Phase

Phase 1/Phase 2

Condition

- Colorectal Cancer
- Colon Cancer
- Rectal Cancer
- Solid Tumor
-

Intervention

Drug: CB-839

Patients will receive CB-839 orally twice daily during each cycle. Each cycle will be 21 days long. Disease assessment will occur after cycle 3.

Drug: Capecitabine

capecitabine will be given orally twice daily for 14-21 days of cycles. Each cycle will be 21 days long. Disease assessment will occur after cycle 3.

Other Names:

Xeloda

Study Arms

Experimental: CB-839 + capecitabine

Patients will receive CB-839 orally twice daily for 21 days (continuous administration) and capecitabine orally twice daily for 14/21 days. In the phase I portion of the study, patients will receive escalating doses of CB-839 and capecitabine and will have day 15 blood samples drawn and archived for as needed assessment of CB-839 pharmacokinetics. In the phase II portion of the study, patients will receiving CB-839 and capecitabine at doses determined in the phase II portion of the study. They will also undergo pre-treatment and post-treatment blood samples and tissue biopsies for evaluation of pharmacodynamic biomarkers.

Recruitment Information

Recruitment Status

Recruiting

Estimated Enrollment

53

Completion Date

July 2020

Primary Completion Date

July 2018

Eligibility Criteria

Inclusion Criteria:

- Phase I
- Patients must have an advanced solid tumors for whom there are no remaining treatment options or colorectal patients who have progressed on front-line fluoropyrimidine containing therapy. Patients with colorectal cancer must have progressed on at least one line of fluoropyrimidine containing therapy. Receipt of either oxaliplatin or irinotecan in combination with a fluoropyrimidine is required in the front line setting for all colorectal cancer patients unless either of these agents are otherwise contraindicated in the opinion of the treating physician. Prior regorafenib or TAS-102 therapy is not required.
- Patients must have an Eastern Cooperative Oncology Group (ECOG) performance status of 0-1
- **Patients must have normal organ and marrow function as defined below:**
- Hemoglobin ≥ 9.0 g/dl
- Leukocytes ≥ 3,000/mcL
- Absolute neutrophil count ≥ 1,500/mcL
- Platelet count ≥ 100,000/mcL
- Serum creatinine ≤ 1.5 X institutional upper limit of normal
- Total bilirubin ≤ 1.5mg/dL
- Aspartate Aminotransferase (AST) serum glutamic oxaloacetic transaminase (SGOT) ≤ 2.5 X institutional upper limit of normal
- Alanine Aminotransferase (ALT) serum glutamic pyruvic transaminase (SGPT) ≤ 2.5 x institutional upper limit of normal
- Patients must be able to swallow pills.
- Patients must have the ability to understand and the willingness to sign a written informed consent document.
- Female patients of childbearing potential must have a negative serum or urine pregnancy test within 3 days prior to the first dose of study drug and agree to use dual methods of contraception during the study and for a minimum of 3 months following the last dose of study drug. Post-menopausal females (>45 years old and without menses for >1 year) and surgically sterilized

females are exempt from these requirements. Male patients must use an effective barrier method of contraception during the study and for a minimum of 3 months following the last dose of study drug if sexually active with a female of childbearing potential.

- Phase II
- Patients must have histologically or cytologically confirmed, phosphatidylinositol-4,5-bisphosphate 3-kinase catalytic subunit alpha (PIK3CA) mutant metastatic colorectal cancer. PIK3CA status must be confirmed by tumor sequencing in a CLIA certified lab.
- Patients must have measurable disease according to Response Evaluation Criteria In Solid Tumors (RECIST) 1.1 criteria that is amenable to biopsy and be willing to undergo preand post-treatment tumor biopsies. Lesions to be biopsied do not have to be those used for measurement.
- Patients must have received and progressed on fluoropyrimidine or fluoropyrimidine based therapy. Receipt of either oxaliplatin or irinotecan in combination with a fluoropyrimidine is required in the front line setting unless either of these agents are otherwise contraindicated in the opinion of the treating physician in which case a fluoropyrimidine only may be used. Prior regorafenib or TAS-102 therapy is not required.
- Patients must have an Eastern Cooperative Oncology Group (ECOG) performance status of 0-1.
- Patients must have normal organ and marrow function as defined below:
- Hemoglobin ≥ 9.0 g/dl
- Leukocytes ≥ 3,000/mcL
- Absolute neutrophil count ≥ 1,500/mcL
- Platelet count ≥ 100,000/mcL
- Serum creatinine within normal institutional limits
- Total bilirubin ≤ 1.5 mg/dL
- AST (SGOT) ≤ 2.5 X institutional upper limit of normal
- ALT (SGPT) ≤ 2.5 x institutional upper limit of normal
- Patients must be able to swallow pills.
- Patients must have the ability to understand and the willingness to sign a written informed consent document.
- Female patients of childbearing potential must have a negative serum or urine pregnancy test within 3 days prior to the first dose of study drug and agree to use dual methods of contraception during the study and for a minimum of 3 months following the last dose of study drug. Post-menopausal females (>45 years old and without menses for >1 year) and surgically sterilized females are exempt from these requirements. Male patients must use an effective barrier method of contraception during the study and for a minimum of 3 months following the last dose of study drug if sexually active with a female of childbearing potential.

Exclusion Criteria:

- Both Phase I and Phase II
- Patients with ongoing toxicities > grade 1 according to National Cancer Institute (NCI) Common Terminology Criteria For Adverse Events (CTCAE) Version 4.0 (excluding alopecia) due to prior anti-cancer therapy.
- Patients receiving any other investigational agents or whom have received recent treatment for colorectal cancer (radiation within the previous two weeks, chemotherapy or investigational therapy within the previous four weeks).
- Patients with untreated brain metastases/central nervous system disease will be excluded due to their poor prognosis and because they often develop progressive neurologic dysfunction that would confound the evaluation of neurologic and other adverse events.
- Patients with a history of allergic reactions attributed to or intolerance to compounds of similar chemical or biologic composition to either CB-839 or capecitabine. If capecitabine has been received previously, must have tolerated at least an equivalent dose to the dose to be administered at their assigned dose level.
- Patients who are unable to swallow pills or who have undergone surgery that prohibits the absorption of pills in the stomach.
- Patients with uncontrolled intercurrent illness including, but not limited to ongoing or active infection, symptomatic congestive heart failure, unstable angina pectoris or myocardial infarction within prior 6 months, cardiac arrhythmia, or psychiatric illness/social situations that would limit compliance with study requirements.
- Patients who are pregnant or breastfeeding will be excluded from the study.
- Patients known to be HIV positive who are not receiving anti-retroviral therapy will be excluded due to the marrow suppressive therapy involved in administration of the study treatment.

■ Sex/Gender

All

■ Ages

19 Years to N/A

■ Accepts Healthy Volunteers

No

■ Contacts

Jennifer Eads, MD   216-844-6031   jennifer.eads@uhhospitals.org

Resection Versus Microwave Ablation for Resectable Colorectal Cancer Liver Metastases

Study ID:

NCT02866344

Sponsor:

Carolinas Healthcare System

Information provided by (Responsible Party):

Carolinas Healthcare System (Carolinas Healthcare System)

Tracking Information

■ **First Submitted Date**

August 10, 2016

■ **Start Date**

August 2016

■ **Primary Completion Date**

January 2019

■ **Last Update Posted Date**

July 19, 2017

■ **Current Primary Outcome Measures**

Local disease control at the site of intervention[Time Frame: 2 years]

Local disease control is measured from time of randomization and is defined as the absence of local recurrence of metastatic adenocarcinoma of the colon or rectum as determined by diagnostic imaging.

■ **Current Secondary Outcome Measures**

Overall survival[Time Frame: 1, 2, 3, 5 years]

Intrahepatic disease-free survival[Time Frame: 1, 2, 3, 5 years]

Postoperative morbidity[Time Frame: 1 month and 3 months]

Postoperative mortality[Time Frame: 1 month and 3 months]

Descriptive Information

■ **Offical Title**

Prospective Randomized Comparison of Resection and Microwave Ablation for Resectable Colorectal Cancer Liver Metastases

■ **Brief Summary**

This single-center, prospective, randomized clinical trial is designed to compare the clinical characteristics and outcomes of hepatic resection and microwave ablation (MWA) to determine the optimal operative intervention for the local treatment of resectable colorectal cancer liver metastases. The primary aim of this study is to test the following hypothesis: 2-year local disease control is equivalent between patients receiving the experimental therapy (MWA) and patients receiving the standard therapy (hepatic resection) as treatment for colorectal cancer liver metastases determined to be resectable by radiographic imaging. Secondarily, the investigators expect that 2-year intrahepatic (regional) and metastatic disease recurrence rates are equivalent between the two treatment arms in this study.

■ **Study Type**

Interventional

■ **Study Phase**

N/A

■ **Condition**

- Colorectal Neoplasms
- Neoplasm Metastasis
- Hepatic Neoplasms

■ **Intervention**

Device: Microwave ablation

Laparoscopic or robot-assisted laparoscopic microwave ablation of cancerous lesions with a 2.45-GHz microwave generator and a 1.8-mm-diameter transcutaneous antenna.

Procedure: Hepatic resection

Laparoscopic or robot-assisted laparoscopic surgical resection of cancerous lesions.

Other Names:
Surgery

Study Arms

Experimental: Microwave ablation

Patients will be given general anesthesia. A laparoscopic trocar and additional ports will be placed under direct visualization and pneumoperitoneum will be established. Once the operating surgeon determines that the lesions as evaluated on intraoperative ultrasound remain amenable to MWA, ablations will be performed with a 2.45-GHz generator with a 1.8-mm-diameter transcutaneous antenna (Acculis pMTA Accu2i; AngioDynamics Inc., Denmead, Hampshire, UK). Additional ablations will be performed sequentially. Laparoscopic core needle biopsy of lesions will be performed and submitted for permanent pathologic sectioning per current treatment standards. At the conclusion of the ablation, a collapsed titanium clip will be inserted into the microwave antenna tract as a radiographic fiducial marker. Hemostasis of the ablation track will be ensured using a combination of microwave energy, monopolar electrocautery, and/or topical hemostatics.

Active Comparator: Hepatic resection

General anesthesia will be induced. A laparoscopic trocar and additional ports will be placed under direct visualization and pneumoperitoneum will be established. The liver will be evaluated with intraoperative ultrasound (BK Medical A/S, Herlev, Denmark). Laparoscopic core needle biopsy of lesions will be performed. Partial hepatectomy may be carried out with parenchymal precoagulation with radiofrequency electrosurgical devices such as the LigaSure™ (Covidien, Medtronic; Minneapolis, MN), Harmonic® (Ethicon Endosurgery; Cincinnati, OH), or saline-coupled radiofrequency ablation device (Aquamantys™; Covidien/Medtronic; Minneapolis, MN); hepatic parenchymal transection can be performed as above or with the use of stapling devices to ligate and divide parenchyma. Hepatic vascular inflow occlusion will be performed at the surgeon's discretion. A topical hemostatic may be used along the transected hepatic parenchyma. Resected specimens will be preserved in formalin for pathology.

Recruitment Information

Recruitment Status

Recruiting

Estimated Enrollment

164

Completion Date

January 2022

Primary Completion Date

January 2019

Eligibility Criteria

Inclusion Criteria:

- Diagnosis of adenocarcinoma of the colon or rectum (diagnosed at the time of colon or rectal resection or on endoscopic biopsy) with liver metastases (by liver biopsy or by history of biopsy-proven colon/rectal cancer with characteristic imaging findings):
- Imaging showing typical features of colorectal cancer liver metastasis;
- Cytologic/histologic diagnosis of colorectal cancer or colorectal cancer liver metastasis.
- No more than 3 hepatic metastatic lesions noted on preoperative imaging
- No lesion greater than 5 cm in maximal dimension
- Adequate clinical condition to undergo laparoscopic or robot-assisted laparoscopic liver resection or microwave ablation as treatment for colorectal cancer liver metastases
- Willing and able to give informed consent

Exclusion Criteria:

- Radiologic (computed tomography or magnetic resonance imaging) evidence of invasion into major portal/hepatic venous branches and no extrahepatic metastases
- Evidence of recurrent disease adjacent to a previous ablation or resection site
- Severe renal dysfunction (creatinine clearance of <40 mL/min)
- Pregnant or nursing women

Sex/Gender

All

Ages

18 Years to 75 Years

Capecitabine and Bevacizumab With or Without Atezolizumab in Treating Patients With Refractory Metastatic Colorectal Cancer

Study ID:

NCT02873195

Sponsor:

Academic and Community Cancer Research United

Information provided by (Responsible Party):

Academic and Community Cancer Research United (Academic and Community Cancer Research United)

Tracking Information

■ **First Submitted Date**

August 16, 2016

■ **Start Date**

July 7, 2017

■ **Primary Completion Date**

November 30, 2020

■ **Last Update Posted Date**

December 18, 2017

■ **Current Primary Outcome Measures**

Progression free survival (PFS) assessed by Response Evaluation Criteria in Solid Tumors (RECIST) version (v) 1.1[Time Frame: From study entry until documented clinical progression, or death from any cause, assessed up to 4 years]

Log rank test will be used to conduct the primary test of hypothesis, superiority PFS for atezolizumab versus placebo. Kaplan-Meier method will be used to estimate PFS within treatment arms. The 95% confidence interval estimates of PFS at 3 months will also be constructed based on the Kaplan-Meier estimate using Greenwood?s formula. The Cox model will be used to study the potential impact of baseline demographics and tumor characteristics on PFS.

■ **Current Secondary Outcome Measures**

Objective response rate defined as partial response plus compete response as assessed using RECIST v 1.1 and immune-related response criteria (irRC)[Time Frame: Up to 4 years]

Will be compared between the two treatment arms (atezolizumab and placebo) using Fisher?s Exact test.

Overall survival (OS)[Time Frame: From study entry until death from any cause, assessed up to 4 years]

Will be compared between the two treatment arms (atezolizumab and placebo). Kaplan-Meier estimates of OS will be provided. The Cox model will be used to study the potential impact of baseline demographics and tumor characteristics on OS.

Descriptive Information

■ **Offical Title**

BACCI: A Phase II Randomized, Double-Blind, Placebo-Controlled Study of Capecitabine Bevacizumab Plus Atezolizumab Versus Capecitabine Bevacizumab Plus Placebo in Patients With Refractory Metastatic Colorectal Cancer

■ **Brief Summary**

This randomized phase II trial studies how well atezolizumab and capecitabine with or without bevacizumab work in treating patients with colorectal cancer that is not responding to treatment and has spread to other places. Monoclonal antibodies, such as atezolizumab and bevacizumab, may interfere with the ability of tumor cells to grow and spread. Drugs used in chemotherapy, such as capecitabine, work in different ways to stop the growth of tumor cells, either by killing the cells, by stopping them from dividing, or by stopping them from spreading. Giving atezolizumab with capecitabine and bevacizumab may be a better way in treating colorectal cancer.

■ **Detailed Description**

PRIMARY OBJECTIVES:

I. To estimate the efficacy of capecitabine/bevacizumab + atezolizumab, as compared with capecitabine/bevacizumab + placebo in refractory metastatic colorectal cancer (mCRC) as measured by progression-free survival (defined as the time of randomization to the first occurrence of progression based on Response Evaluation Criteria in Solid Tumors version 1.1, clinical

336

progression, or death from any cause on study as determined by the investigator).

SECONDARY OBJECTIVES:

I. To estimate the efficacy of capecitabine/bevacizumab + atezolizumab, as compared with capecitabine/bevacizumab + placebo in refractory mCRC as measured by objective response rate (defined as partial response plus complete response) as determined by the investigator using Response Evaluation Criteria in Solid Tumors version 1.1 and immune-related response criteria (irRC).

II. To estimate the efficacy of capecitabine/bevacizumab + atezolizumab as compared with capecitabine/bevacizumab + placebo in refractory mCRC as measured by overall survival (defined as death from any cause from the time of randomization until study completion).

III. To evaluate the safety and tolerability of atezolizumab in combination with bevacizumab and capecitabine in refractory mCRC as measured by the serious adverse events and adverse events >= grade 3 according to National Cancer Institute Common Terminology Criteria for Adverse Events version 4.0.

TERTIARY OBJECTIVES:

I. To explore any correlation between tissue and blood based biomarkers and clinical outcomes.

OUTLINE: Patients are randomized 2:1 to Arm I:Arm II.

ARM I (ATEZOLIZUMAB, BEVACIZUMAB, CAPECITABINE): Patients receive atezolizumab intravenously (IV) over 60 minutes on day 1, bevacizumab IV over 30-90 minutes on day 1, and capecitabine orally (PO) twice daily (BID) on days 1-14. Courses repeat every 21 days in the absence of disease progression or unacceptable toxicity.

ARM II (PLACEBO, BEVACIZUMAB, CAPECITABINE): Patients receive placebo IV over 60 minutes on day 1, bevacizumab IV over 30-90 minutes on day 1, and capecitabine PO BID on days 1-14. Courses repeat every 21 days in the absence of disease progression or unacceptable toxicity.

After completion of study treatment, patients are followed up at 30 days and every 12 weeks thereafter.

▨ **Study Type**

Interventional

▨ **Study Phase**

Phase 2

▨ **Condition**

- Recurrent Colorectal Carcinoma
- Stage IV Colorectal Cancer AJCC v7
- Stage IVA Colorectal Cancer AJCC v7
- Stage IVB Colorectal Cancer AJCC v7
-

▨ **Intervention**

Drug: Atezolizumab
   Given IV

Other Names:
   MPDL 3280A

   MPDL 328OA

   MPDL-3280A

   MPDL3280A

   MPDL328OA

   RG7446

   RO5541267

   Tecentriq

Biological: Bevacizumab
   Given IV

Other Names:
   Anti-VEGF

   Anti-VEGF Humanized Monoclonal Antibody

   Anti-VEGF rhuMAb

   Avastin

   Bevacizumab Biosimilar BEVZ92

Bevacizumab Biosimilar BI 695502

Bevacizumab Biosimilar CBT 124

Bevacizumab Biosimilar FKB238

Immunoglobulin G1 (Human-Mouse Monoclonal rhuMab-VEGF Gamma-Chain Anti-Human Vascular Endothelial Growth Factor), Disulfide With Human-Mouse Monoclonal rhuMab-VEGF Light Chain, Dimer

Recombinant Humanized Anti-VEGF Monoclonal Antibody

rhuMab-VEGF

Drug: Capecitabine
Given PO

Other Names:
Ro 09-1978/000

Xeloda

Other: Laboratory Biomarker Analysis
Correlative studies

Other: Placebo
Given IV

Other Names:
placebo therapy

PLCB

sham therapy

Study Arms

Experimental: Arm I (atezolizumab, bevacizumab, capecitabine)

Patients receive atezolizumab IV over 60 minutes on day 1, bevacizumab IV over 30-90 minutes on day 1, and capecitabine PO BID on days 1-14. Courses repeat every 21 days in the absence of disease progression or unacceptable toxicity.

Active Comparator: Arm II (placebo, bevacizumab, capecitabine)

Patients receive placebo IV over 60 minutes on day 1, bevacizumab IV over 30-90 minutes on day 1, and capecitabine PO BID on days 1-14. Courses repeat every 21 days in the absence of disease progression or unacceptable toxicity.

Recruitment Information

Recruitment Status

Recruiting

Estimated Enrollment

135

Completion Date

November 30, 2020

Primary Completion Date

November 30, 2020

Eligibility Criteria

Inclusion Criteria:

- Histologically confirmed metastatic colorectal cancer that has progressed on regimens containing a fluoropyrimidine (e.g., 5-fluorouracil or capecitabine), oxaliplatin, irinotecan, bevacizumab and an anti-EGFR antibody (if tumor is RAS wild-type), or where the treatment was not tolerated or contraindicated
- Measurable disease; Note: previously irradiated sites can be included if there is documented disease progression in that site
- Capecitabine and bevacizumab considered appropriate treatment for the patient
- Eastern Cooperative Oncology Group (ECOG) performance status (PS) 0-1
- Absolute neutrophil count >= 1,500/uL obtained =< 7 days prior to randomization
- Platelets >= 100,000/uL obtained =< 7 days prior to randomization
- Total bilirubin =< 1.5 X upper limit of normal (ULN) obtained =< 7 days prior to randomization; patients with known Gilbert?s syndrome who have serum bilirubin =< 3 X ULN may enroll
- Aspartate aminotransferase (AST)/alanine aminotransferase (ALT) =< 1.5 X ULN; < 3 X ULN if known hepatic metastases
- Hemoglobin >= 9 g/dL continuation of erythropoietin products is permitted obtained =< 7 days prior to randomization; hemoglobin must be stable >= 9 g/dL >= 14 days without blood transfusion to maintain hemoglobin level
- Calculated creatinine clearance must be >= 50 ml/min using the Cockcroft-Gault formula or a 24 hour urine obtained =< 7 days prior to randomization
- The following laboratory values obtained =< 14 days prior to randomization

- Prothrombin time (PT)/partial thromboplastin time (PTT)/international normalized ratio (INR) =< 1.5 X ULN if not anticoagulated; within local institutional guidelines per local physician if anticoagulated
- Negative pregnancy test done =< 7 days prior to randomization, for women of childbearing potential only
- Provide informed written consent
- Willingness to return to enrolling institution for follow-up (during the active monitoring phase of the study)
- Willingness to provide tissue and blood samples for correlative research purposes
- Life expectancy of >= 3 months

Exclusion Criteria:
- Any of the following:
- Pregnant women
- Nursing women
- Women of child-bearing potential must agree to use two forms of adequate contraception from time of initial consent, for the duration of study participation, and for >= 6 months after the last dose of study drug; medically acceptable contraceptives include: (1) surgical sterilization (such as a tubal ligation or hysterectomy), (2) approved hormonal contraceptives (such as birth control pills, patches, implants or injections), (3) barrier methods (such as a condom or diaphragm) used with a spermicide, or (4) an intrauterine device (IUD); contraceptive measures such as Plan B, sold for emergency use after unprotected sex, are not acceptable methods for routine use; postmenopausal woman must have been amenorrheic for at least 2 years to be considered of non-childbearing potential; sexually active men must use at least one form of adequate contraception from time of initial consent, for the duration of study participation, and for >= 6 months after the last dose of study drug
- Chemotherapy, biologic anti-cancer therapy, or central field radiation therapy =< 28 days prior to randomization; Note: local or stereotactic radiation =< 14 days prior to randomization
- Any investigational agent =< 28 days or 5 half-lives prior to randomization (whichever is longer)
- Prior treatment with atezolizumab or another PD-L1/PD-1 therapy
- History of allergic reactions attributed to therapeutic antibodies; Note: patients with reactions to chimeric antibodies may be permitted on a case by case basis with approval by study chair by contacting the data manager
- Known untreated central nervous system (CNS) metastases; Note: patients with radiated or resected lesions are permitted, provided the lesions are fully treated and inactive, patients are asymptomatic, and no steroids have been administered for this purpose =< 30 days prior to randomization
- Inadequately controlled hypertension (defined as average systolic blood pressure > 150 mmHg and/or diastolic blood pressure > 100 mmHg)
- History of hypertensive crisis or hypertensive encephalopathy
- New York Heart Association (NYHA) grade II or greater congestive heart failure
- History of myocardial infarction, unstable angina, cardiac or other vascular stenting, angioplasty, or surgery =< 12 months prior to randomization
- Active coronary heart disease evidenced as angina or requiring medications to prevent angina
- History of stroke or transient ischemic attack, or other arterial thrombosis =< 12 months prior to randomization
- Symptomatic peripheral vascular disease
- Any other significant vascular disease (e.g., aortic aneurysm, aortic dissection, or carotid stenosis that requires medical or surgical intervention, including angioplasty or stenting)
- Any previous National Cancer Institute (NCI) Common Terminology Criteria for Adverse Events (CTCAE) grade 4 venous thromboembolism
- Clinically-significant evidence of bleeding diathesis or coagulopathy as so judged by the treating physician
- History of active gastrointestinal (GI) bleeding or other major bleeding =< 12 months prior to randomization; Note: patients who do not have resolution of the predisposing risk factor (e.g., resection of a bleeding tumor, treatment and endoscopic documentation of a resolved ulcer) will also be excluded
- Major surgical procedure, open biopsy, or significant traumatic injury =< 56 days prior to randomization
- Anticipation of need for major surgical procedure =< 6 months after randomization
- Minor surgical procedure =< 7 days prior to randomization; exception: insertion of an indwelling catheter or percutaneous needle biopsy =< 48 hours prior to randomization
- History of intra-abdominal abscess =< 6 months prior to randomization; Note: if the affected area was surgically resected, and there is no further risk to the area, patients may enroll
- History of abdominal or other significant fistula, gastrointestinal or other organ perforation; Note: if the affected area was surgically resected, and there is no further risk to the area, patients may enroll
- Serious, non-healing wound, ulcer, or bone fracture as so judged by the treating physician
- Known proteinuria defined by >= 2+ protein by urinalysis (UA) or >= 1 gram protein by 24 hour urine collection
- Intolerance to bevacizumab defined as any NCI CTCAE grade 3 or grade 4 toxicity attributed to this agent that required discontinuation of bevacizumab (e.g., arterial thromboembolism [ATE], perforation, wound healing difficulty, proteinuria, reversible posterior leukoencephalopathy syndrome [RPLS]); Note: patients with prior grade 3 bevacizumab-related hypertension may be permitted if hypertension was manageable with standard oral antihypertensives as so judged by the treating physician

- Known dihydropyrimidine dehydrogenase (DPD) deficiency
- Impairment of GI function or GI disease that may significantly alter capecitabine drug absorption
- Active inflammatory bowel disease
- History of diverticulitis, chronic ulcerative lower GI disease such as Crohn?s disease or ulcerative colitis, or other symptomatic lower GI conditions that might predispose to perforations
- History of autoimmune disease including, but not limited to, systemic lupus erythematosus, rheumatoid arthritis, inflammatory bowel disease, vascular thrombosis associated with antiphospholipid syndrome, Wegener?s granulomatosis, Sjogren?s syndrome, Bell?s palsy, Guillain-Barre syndrome, multiple sclerosis, autoimmune thyroid disease, vasculitis, or glomerulonephritis; Note: patients with a history of autoimmune-related hypothyroidism on a stable dose of thyroid replacement hormone may be eligible for this study
- Active current infection or history of recurrent bacterial, viral, fungal, mycobacterial or other infections, including but not limited to tuberculosis and atypical mycobacterial disease, hepatitis B and C, herpes zoster, and HIV, but excluding fungal infections of nail beds
- Vaccination with a live or attenuated vaccine =< 28 days prior to randomization; Note: other types of vaccines, including inactivated/killed, toxoid (inactivated toxoid), and subunit/conjugate are all permitted at any time
- Any reversible treatment-related toxicity that has not resolved to NCI CTCAE grade =< 1 except neuropathy
- Other concurrent severe and/or uncontrolled medical disease, psychiatric illness, or social situation, which could compromise safety of treatment as so judged by the treating physician; Note: this includes but is not limited to: severely impaired lung function, uncontrolled diabetes (history of consistent blood glucose readings above 300 mg/dL or less than 50 mg/dL), severe infection, severe malnutrition, ventricular arrhythmias, known active vasculitis of any cause, tumor invasion of any major blood vessel, chronic liver or renal disease, and active upper GI tract ulceration
- Unwilling to or unable to comply with the protocol
- Current or recent (=< 10 days prior to randomization) use of aspirin (> 325 mg/day), or clopidogrel (> 75 mg/day)
- Current or recent (=< 10 days prior to randomization) use of therapeutic oral or parenteral anticoagulants or thrombolytic agents for therapeutic purposes, unless the patient has been on a stable dose of anticoagulants for at least 2 weeks at the time of randomization; Note: the use of full-dose oral or parenteral anticoagulants is permitted as long as the INR or activated partial thromboplastin time (aPTT) is within therapeutic limits (according to the medical standard of the institution) and the patient has been on a stable dose of anticoagulants >= 14 days at the time of randomization; prophylactic use of anticoagulants is allowed
- History or recent diagnosis of demyelinating disease
- History of other carcinoma =< 3 years; exception: if risk of recurrence is known to be under 5% at time of randomization
- Current or recent (=< 90 days prior to randomization) endoluminal stent in the stomach, bowel, colon or rectum
- Colonoscopy, sigmoidoscopy, or proctoscopy =< 7 days prior to randomization
- Current or recent (=< 28 days prior to randomization) use of sorivudine, brivudine, and St. John?s wort
- Primary or secondary immunodeficiency (history of or currently active) unless related to primary disease under investigation
- Prior allogeneic bone marrow transplantation or prior solid organ transplantation
- Treatment with systemic immunosuppressive medications (including but not limited to prednisone, cyclophosphamide, azathioprine, methotrexate, thalidomide, and anti-tumor necrosis factor [anti-TNF] agents) =< 14 days prior to randomization; exception: patients who have received acute, low-dose, systemic immunosuppressant medications (e.g. a one-time dose of dexamethasone for nausea) are eligible; the use of inhaled corticosteroids and mineral-corticoids (e.g. fludrocortisone) for patients with orthostatic hypotension or adrenocortical insufficiency is allowed

■ Sex/Gender

All

■ Ages

18 Years to N/A

■ Accepts Healthy Volunteers

No

Study of Cobimetinib in Combination With Atezolizumab and Bevacizumab in Participants With Gastrointestinal and Other Tumors

Study ID:

NCT02876224

Sponsor:

Hoffmann-La Roche

Information provided by (Responsible Party):

Hoffmann-La Roche (Hoffmann-La Roche)

Tracking Information

First Submitted Date

August 18, 2016

Start Date

September 30, 2016

Primary Completion Date

December 15, 2018

Last Update Posted Date

December 18, 2017

Current Primary Outcome Measures

Percentage of Participants with Adverse Events[Time Frame: Baseline up to approximately 12 months]

Current Secondary Outcome Measures

Plasma Maximum Concentration (Cmax) of Cobimetinib[Time Frame: Safety run-in phase and expansion cohort: Predose (0 hours) on Cycle 1 Day 15 and Cycle 3 Day 15; 2 to 4 hours postdose on Cycle 1 Day 1 and Cycle 3 Day 15. Biopsy cohort: 0-2 hours predose and 2-4 hours postdose on Cycle 2 Day 1. Each cycle is 28 days.]

Plasma Minimum Concentration (Cmin) of Cobimetinib[Time Frame: Safety run-in phase and expansion cohort: Predose (0 hours) on Cycle 1 Day 15 and Cycle 3 Day 15; 2 to 4 hours postdose on Cycle 1 Day 1 and Cycle 3 Day 15. Biopsy cohort: 0-2 hours predose and 2-4 hours postdose on Cycle 2 Day 1. Each cycle is 28 days.]

Serum Cmax of Atezolizumab[Time Frame: Baseline up to approximately 12 months (detailed sample collection timepoints are provided in outcome measure description field)]

Safety run-in phase and expansion cohort: Prior to the infusion (0 hours) on Day 1 of Cycles 1, 2, 4, 8, every 8 cycles thereafter (maximum up to 12 months) and on Day 15 of Cycle 3; 30 minutes after end of infusion (infusion duration 30-60 minutes) on Cycle 1 Day 1 and Cycle 3 Day 15; at treatment discontinuation visit (up to 12 months). Biopsy cohort: prior to the infusion (0 hours) on Day 1 of Cycles 3, 5, 9, every 8 cycles thereafter (maximum up to 12 months) and on Day 15 of Cycle 4; 30 minutes after end of infusion on Day 15 of Cycle 4; at treatment discontinuation visit (up to 12 months). Each cycle is 28 days.

Serum Cmin of Atezolizumab[Time Frame: Baseline up to approximately 12 months (detailed sample collection timepoints are provided in outcome measure description field)]

Safety run-in phase and expansion cohort: Prior to the infusion (0 hours) on Day 1 of Cycles 1, 2, 4, 8, every 8 cycles thereafter (maximum up to 12 months) and on Day 15 of Cycle 3; 30 minutes after end of infusion (infusion duration 30-60 minutes) on Cycle 1 Day 1 and Cycle 3 Day 15; at treatment discontinuation visit (up to 12 months). Biopsy cohort: prior to the infusion (0 hours) on Day 1 of Cycles 3, 5, 9, every 8 cycles thereafter (maximum up to 12 months) and on Day 15 of Cycle 4; 30 minutes after end of infusion on Day 15 of Cycle 4; at treatment discontinuation visit (up to 12 months). Each cycle is 28 days.

Serum Cmin of Bevacizumab[Time Frame: Safety run-in phase and expansion cohort: prior to the infusion (0 hours) on Cycle 3 Day 15. Biopsy cohort: prior to the infusion (0 hours) on Cycle 3 Day 1. Each cycle is 28 days.]

Percentage of Participants with Anti-therapeutic Antibodies (ATAs) Response to Atezolizumab[Time Frame: Baseline up to approximately 12 months (detailed sample collection timepoints are provided in outcome measure description field)]

Safety run-in phase and expansion cohort: Prior to the infusion (0 hours) on Day 1 of Cycle 1, 2, 4, 8, and every 8 cycles thereafter (maximum up to 12 months) and on Day 15 of Cycle 3; 30 minutes after end of infusion (infusion duration 30-60 minutes) on Cycle 3 Day 15; at treatment discontinuation visit (up to 12 months). Biopsy cohort: prior to the infusion (0 hours) on Day 1 of Cycles 3, 5, 9, every 8 cycles thereafter (maximum up to 12 months) and on Day 15 of Cycle 4; 30 minutes after end of infusion on Day 15 of Cycle 4; at treatment discontinuation visit (up to 12 months). Each cycle is 28 days.

Descriptive Information

Offical Title

A Phase Ib Open-Label Study Evaluating the Safety, Tolerability and Pharmacokinetics of Cobimetinib in Combination With Bevacizumab and Immunotherapy When Administered in Patients With Gastrointestinal and Other Tumors

Brief Summary

This is an open-label, multicenter, single-arm, two-stage, Phase Ib study designed to assess the safety, tolerability, and pharmacokinetics of oral cobimetinib with intravenous (IV) atezolizumab and bevacizumab in participants with metastatic colorectal cancer (mCRC) who have received and progressed on at least one prior line of therapy that contained a fluoropyrimidine and oxaliplatin or irinotecan. There are two stages in this study: Stage 1 (safety run-in phase) and Stage 2 (dose expansion phase with two cohorts, an expansion cohort and a biopsy cohort).

Study Type

Interventional

Study Phase

Phase 1

Condition

- Colorectal Cancer

Intervention

Drug: Atezolizumab

Atezolizumab 840 mg will be administered by IV infusion on Days 1 and 15 of each 28-day cycle.

Other Names:

RO5541267

Drug: Bevacizumab

Bevacizumab 5 mg/kg will be administered by IV infusion on Days 1 and 15 of each 28-day cycle.

Other Names:

RO4876646

Drug: Cobimetinib

Cobimetinib 60 mg or at dose determined during safety run-in phase will be administered orally once daily for 21 days of each 28-day cycle as specified in the arm descriptions.

Other Names:

RO5514041

Study Arms

Experimental: Cobimetinib + Bevacizumab + Atezolizumab (Stage 1: SRP)

Stage 1 Safety Run-in Phase (SRP): Approximately 12 participants will receive cobimetinib 60 milligrams (mg) orally once daily for Days 1-21 with atezolizumab 840 mg and bevacizumab 5 milligrams per kilogram (mg/kg) administered by IV infusion on Days 1 and 15 of each 28-day cycle. Atezolizumab will be administered first, followed by bevacizumab, with a minimum of 60 minutes between dosing. Upon determination of the safety and tolerability of the treatment regimen, the study will proceed to Stage 2: dose expansion phase. If the results from the safety run-in phase require dose reduction in cobimetinib, then an additional Stage 1 cohort will be opened. Treatment will continue until the participant has disease progression according to Response Evaluation Criteria in Solid Tumors Version 1.1 (RECIST v1.1), unacceptable toxicity, death, participant or physician decision to withdraw, or pregnancy, whichever occurs first.

Experimental: Cobimetinib + Bevacizumab + Atezolizumab (Stage 2: BC)

Stage 2 Biopsy Cohort (BC): Approximately 7 evaluable participants in the biopsy cohort in expansion phase will receive bevacizumab 5 mg/kg IV on Cycle 1 Days 1 and 15 (tumor biopsy on Cycle 1 Day 8) and cobimetinib (at dose determined during safety run-in phase) orally on Cycle 1 Day 15 to Cycle 2 Day 14 (tumor biopsy on Cycle 1 Day 22). From Cycle 2 onwards, participants will follow the same treatment regimen for bevacizumab and atezolizumab (optional tumor biopsy on Cycle 2 Day 22) as those in the safety run-in phase and expansion cohort, and for cobimetinib cycles start at Day 15 and will continue 21 days to Day 7 of next cycle. Atezolizumab will be administered first, followed by bevacizumab, with a minimum of 60 minutes between dosing. Biopsies must be collected before the initiation of cobimetinib and atezolizumab. Treatment will continue until disease progression according to RECIST v1.1, unacceptable toxicity, death, decision to withdraw, or pregnancy, whichever occurs first.

Experimental: Cobimetinib + Bevacizumab + Atezolizumab (Stage 2: EC)

Stage 2 Expansion Cohort (EC): Approximately 14 participants will receive cobimetinib (at dose determined during safety run-in phase) orally once daily for Days 1-21 with atezolizumab 840 mg and bevacizumab 5 mg/kg administered by IV infusion on Days 1 and 15 of each 28-day cycle. Atezolizumab will be administered first, followed by bevacizumab, with a minimum of 60 minutes between dosing. Treatment will continue until the participant has disease progression according to RECIST v1.1, unacceptable toxicity, death, participant or physician decision to withdraw, or pregnancy, whichever occurs first.

Recruitment Information

Recruitment Status

Recruiting

Estimated Enrollment

48

Completion Date

February 14, 2020

Primary Completion Date

December 15, 2018

Eligibility Criteria

Inclusion Criteria:

- Eastern Cooperative Oncology Group performance status of 0 or 1
- Histologically confirmed unresectable metastatic colorectal adenocarcinoma
- Life expectancy at least 12 weeks

- Progression on a prior line of therapy that contained a fluoropyrimidine and oxaliplatin or irinotecan for unresectable metastatic colorectal adenocarcinoma
- Measurable disease per RECIST v1.1
- Adequate hematologic and end organ function
- Creatinine clearance greater than or equal to (>=) 30 milliliters per minute (mL/min)
- For biopsy cohort, participants must be bevacizumab naive or received the last bevacizumab treatment at least 12 months prior to Cycle 1 Day 1 and according to the investigator's judgment the planned biopsies would not expose participants to substantially increased risk of complications
- For women of childbearing potential, agreement to remain abstinent (refrain from heterosexual intercourse) or use of contraceptive methods that result in a failure rate of less than (<) 1 percent (%) per year during the treatment period and for at least 180 days after the last study treatment
- For men, agreement to remain abstinent (refrain from heterosexual intercourse) or use contraceptive measures, and agreement to refrain from donating sperm

Exclusion Criteria:

- More than one prior line of systemic therapy for advanced CRC
- Participants with known microsatellite (MSI)-high status
- Major surgery or significant traumatic injury within 60 days prior to enrollment
- Minor surgical procedure within 15 days of study Cycle 1 Day 1
- Untreated central nervous system (CNS) metastases
- Treatment with any investigational agent or approved therapy within 28 days
- Malignancies other than colorectal cancer within 5 years prior to Cycle 1 Day 1
- Prior radiation therapy within 30 days prior to study Cycle 1 Day 1 and/or persistence of radiation-related adverse effects
- Prior allogeneic bone marrow transplantation or solid organ transplant for another malignancy in the past
- Spinal cord compression not definitively treated with surgery and/or radiation
- Uncontrolled pleural effusion, pericardial effusion, or ascites requiring recurrent drainage procedures
- Current or recent use of therapeutic oral or parenteral anticoagulants or thrombolytic agents
- Intake of St. John's wort or hyperforin (potent cytochrome P450 [CYP] 3A4 enzyme inducer) or grapefruit juice (potent CYP3A4 enzyme inhibitor) within 7 days prior to initiation of study treatment
- History of severe allergic, anaphylactic, or other hypersensitivity reactions to chimeric or humanized antibodies or fusion proteins
- Known hypersensitivity or allergy to biopharmaceuticals produced in Chinese hamster ovary cells or any components of cobimetinib, atezolizumab, or bevacizumab formulations
- Prior treatment with clusters of differentiation (CD) 137 (CD137) agonists or immune checkpoint blockage therapies, anti-programmed death protein-1, anti-program death-ligand 1, mitogen-activated protein kinase (MEK) inhibitor
- Proteinuria value > 1.0 g at screening
- Uncontrolled glaucoma with intraocular pressure ≥ 21 mmHg
- Hyperglycemia (fasting) ≥ Grade 2
- Human Immunodeficiency Virus (HIV) infection
- Active hepatitis B or hepatitis C
- History of autoimmune disease, clinically significant cardiac or pulmonary dysfunction
- Administration of a live, attenuated vaccine within 4 weeks prior to Cycle 1 Day 1 or at any time during the study and for at least 5 months after the last dose of study drug
- History of or evidence of retinal pathology on ophthalmologic examination that is considered a risk factor for neurosensory retinal detachment/central serous chorioretinopathy, retinal vein occlusion, or neovascular macular degeneration
- History of idiopathic pulmonary fibrosis, organizing pneumonia, drug-induced pneumonitis, or idiopathic pneumonitis
- Uncontrolled tumor pain

Sex/Gender

All

Ages

18 Years to N/A

Accepts Healthy Volunteers

No

Contacts

Reference Study ID Number: CO39083 www.roche.com/about roche/roche worldwide.htm 888-662-6728 (U.S. and Canada) global-roche-genentech-trials@gene.com

Durvalumab and Tremelimumab With or Without High or Low-Dose Radiation Therapy in Treating Patients With Metastatic Colorectal or Non-small Cell Lung Cancer

Study ID:

NCT02888743

Sponsor:

National Cancer Institute (NCI)

Information provided by (Responsible Party):

National Cancer Institute (NCI) (National Cancer Institute (NCI))

Tracking Information

▦ **First Submitted Date**

August 31, 2016

▦ **Start Date**

June 6, 2017

▦ **Primary Completion Date**

December 31, 2020

▦ **Last Update Posted Date**

January 29, 2018

▦ **Current Primary Outcome Measures**

Overall response rate as determined by Response Evaluation Criteria in Solid Tumors (RECIST) 1.1[Time Frame: Up to 2 years]

The proportion of patients with response (complete response or partial response according to RECIST) will be compared for each pair-wise comparison of radiotherapy (RT)-containing therapy and control using chisquared tests. The difference between the proportions responding will be presented with a 90% confidence interval. For colorectal cancer, response rates within each two-stage design will be calculated and presented with 90% confidence intervals estimated using the method of Atkinson and Brown, which allows for the two-stage design.

▦ **Current Secondary Outcome Measures**

Incidence of adverse events assessed by Common Terminology Criteria for Adverse Events version 4.0[Time Frame: Up to 2 years]

Safety data will be summarized for each treatment arm within each cohort. The proportions of subjects with grade-3 or higher adverse events will be presented with exact binomial confidence intervals.

Local control rate and abscopal response rates[Time Frame: Up to 2 years]

The proportions of patients with local control within the irradiated field will be reported within each RT treatment arm and presented with 90% exact binomial confidence intervals. Similar presentations will be used for abscopal response rates. For cohort sizes of 30 (cohort 2) and 40 patients (cohort 1), the confidence intervals will be no wider than 0.32 and 0.28, respectively.

Objective response per immune-related response criteria[Time Frame: Up to 2 years]

Will be presented with 90% exact binomial confidence intervals. For cohort sizes of 30 (cohort 2) and 40 patients (cohort 1), the confidence intervals will be no wider than 0.32 and 0.28, respectively. For cohort 1, the pairwise comparisons of irORR between RT and the control arm will be conducted using chi-squared tests.

Overall survival (OS)[Time Frame: From time of randomization to death from any cause, assessed up to 2 years]

Distributions will be summarized using the Kaplan-Meier method. Median times for each therapy arm will be accompanied by 90% confidence intervals based on log(-log(endpoint)) methodology. For cohort 1, the pairwise comparisons between the durvalumab/tremelimumab alone and durvalumab/tremelimumab with RT arms will be conducted using log-rank tests.

Prognostic effect of PD-L1 expression[Time Frame: Up to 2 years]

Clinical response will be compared according to PD-L1 expression using Fisher's exact tests.

Prognostic effect of T-cell infiltration[Time Frame: Up to 2 years]

Clinical response will be compared according to infiltration using Fisher's exact tests.

Progression-free survival (PFS)[Time Frame: From date of randomization until objective disease progression or death, whichever occurs first, assessed up to 2 years]

Distributions will be summarized using the Kaplan-Meier method. Median times for each therapy arm will be accompanied by 90% confidence intervals based on log(-log(endpoint)) methodology. For cohort 1, the pairwise comparisons between the durvalumab/tremelimumab alone and durvalumab/tremelimumab with RT arms will be conducted using log-rank tests.

Descriptive Information

▦ **Offical Title**

A Phase 2 Study of MEDI4736 (Durvalumab) and Tremelimumab Alone or in Combination With High or Low-Dose Radiation in Metastatic Colorectal and NSCLC

Brief Summary

This randomized phase II trial studies the side effects of durvalumab and tremelimumab and to see how well they work with or without high or low-dose radiation therapy in treating patients with colorectal or non-small cell lung cancer that has spread to other parts of the body. Monoclonal antibodies, such as durvalumab and tremelimumab, may interfere with the ability of tumor cells to grow and spread. Radiation therapy uses high energy x-rays to kill tumor cells and shrink tumors. Giving durvalumab and tremelimumab with radiation therapy may work better in treating patients with colorectal or non-small cell lung cancer.

Detailed Description

PRIMARY OBJECTIVES:

I. To assess safety and tolerability of combined checkpoint blockade with MEDI4736 (durvalumab) and tremelimumab alone or with high or low-dose radiation in non-small cell lung cancer (NSCLC). (NSCLC Cohort) II. To compare the overall response (excluding the irradiated lesion[s]) between combined checkpoint blockade with MEDI4736 and tremelimumab alone or combined checkpoint blockade with low or high dose radiation. (NSCLC Cohort) III. To assess safety and tolerability of combined checkpoint blockade with MEDI4736 and tremelimumab with high or low-dose radiation. (Colorectal Cohort) IV. To determine the overall response rate (excluding the irradiated lesion[s]) with combined checkpoint blockade with MEDI4736 and tremelimumab with either low or high dose radiation. (Colorectal Cohort)

SECONDARY OBJECTIVES:

I. To estimate median progression-free survival and overall survival. (NSCLC Cohort) II. To determine local control within the irradiated field(s) and abscopal response rates. (NSCLC Cohort) III. To evaluate associations between PD-L1 expression as well as levels of infiltrating CD3+, CD8+ T-cells and overall response. (NSCLC Cohort) IV. To explore changes in PD-L1 expression, circulating T-cell populations, T-cell infiltration, ribonucleic acid (RNA) expression, spatial relationship of immune markers, and mutational burden as a result of low or high dose radiation. (NSCLC Cohort) V. To estimate median progression-free survival and overall survival. (Colorectal Cohort) VI. To determine local control within the irradiated field and abscopal response rates. (Colorectal Cohort) VII. To evaluate associations between PD-L1 expression as well as levels of infiltrating CD3+ CD8+ T-cells and overall response. (Colorectal Cohort) VIII. To evaluate changes between PD-L1 expression as well as levels of infiltrating CD3+, CD8+ T-cells induced by targeted low or high dose radiation. (Colorectal Cohort) IX. To explore changes in circulating T-cell populations, T-cell infiltration, RNA expression, spatial relationship of immune markers, and mutational burden as a result of low or high dose radiation.

OUTLINE: Patients with NSCLC are randomized to Arm A, B, or C. Patients with colorectal cancer are randomized to Arm B or C.

COHORT 1: Patients with NSCLC are randomized to 1 of 3 arms.

ARM A: Patients receive tremelimumab intravenously (IV) and durvalumab IV over 60 minutes every 4 weeks for up to 16 weeks in the absence of disease progression or unacceptable toxicity. Patients then receive durvalumab IV over 60 minutes 4 weeks after last combination dose for up to 9 additional doses.

ARM B: Patients receive tremelimumab and durvalumab and as in Arm A. Beginning at week 2, patients receive high dose radiation therapy once per day (QD) over 10 days for up to 3 fractions.

ARM C: Patients receive tremelimumab and durvalumab and as in Arm A. Beginning at week 2, patients receive low dose radiation therapy every 6 hours twice per day (BID) on weeks 2, 6, 10 and 14.

After completion of study treatment, patients are followed for up to 12 weeks.

Study Type

Interventional

Study Phase

Phase 2

Condition

- Microsatellite Stable
- Stage IV Colorectal Cancer AJCC v7
- Stage IV Non-Small Cell Lung Cancer AJCC v7
- Stage IVA Colorectal Cancer AJCC v7
- Stage IVB Colorectal Cancer AJCC v7

Intervention

Biological: Durvalumab

Given IV

Other Names:

Imfinzi

Immunoglobulin G1, Anti-(Human Protein B7-H1) (Human Monoclonal MEDI4736 Heavy Chain), Disulfide with Human Monoclonal MEDI4736 Kappa-chain, Dimer

MEDI-4736

MEDI4736

Other: Laboratory Biomarker Analysis

Correlative studies

Radiation: Radiation Therapy
Undergo radiation therapy

Other Names:

Cancer Radiotherapy

Irradiate

Irradiated

irradiation

RADIATION

Radiotherapeutics

radiotherapy

RT

Therapy, Radiation

Biological: Tremelimumab

Given IV

Other Names:

Anti-CTLA4 Human Monoclonal Antibody CP-675,206

CP-675

CP-675,206

CP-675206

Ticilimumab

■ **Study Arms**

Experimental: Arm A (tremelimumab, durvalumab)

Patients receive tremelimumab IV and durvalumab IV over 60 minutes every 4 weeks for up to 16 weeks in the absence of disease progression or unacceptable toxicity. Patients then receive durvalumab IV over 60 minutes 4 weeks after last combination dose for up to 9 additional doses.

Experimental: Arm B (tremelimumab, Durvalumab, RT)

Patients receive tremelimumab and durvalumab and as in Arm A. Beginning at week 2, patients receive high dose radiation therapy QD over 10 days for up to 3 fractions.

Experimental: Arm C (tremelimumab, durvalumab, and RT)

Patients receive tremelimumab and durvalumab and as in Arm A. Beginning at week 2, patients receive low dose radiation therapy every 6 hours BID on weeks 2, 6, 10 and 14.

Recruitment Information

■ **Recruitment Status**

Recruiting

■ **Estimated Enrollment**

180

■ **Eligibility Criteria**

Inclusion Criteria:

- Patients must have histologically or cytologically confirmed non-small cell lung cancer (cohort 1) or colorectal cancer (cohort 2)

- Patients must have measurable disease, defined as at least one lesion that can be accurately measured in at least one dimension (longest diameter to be recorded for non-nodal lesions and short axis for nodal lesions) as >= 20 mm (>= 2 cm) with conventional techniques or as >= 10 mm (>= 1 cm) with spiral computed tomography (CT) scan, magnetic resonance imaging (MRI), or calipers by clinical exam

■ **Completion Date**

December 31, 2020

■ **Primary Completion Date**

December 31, 2020

- Patients in both cohorts must have progressive disease following prior therapy; specifically:
- Cohort 1 (NSCLC): Patients must have evidence of radiologic or clinical disease progression during previous treatment with systemic PD-1 directed therapy and/or have been deemed not to derive clinical benefit from PD-1 directed treatment; this includes patients who demonstrated an initial response and subsequent progression; no prior treatment with chemotherapy or targeted agents are required; intervening therapy is allowed between previous PD-1 directed treatment and there is no required interval from prior PD-1 treatment required; PD-1 directed treatment includes treatment with antibodies targeting the PD-1 receptor such as pembrolizumab or nivolumab, as well as PD-L1 targeted antibodies such as MEDI4736 (durvalumab), atezolizumab and avelumab; these agents may have been administered as part of a clinical trial
- Cohort 2 (colorectal cancer): Patients must have progressed on first-line chemotherapy
- At least 21 days must have elapsed from prior therapy (chemotherapy or radiation)
- Eastern Cooperative Oncology Group (ECOG) performance status =< 1 (Karnofsky >= 60%) and life expectancy greater than 6 months; furthermore, enrollment of patients with greater than 10 measurable lesions is discouraged
- Patients must have normal organ and marrow function independent of transfusion for at least 7 days prior to screening and independent of growth factor support for at least 14 days prior to screening
- Hemoglobin (Hgb) >= 9 g/dl
- Absolute neutrophil count >= 1,500/mcL
- Platelets >= 100,000/mcL
- Total bilirubin =< 1.5 x normal institutional limits; this will not apply to patients with confirmed Gilbert's syndrome (persistent or recurrent hyperbilirubinemia [predominantly unconjugated bilirubin] in the absence of evidence of hemolysis or hepatic pathology), who will be allowed in consultation with their physician
- Aspartate aminotransferase (AST) (serum glutamic-oxaloacetic transaminase [SGOT])/alanine aminotransferase (ALT) (serum glutamate pyruvate transaminase [SGPT]) = < 2.5 x institutional upper limit of normal; for patients with hepatic metastases, ALT and AST =< 5 x ULT
- Measured creatinine clearance (CL) > 40 mL/min OR calculated creatinine clearance (CL) >40 mL/min as determined by Cockcroft-Gault (using actual body weight)
- Patients must have at least one lesion that has not previously been irradiated (and is not within a previously radiated field) and for which palliative radiation is potentially indicated and could be safely delivered at the radiation doses specified in this protocol; this lesion must not be the only measurable lesion so that it is still possible to determine the response rate outside of the radiation treatment field; this lesion must not be within the central nervous system (CNS) (brain or spinal cord) or requiring urgent or emergent palliative radiation given the timing of radiation specified on this protocol; furthermore, this lesion:
- For cohort 1 (NSCLC cohort) the lesion to be irradiated must be in the lung, lymph nodes of the neck, adrenal gland or liver
- For cohort 2 (colorectal cohort) the lesion to be irradiated must be in the liver
- Evidence of post-menopausal status or negative urinary or serum pregnancy test for female pre-menopausal patients is required; women will be considered post-menopausal if they have been amenorrheic for 12 months without an alternative medical cause; the following age-specific requirements apply:
- Women < 50 years of age would be considered post-menopausal if they have been amenorrheic for 12 months or more following cessation of exogenous hormonal treatments and if they have luteinizing hormone and follicle stimulating hormone levels in the post-menopausal range for the institution or underwent surgical sterilization (bilateral oophorectomy or hysterectomy)
- Women >= 50 years of age would be considered post-menopausal if they have been amenorrheic for 12 months or more following cessation of all exogenous hormonal treatments, had radiation-induced oophorectomy with last menses > 1 year ago, had chemotherapy-induced menopause with > 1 year interval since last menses, or underwent surgical sterilization (bilateral oophorectomy or hysterectomy)
- Females of childbearing potential who are sexually active with a non sterilized male partner must use at least 1 highly effective method of contraception from the time of screening and must agree to continue using such precautions for 180 days after the last dose of durvalumab + tremelimumab combination therapy or 90 days after the last dose of durvalumab monotherapy; non-sterilised male partners of a female patient must use male condom plus spermicide throughout this period; cessation of birth control after this point should be discussed with a responsible physician; not engaging in sexual activity for the total duration of the drug treatment and the drug washout period is an acceptable practice; however, periodic abstinence, the rhythm method, and the withdrawal method are not acceptable methods of birth control; female patients should also refrain from breastfeeding throughout this period
- Non-sterilized males who are sexually active with a female partner of childbearing potential must use a male condom plus spermicide from screening through 180 days after receipt of the final dose of durvalumab + tremelimumab combination therapy or 90 days after receipt of the final dose of durvalumab monotherapy; not engaging in sexual activity is an acceptable practice; however, occasional abstinence, the rhythm method, and the withdrawal method are not acceptable methods of contraception; male patients should refrain from sperm donation throughout this period
- Female partners (of childbearing potential) of male patients must also use a highly effective method of contraception throughout this period
- Should a woman become pregnant or suspect she is pregnant while she or her partner is participating in this study, she should inform her treating physician immediately
- Ability to understand and the willingness to sign a written informed consent document
- Body weight > 30 kg

- Cohort 1 (NSCLC cohort)
- Ability to undergo a fresh tumor biopsy for the purpose of screening for this clinical trial (including able and willing to give valid written consent) to ability or to provide an available archival tumor sample taken less than 3 months prior to study enrollment (and not obtained prior to progression on a PD-1/PD-L1 inhibitor) if a fresh tumor biopsy is not feasible with an acceptable clinical risk; tumor lesions used for fresh biopsies should be the same lesions to be irradiated when possible and should not be the same lesions used as Response Evaluation Criteria in Solid Tumors (RECIST) target lesions, unless there are no other lesions accessible; additional, optional archival tumor tissue is also requested from before the prior PD-1 directed therapy
- Cohort 2 (colorectal cohort)
- Ability to undergo a fresh tumor biopsy for the purpose of screening for this clinical trial (including able and willing to give valid written consent) to ability or to provide an available archival tumor sample taken less than 3 months prior to study enrollment if a fresh tumor biopsy is not feasible with an acceptable clinical risk; tumor lesions used for fresh biopsies should be the same lesions to be irradiated when possible and should not be the same lesions used as RECIST target lesions, unless there are no other lesions accessible
- **Microsatellite stable (MSS) tumor as documented by either:**
- Immunohistochemistry (IHC) testing that does not suggest loss of MLH-1, MSH-2, PMS2 or MSH6
- Polymerase chain reaction (PCR) testing that does not suggest microsatellite instability (MSI)

Exclusion Criteria:
- Patients who have had chemotherapy or radiotherapy within 3 weeks (6 weeks for nitrosoureas or mitomycin C) prior to entering the study
- Receipt of prior radiotherapy or condition for any reason that would contribute radiation dose that would exceed tolerance of normal tissues, at the discretion of the treating physician
- Patients who have not recovered from adverse events due to prior anti-cancer therapy (i.e., have residual toxicities > grade 1)
- Patients who are receiving any other investigational agents
- Patients with untreated brain metastases, spinal cord compression, or leptomeningeal carcinomatosis should be excluded from this clinical trial; patients whose brain metastases have been treated may participate provided they show radiographic stability (defined as 2 brain images, both of which are obtained after treatment to the brain metastases; these imaging scans should both be obtained at least four weeks apart and show no evidence of intracranial progression); in addition, any neurologic symptoms that developed either as a result of the brain metastases or their treatment must have resolved or be stable either, without the use of steroids, or are stable on a steroid dose of =< 10 mg/day of prednisone or its equivalent (and anti-convulsants) for at least 14 days prior to the start of treatment
- History of allergic reactions attributed to compounds of similar chemical or biologic composition to tremelimumab and MEDI4736 or previous toxicity attributed to MEDI4736 or other PD-1 or PD-L1 directed therapy that led to drug discontinuation
- Prior exposure to immune-mediated therapy, except for anti-PD-1 or anti-PD-L1 therapy in NSCLC patients; this includes anti-CTLA-4 agents (prior treatment with these agents is NOT allowed in either cohort) and, excludes therapeutic anticancer vaccines, excluding therapeutic anticancer vaccines; exposure to other investigational agents may be permitted after discussion with the study principal investigator (PI)
- Uncontrolled intercurrent illness including, but not limited to, ongoing or active infection, symptomatic congestive heart failure, unstable angina pectoris, cardiac arrhythmia, or psychiatric illness/social situations that would limit compliance with study requirements
- Pregnant women are excluded from this study; breastfeeding should be discontinued if the mother is treated with MEDI4736 (durvalumab), tremelimumab and radiation
- Female patients who are pregnant or breastfeeding or male or female patients of reproductive potential who are not willing to employ effective birth control from screening to 90 days after the last dose of durvalumab monotherapy or 180 days after the last dose of durvalumab + tremelimumab combination therapy, whichever is later
- Human immunodeficiency virus (HIV)-positive patients are ineligible; appropriate studies will be undertaken in patients receiving combination antiretroviral therapy when indicated
- Any concurrent chemotherapy, immune therapy, biologic, hormonal therapy for cancer treatment
- **Current or prior use of immunosuppressive medication within 14 days before the first dose of their assigned IP; the following are exceptions to this criterion:**
- Intranasal, inhaled, topical steroids, or local steroid injections (e.g., intra-articular injection)
- Systemic corticosteroids at physiologic doses not to exceed 10 mg/day of prednisone or its equivalent
- Steroids as pre-medication for hypersensitivity reactions (e.g., CT scan pre-medication)
- Major surgical procedure (as defined by the investigator) within 28 days prior to the first dose of IP; Note: local surgery of isolated lesions for palliative intent is acceptable
- History of allogeneic organ transplantation
- **Active or prior documented autoimmune or inflammatory disorders (including inflammatory bowel disease, diverticulitis [with the exception of diverticulosis]; sarcoidosis syndrome, or other serious gastrointestinal [GI] chronic conditions associated with diarrhea; systemic lupus erythematosus; Wegener syndrome [granulomatosis with polyangiitis]; myasthenia gravis; Graves disease; rheumatoid arthritis; hypophysitis; uveitis, sarcoidosis syndrome, etc.) within the past 3 years prior to the start of treatment; the following are exceptions to this criterion:**

- Patients with vitiligo or alopecia
- Patients with hypothyroidism (e.g., following Hashimoto syndrome) stable on hormone replacement or psoriasis not requiring systemic treatment
- Any chronic skin condition that does not require systemic therapy
- Patients without active disease in the last 5 years may be included but only after consultation with the study physician
- Patients with celiac disease controlled by diet alone
- History of another primary malignancy except for
- Malignancy treated with curative intent and with no known active disease >= 5 years before the first dose of study drug and of low potential risk for recurrence
- Adequately treated non-melanoma skin cancer or lentigo maligna without evidence of disease
- Adequately treated carcinoma in situ without evidence of disease (e.g., cervical cancer in situ)
- Mean QT interval corrected for heart rate (QTc) >= 470 ms calculated from 3 electrocardiograms (ECGs) using Fridericia's correction
- History of active primary immunodeficiency
- Known history of previous clinical diagnosis of tuberculosis
- Active infection including hepatitis B (known positive hepatitis B virus [HBV] surface antigen [HBsAg]) result or, hepatitis C; patients with a past or resolved HBV infection (defined as the presence of hepatitis B core antibody [anti-HBc] and absence of HBsAg) are eligible; patients positive for hepatitis C (HCV) antibody are eligible only if polymerase chain reaction is negative for HCV ribonucleic acid (RNA)
- Receipt of live, attenuated vaccine within 30 days prior to the first dose of investigational treatment; Note: patients, if enrolled, should not receive live vaccine during the study and up to 30 days after the last dose of investigational treatment
- Any condition that, in the opinion of the investigator, would interfere with evaluation of the investigational treatment or interpretation of patient safety or study results
- Cohort 1 (NSCLC cohort)
- **In regards to administration of prior anti-PD-1 or anti PD-L1 antibodies, a patients:**
- Must not have experienced a toxicity that led to permanent discontinuation of prior immunotherapy

▨ Sex/Gender

All

▨ Ages

18 Years to N/A

▨ Accepts Healthy Volunteers

No

A Study of PDR001 in Combination With LCL161, Everolimus or Panobinostat

Study ID:

NCT02890069

Sponsor:

Novartis Pharmaceuticals

Information provided by (Responsible Party):

Novartis (Novartis Pharmaceuticals)

Tracking Information

▨ First Submitted Date

May 9, 2016

▨ Start Date

October 14, 2016

▨ Primary Completion Date

May 12, 2019

▨ Last Update Posted Date

December 5, 2017

▨ Current Primary Outcome Measures

Phase 1: Incidence of dose limiting toxicities (DLTs)[Time Frame: During the first two cycles]
    cycle = 28 days

Frequency of dose interruptions and reductions[Time Frame: Through study completion, an average of 6 months]

Frequency and severity of treatment-emergent adverse events (AEs) and serious adverse events (SAEs)[Time Frame: Through study completion, an average of 6 months]

Changes between baseline and post-baseline laboratory parameters and vital signs[Time Frame: Through study completion, an average of 6 months]

Dose intensities[Time Frame: Through study completion, an average of 6 months]

Current Secondary Outcome Measures

Quantification of Tumor Infiltrating Lymphocytes (TILs) by Hematoxylin[Time Frame: Baseline and approximately after 2 cycles of treatment and at disease progression (an average of 6 months)]

cycle = 28 days

Changes from baseline in ECG parameters in patients recieving PDR001 in combination with Panobinostat[Time Frame: Baseline and end of treatment, an average of 6 months]

Best overall response (BOR)[Time Frame: T1: Every 2 cycles until the start of T2; T2: every 2 cycles till cycle 5, and every 3 cycles till the patient progresses or is withdrawn from study, an average of 6 months]

cycle = 28 days T1: treatment period 1 (6 cycles of treatment) T2: treatment period 2

Time to reach max concentration (Tmax) for PDR001[Time Frame: Cycle 1 through cycle 6 in treatment period 1 and 2, an average of 6 months]

T1: treatment period 1 (6 cycles of treatment) T2: treatment period 2

Presence of anti-PDR001 antibodies[Time Frame: Cycle 1 through cycle 6 in treatment period 1 and 2, an average of 6 months]

T1: treatment period 1 (6 cycles of treatment) T2: treatment period 2

Progression free survival (PFS) per RECIST v1.1[Time Frame: T1: Every 2 cycles until the start of T2; T2: every 2 cycles till cycle 5, and every 3 cycles till the patient progresses or is withdrawn from study, an average of 6 months]

cycle = 28 days T1: treatment period 1 (6 cycles of treatment) T2: treatment period 2

Treatment Free Survival (TFS)[Time Frame: T1: Every 2 cycles until the start of T2; T2: every 2 cycles till cycle 5, and every 3 cycles till the patient progresses or is withdrawn from study, an average of 6 months]

cycle = 28 days T1: treatment period 1 (6 cycles of treatment) T2: treatment period 2

Maximum and minimum plasma concentrations of LCL161 (Cmax and Cmin)[Time Frame: Cycle 1 through cycle 6 in treatment period 1 and 2, an average of 6 months]

T1: treatment period 1 (6 cycles of treatment) T2: treatment period 2

Maximum and minimum Plasma concentrations of everolimus (Cmax and Cmin)[Time Frame: Cycle 1 through cycle 6 in treatment period 1 and 2, an average of 6 months]

T1: treatment period 1 (6 cycles of treatment) T2: treatment period 2

Maximum and minimum plasma concentrations of panobinostat (Cmax and Cmin)[Time Frame: Cycle 1 through cycle 6 in treatment period 1 and 2, an average of 6 months]

T1: treatment period 1 (6 cycles of treatment) T2: treatment period 2

Concentration of anti-PDR001 antibodies[Time Frame: Cycle 1 through cycle 6 in treatment period 1 and 2, an average of 6 months]

T1: treatment period 1 (6 cycles of treatment) T2: treatment period 2

Characterization of TILs and myeloid cell infiltrate by IHC (such as CD8, FoxP3 and myeloid markers as appropriate)[Time Frame: Baseline and approximately after 2 cycles of treatment and at disease progression (an average of 6 months)]

Cycle = 28 days

Quantification of Tumor Infiltrating Lymphocytes (TILs) by eosin (H&E) stain[Time Frame: Baseline and approximately after 2 cycles of treatment and at disease progression (an average of 6 months)]

cycle = 28 days

Maximum and minimum serum concentration of PDR001 (Cmax and Cmin)[Time Frame: Cycle 1 through cycle 6 in treatment period 1 and 2, an average of 6 months]

T1: treatment period 1 (6 cycles of treatment) T2: treatment period 2

Area under the concentration-time curve calculated to the last concentration point (AUClast) for PDR001, as applicable[Time Frame: Cycle 1 through cycle 6 in treatment period 1 and 2, an average of 6 months]

T1: treatment period 1 (6 cycles of treatment) T2: treatment period 2

Progression free survival (PFS) per irRC[Time Frame: T1: Every 2 cycles until the start of T2; T2: every 2 cycles till cycle 5, and every 3 cycles till the patient progresses or is withdrawn from study, an average of 6 months]

cycle = 28 days T1: treatment period 1 (6 cycles of treatment) T2: treatment period 2

Area under the concentration-time curve calculated to the last concentration point (AUClast) for LCL161, as applicable[Time

Frame: Cycle 1 through cycle 6 in treatment period 1 and 2, an average of 6 months]

T1: treatment period 1 (6 cycles of treatment) T2: treatment period 2

Time to reach max concentration (Tmax) for LCL161[Time Frame: Cycle 1 through cycle 6 in treatment period 1 and 2, an average of 6 months]

T1: treatment period 1 (6 cycles of treatment) T2: treatment period 2

Time to reach max concentration (Tmax) for Everolimus[Time Frame: Cycle 1 through cycle 6 in treatment period 1 and 2, an average of 6 months]

Cycle 1 through cycle 6 in treatment period 1 and 2, an average of 6 months

Time to reach max concentration (Tmax) for Panobinostat[Time Frame: Cycle 1 through cycle 6 in treatment period 1 and 2, an average of 6 months]

T1: treatment period 1 (6 cycles of treatment) T2: treatment period 2

Area under the concentration-time curve calculated to the last concentration point (AUClast) for Everolimus, as applicable[Time Frame: Cycle 1 through cycle 6 in treatment period 1 and 2, an average of 6 months]

T1: treatment period 1 (6 cycles of treatment) T2: treatment period 2

Area under the concentration-time curve calculated to the last concentration point (AUClast) for Panobinostat, as applicable[Time Frame: Cycle 1 through cycle 6 in treatment period 1 and 2, an average of 6 months]

T1: treatment period 1 (6 cycles of treatment) T2: treatment period 2

Descriptive Information

▣ Offical Title

Phase Ib, Open-label, Multi-center Study to Characterize the Safety, Tolerability and Pharmacodynamics (PD) of PDR001 in Combination With LCL161, Everolimus (RAD001) or Panobinostat (LBH589)

▣ Brief Summary

The purpose of this study is to combine the PDR001 checkpoint inhibitor with several agents with immunomodulatory activity to identify the doses and schedule for combination therapy and to preliminarily assess the safety, tolerability, pharmacological and clinical activity of these combinations.

▣ Study Type

Interventional

▣ Study Phase

Phase 1

▣ Condition

- Colorectal Cancer, Non-small Cell Lung Carcinoma (Adenocarcinoma), Triple Negative Breast Cancer

▣ Intervention

Biological: PDR001

anti-PD1 antibody

Drug: LCL161

Drug: Everolimus

Other Names:

RAD001

Drug: Panobinostat

Other Names:

LBH589

▣ Study Arms

- Experimental: CRC PDR001 + LCL161
- Experimental: NSCLC PDR001 + LCL161
- Experimental: TNBC PDR001 + LCL161
- Experimental: CRC PDR001+ Everolimus
- Experimental: NSCLC PDR001+ Everolimus
- Experimental: TNBC PDR001+ Everolimus
- Experimental: CRC PDR001 + Panobinostat

- Experimental: NSCLC PDR001 + Panobinostat
- Experimental: TNBC PDR001 + Panobinostat

Recruitment Information

▥ Recruitment Status
Recruiting

▥ Estimated Enrollment
350

▥ Completion Date
May 12, 2019

▥ Primary Completion Date
May 12, 2019

▥ Eligibility Criteria

Inclusion Criteria:

- Written informed consent prior to any procedure
- Patients with advanced/metastatic cancer, with measurable disease as determined by RECIST version 1.1, who have progressed despite standard therapy or are intolerant to SOC, or for whom no standard therapy exists. Patients must fit into one of the following groups:
- CRC •NSCLC • TNBC
- ECOG ≤ 2
- Patient must have a site of disease for biopsy, and be a candidate for tumor biopsy according to the institution's guidelines. Patient must be willing to undergo a new tumor biopsy at screening, and again during therapy on this study.
- Prior therapy with PD-1/PDL-1 inhibitors is allowed provided any toxicity attributed to prior PD-1or PD-L1-directed therapy did not lead to discontinuation of therapy.

Exclusion Criteria:

- Presence of symptomatic central nervous system (CNS) metastases, or CNS metastases that require local CNS-directed therapy within prior 2 weeks.
- Patients with known hypersensitivity to any of the components of an investigational treatment will be excluded from participation in the corresponding arm but are eligible for participation in other study arm; Patients that have a history of hypersensitivity to rapamycin derivatives will be excluded from participation in the everolimus arm
- History of or current drug-induced interstitial lung disease or pneumonitis grade ≥2
- Out of range lab values as defined in protocol
- Impaired cardiac function or clinically significant cardiac disease
- Active, known or suspected autoimmune disease
- Human Immunodeficiency Virus (HIV), or active Hepatitis C (HCV) virus. Escalation: active Hepatitis B (HBV); Expansion: Patients with Chronic HBV currently on medication will not be excluded.
- Impairment of gastrointestinal (GI) function
- Malignant disease, other than that being treated in this study
- Systemic anti-cancer therapy within 2 weeks of the first dose of study treatment. For cytotoxic agents that have major delayed toxicity and washout period is 6 weeks; prior immunotherapy washout is 4 weeks
- Active infection requiring systemic antibiotic therapy.
- Patients requiring chronic treatment with systemic steroid therapy, other than replacement dose steroids or treatment with low, stable dose of steroid (<10 mg/day prednisone or equivalent) for stable CNS metastatic disease.
- Patients receiving systemic treatment with any immunosuppressive medication.
- Major surgery within 2 weeks of the first dose of study treatment
- Radiotherapy within 2 weeks of the first dose of study drug
- Participation in an interventional, investigational study within 2 weeks of the first dose of study treatment.
- Presence of ≥ CTCAE grade 2 toxicity (except alopecia, peripheral neuropathy and ototoxicity, which are excluded if ≥ CTCAE grade 3) due to prior therapy.
- Use of hematopoietic colony stimulating growth factors </= 3 weeks prior to first dose

Additional exclusion criteria for PDR001/LCL161

- Patients requiring medications metabolized through CYP3A4/5 and have a narrow therapeutic index or medications that are CYP3A4 substrates that cause QT prolongation
- Patients requiring treatment with strong CYP2C8 inhibitors

Additional exclusion criteria for PDR001/Everolimus

- Patients requiring treatment with moderate CYP3A4 inhibitors
- Patients requiring treatment with a strong CYP3A4 inhibitor or inducer

Additional exclusion criteria for PDR001/Panobinostat-

- Patient who received DAC inhibitors
- Patient needing valproic acid during the study or within 5 days prior to first dose

- Patients requiring medications that are sensitive CYP2D6 substrates areCYP2D6 substrates with a narrow therapeutic index or are anti-arrhythmic drugs/drugs with QT-prolongation risks
- Patients requiring a strong inhibitor or inducer of CYP3A4
- Clinically significant, uncontrolled heart disease and/or recent cardiac event within 6 months prior to study
- Unresolved diarrhea ≥ CTCAE grade 2 or a medical condition associated with chronic diarrhea
- Taking medications with QT prolongation risk or interval or inducing Torsade de pointes

Other protocol-defined inclusion exclusion criteria may apply.

Sex/Gender

All

Ages

18 Years to N/A

Accepts Healthy Volunteers

No

Contacts

Novartis Pharmaceuticals   1-888-669-6682   Novartis.email@novartis.com

Novartis Pharmaceuticals   +41613241111

Phase I Trial of Universal Donor NK Cell Therapy in Combination With ALT803

Study ID:

NCT02890758

Sponsor:

David Wald

Information provided by (Responsible Party):

Case Comprehensive Cancer Center (David Wald)

Tracking Information

First Submitted Date

September 1, 2016

Start Date

January 10, 2018

Primary Completion Date

August 2019

Last Update Posted Date

January 23, 2018

Current Primary Outcome Measures

Number of patients without Graft Versus Host Disease (GVHD)[Time Frame: up to 28 days after beginning treatment]
  Measure of safety of natural killer (NK) cells in the absence of HLA matching

Current Secondary Outcome Measures

Number of patients with hematological response[Time Frame: Up to 12 months after beginning treatment]

  Complete Remission (CR): Bone marrow blasts <5%; absence of blasts with Auer rods; absence of extramedullary disease; absolute neutrophil count >1.0x10^9/L; platelet count >100x10^9/L.

  CR with incomplete recovery (CRi): All CR criteria except residual neutropenia or thrombocytopenia.

  Partial Remission (PR):Hematologic criteria of CR; decrease of bone marrow blast percentage to 5-25%; and decrease of pretreatment bone marrow blast percentage by ≥50%.

  Cytogenetic CR (CRc): Reversion to normal karyotype at the time of morphologic CR.

  Resistant disease (RD): Failure to achieve CR, CRi, or PR. Death in aplasia: Deaths occurring ≥7 days after initial treatment. Death from indeterminate cause: Deaths before completing therapy, or <7 days following completion; or deaths occurring ≥7 days after therapy with no blasts in the blood Relapse: Bone marrow blasts ≥ 5%; or reappearance of blasts in the blood; or development of extramedullary disease

Patients response for radiographically measurable lesions[Time Frame: Up to 12 months after beginning treatment]
  Measurable disease: at least one measurable lesion.

Measurable lesions: those that can be measured in at least one dimension as >20 mm with conventional techniques or as >10 mm with spiral CT scan.

Non-measurable lesions: all other lesions, including small lesions that are not confirmed and followed by imaging techniques.

Baseline documentation of "Target" lesions: all measurable lesions up to a maximum of five lesions per organ and 10 lesions in total. Target lesions should be selected on the basis of their size and their suitability for accurate repeated measurements.

Non-target lesions: all other lesions should be identified as non-target lesions. Non-target lesions include measurable lesions that exceed the maximum numbers per organ or total of all involved organs as well as non-measurable lesions.

Patients with malignant lymphoma response[Time Frame: Up to 12 months after beginning treatment]

Lymphoma response of Complete remission, partial remission, relapsed disease, stable disease, progressive disease and best response based on the Journal of Clinical Oncology criteria defined by Cheson in 2014

Patients response for Waldenstrom's macroglobulinemia (WM)[Time Frame: Up to 12 months after beginning treatment]

Complete response (CR): complete disappearance of disease at and negative serum immunofixation.

Partial response (PR): >50% reduction of serum monoclonal protein concentration with >50% reduction of tumor infiltrate and resolution of symptoms attributable to WM.

Minor response (MR): > 25% but l<50% reduction of serum monoclonal immunoglobulin M (IgM) determined by protein electrophoresis and no new symptoms or signs of active disease.

Stable disease: < 25% reduction and <25% increase of serum monoclonal IgM without progression of adenopathy, organomegaly, cytopenias, or clinically significant symptoms caused by disease and/or signs of WM.

Progressive disease: fails to meet criteria for response or stable disease. Progression also requires at least a 25% increase of serum monoclonal protein from the lowest value or worsening of cytopenias, lymphadenopathy, or organomegaly, or appearance of disease-related complications.

Patients response for cutaneous lymphomas[Time Frame: Up to 12 months after beginning treatment]

CR/CCR

Complete resolution of skin patches, plaques and tumors (or erythroderma)

No evidence of abnormal lymph nodes

Absence of circulating Sézary cells

No evidence of new tumor (CCR) plus confirmation by skin biopsy (CR) PR

≥50% improvement in the summation of (Δ Skin + Δ Lymph Node + Δ Peripheral Blood) with at least ≥30% improvement in Δ Skin

No worsening in Lymph Node or Sézary cells

No evidence of new tumors (cutaneous or non-cutaneous)

Stable Disease at 90 Days (SD90)

• Fails to meet criteria for PR or CR but absence of new cutaneous or non-cutaneous disease over 90 days

Progressive Disease (PD)

≥ 50% increase from nadir or baseline in styrylpyridine derivative (SPD) or any node or lesion

≥ 50% increase from nadir in gestational trophoblastic disease (GTD) of any node previously >1cm in shortest diameter

Appearance of any new cutaneous or non-cutaneous lesion during or at the end of therapy.

Patients response for multiple myeloma[Time Frame: Up to 12 months after beginning treatment]

Stringent Complete Response (sCR)

CR as defined below plus:

• Normal FLC ratio and Absence of clonal cells in bone marrow CR

Negative immunofixation on the serum and urine and:

Disappearance of any soft tissue plasmacytomas

≤5% plasma cells in bone marrow Very good partial response (VGPR)

Serum and urine M-protein detectable by immunofixation but not on electrophoresis or 90% or greater reduction in serum M-protein plus urine M-protein level <100mg per 24h PR

≥ 50% reduction of serum M-protein and reduction in 24-h urinary M-protein by ≥ 90% or to <200 mg per 24h

If the serum and urine protein are unmeasurable, ≥ 50% decrease in the difference between involved and uninvolved FLC levels is required

If the serum and urine protein are unmeasurable, and serum free light assay is also unmeasurable, ≥ 50% decrease in plasmacells is required SD

Not meeting criteria for CR, VGPR, PR, or progressive disease

Patients response for chronic myeloid leukemia (CML)[Time Frame: Up to 12 months after beginning treatment]

Complete hematologic response

• White blood cell count <10,000/microL with no immature granulocytes and <5 percent basophils on differential, platelet count <450,000/microL, and spleen not palpable.

Cytogenetic responses

Complete cytogenetic response: No Philadelphia chromosome positive cells present.

Partial cytogenetic response: 1 to 35 percent Philadelphia chromosome positive cells present.

Major cytogenetic response includes patients with complete and partial cytogenetic response (ie, 0 to 35 percent Philadelphia chromosome positive cells present).

Minor-minimal cytogenetic response: 36 to 95 percent Philadelphia chromosome positive cells present.

Molecular response:

Complete molecular response: break cluster region Abelson family kinases (BCR-ABL) transcript nondetectable and nonquantifiable in an assay that has at least 4 to 5 log range.

Major molecular response: An at least three log reduction in BCR-ABL transcript levels from baseline.

Patients response for metastatic colon/rectal carcinoma and soft tissue sarcomas[Time Frame: Up to 12 months after beginning treatment]

Complete Response: Disappearance of all target lesions. Any pathological lymph nodes (whether target or non-target) must have reduction in short axis to < 10 mm (the sum may not be "0" if there are target nodes). Partial Response: At least a 30% decrease in the sum of the diameters of target lesions, taking as reference the baseline sum diameters.

Progressive Disease: At least a 20% increase in the sum of diameters of target lesions, taking as reference the smallest sum on study (this includes the baseline sum if that is the smallest on study). In addition to the relative increase of 20%, the sum must also demonstrate an absolute increase of at least 5 mm. The appearance of one or more new lesions may be considered progression).

Stable Disease: Neither sufficient shrinkage to qualify for PR nor sufficient increase to qualify for PD, taking as reference the smallest sum of diameters while on study.

Average duration of response[Time Frame: Up to 12 months after beginning treatment]

The duration of overall response is measured from the time of NK Cell infusion until the first date that recurrent or progressive disease is objectively documented (taking as reference for progressive disease the smallest measurements recorded since the treatment started).

Average duration of Overall Survival[Time Frame: Up to 12 months after beginning treatment]

Overall survival is measured from the date of first infusion of NK cells to the date of death from any cause; patients not known to have died at last follow up are censored on the date they were last known to be alive.

Average duration of relapse free survival[Time Frame: Up to 12 months after beginning treatment]

Only those patients achieving complete response (CR) or complete response with incomplete recovery (CRI). It is measured from the date of infusion of NK cells until the date of relapse or death from any cause; patients not known to have relapsed or died at last follow up are censored on the date they were last examined.

in vivo Natural Killer (NK) levels[Time Frame: up to 28 days after beginning treatment]

Measurement of in vivo NK cell levels following cell product infusion will be done on peripheral blood by flow cytometry (CD3CD56+ positive cells). This will be done on peripheral blood samples of patients. Measurement of successful donor NK cell persistence (absence of cell product rejection) will be defined as measurement of >100 NK cell/µL

Descriptive Information

Offical Title

Phase I Trial of Universal Donor NK Cell Therapy in Combination With ALT-803

Brief Summary

The purpose of this study is to find the number of natural killer (NK) cells from non-HLA matched donors that can be safely infused into patients with cancer. NK cells are a form of lymphocytes that defend against cancer cells. NK cells in cancer patients do not work well to fight cancer. In this study, the NK cells are being donated by healthy individuals without cancer who are not "matched" by human leukocyte antigen (HLA) genes to patients. After receiving these NK cells, patients may also be given a drug called ALT803. ALT803 is a protein that keeps NK cells alive, helps them grow in number and supports their cancer-fighting characteristics. HLA-unmatched NK cell infusion is investigational (experimental) because the process has not approved by the Food and Drug Administration (FDA).

Detailed Description

Primary Objective:

To determine the maximum tolerated dose of ex vivo expanded non-HLA matched donor NK cells in combination with ALT-803

Secondary Objectives:

- Describe safety profile / toxicity of combining ALT-803 with NK cell adoptive therapy.
- Determine antitumor activity of allogeneic NK cells with ALT-803 support.
- Determine if a lymphocyte depleting regimen is adequate for preventing early elimination of HLA-mismatched donor NK cells by host T-cells.

Study Design:

This is a phase I study with "3+3" design with three planned dose levels of NK cells and a fixed dose of ALT-803. Three patients will be enrolled sequentially to each dose level, starting with dose level 1. Patients will be segregated to either receive ALT803 as cytokine support after NK cell infusion (starting with same dose level as Level 1) or no cytokine administration. Patients in the arm receiving ALT803 will be either hematologic malignancy patients (Cohort A) or Colon/Soft tissue sarcoma patients (Cohort B). Absence of dose limiting toxicity (DLT) in the DLT assessment period of 28 days must be documented for all patients enrolled a cell dose without ALT803 before the next cohort of patients to receive cytokines at that dose level can be enrolled. Patients can also be enrolled in parallel to the next cell dose level without cytokines.

Study Type

Interventional

Study Phase

Phase 1

Condition

- Acute Myeloid Leukemia
- Myelodysplastic Syndrome
- Acute Lymphoblastic Leukemia
- Chronic Myeloid Leukemia
- Chronic Lymphocytic Leukemia
- Non Hodgkin Lymphoma
- Hodgkin Lymphoma
- Myeloproliferative Syndromes
- Plasma Cell Myeloma
- Colon Carcinoma
- Adenocarcinoma of Rectum
- Soft Tissue Sarcoma
- Ewing's Sarcoma
- Rhabdomyosarcoma

Intervention

Biological: Natural Killer (NK) Cells

dose escalation of Natural Killer (NK) Cells from two infusion of 10 x 10^6 cells/kg to 1000 x 10^6 cells/kg dependent on dose limited toxicity

Biological: ALT803

given at 6mcg/kg weekly for four weeks

Other Names:

Cytokine

Study Arms

Experimental: Cytokine Arm

Two infusions of Natural Killer (NK) cells and ALT803

Active Comparator: No Cytokine Arm

Two infusions of Natural Killer (NK) Cells

Recruitment Information

Recruitment Status

Recruiting

Estimated Enrollment

54

Completion Date

August 2019

Primary Completion Date

August 2019

Eligibility Criteria

Inclusion Criteria:

- Patients must have histologic confirmation of relapsed and or refractory hematologic malignancy, locally advanced or metastatic colon/rectal carcinoma, or refractory and/or relapsed soft tissue sarcomas and have failed at least one standard line of therapy.
- Patients will be eligible if they have either declined standard treatment regimens or if there is no standard approach to curative salvage therapy per National Comprehensive Cancer Network (NCCN) guidelines in the setting of relapsed/refractory disease.
- In addition, patients for whom a potential 29-day delay in treatment will not interfere with the subject's potential therapeutic options can be eligible per the treating physician's discretion.

Malignancies can include:

- Acute myeloid leukemia
- Myelodysplastic syndrome
- Acute lymphoblastic leukemia
- Chronic myeloid leukemia
- Chronic lymphocytic leukemia
- Non Hodgkin Lymphoma
- Hodgkin Lymphoma
- Myeloproliferative syndromes
- Plasma cell myeloma
- Colon/rectal carcinoma
- Soft tissue sarcomas including but not limited to Ewing's sarcoma and Rhabdomyosarcoma
- Patients must have recovered from acute toxicities of prior chemotherapy or stem cell transplant. Any prior non-hematologic vital organ toxicity (cardiac, pulmonary, hepatic, renal) of previous therapy must have resolved to grade 1 or less.
- All previous chemotherapy or radiation must be completed at least 3 weeks prior to study entry. Immunologic therapy must be completed at least 1 week prior to study entry. Patients with prior stem cell transplant must be greater than 365 days post-transplant.
- Eastern Cooperative Oncology Group (ECOG) performance status ≤2
- Organ function criteria (There is no exclusion for the presence of cytopenias),
- Serum total bilirubin <2 mg/dl (except if known Gilbert syndrome and normal transaminases)
- Aspartate aminotransferase (AST) (SGOT) < 2.5 X institutional upper limit of normal
- Alanine aminotransferase (ALT) (SGPT) < 2.5 X institutional upper limit of normal
- Pulmonary function (DLCO) >40% of the expected value corrected for alveolar volume and hemoglobin
- Serum Creatinine ≤ 1.5 X institutional upper limit of normal
- Subjects must have the ability to understand and the willingness to sign a written informed consent document.
- Women of child-bearing potential and men must agree to use adequate contraception (double barrier method of birth control or abstinence) 4 weeks prior to study entry and for the duration of study participation. Women of child-bearing age must have documented negative pregnancy test prior to start of lympho-depleting regimen.

Exclusion Criteria:

- Subjects receiving any other investigational agents.
- Subjects for whom a potential 29-day delay in treatment will interfere with the subject's potential therapeutic options.
- Patients with untreated malignant involvement of the central nervous system (CNS) should be excluded from this clinical trial because of their poor prognosis and because they often develop progressive neurologic dysfunction that would confound the evaluation of neurologic and other adverse events. Head imaging will be necessary to document absence of CNS involvement in patients with colon/rectal cancer and soft tissue sarcomas. Patients with hematologic malignancies who have undergone treatment for malignant involvement of the CNS must have no evidence of residual disease by imaging or CSF sampling prior to study enrollment.
- History of allergic reactions to chemotherapy agents used in this protocol as part of lymphodepletion regimen (Fludarabine and Cyclophosphamide)
- Patients with uncontrolled intercurrent illness including, but not limited to ongoing active uncontrolled infection, symptomatic congestive heart failure, unstable angina pectoris, cardiac arrhythmia, or psychiatric illness/social situations that would limit compliance with study requirements.
- Pregnant or breastfeeding women are excluded from this study.
- HIV-positive patients on combination antiretroviral therapy are ineligible because of the potential for pharmacokinetic interactions with chemotherapeutic agents. In addition, these patients are at increased risk of lethal infections when treated with marrow suppressive therapy. Appropriate studies will be undertaken in patients receiving combination antiretroviral therapy when indicated.

- Chronic active untreated hepatitis B or C infection.
- Recipients of previous allogeneic transplants who have rash involving more than 10% body surface area attributed to graft versus host disease (GVHD) (> Grade 1 GVHD of skin). Stem cell transplant recipients will be excluded if they are still receiving immunosuppression including steroids for GVHD or have active GVHD in any organ (except for Grade 1 only of skin, not requiring treatment).

Sex/Gender

All

Ages

18 Years to N/A

Accepts Healthy Volunteers

No

Contacts

Folashade Otegbeye, MD   216-286-4443   folashade.otegbeye@uhhospitals.org

Chemopreventive Effects of Epigallocatechin Gallate (EGCG) in Colorectal Cancer (CRC) Patients

Study ID:

NCT02891538

Sponsor:

The University of Texas Health Science Center at San Antonio

Information provided by (Responsible Party):

The University of Texas Health Science Center at San Antonio (The University of Texas Health Science Center at San Antonio)

Tracking Information

First Submitted Date

August 31, 2016

Start Date

January 31, 2017

Current Primary Outcome Measures

Primary Completion Date

November 2019

Last Update Posted Date

September 14, 2017

Change in methylation from baseline when compared to the control arm[Time Frame: 1 year]

Descriptive Information

Offical Title

A Pilot Study to Evaluate the Chemopreventive Effects of Epigallocatechin Gallate (EGCG) in Colorectal Cancer (CRC) Patients With Curative Resections.

Brief Summary

This will be a randomized, controlled pilot trial of patients with histological documentation of primary colon or rectal adenocarcinoma with resectable cancer, who have not received any treatments for cancer. If patient is a candidate for surgical resection, with no planned neoadjuvant chemotherapy, then the patient is eligible. All eligible subjects will be consented prior to surgery.

Detailed Description

Part 1: Blood draw prior to surgery, followed by surgical resection, and surgical pathologic specimen will be archived. After surgery, patient will be seen in 4-12 weeks to determine if adjuvant chemotherapy is indicated, in which case patient will receive adjuvant therapy. At this visit a blood draw will be done.

Part 2: If the patient is stage 0/1/2 and no plan for adjuvant treatments, then the patient will be randomized in a 2:1 manner to EGCG 900 mg daily vs observation (standard of care) for 1 year. Patients randomized to the EGCG arm, will start EGCG within 4-12 weeks of surgery and take EGCG 450 mg PO twice a day. Blood draw will be done at 0, 3, 6, 9, 12, 15, 18 months. Colonoscopy will be done at 1 year from diagnosis, at which time normal colonic tissue biopsies as well as any resected polyps will be collected.

Study Type

Interventional

Study Phase

Early Phase 1

Condition

- Colon Cancer

Intervention

Drug: Epigallocatechin gallate (EGCG)

Teavigo™ is a natural, caffeine-free, highly purified and refined green tea extract providing 94% epigallocatechin gallate (EGCG).

Other Names:

Green Tea Extract

Study Arms

Experimental: epigallocatechin gallate (EGCG)

Patients randomized to the EGCG arm, will start EGCG within 4-12 weeks of surgery and take EGCG 450 mg PO twice a day.

No Intervention: Observation Only

Standard of care surgical resection followed by standard of care colonoscopy at year.

Recruitment Information

Recruitment Status

Recruiting

Estimated Enrollment

50

Eligibility Criteria

Inclusion Criteria:

- Cytologically or histologically confirmed of primary colon or rectal adenocarcinoma with resectable cancer, who have not received any treatments for cancer.
- Age 18 years and above
- Eastern Cooperative Oncology Group (ECOG) performance status of 0-2
- The patient is a candidate for surgical resection, with no planned neoadjuvant chemotherapy, and there is a planned surgery for the primary colorectal cancer.
- For women who are not postmenopausal (12 months of amenorrhea) or surgically sterile (absence of ovaries and/or uterus): agreement to use two adequate methods of contraception. For men: agreement to use a barrier method of contraception during the treatment period
- Hematologic, Biochemical, and Organ Function within 7 days prior to Cycle 1 Day 1: Granulocyte count > 1000/mm3, Platelet count > 50,000/ mm3, Hemoglobin > 7 g/dL; Total bilirubin < 2.0; Albumin > 2.8g/dl; aspartate aminotransferase (AST) (SGOT) and alanine aminotransferase (ALT) (SGPT) < 5 x upper limit of normal (ULN); Serum creatinine< 2 x ULN

Exclusion Criteria:

- Patients receiving prior chemotherapy.
- Patients with metastatic disease.
- Patients may not be receiving any other investigational agents.
- History of allergic reactions attributed to compounds of similar chemical or biologic composition to green tea or EGCG.
- Uncontrolled intercurrent illness including, but not limited to, ongoing or active infection, symptomatic congestive heart failure, unstable angina pectoris, cardiac arrhythmia, or psychiatric illness/social situations that would limit compliance with study requirements
- Gastrointestinal tract disease resulting in an inability to take oral medication or a requirement for IV alimentation, prior surgical procedures affecting absorption, or active peptic ulcer disease. Patients with nasogastric tube (NG-tube), J-tube, or G-tube will not be allowed to participate.
- Pregnant women are excluded from this study because of unknown effects of EGCG on teratogenic or abortifacient effects. For this reason, women of childbearing potential and men must also agree to use adequate contraception (hormonal or barrier method of birth control) prior to study entry and for the duration of study participation.
- Should a woman become pregnant or suspect she is pregnant while participating in this study, she should inform her treating physician immediately. Because there is an unknown but potential risk for adverse events in nursing infants secondary to treatment of the mother with EGCG, breastfeeding should be discontinued.

Completion Date

November 2019

Primary Completion Date

November 2019

- Informed Consent No study specific procedures will be performed without a written and signed informed consent document. Patients who do not demonstrate the ability to understand or the willingness to sign the written informed consent document will be excluded from study entry.

■ **Sex/Gender**

All

■ **Ages**

18 Years to N/A

■ **Accepts Healthy Volunteers**

No

■ **Contacts**

Epp Goodwin   210-450-5798   ctrcreferral@uthscsa.edu

Jay L Morris, PhD   210-567-8389   morrisjl@uthscsa.edu

Palbociclib With Cisplatin or Carboplatin in Advanced Solid Tumors

Study ID:

NCT02897375

Sponsor:

Emory University

Information provided by (Responsible Party):

Emory University (Emory University)

Tracking Information

■ **First Submitted Date**

August 30, 2016

■ **Start Date**

October 2016

■ **Primary Completion Date**

February 2019

■ **Last Update Posted Date**

November 27, 2017

■ **Current Primary Outcome Measures**

Incidence of adverse events according to National Cancer Institute Common Terminology Criteria for Adverse Events version 4.0[Time Frame: study completion, an average of 2 years]

Incidence of dose limiting toxicities defined as grade 3 or higher toxicity[Time Frame: up to 4 weeks]

Recommended phase 2 dose (RP2D) as the highest doses of palbociclib and cisplatin or palbociclib and carboplatin[Time Frame: study completion, an average of 2 years]

■ **Current Secondary Outcome Measures**

Overall response rate (complete response + partial response) assessed by Response Evaluation Criteria in Solid Tumors 1.1 criteria[Time Frame: Up to 3 years]

Will be summarized and presented along with 95% exact confidence intervals.

Pharmacokinetic (PK) characteristics of carboplatin including maximum concentration (Cmax)[Time Frame: Up to 4 weeks]

Within-subject and between-cohort comparisons of Cmax will be performed using Wilcoxon (non-parametric) test.

Pharmacokinetic (PK) characteristics of cisplatin including maximum concentration (Cmax)[Time Frame: Up to 4 weeks]

Within-subject and between-cohort comparisons of Cmax will be performed using Wilcoxon (non-parametric) test.

Descriptive Information

■ **Offical Title**

A Phase 1 Study of Palbociclib in Combination With Cisplatin or Carboplatin in Advanced Solid Malignancies

■ **Brief Summary**

This phase I trial studies the side effects and best dose of palbociclib with cisplatin or carboplatin in treating patients with solid tumors that have spread to other places and usually cannot be cured or controlled with treatment. Palbociclib may stop the growth of tumor cells by blocking some of the enzymes needed for cell growth. Drugs used in chemotherapy, such as cisplatin and carboplatin, work in different ways to stop the growth of tumor cells, either by killing the cells, by stopping them from dividing, or by stopping them from spreading. Giving palbociclib with cisplatin or carboplatin may help stop tumor growth in patients with advanced solid tumors.

Detailed Description

PRIMARY OBJECTIVES:

I. Assess the safety and tolerability of palbociclib when administered along with cisplatin or carboplatin.

II. Establish the recommended phase 2 dose (RP2D) of the tested combinations.

SECONDARY OBJECTIVES:

I. Characterize the pharmacokinetic (PK) profiles of cisplatin, carboplatin.

II. Obtain preliminary evidence of anti-tumor efficacy of the tested combination regimens.

III. Conduct PK/pharmacodynamics (PD) correlative analyses using palbociclib trough concentration and cyclin-dependent kinase 4 (CDK4) inhibition read-outs in tumor and surrogate samples collected on course 1 day 22 (C1D22).

IV. Assess potential association between tissue-based biomarkers and efficacy.

OUTLINE: This is a dose-escalation study. Patients are assigned to 1 of 2 arms.

ARM A: Patients receive cisplatin intravenously (IV) over 30-60 minutes on day 1 and palbociclib orally (PO) once daily (QD) on days 2-22. Treatment repeats every 28 days for up to 6 courses in the absence of disease progression or unacceptable toxicity.

ARM B: Patients receive carboplatin IV over 30-60 minutes on day 1 and palbociclib PO QD on days 2-22. Treatment repeats every 28 days for up to 6 courses in the absence of disease progression or unacceptable toxicity.

After completion of study treatment, patients are followed for up to 4 weeks.

Study Type

Interventional

Study Phase

Phase 1

Condition

- Solid Neoplasm
- Stage III Pancreatic Cancer
- Stage IIIA Breast Cancer
- Stage IIIA Non-Small Cell Lung Cancer
- Stage IIIB Breast Cancer
- Stage IIIB Non-Small Cell Lung Cancer
- Stage IIIC Breast Cancer
- Stage IV Breast Cancer
- Stage IV Non-Small Cell Lung Cancer
- Stage IVA Pancreatic Cancer
- Stage IVB Pancreatic Cancer
- Sarcoma
- Colorectal Cancer
- Head and Neck Cancer
- Cancer of Unknown Primary
- Bladder Cancer
- Ovarian Cancer

Intervention

Drug: Carboplatin

Given IV

Other Names:

Paraplatin

Drug: Cisplatin

Given IV

Other Names:

CDDP

Cis-diamminedichloridoplatinum

Cisplatinum

Cismaplat

Neoplatin

Drug: Palbociclib

Given PO

Other Names:

Ibrance

PD-0332991

Study Arms

Experimental: Arm A (palbociclib, cisplatin)

Patients receive cisplatin IV over 30-60 minutes on day 1 and palbociclib PO QD on days 2-22. Treatment repeats every 28 days for up to 6 courses in the absence of disease progression or unacceptable toxicity.

Experimental: Arm B (palbociclib, carboplatin)

Patients receive carboplatin IV over 30-60 minutes on day 1 and palbociclib PO QD on days 2-22. Treatment repeats every 28 days for up to 6 courses in the absence of disease progression or unacceptable toxicity.

Recruitment Information

Recruitment Status

Recruiting

Estimated Enrollment

90

Completion Date

February 2021

Primary Completion Date

February 2019

Eligibility Criteria

Inclusion Criteria:

- Patients must have histologically or cytologically confirmed solid organ malignancy
- Patients enrolled in the expansion cohort must have histologically or cytologically confirmed squamous non-small cell lung cancer (NSCLC), breast or pancreaticobiliary tract cancer
- Eastern Cooperative Oncology Group (ECOG) performance status ≤ 2
- Patients must have measurable disease, defined as at least one lesion that can be accurately measured in at least one dimension (longest diameter to be recorded for non-nodal lesions and short axis for nodal lesions) as ≥ 20 mm (≥ 2 cm) with conventional techniques or as ≥ 10 mm (≥ 1 cm) with spiral computed tomography (CT) scan, magnetic resonance imaging (MRI), or calipers by clinical exam
- Leukocytes ≥ 3,000/mL
- Absolute neutrophil count ≥ 1,500/mL
- Platelets ≥ 100,000/mL
- Hemoglobin ≥ 10
- Total bilirubin ≤ 1.5 × institutional upper limit of normal (except for patients with Gilbert disease)
- Aspartate aminotransferase (AST) (serum glutamic-oxaloacetic transaminase [SGOT])/ alanine aminotransferase (ALT) (serum glutamate pyruvate transaminase [SGPT]) ≤ 2.5 × institutional upper limit of normal (up to 5 X upper limit of normal [ULN] for patients with liver metastasis)
- Creatinine within normal institutional limits OR creatinine clearance ≥ 60 mL/min/1.73 m² for patients with creatinine levels above institutional normal
- Women of child-bearing potential and men must agree to use adequate contraception (hormonal or barrier method of birth control; abstinence) prior to study entry and for the duration of study participation; should a woman become pregnant or suspect she is pregnant while she or her partner is participating in this study, she should inform her treating physician immediately; men treated or enrolled on this protocol must also agree to use adequate contraception prior to the study, for the duration of study participation, and for 6 months after completion of study drug administration
- Ability to understand and the willingness to sign a written informed consent document

Exclusion Criteria:

- Patients who have had cytotoxic anticancer chemotherapy or immune checkpoint inhibitor within 4 weeks (6 weeks for nitrosoureas or mitomycin C) or palliative radiation within 2 weeks (stereotactic radiation therapy [SRS] for brain metastasis within 48 hours) prior to entering the study or those who have not recovered from adverse events due to agents administered more than 4 weeks earlier
- Patients receiving cytotoxic agent as immunomodulatory therapy for a non neoplastic indication (e.g. methotrexate for rheumatoid arthritis) and who are unable to discontinue such agents within 2 weeks prior to starting treatment
- Oral targeted therapy within five days or five half-lives, whichever is longer, prior to initiating protocol therapy treatment

- Patients who are receiving any other investigational agents
- Use of strong cytochrome P450, family 3, subfamily A (CYP3A) inhibitors and inducers
- Patients with symptomatic uncontrolled brain metastases are excluded; (patients with stable treated or asymptomatic untreated brain metastasis not requiring glucocorticoids are allowed)
- History of allergic reactions attributed to compounds of similar chemical or biologic composition to palbociclib, carboplatin or cisplatin
- Concurrent administration of strong inducers and inhibitors of CYP3A enzyme or CYP3A substrates with narrow therapeutic window
- Uncontrolled intercurrent illness including, but not limited to:
- Ongoing or active infection requiring intravenous antibiotics at the time of treatment initiation
- Symptomatic congestive heart failure (requiring hospital stay within the last 6 months)
- Myocardial infarction within the last 6 months
- Unstable angina pectoris, cardiac arrhythmia
- Psychiatric illness
- Social situations or circumstances that would limit compliance with study requirements
- Pregnant women are excluded from this study; breastfeeding should be discontinued if the mother is treated with palbociclib
- Human immunodeficiency virus (HIV)-positive patients on combination antiretroviral therapy are ineligible

Sex/Gender

All

Ages

18 Years to N/A

Accepts Healthy Volunteers

No

Contacts

Taofeek Owonikoko, MD, PhD   404-778-1802   towonik@emory.edu

A Study of PDR001 in Combination With CJM112, EGF816, Ilaris® (Canakinumab) or Mekinist® (Trametinib)

Study ID:

NCT02900664

Sponsor:

Novartis Pharmaceuticals

Information provided by (Responsible Party):

Novartis (Novartis Pharmaceuticals)

Tracking Information

First Submitted Date

May 17, 2016

Start Date

August 23, 2016

Primary Completion Date

January 31, 2019

Last Update Posted Date

February 8, 2018

Current Primary Outcome Measures

Frequency of treatment-emergent Adverse Events (AEs) and Serious Adverse Events (SAEs) as a measure of safety[Time Frame: Throughout the study at every visit, an average of 1 year]

Changes between baseline and post-baseline laboratory parameters and vital signs.[Time Frame: Baseline and throughout the study at every visit, an average of 1 year]

Incidence of dose limiting toxicities (DLTs) of treatment (Escalation only)[Time Frame: During the first two cycles; Cycle = 28 days]

Frequency of dose interruptions[Time Frame: Throughout the study at every visit, an average of 1 year]

Dose intensities[Time Frame: Throughout the study at every visit, an average of 1 year]

Severity of treatment-emergent Adverse Events (AEs) and Serious Adverse Events (SAEs) as a measure of safety[Time Frame: Throughout the study at every visit, an average of 1 year]

Frequency of dose reductions[Time Frame: Throughout the study at every visit, an average of 1 year]

Current Secondary Outcome Measures

Key secondary: Histopathology of tumor infiltrating lymphocytes (TILs)[Time Frame: Baseline and approximately after 2 cycles of treatment and at disease progression; Cycle = 28 days]

Changes from baseline in electrocardiogram (ECG) parameters[Time Frame: Baseline and end of treatment, an average of 1 year]

Best overall response (BOR)[Time Frame: T1: Every 2 cycles until the start of T2. T2: Every 2 cycles until cycle 3 and then every 3 cycles until PD; cycle = 28 days]

T1: treatment period 1 (6 cycles of treatment) T2: treatment period 2

Progression free survival (PFS) per irRC and RECIST v1.1[Time Frame: T1: Every 2 cycles until the start of T2. T2: Every 2 cycles until cycle 3 and then every 3 cycles until PD; cycle = 28 days]

T1: treatment period 1 (6 cycles of treatment) T2: treatment period 2

Treatment Free Survival (TFS)[Time Frame: T1: Every 2 cycles until the start of T2. T2: Every 2 cycles until cycle 3 and then every 3 cycles until PD; cycle = 28 days]

T1: treatment period 1 (6 cycles of treatment) T2: treatment period 2

Presence and/or concentration of anti-PDR001 antibodies.[Time Frame: Cycle 1 through cycle 6 in treatment period 1 and 2 (an average of 1 year)]

T1: treatment period 1 (6 cycles of treatment) T2: treatment period 2

Serum concentration of PDR001, canakinumab, CJM112[Time Frame: Cycle 1 through cycle 6 in treatment period 1 and 2 (an average of 1 year)]

T1: treatment period 1 (6 cycles of treatment) T2: treatment period 2

Plasma concentrations of trametinib and EGF816[Time Frame: Cycle 1 through cycle 6 in treatment period 1 and 2 (an average of 1 year)]

T1: treatment period 1 (6 cycles of treatment) T2: treatment period 2

Key secondary: Histopathology of myeloid cell infiltrate by IHC (such as CD8, FoxP3 and myeloid markers as appropriate).[Time Frame: Baseline and approximately after 3 cycles of treatment and at disease progression; cycle = 28 days]

PK parameters (Eg. TMax) of EGF816[Time Frame: Cycle 1 through cycle 6 in treatment period 1 and 2 (an average of 1 year)]

T1: treatment period 1 (6 cycles of treatment) T2: treatment period 2

PK parameters (Eg. TMax) of trametinib[Time Frame: Cycle 1 through cycle 6 in treatment period 1 and 2 (an average of 1 year)]

T1: treatment period 1 (6 cycles of treatment) T2: treatment period 2

PK parameter (Eg. TMax) of PDR001[Time Frame: Cycle 1 through cycle 6 in treatment period 1 and 2 (an average of 1 year)]

T1: treatment period 1 (6 cycles of treatment) T2: treatment period 2

PK parameters (Eg. TMax) of canakinumab[Time Frame: Cycle 1 through cycle 6 in treatment period 1 and 2 (an average of 1 year)]

T1: treatment period 1 (6 cycles of treatment) T2: treatment period 2

PK parameters (Eg. TMax) of CJM112[Time Frame: Cycle 1 through cycle 6 in treatment period 1 and 2 (an average of 1 year)]

T1: treatment period 1 (6 cycles of treatment) T2: treatment period 2

Presence and/or concentration of anti-canakinumab antibodies.[Time Frame: Cycle 1 through cycle 6 in treatment period 1 and 2 (an average of 1 year)]

T1: treatment period 1 (6 cycles of treatment) T2: treatment period 2

Presence and/or concentration of anti-CJM112 antibodies.[Time Frame: Cycle 1 through cycle 6 in treatment period 1 and 2 (an average of 1 year)]

T1: treatment period 1 (6 cycles of treatment) T2: treatment period 2

Descriptive Information

Offical Title

Phase Ib, Open-label, Multi-center Study to Characterize the Safety, Tolerability and Pharmacodynamics (PD) of PDR001 in Combination With CJM112, EGF816, Ilaris® (Canakinumab) or Mekinist® (Trametinib)

Brief Summary

The purpose of this study is to combine the PDR001 checkpoint inhibitor with each of four agents with immunomodulatory activity to identify the doses and schedule for combination therapy and to preliminarily assess the safety, tolerability, pharmacological and clinical activity of these combinations.

Study Type

Interventional

Study Phase

Phase 1

Condition

- Colorectal Cancer, Triple Negative Breast Cancer, NSCLC Adenocarcinoma

Intervention

Biological: PDR001

    Powder for solution for infusion

    Biological: ACZ885

    Solution for injection

Other Names:

    canakinumab

    Biological: CJM112

    Solution for infusion

Drug: TMT212

    Tablets

Other Names:

    trametinib

    Drug: EGF816

    Tablets

Study Arms

Experimental: PDR001+canakinumab in TNBC
Experimental: PDR001+CJM112 in TNBC
Experimental: PDR001+trametinib in TNBC
Experimental: PDR001+EGF816 in TNBC
Experimental: PDR001+canakinumab in NSCLC
Experimental: PDR001+CJM112 in NSCLC
Experimental: PDR001+ trametinib in NSCLC
Experimental: PDR001+EGF816 in NSCLC
Experimental: PDR001+canakinumab in CRC
Experimental: PDR001+ CJM112 in CRC
Experimental: PDR001+trametinib in CRC
Experimental: PDR001+ EGF816 in CRC

Recruitment Information

Recruitment Status

Recruiting

Estimated Enrollment

432

Completion Date

January 31, 2020

Primary Completion Date

January 31, 2019

Eligibility Criteria

Inclusion Criteria:

- Patients with advanced/metastatic cancer, with measurable disease as determined by RECIST version 1.1, who have progressed despite standard therapy or are intolerant to standard therapy, and for whom no effective therapy is available.

Patients must fit into one of the following groups:

- Colorectal cancer (CRC) (not mismatch repair deficient by local assay including PCR and/or immunohistochemistry)
- Non-small cell lung cancer (NSCLC) (adenocarcinoma)
- Triple Negative Breast Cancer (TNBC) (D

- ECOG Performance Status ≤ 2
- Patient must have a site of disease amenable to biopsy, and be a candidate for tumor biopsy according to the treating institution's guidelines. Patient must be willing to undergo a new tumor biopsy at baseline, and again during therapy on this study.
- Prior therapy with PD-1/PDL-1 inhibitors is allowed provided any toxicity attributed to prior PD-1or PD-L1-directed therapy did not lead to discontinuation of therapy.
- Written informed consent must be obtained prior to any screening procedures other than procedures performed as part of standard of care.

Other protocol-defined inclusion criteria may apply.

Exclusion Criteria:

- Presence of symptomatic central nervous system (CNS) metastases, or CNS metastases that require local CNS-directed therapy, or increasing doses of corticosteroids within the prior 2 weeks.
- History of severe hypersensitivity reactions to other monoclonal antibodies.
- Out of range laboratory values for measures of hepatic and renal function, electrolytes and blood counts
- Impaired cardiac function or clinically significant cardiac disease.
- Patients with active, known or suspected autoimmune disease.
- Human Immunodeficiency Virus infection at screening.
- Escalation part: Active Hepatitis B (HBV) or Hepatitis C (HCV) virus infection at screening.

Expansion part: Patients with active HBV or HCV are excluded, excepting those patients undergoing treatment for HBV or HCV.

- Malignant disease, other than that being treated in this study.
- Recent systemic anti-cancer therapy
- Active infection requiring systemic antibiotic therapy.
- Patients requiring chronic treatment with systemic steroid therapy, other than replacement dose steroids in the setting of adrenal insufficiency or treatment with low, stable dose of steroid (<10mg/ day prednisone or equivalent) for stable CNS metastatic disease.
- Patients receiving systemic treatment with any immunosuppressive medication, excepting the above
- Use of any live vaccines against infectious diseases (e.g. influenza, varicella, pneumococcus) within 4 weeks of initiation of study treatment.
- Participation in an interventional, investigational study within 2 weeks of the first dose of study treatment.
- Presence of ≥ CTCAE grade 2 toxicity (except alopecia and ototoxicity, which are excluded if ≥ CTCAE grade 3) due to prior cancer therapy.
- Recent use of hematopoietic colony-stimulating growth factors (e.g. G-CSF, GMCSF, M-CSF)

Additional exclusion criteria for Combination arm PDR001+canakinumab

- Patients with tuberculosis (TB). Note: Patient with latent TB may be eligible based on the investigator's benefit-risk assessment.
- Patients who have been infected with HBV or HCV including those with inactive disease.

Additional exclusion criteria for Combination arm PDR001+CJM112

- Patients with TB. Note: Patient with latent TB may be eligible based on the investigator's benefit-risk assessment.
- Patients with history of and/or active inflammatory bowel disease.
- Active skin or soft tissue infection including cellulitis, erysipelas, impetigo, furuncle,carbuncle, abscess, or fasciitis.
- Active candida infection, including mucocutaneous infection or history of invasive candidiasis.

Additional exclusion criteria for Combination arm PDR001+trametinib

- Patients with history of retinal vein oclusion.
- Patients with history of interstitial lung disease or pneumonitis.
- Patients with cardiomyopathy and/or LVEF < LLN.
- Impairment of gastrointestinal function or GI disease that may significantly alter the absorption of oral combination partners.
- Hemoglobin (Hgb) < 9 g/dL without growth factor or transfusion support
- Women of child-bearing potential using hormonal contraception, unless an additional contraception method is also used according to the Mekinist® label.

Additional exclusion criteria for Combination arm PDR001+EGF816

- NSCLC patients with EGFR mutant tumors.
- Strong inhibitors and strong inducers of CYP3A4 should not be used concomitantly.
- Patients with history of interstitial lung disease.
- Patients who have been infected with HBV or HCV including those with inactive disease.
- Impairment of gastrointestinal function or GI disease that may significantly alter the absorption of oral combination partners
- Patients cannot have received radiotherapy to lung fields within 6 months of study treatment start.

Other protocol-defined exclusion criteria may apply.

- **Sex/Gender**

  All

- **Ages**

  18 Years to N/A

- **Accepts Healthy Volunteers**

  No

- **Contacts**

  Novartis Pharmaceuticals 1-888-669-6682 Novartis.email@novartis.com

  Novartis Pharmaceuticals +41613241111

Arginase Inhibitor INCB001158 as a Single Agent and in Combination With Immune Checkpoint Therapy in Patients With Advanced/Metastatic Solid Tumors

Study ID:

NCT02903914

Sponsor:

Incyte Corporation

Information provided by (Responsible Party):

Incyte Corporation (Incyte Corporation)

Tracking Information

- **First Submitted Date**

  September 9, 2016

- **Start Date**

  September 2016

- **Primary Completion Date**

  May 2019

- **Last Update Posted Date**

  November 6, 2017

- **Current Primary Outcome Measures**

  Safety and Tolerability of INCB001158 as a single agent and in combination with Pembrolizumab: Incidence of Adverse Events[Time Frame: Every 28 days (single agent INCB001158) or 21 days (INCB001158 in combination with Pembrolizumab) from study start until disease progression or unacceptable toxicity, assessed for an expected average of 6 months]

  Evaluation of adverse events (AEs) and changes in laboratory values, vital signs, and physical examinations.

- **Current Secondary Outcome Measures**

  Recommended Phase 2 Dose (RP2D) of INCB001158[Time Frame: 12 Weeks]

  Up to 42 patients with advanced/metastatic solid tumors will be enrolled in Dose Escalation to determine the RP2D of INCB001158 as monotherapy.

  RP2D of INCB001158 with Pembrolizumab[Time Frame: 12 Weeks]

  Up to 42 patients with advanced/metastatic solid tumors will be enrolled in Dose Escalation to determine the RP2D of INCB001158 with Pembrolizumab.

  Plasma pharmacokinetic (PK) profile of INCB001158 alone and in combination with Pembrolizumab[Time Frame: 12 Weeks]

  Non-compartmental method of analysis will be used to analyze the plasma concentrations of INCB001158.

  Anti-tumor Activity of INCB001158 as Monotherapy and in Combination with Pembrolizumab for patients with advanced/metastatic solid tumors[Time Frame: Until disease progression/study discontinuation up to 24 months]

  Assessment of anti-tumor activity per RECIST Criteria (v1.1) and immune-related RECIST (irRECIST) criteria.

Descriptive Information

- **Offical Title**

  Safety, Pharmacokinetics, and Pharmacodynamics of Escalating Oral Doses of the Arginase Inhibitor INCB001158 (Formerly Known as CB1158) as a Single Agent and in Combination With Immune Checkpoint Therapy in Patients With Advanced/

Metastatic Solid Tumors

▨ Brief Summary

This study is an open-label Phase 1/Phase 2 evaluation of INCB001158 as a single agent and in combination with immune checkpoint therapy in patients with advanced/metastatic solid tumors.

▨ Detailed Description

This study is an open-label Phase 1 evaluation of INCB001158 as a single agent and in combination with immune checkpoint therapy in patients with advanced/metastatic solid tumors.

Single Agent INCB001158:

Patients with advanced/metastatic solid tumors will be enrolled into escalating monotherapy dose cohorts to determine the Recommended Phase 2 Dose (RP2D) of INCB001158. Additional patients with NSCLC, Colorectal Cancer (CRC), and other tumors including SCCHN, RCC, Gastric, Bladder and Melanoma will be enrolled at the single agent RP2D.

Combination Treatment:

Patients with advanced/metastatic NSCLC, Melanoma, Urothelial, Microsatellite Instability (MSI)/ Microsatellite Stable (MSS) CRC, Gastric, SCCHN and Mesothelioma will be enrolled into separate cohorts of combination therapy (INCB001158 and Pembrolizumab) to determine the RP2D.

In the dose expansion phase, additional patients with NSCLC, Melanoma, Urothelial, MSI/MSS CRC, Gastric, SCCHN and Mesothelioma will be treated with the combination of INCB001158 and Pembrolizumab at the RP2D.

All patients will be assessed for safety, pharmacokinetics, biomarkers and tumor response.

▨ Study Type

Interventional

▨ Study Phase

Phase 1/Phase 2

▨ Condition

- Metastatic Cancer
- Solid Tumors
- Non-small Cell Lung Cancer
- Colorectal Cancer
- Gastric Cancers
- Renal Cell Carcinoma
- Squamous Cell Carcinoma of the Head and Neck
- Bladder Cancer
- Urothelial Carcinoma
- Mesothelioma

▨ Intervention

Drug: INCB001158

  Arginase Inhibitor

Other Names:

  CB-1158

  Drug: Pembrolizumab

  PD-1 Inhibitor

Other Names:

  Keytruda

▨ Study Arms

Experimental: Monotherapy Dose Escalation Solid Tumors

  Monotherapy Part 1a: INCB001158 administered orally in patients with advanced/metastatic solid tumors. Escalating doses will be explored to determine the recommended phase 2 dose (RP2D).

Experimental: INCB001158 as Monotherapy in NSCLC

  Monotherapy Part 2a: INCB001158 administered orally at the RP2D in patients with advanced/metastatic NSCLC (EGFR and Anaplastic Lymphoma Kinase (ALK) negative) previously treated with Standard of Care (SOC).

Experimental: INCB001158 as Monotherapy in CRC

  Monotherapy Part 2b: INCB001158 administered orally at the RP2D in patients with advanced/metastatic CRC previously treated with SOC.

Experimental: INCB001158 as Monotherapy in Solid Tumors

Monotherapy Part 2c: INCB001158 administered orally at the RP2D in patients with Bladder Cancer, Gastric or Gastroesophageal Junction (GEJ) Cancer, Renal Cell Cancer (RCC), Squamous Cell Carcinoma of the Head and Neck (SCCHN), Urothelial Cell Cancer (UCC), or Melanoma, previously treated with SOC.

Experimental: INCB001158 and anti-PD-1 in Combination Dose Escalation

Combination Part 1b: INCB001158 and Pembrolizumab administered in patients with advanced/metastatic NSCLC, Melanoma, Urothelial Cell Cancer, MSI CRC, MSS CRC, Gastric or Gastroesophageal Junction (GEJ) Cancer, SCCHN and Mesothelioma. Multiple dose levels will be explored to determine the recommended phase 2 dose (RP2D).

Experimental: INCB001158 and anti-PD-1 in NSCLC

Part 3a: INCB001158 and Pembrolizumab the combination RP2D in patients with advanced/metastatic NSCLC (EGFR and ALK negative) with disease progression on anti-PD-1 therapy or prolonged stable disease on Pembrolizumab in the immediate prior line of therapy.

Experimental: INCB001158 and anti-PD-1 in Melanoma

Part 3b: INCB001158 and Pembrolizumab at the combination RP2D administered in patients with advanced/metastatic Melanoma with disease progression on anti-PD-1 therapy or prolonged stable disease on Pembrolizumab in the immediate prior line of therapy.

Experimental: INCB001158 and anti-PD-1 in Urothelial Carcinoma

Part 3c: INCB001158 and Pembrolizumab at the combination RP2D administered in patients with advanced/metastatic Urothelial Carcinoma with disease progression on anti-PD-1 therapy or prolonged stable disease on Pembrolizumab in the immediate prior line of therapy.

Experimental: INCB001158 and anti-PD-1 in MSI CRC

Part 3d: INCB001158 and Pembrolizumab at the combination RP2D administered in patients with advanced/metastatic MSI CRC with disease progression on anti-PD-1 therapy or prolonged stable disease on Pembrolizumab in the immediate prior line of therapy.

Experimental: INCB001158 and anti-PD-1 in MSS CRC

Part 3e: INCB001158 and Pembrolizumab at the combination RP2D administered in patients with advanced/metastatic MSS CRC that have received at least 1 prior 5-FU containing therapy and must not have had any prior checkpoint inhibitor therapy.

Experimental: INCB001158 and anti-PD-1 in Gastric/GE Junction

Part 3f: INCB001158 and Pembrolizumab at the combination RP2D administered in patients with advanced/metastatic Gastric/GE Junction that have never received prior checkpoint inhibitor therapy.

Experimental: INCB001158 and anti-PD-1 in SCCHN

Part 3g: INCB001158 and Pembrolizumab at the combination RP2D administered in patients with advanced/metastatic SCCHN that have never received prior checkpoint inhibitor therapy.

Experimental: INCB001158 and anti-PD-1 in Mesothelioma

Part 3h: INCB001158 and Pembrolizumab at the combination RP2D administered in patients with advanced/metastatic mesothelioma that have received or were unable to receive standard front line standard therapy and have never received prior checkpoint inhibitor therapy.

Recruitment Information

Recruitment Status

Recruiting

Estimated Enrollment

346

Completion Date

May 2019

Primary Completion Date

May 2019

Eligibility Criteria

Additional cohort specific criteria may apply

Inclusion Criteria:

- Must be age 18 or older
- Ability to provide written informed consent in accordance with federal, local, and institutional guidelines
- Histological or cytological diagnosis of metastatic cancer or locally advanced cancer that is not amenable to local therapy
- Eastern Cooperative Oncology Group (ECOG) Performance Status of 0-1
- Life Expectancy of at least 3 months
- Adequate hepatic, renal, cardiac, and hematologic function
- Measurable disease by RECISTv1.1 criteria
- Resolution of treatment-related toxicities

- Willingness to avoid pregnancy or fathering children
- Prior anti-PD-1 treatment for combination dose expansion cohorts 3a 3d

Exclusion Criteria:

- Currently pregnant or lactating
- Unable to receive oral medications
- Unable to receive oral or IV hydration
- Intolerance to prior anti-PD-1/PD-L1 therapy
- Prior anti-PD-1 treatment for combination dose expansion cohorts 3e 3h
- Prior severe hypersensitivity reaction to another monoclonal antibody (mAb)
- Any other current or previous malignancy within 3 years except protocol allowed malignancies
- Chemotherapy, Tyrosine Kinase Inhibitor therapy, radiation therapy or hormonal therapy within 2 weeks
- Immunotherapy or biological therapy, or investigational agent within 3 weeks (Note: some cohort exceptions allow anti-PD-1 therapy)
- Active known or suspected exclusionary autoimmune disease
- Any condition requiring systemic treatment with either corticosteroids (> 10 mg daily prednisone equivalent) or other systemic immunosuppressive medications within 2 weeks
- Concomitant therapy with valproic acid/valproate-containing therapies
- Concomitant therapy with allopurinol and other xanthine oxidase inhibitors
- History of known risks factors for bowel perforation
- Symptomatic ascites or pleural effusion
- Major surgery within 28 days before Cycle 1 Day 1
- Active infection requiring within 2 weeks prior to first dose of study drug
- Patients who have HIV, Hepatitis B or C
- Conditions that could interfere with treatment or protocol-related procedures
- Active, non-stable brain metastases or CNS disease
- Known deficiencies or suspected defect in the urea cycle
- Received live-virus vaccination within 30 days (seasonal flu vaccine allowed if non-live virus)
- NSCLC with EGFR or ALK mutation

Sex/Gender

All

Ages

18 Years to N/A

Accepts Healthy Volunteers

No

Contacts

Incyte Corporation Call Center (US)   1.855.463.3463   medinfo@incyte.com

Study of Irinotecan and AZD1775, a Selective Wee 1 Inhibitor, in RAS or BRAF Mutated, Second-line Metastatic Colorectal Cancer

Study ID:

NCT02906059

Sponsor:

New York University School of Medicine

Information provided by (Responsible Party):

New York University School of Medicine (New York University School of Medicine)

Tracking Information

First Submitted Date

September 9, 2016

Start Date

September 2016

Primary Completion Date

September 2018

Last Update Posted Date

November 22, 2017

Current Primary Outcome Measures

Number of participants dose limiting toxicities with treatment-related adverse events as assessed by common terminology criteria for adverse events (CTCAE), version 4.[Time Frame: Up to 12 months]

Current Secondary Outcome Measures

Tumor assessment by imaging techniques using Response Evaluation Criteria in Solid Tumors (RECIST), version 1.1[Time Frame: From baseline to every 8 weeks up to 12 months]

Descriptive Information

Offical Title

A Phase Ib Study Combining Irinotecan With AZD1775, a Selective Wee 1 Inhibitor, in RAS (KRAS or NRAS) or BRAF Mutated Metastatic Colorectal Cancer Patients Who Have Progressed on First Line Therapy

Brief Summary

The purpose of this study is to determine whether combination therapy of irinotecan with AZD1775 is safe and effective in treating mutated metastatic colorectal cancer patients.

Study Type

Interventional

Study Phase

Phase 1

Condition

- Metastatic Colorectal Cancer

Intervention

Drug: AZD1775

Drug: Irinotecan

Other Names:

Camptosar, Campto

Study Arms

Experimental: AZD1775 & Irinotecan

Group AZD1775 (study drug); Irinotecan (chemotherapy)

1) 125 mg two times a day (BID) for 3 days every 2 weeks; 180mg/m2 every 2 weeks

2A) 150 mg BID for 3 days every 2 weeks; 180mg/m2 every 2 weeks

2B) 125 mg BID for 5 days every 2 weeks; 180mg/m2 every 2 weeks

3) 150 mg BID for 5 days every 2 weeks ; 180mg/m2 every 2 weeks

Recruitment Information

Recruitment Status

Recruiting

Estimated Enrollment

32

Eligibility Criteria

Inclusion Criteria:

- Provide signed and dated informed consent prior to any study specific procedures
- Age 18 years or older

Completion Date

September 2019

Primary Completion Date

September 2018

- Histological or cytological confirmation of Colorectal Cancer (CRC) with available tissue, currently stage IV
- Failure of first-line anti-cancer therapy with an oxaliplatin and bevacizumab based regimen (either radiological documentation of disease progression or due to toxicity) or subsequent relapse of disease following first-line therapy. Patients relapsing within 12 months of completing adjuvant FOLFOX will also be considered eligible.
- Eastern Cooperative Oncology Group (ECOG) Performance Status 0 1
- At least one lesion, not previously irradiated, that can be accurately measured as ≥ 10 mm in the longest diameter (LD) with spiral computed tomography (CT) scan or as ≥ 20 mm with conventional techniques (conventional CT, MRI) and which is suitable for accurate repeated measurements
- Tumor sample confirmed as KRAS or NRAS [codons 12 and 13 (exon 2), 59 and 61 (exon 3), and 117 and 146 (exon 4)] or BRAF [codon 600 (exon 15)] mutation positive.
- Patients must be able to swallow AZD1775 capsules

Exclusion Criteria:

- Treatment within 14 days prior to first study treatment with conventional therapy or treatment within 28 days prior to first study treatment with an investigational drug
- Received more than 1 line of systemic treatment for advanced/metastatic CRC and/or a patient whose first line therapy did not contain oxaliplatin and bevacizumab
- Prior treatment with a Wee1 inhibitor or any irinotecan containing regimen
- Any unresolved toxicity ≥ CTCAE Grade 2 from previous anti-cancer therapy, except for alopecia and neurotoxicity.
- The last radiation therapy within 4 weeks prior to starting study treatment, or limited field of radiation for palliation within 2 weeks of the first dose of study treatment
- Recent major surgery within 4 weeks prior to entry into the study (excluding the placement of vascular access) which would prevent administration of study treatment
- History of hypersensitivity to AZD1775, irinotecan, or any excipients of these agents
- Brain metastases or spinal cord compression unless asymptomatic, treated and stable off steroids and anti-convulsants for at least 3 months
- Laboratory values as listed below (from laboratory results during screening):
- Absolute Neutrophil Count (ANC) <1.5 x 10^9/L (1500 per mm3)
- Platelets < 100 x 109/L (100,000 per mm3)
- Hemoglobin <9.0 g/dL
- Serum bilirubin >Upper Limit of Normal (ULN)
- Aspartate aminotransferase (AST) or Alanine aminotransferase (ALT):
- > 2.5 x ULN
- > 5 x ULN, if liver metastasis present
- Creatinine clearance < 50 cc/min measured or calculated by Cockcroft Gault equation Cardiac conditions as follows:
- Uncontrolled hypertension (BP ≥ 170/100 despite optimal therapy)
- Heart failure New York Heart Association (NYHA) Class II or above
- Prior or current cardiomyopathy
- If NYHA Class I heart failure, Left Ventricular Ejection Fraction (LVEF) by Multi Gated Acquisition Scan (MUGA) or Echocardiogram (ECHO) is less than 50%
- Unstable ischemic heart disease (myocardial infarction within 6 months prior to starting treatment, or angina requiring use of nitrates more than once weekly)
- Mean resting corrected QT (QTc) interval using the Fridericia formula (QTcF) > 450 msec/male and > 470 msec/female (as calculated per institutional standards) obtained from 3 electrocardiograms (ECGs) 2-5 minutes apart at study entry, or congenital long QT syndrome
- Patients with significant ventricular or supraventricular arrhythmias and patients with cardiac conduction abnormalities that are not controlled (e.g. with a pacemaker or medication).
- Any evidence of severe or uncontrolled systemic disease, active infection, active bleeding diatheses or renal transplant, including any patient known to have hepatitis B, hepatitis C or human immunodeficiency virus (HIV)
- Refractory nausea and vomiting, chronic gastrointestinal diseases (e.g., inflammatory bowel disease), or significant bowel resection that would preclude adequate ingestion and absorption of an oral agent
- Clinical evidence of bowel obstruction at the time of study entry
- Female patients who are pregnant or breast-feeding, or male or female patients of reproductive potential who are not employing an effective method of birth control
- History of another primary malignancy within 5 years prior to starting study treatment, except for adequately treated basal or squamous cell carcinoma of the skin or cancer of the cervix in situ. Patients with an early stage cancer, now off therapy for at least 3 years may be enrolled with permission of the PI if that disease is unlikely to interfere with the primary endpoints of this study.

■ Sex/Gender

All

Combination Chemotherapy With or Without Atezolizumab in Treating Patients With Stage III Colon Cancer and Deficient DNA Mismatch Repair

Study ID:

NCT02912559

Sponsor:

National Cancer Institute (NCI)

Information provided by (Responsible Party):

National Cancer Institute (NCI) (National Cancer Institute (NCI))

Tracking Information

■ **First Submitted Date**

September 22, 2016

■ **Start Date**

September 12, 2017

■ **Primary Completion Date**

July 1, 2020

■ **Last Update Posted Date**

February 12, 2018

■ **Current Primary Outcome Measures**

Disease free survival (DFS)[Time Frame: From the time from randomization to first documentation of disease recurrent or death, assessed up to 5 years]

DFS will be compared between treatment arms using the stratified log rank test at one-sided level 0.025. The hazard ratio (HR) for DFS will be estimated using a stratified Cox proportional hazards model and the 95% confidence interval (CI) for the HR will be provided. Results from an unstratified analysis will also be provided. Kaplan-Meier methodology will be used to estimate the median DFS for each treatment arm, and Kaplan-Meier curves will be produced. Brookmeyer Crowley methodology will be used to construct the 95% CI for the median DFS for each treatment arm.

■ **Current Secondary Outcome Measures**

Incidence of adverse events assessed by Common Terminology Criteria for Adverse Events version 4.0[Time Frame: Up to 30 days after last treatment]

Frequency tables will be reviewed to determine the patterns. The overall adverse event rates will be compared between treatment arms using Chi-square test (or Fisher's exact test if the data in contingency table is sparse).

Overall survival[Time Frame: From the time from randomization to death, from any cause, assessed up to 5 years]

The distribution of overall survival will be estimated using the method of Kaplan-Meier. Overall survival will be compared between treatment arms using the log-rank test.

Descriptive Information

■ **Offical Title**

Randomized Trial of Standard Chemotherapy Alone or Combined With Atezolizumab as Adjuvant Therapy for Patients With Stage III Colon Cancer and Deficient DNA Mismatch Repair

■ **Brief Summary**

This randomized phase III trial studies combination chemotherapy and atezolizumab to see how well it works compared with combination chemotherapy alone in treating patients with stage III colon cancer and deficient deoxyribonucleic acid (DNA) mismatch repair. Drugs used in combination chemotherapy, such as oxaliplatin, leucovorin calcium, and fluorouracil, work in different ways to stop the growth of tumor cells, either by killing the cells, by stopping them from dividing, or by stopping them from spreading. Monoclonal antibodies, such as atezolizumab, may interfere with the ability of tumor cells to grow and spread. Giving combination chemotherapy with atezolizumab may work better than combination chemotherapy alone in treating patients with colon cancer.

Detailed Description

PRIMARY OBJECTIVES:

I. To determine whether atezolizumab combined with oxaliplatin, leucovorin calcium, and fluorouracil (FOLFOX) and its continuation as monotherapy can significantly improve disease-free survival (DFS) compared to FOLFOX alone in patients with stage III colon cancers and deficient DNA mismatch repair (dMMR).

SECONDARY OBJECTIVES:

I. To determine whether atezolizumab combined with FOLFOX and its continuation as monotherapy can significantly improve overall survival compared to FOLFOX alone in patients with stage III colon cancers and dMMR.

II. To assess the adverse events (AE) profile and safety of each treatment arm, using the Common Terminology Criteria for Adverse Events (CTCAE) and patient related outcomes (PRO)-CTCAE.

TERTIARY OBJECTIVES:

I. To determine the impact of the addition of atezolizumab to FOLFOX on patient-reported neuropathy, health-related quality of life (QOL), and functional domains of health-related QOL.

II. To determine if the "immunoscore" can predict the efficacy of atezolizumab for disease-free survival among patients with stage III colon cancer.

III. To assess whether circulating immune cell populations can predict the efficacy of atezolizumab as adjuvant therapy for stage III colon cancer.

IV. To explore the associations of genomic alterations identified in cell-free (cf)DNA with DFS in patients treated with FOLFOX with or without atezolizumab.

V. To assess whether soluble markers of systemic inflammation in blood can predict the efficacy of atezolizumab as adjuvant therapy for stage III colon cancer.

- VI. To assess the relationship between baseline plasma 25(OH) D levels, change in 25(OH)D levels, and DFS and overall survival (OS) in patients with stage III colon cancer receiving FOLFOX +/atezolizumab.

VII. To determine the ability of using fecal microbiota and their metabolic products to predict survival benefit from anti-PD-L1 antibody therapy in dMMR colon cancer patients.

VIII. To determine if hypermutation or hyper-indel status is associated with response to atezolizumab.

IX. To determine if unique messenger ribonucleic acid (mRNA) expression signatures are predictive of disease-free survival among patients receiving adjuvant chemotherapy for stage III colon cancer.

X. To determine if the efficacy of atezolizumab differs among dMMR cancers due to germline MMR mutation (MLH1, MSH2, MSH6, PMS2) versus those with MLH1 hypermethylation and CIMP in patients with stage III colon cancer.

XI. To identify overall mutational burden and number of putative tumor neoantigens in colon carcinoma specimens.

OUTLINE: Patients are randomized to 1 of 2 arms.

ARM I: Patients receive oxaliplatin intravenously (IV) over 2 hours and leucovorin calcium IV over 2 hours on day 1, and fluorouracil IV as a bolus on day 1, then continuously over 46 hours on days 1-3. Treatment repeats every 14 days for up to 12 courses in the absence of disease progression or unacceptable toxicity. Patients also receive atezolizumab IV over 30-60 minutes starting on day 1 of course 1 or 2. Treatment repeats every 14 days for up to 25 courses in the absence of disease progression or unacceptable toxicity.

ARM II: Patients receive oxaliplatin IV over 2 hours and leucovorin calcium IV over 2 hours on day 1, and fluorouracil IV as a bolus on day 1, then continuously over 46 hours on days 1-3. Treatment repeats every 14 days for up to 12 courses in the absence of disease progression or unacceptable toxicity.

After completion of study treatment, patients are followed up for recurrence every 6 months for 2 years, then annually for 3 years. Patients are also followed up for survival every 6 months for up to 8 years.

Study Type

Interventional

Study Phase

Phase 3

Condition

- Colon Adenocarcinoma
- DNA Repair Disorder
- Lynch Syndrome
- Stage III Colon Cancer AJCC v7
- Stage IIIA Colon Cancer AJCC v7
- Stage IIIB Colon Cancer AJCC v7
- Stage IIIC Colon Cancer AJCC v7

■ **Intervention**

Drug: Atezolizumab
  Given IV

Other Names:
  MPDL 3280A

  MPDL 328OA

  MPDL-3280A

  MPDL3280A

  MPDL328OA

  RG7446

  RO5541267

  Tecentriq

Drug: Fluorouracil
  Given IV

Other Names:
  5-Fluoro-2,4(1H, 3H)-pyrimidinedione

  5-Fluorouracil

  5-Fluracil

  5-FU

  AccuSite

  Carac

  Fluoro Uracil

  Fluouracil

  Flurablastin

  Fluracedyl

  Fluracil

  Fluril

  Fluroblastin

  Ribofluor

  Ro 2-9757

  Ro-2-9757

Other: Laboratory Biomarker Analysis
  Correlative studies

Drug: Leucovorin Calcium
  Given IV

Other Names:
  Adinepar

  Calcifolin

  Calcium (6S)-Folinate

  Calcium Folinate

  Calcium Leucovorin

  Calfolex

  Calinat

  Cehafolin

  Citofolin

Citrec

citrovorum factor

Cromatonbic Folinico

Dalisol

Disintox

Divical

Ecofol

Emovis

Factor, Citrovorum

Flynoken A

Folaren

Folaxin

FOLI-cell

Foliben

Folidan

Folidar

Folinac

Folinate Calcium

folinic acid

Folinic Acid Calcium Salt Pentahydrate

Folinoral

Folinvit

Foliplus

Folix

Imo

Lederfolat

Lederfolin

Leucosar

leucovorin

Rescufolin

Rescuvolin

Tonofolin

Wellcovorin

Drug: Oxaliplatin
Given IV

Other Names:
1-OHP

Ai Heng

Aiheng

Dacotin

Dacplat

Diaminocyclohexane Oxalatoplatinum

Eloxatin

Eloxatine

JM-83

Oxalatoplatin

Oxalatoplatinum

RP 54780

RP-54780

SR-96669

Other: Quality-of-Life Assessment
   Ancillary studies

Other Names:
   Quality of Life Assessment

▦ Study Arms

Experimental: Arm I (combination chemotherapy, atezolizumab)

   Patients receive oxaliplatin IV over 2 hours and leucovorin calcium IV over 2 hours on day 1, and fluorouracil IV as a bolus on day 1, then continuously over 46 hours on days 1-3. Treatment repeats every 14 days for up to 12 courses in the absence of disease progression or unacceptable toxicity. Patients also receive atezolizumab IV over 30-60 minutes starting on day 1 of course 1 or 2. Treatment repeats every 14 days for up to 25 courses in the absence of disease progression or unacceptable toxicity.

Active Comparator: Arm II (combination chemotherapy)

   Patients receive oxaliplatin IV over 2 hours and leucovorin calcium IV over 2 hours on day 1, and fluorouracil IV as a bolus on day 1, then continuously over 46 hours on days 1-3. Treatment repeats every 14 days for up to 12 courses in the absence of disease progression or unacceptable toxicity.

Recruitment Information

▦ Recruitment Status
Recruiting

▦ Estimated Enrollment
700

▦ Completion Date
July 1, 2020

▦ Primary Completion Date
July 1, 2020

▦ Eligibility Criteria

Inclusion Criteria:

- Histologically proven stage III colon adenocarcinoma (any T [Tx, T1, T2, T3, or T4], N1-2M0; includes N1C)
- Presence of deficient (d) DNA mismatch repair (dMMR); MMR status must be assessed by immunohistochemistry (IHC) for MMR protein expression (MLH1, MSH2, MSH6, PMS2) where loss of one or more proteins indicates dMMR; dMMR may be determined either locally or by site-selected reference lab; Note: loss of MLH1 and PMS2 commonly occur together; formalin-fixed paraffin-embedded (FFPE) tumor tissue is required for subsequent retrospective central confirmation of dMMR status
- Patients with testing that did not show dMMR (loss of MMR protein) are not eligible to participate; patients whose tumors show MSI-H by polymerase chain reaction (PCR)-based assay are not eligible to participate unless they also have MMR testing by IHC and are found to have dMMR (i.e. loss of one or more MMR proteins)
- Patients who are known to have Lynch syndrome and have been found to carry a specific germline mutation in an MMR gene (MLH1, MSH2, MSH6, PMS2) are eligible to participate
- Tumors must have been completely resected; in patients with tumor adherent to adjacent structures, en bloc R0 resection must be documented; positive radial margins are not excluded as long as en bloc resection was performed; proximal or distal margin positivity is excluded
- Entire tumor must be in the colon (rectal involvement is an exclusion); surgeon confirmation that entire tumor was located in the colon is required only in cases where it is important to establish if the tumor is a colon versus (vs.) rectal primary
- Based upon the operative report and other source documentation, the location of the primary tumor will be categorized as proximal or distal to the splenic flexure (distal includes), and further categorization will be as follows: cecum/ascending, descending, sigmoid colon, or rectosigmoid colon
- No evidence of residual involved lymph node disease or metastatic disease at the time of registration based on clinician assessment of imaging; the treating physician will determine if incidental lesions on imaging require workup to exclude metastatic disease; if based on review of images, the treating physician determines the patient to be stage III, then the patient is eligible
- No prior medical therapy (chemotherapy, immunotherapy, biologic or targeted therapy) or radiation therapy for colon cancer except for one cycle of mFOLFOX6
- Eastern Cooperative Oncology Group (ECOG) performance status =< 2
- For women of childbearing potential only, a negative pregnancy test done =< 7 days prior to registration is required; a female of childbearing potential is a sexually mature female who:

- Has not undergone a hysterectomy or bilateral oophorectomy; or
- Has not been naturally postmenopausal for at least 12 consecutive months (i.e. has had menses at any time in the preceding 12 consecutive months)
- Absolute neutrophil count (ANC) >= 1500 mm^3
- Platelet count >= 100,000 mm^3; platelets >= 75,000 required for patients who received cycle 1 of mFOLFOX6 prior to registration
- Creatinine =< 1.5 x upper limit of normal (ULN) or
- Calculated creatinine clearance >= 45 mL/min by Cockcroft-Gault equation
- Total bilirubin =< 1.5 x upper limit of normal (ULN) except in the case of Gilbert disease
- Aspartate aminotransferase (AST)/alanine aminotransferase (ALT) =< 2.5 x upper limit of normal (ULN)
- Thyroid-stimulating hormone (TSH) within normal limits (WNL); supplementation is acceptable to achieve a TSH WNL; in patients with abnormal TSH, if free T4 is normal and patient is clinically euthyroid, patient is eligible
- No active known autoimmune disease, including colitis, inflammatory bowel disease (i.e. ulcerative colitis or Crohn's disease), rheumatoid arthritis, panhypopituitarism, adrenal insufficiency
- No known active hepatitis B or C
- Active hepatitis B can be defined as:
- Hepatitis B virus surface antigen (HBsAg) detectable for > 6 months;
- Serum hepatitis B virus (HBV) DNA 20,000 IU/ml (105 copies/ml); lower values 2,000-20,000 IU/ml (104-105 copies/ml) are often seen in hepatitis B virus e antigen (HBeAg)-negative chronic hepatitis B
- Persistent or intermittent elevation in ALT/AST levels
- Liver biopsy showing chronic hepatitis with moderate or severe necroinflammation
- Active hepatitis C can be defined as:
- Hepatitis C antibody (AB) positive AND
- Presence of hepatitis C virus (HCV) RNA
- Excluded if known active pulmonary disease with hypoxia defined as:
- Oxygen saturation < 85% on room air, or
- Oxygen saturation < 88% despite supplemental oxygen
- No grade >= 2 peripheral motor or sensory neuropathy
- Patients positive for human immunodeficiency virus (HIV) are eligible only if they meet all of the following:
- A stable regimen of highly active anti-retroviral therapy (HAART)
- No requirement for concurrent antibiotics or antifungal agents for the prevention of opportunistic infections
- A CD4 count above 250 cells/mcL, and an undetectable HIV viral load on standard PCR-based tests
- No other planned concurrent investigational agents or other tumor directed therapy (chemotherapy, radiation) while on study
- No systemic daily treatment with either corticosteroids (> 10 mg daily prednisone equivalents) or other immunosuppressive medications within 7 days of registration
- No known history of severe allergic anaphylactic reactions to chimeric, human or humanized antibodies, or fusion proteins
- No known hypersensitivity to Chinese hamster ovary (CHO) cell products or any component of the atezolizumab formulation
- No known allergy to 5-fluorouracil, oxaliplatin, or leucovorin

Sex/Gender

All

Ages

18 Years to N/A

Accepts Healthy Volunteers

No

Study of Encorafenib + Cetuximab Plus or Minus Binimetinib vs. Irinotecan/Cetuximab or Infusional 5-Fluorouracil (5-FU)/Folinic Acid (FA)/Irinotecan (FOLFIRI)/Cetuximab With a Safety Lead-in of Encorafenib + Binimetinib + Cetuximab in Patients With BRAF V600E-mutant Metastatic Colorectal Cancer

Study ID:

NCT02928224

Sponsor:

Array BioPharma

Information provided by (Responsible Party):

Array BioPharma (Array BioPharma)

Tracking Information

▦ **First Submitted Date**

August 16, 2016

▦ **Start Date**

August 2016

▦ **Primary Completion Date**

July 2019

▦ **Last Update Posted Date**

February 12, 2018

▦ **Current Primary Outcome Measures**

(Safety Lead-in) Incidence of dose-limiting toxicities (DLTs)[Time Frame: Cycle 1 (up to 28 days)]

   (Safety Lead-in) Incidence and severity of adverse events (AEs) and changes in clinical laboratory parameters, vital signs, electrocardiograms (ECGs), echocardiogram (ECHO)/multi-gated acquisition (MUGA) scans and ophthalmic examinations[Time Frame: Duration of safety lead-in, approximately 6 months (up to 28 days per cycle)]

(Safety Lead-in) Incidence of dose interruptions, dose modifications and discontinuations due to adverse events (AEs)[Time Frame: Duration of safety lead-in, approximately 6 months (up to 28 days per cycle)]

(Phase 3) Overall Survival (OS) of Triplet Arm vs. Control Arm[Time Frame: Duration of Phase 3, approximately 6 months (up to 28 days per cycle)]

▦ **Current Secondary Outcome Measures**

(Safety Lead-in) Response Rate (ORR)[Time Frame: Duration of safety lead-in, approximately 6 months (up to 28 days per cycle)]

   (Safety Lead-in) Duration of Response (DOR)[Time Frame: Duration of safety lead-in, approximately 6 months (up to 28 days per cycle)]

   (Safety Lead-in) Time to Response[Time Frame: Duration of safety lead-in, approximately 6 months (up to 28 days per cycle)]

   (Phase 3) Overall Survival (OS) in Doublet Arm vs. Control Arm and Triplet Arm vs. Doublet Arm[Time Frame: Duration of Phase 3, approximately 6 months (up to 28 days per cycle)]

   (Phase 3) Comparison of Progression-free Survival (PFS) in study arms[Time Frame: Duration of Phase 3, approximately 6 months (up to 28 days per cycle)]

   (Phase 3) Comparison of Objective Response Rate (ORR) in study arms[Time Frame: Duration of Phase 3, approximately 6 months (up to 28 days per cycle)]

   (Phase 3) Comparison of Duration of Response (DOR) in study arms[Time Frame: Duration of Phase 3, approximately 6 months (up to 28 days per cycle)]

   (Phase 3) Comparison of Time to Response in study arms[Time Frame: Duration of Phase 3, approximately 6 months (up to 28 days per cycle)]

(Phase 3) Incidence and severity of adverse events (AEs) and changes in clinical laboratory parameters, vital signs, electrocardiograms (ECGs), echocardiogram (ECHO)/multi-gated acquisition (MUGA) scans and ophthalmic examinations[Time Frame: Duration of Phase 3, approximately 6 months (up to 28 days per cycle)]

   (Phase 3) Comparison of the Quality of Life in study arms[Time Frame: Duration of Phase 3, approximately 6 months (up to 28 days per cycle)]

   (Safety Lead-in) Evaluation of the area under the concentration-time curve (AUC) for cetuximab, encorafenib, binimetinib, and a metabolite of binimetinib[Time Frame: Predose and 1, 2, 4 and 6 hours post-dose on Day 1 of Cycles 1 and 2]

(Safety Lead-in) Evaluation of the maximum concentration (Cmax) for cetuximab, encorafenib, binimetinib, and a metabolite of binimetinib[Time Frame: Predose and 1, 2, 4 and 6 hours post-dose on Day 1 of Cycles 1 and 2]

(Safety Lead-in) Evaluation of the time of maximum observed concentration (Tmax) for cetuximab, encorafenib, binimetinib, and a metabolite of binimetinib[Time Frame: Predose and 1, 2, 4 and 6 hours post-dose on Day 1 of Cycles 1 and 2]

(Safety Lead-in) Evaluation of the steady-state concentration measured just before the next dose of study drug (Ctrough) for cetuximab, encorafenib, binimetinib, and a metabolite of binimetinib[Time Frame: Predose and 1, 2, 4 and 6 hours post-dose on Day 1 of Cycles 1 and 2]

Descriptive Information

▣ Offical Title

- A Multicenter, Randomized, Open-label, 3-Arm Phase 3 Study of Encorafenib + Cetuximab Plus or Minus Binimetinib vs. Irinotecan/Cetuximab or Infusional 5Fluorouracil (5-FU)/Folinic Acid (FA) /Irinotecan (FOLFIRI)/Cetuximab With a Safety Lead-in of Encorafenib + Binimetinib + Cetuximab in Patients With BRAF V600E-mutant Metastatic Colorectal Cancer

▣ Brief Summary

This is a multicenter, randomized, open-label, 3-arm Phase 3 study to evaluate encorafenib + cetuximab plus or minus binimetinib versus Investigator's choice of either irinotecan/cetuximab or FOLFIRI/cetuximab, as controls, in patients with BRAFV600E mCRC whose disease has progressed after 1 or 2 prior regimens in the metastatic setting. The study contains a Safety Lead-in Phase in which the safety and tolerability of encorafenib + binimetinib + cetuximab will be assessed prior to the Phase 3 portion of the study.

▣ Study Type

Interventional

▣ Study Phase

Phase 3

▣ Condition

- BRAF V600E-mutant Metastatic Colorectal Cancer

▣ Intervention

Drug: Encorafenib
    Orally, once daily.

    Drug: Binimetinib

    Orally, twice daily.

Drug: Cetuximab
    Standard of care.

    Drug: Irinotecan

    Standard of care.

Drug: Folinic Acid
    Standard of care.

Other Names:
    FA

    Drug: 5-Fluorouracil

    Standard of care.

Other Names:
    5-FU

▣ Study Arms

Experimental: Safety Lead-in, Triplet Arm
    Encorafenib + binimetinib + cetuximab.

Experimental: Doublet Arm
    Encorafenib + cetuximab.

Active Comparator: Control Arm
    Investigator's choice of either irinotecan/cetuximab or FOLFIRI/cetuximab.

Recruitment Information

Recruitment Status
Recruiting

Completion Date
July 2019

Estimated Enrollment
645

Primary Completion Date
July 2019

Eligibility Criteria

Key Inclusion Criteria:
- Age ≥ 18 years at time of informed consent
- Histologicallyor cytologically-confirmed CRC that is metastatic
- Presence of BRAFV600E in tumor tissue as previously determined by a local assay at any time prior to Screening or by the central laboratory
- Progression of disease after 1 or 2 prior regimens in the metastatic setting
- Evidence of measurable or evaluable non-measurable disease per RECIST, v1.1
- Adequate bone marrow, cardiac, kidney and liver function
- Able to take oral medications
- Female patients are either postmenopausal for at least 1 year, are surgically sterile for at least 6 weeks, or must agree to take appropriate precautions to avoid pregnancy from screening through follow-up if of childbearing potential
- Males must agree to take appropriate precautions to avoid fathering a child from screening through follow-up

Key Exclusion Criteria:
- Prior treatment with any RAF inhibitor, MEK inhibitor, cetuximab, panitumumab or other EGFR inhibitors
- Prior irinotecan hypersensitivity or toxicity that would suggest an inability to tolerate irinotecan 180 mg/m2 every 2 weeks
- Symptomatic brain metastasis or leptomeningeal disease
- History or current evidence of retinal vein occlusion or current risk factors for retinal vein occlusion (e.g., uncontrolled glaucoma or ocular hypertension, history of hyperviscosity or hypercoagulability syndromes)
- Known history of acute or chronic pancreatitis
- History of chronic inflammatory bowel disease or Crohn's disease requiring medical intervention (immunomodulatory or immunosuppressive medications or surgery) ≤12 months prior to randomization
- Uncontrolled blood pressure despite medical treatment
- Impaired GI function or disease that may significantly alter the absorption of encorafenib or binimetinib (e.g., ulcerative diseases, uncontrolled vomiting, malabsorption syndrome, small bowel resection with decreased intestinal absorption)
- Concurrent or previous other malignancy within 5 years of study entry, except cured basal or squamous cell skin cancer, superficial bladder cancer, prostate intraepithelial neoplasm, carcinoma in-situ of the cervix, or other noninvasive or indolent malignancy
- History of thromboembolic or cerebrovascular events ≤ 6 months prior to starting study treatment, including transient ischemic attacks, cerebrovascular accidents, deep vein thrombosis or pulmonary emboli
- Concurrent neuromuscular disorder that is associated with the potential of elevated CK (e.g., inflammatory myopathies, muscular dystrophy, amyotrophic lateral sclerosis, spinal muscular atrophy)
- Residual CTCAE ≥ Grade 2 toxicity from any prior anticancer therapy, with the exception of Grade 2 alopecia or Grade 2 neuropathy
- Known history of HIV infection
- Active hepatitis B or hepatitis C infection
- Known history of Gilbert's syndrome
- Known contraindication to receive cetuximab or irinotecan at the planned doses

Sex/Gender
All

Ages
18 Years to N/A

Accepts Healthy Volunteers
No

Contacts
Array BioPharma, Inc.   303-381-6604   clinicaltrials@arraybiopharma.com

Phase I/Ib Study of NIS793 in Combination With PDR001 in Patients With Advanced Malignancies.

Study ID:

NCT02947165

Sponsor:

Novartis Pharmaceuticals

Information provided by (Responsible Party):

Novartis (Novartis Pharmaceuticals)

Tracking Information

▨ **First Submitted Date**

October 18, 2016

▨ **Start Date**

April 25, 2017

▨ **Primary Completion Date**

January 12, 2020

▨ **Last Update Posted Date**

January 4, 2018

▨ **Current Primary Outcome Measures**

Incidence of DLTs, AEs, SAEs and dose reductions / interruptions for NIS793[Time Frame: Up to 90 days after end of treatment]

Incidence of DLTs, AEs, SAEs and dose reductions/interruptions for NIS793 in combination with PDR001[Time Frame: Up to 150 days after end of treatment]

▨ **Current Secondary Outcome Measures**

Best overall response (BOR)[Time Frame: 37 months]

Evaluate the anti-tumor activity per RECIST as well as per immune related Response Criteria (irRC) of NIS793 as single agent and in combination with PDR001 every 6 weeks (1 cycle = 3 weeks) from start of treatment until cycle 9 then every 9 weeks until end of treatment (if applicable).

Disease control rate (DCR)[Time Frame: 37 months]

Evaluate the anti-tumor activity per RECIST as well as per immune related Response Criteria (irRC) of NIS793 as single agent and in combination with PDR001every 6 weeks (1 cycle = 3 weeks) from start of treatment until cycle 9 then every 9 weeks until end of treatment (if applicable).

Overall response rate (ORR)[Time Frame: 37 months]

Evaluate the anti-tumor activity per RECIST as well as per immune related Response Criteria (irRC) of NIS793 as single agent and in combination with PDR001 every 6 weeks (1 cycle = 3 weeks) from start of treatment until cycle 9 then every 9 weeks until end of treatment (if applicable).

Progression free survival (PFS)[Time Frame: 37 months]

Evaluate the anti-tumor activity per RECIST as well as per immune related Response Criteria (irRC) of NIS793 as single agent and in combination with PDR001 every 6 weeks from start of treatment until cycle 9 then every 9 weeks until end of treatment. During disease progression f/u, every 8 weeks for 40 weeks, then every 12 weeks.

Duration of response (DOR)[Time Frame: 37 months]

Evaluate the anti-tumor activity per RECIST as well as per immune related Response Criteria (irRC) of NIS793 as single agent and in combination with PDR001 every 6 weeks (1 cycle = 3 weeks) from start of treatment until cycle 9 then every 9 weeks until end of treatment (if applicable).

Serum concentration-time profiles of NIS793 single agent and NIS793 in combination with PDR001[Time Frame: 37 months]

Evaluate serum concentration of NIS793 and PDR001 every 3 weeks up to 24 weeks after start of treatment and at end of treatment.

Presence of anti-NIS793 and anti-PDR001 antibodies[Time Frame: 37 months]

Assess the emergence of anti-NIS793 and anti-PDR001 antibodies every 3 weeks up to 24 weeks after start of treatment and at end of treatment.

Concentration of anti-NIS793 and anti-PDR001 antibodies[Time Frame: 37 months]

Assess the concentration of anti-NIS793 and anti-PDR001 antibodies every 3 weeks up to 24 weeks after start of treatment and at end of treatment.

Area under the curve (AUC) for NIS793 single agent and NIS793 in combination with PDR001.[Time Frame: 37 months]

Characterize the pharmacokinetic properties of NIS793 given alone and in combination with PDR001.

Cmax for NIS793 single agent and NIS793 in combination with PDR001.[Time Frame: 37 months]

Characterize the pharmacokinetic properties of NIS793 given alone and in combination with PDR001.

Tmax for NIS793 single agent and NIS793 in combination with PDR001.[Time Frame: 37 months]

Characterize the pharmacokinetic properties of NIS793 given alone and in combination with PDR001.

Half life of NIS793 as single agent and in combination with PDR001.[Time Frame: 37 months]

Characterize the pharmacokinetic properties of NIS793 given alone and in combination with PDR001.

Characterization of tumor infiltrating lymphocytes (TILs) by H&E[Time Frame: 37 months]

Assess change from baseline of immune infiltrates in tumor biopsies after 3 cycles of treatment.

Characterization of tumor infiltrating lymphocytes by immunohistochemistry (CD8, FOXP3, PD-L1, TIM-3, LAG-3)[Time Frame: 37 months]

Assess change from baseline in immunological markers in tumor biopsies after 3 cycles of treatment.

Descriptive Information

▦ Offical Title

A Phase I/Ib, Open-label, Multi-center Dose Escalation Study of NIS793 in Combination With PDR001 in Adult Patients With Advanced Malignancies

▦ Brief Summary

To characterize the safety and tolerability of NIS793 as single agent and in combination with PDR001 and to identify recommended doses for future studies.

▦ Study Type

Interventional

▦ Study Phase

Phase 1

▦ Condition

- Breast Cancer
- Lung Cancer
- Hepatocellular Cancer
- Colorectal Cancer
- Pancreatic Cancer
- Prostate Cancer
- Renal Cancer

▦ Intervention

Drug: NIS793

Anti-TGF beta antibody

Drug: PDR001

Anti-PD-1 antibody

▦ Study Arms

Experimental: NIS793
Experimental: NIS793 + PDR001

Recruitment Information

▦ Recruitment Status

Recruiting

▦ Estimated Enrollment

160

▦ Eligibility Criteria

Inclusion Criteria:

1. Written informed consent must be obtained prior to any screening procedures.

2. Patient (male or female) ≥ 18 years of age.

3. Escalation: Patients with advanced/metastatic solid tumors, with measurable or non-measurable disease as determined by RECIST version 1.1 who have progressed despite standard therapy or are intolerant of standard therapy, or for whom no standard therapy exists.

▦ Completion Date

January 12, 2020

▦ Primary Completion Date

January 12, 2020

4. Expansion: Patients with advanced/metastatic solid tumors, with at least one measurable lesion as determined by RECIST version 1.1, who have progressed despite standard therapy following their last prior therapy or are intolerant to standard therapy and fit into one of the following groups: Group 1: NSCLC; Group 2: TNBC; Group 3: HCC; Group 4: MSS-CRC; Group 5: pancreatic, prostate and ccRCC.

5. ECOG Performance Status ≤ 2.

6. Patients must have a site of disease amenable to biopsy, and be a candidate for tumor biopsy. Patient must be willing to undergo a new tumor biopsy at screening, and during therapy on this study. Exceptions may be made on a case by case basis after documented discussion with Novartis.

Exclusion Criteria:

1. History of severe hypersensitivity reactions to study treatment ingredients or other monoclonal antibodies and components of study drug.

2. Patients with active, known or suspected autoimmune disease. Note: Patients with vitiligo, type I diabetes mellitus, residual hypothyroidism only requiring hormone replacement, psoriasis not requiring systemic treatment, or conditions not expected to recur in the absence of an external trigger are permitted to enroll.

3. HIV infection.

4. Active HBV or HCV infection.

Other protocol-defined inclusion/exclusion criteria may apply.

◼ **Sex/Gender**

All

◼ **Ages**

18 Years to N/A

◼ **Accepts Healthy Volunteers**

No

◼ **Contacts**

Novartis Pharmaceuticals   1-888-669-6682   Novartis.email@novartis.com
Novartis Pharmaceuticals   +41613241111

Trial of Hu5F9-G4 in Combination With Cetuximab in Patients With Solid Tumors and Advanced Colorectal Cancer

Study ID:
NCT02953782

Sponsor:
Forty Seven, Inc.

Information provided by (Responsible Party):
Forty Seven, Inc. (Forty Seven, Inc.)

Tracking Information

◼ **First Submitted Date**

November 1, 2016

◼ **Start Date**

November 2016

◼ **Primary Completion Date**

May 2018

◼ **Last Update Posted Date**

September 25, 2017

◼ **Current Primary Outcome Measures**

Dose-limiting toxicities (Number of participants with a DLT)[Time Frame: 28 days]
   Dose-limiting toxicities (DLTs) (Phase 1b only) Number of participants with a DLT

Objective response rate (as defined by RECIST Version 1.1)[Time Frame: 8 weeks]
   Phase 2: Objective response as defined by RECIST Version 1.1

Descriptive Information

Offical Title

A Phase 1b/2 Trial of Hu5F9-G4 in Combination With Cetuximab in Patients With Solid Tumors and Advanced Colorectal Cancer

Brief Summary

This trial will evaluate Hu5F9-G4 in combination with cetuximab. Hu5F9-G4 is a monoclonal antibody which is designed to block a protein called CD47, which is widely expressed on human cancer cells. Blocking CD47 with Hu5F9-G4 may enable the body's immune system to find and destroy the cancer cells. Cetuximab is a monoclonal antibody drug that is used for treatment of certain types of colorectal cancer as well as head and neck cancer.

The major aims of the study are: (Phase 1b) to define the safety profile and to determine a recommended Phase 2 dose for Hu5F9-G4 in combination with cetuximab, and (Phase 2) to evaluate the objective response rate of Hu5F9-G4 in combination with cetuximab in patients with advanced colorectal cancer.

Study Type

Interventional

Study Phase

Phase 1/Phase 2

Condition

- Colorectal Neoplasms
- Solid Tumors

Intervention

Drug: Hu5F9-G4

  Hu5F9-G4 will be administered weekly.

  Drug: Cetuximab

  Cetuximab will be administered weekly.

Other Names:
  ERBITUX®

Study Arms

Experimental: Phase 1b dose escalation

  In Phase 1b, patients with advanced solid tumors will receive escalating doses of Hu5F9-G4 in combination with cetuximab.

Experimental: Phase 2 KRAS mutant

  In Phase 2, patients with advanced KRAS mutant colorectal cancer will receive Hu5F9-G4 in combination with cetuximab.

Experimental: Phase 2 KRAS wild-type

  In Phase 2, patients with advanced KRAS wild-type colorectal cancer will receive Hu5F9-G4 in combination with cetuximab.

Recruitment Information

Recruitment Status

Recruiting

Estimated Enrollment

112

Completion Date

March 2023

Primary Completion Date

May 2018

Eligibility Criteria

Inclusion Criteria:

- Histological Diagnosis
- Phase 1b only: Advanced solid malignancy with an emphasis on colorectal, head and neck, breast, pancreatic and ovarian cancers who have been treated with at least one regimen of prior systemic therapy, or who refuse systemic therapy, and for which there is no curative therapy available.
- Phase 2:
- KRAS Mutant CRC: Advanced KRAS mutant CRC who have progressed or are ineligible for both irinotecan and oxaliplatin based chemotherapy
- KRAS Wild Type CRC: Advanced KRAS wild type CRC who have progressed or are ineligible for both irinotecan and oxaliplatin based chemotherapy and who are relapsed or refractory to at least 1 prior systemic therapy that included an anti-EGFR antibody, such as cetuximab, panitumumab or others.

- Adequate performance status and hematological, liver, and kidney function
- Phase 2 only: Willing to consent to 1 mandatory pre-treatment and 1 on-treatment tumor biopsy

Exclusion Criteria:
- Active brain metastases
- Prior treatment with CD47 or signal regulatory protein alpha (SIRPα) targeting agents.
- Phase 2 only: second malignancy within the last 3 years.
- Known active or chronic hepatitis B or C infection or HIV
- Pregnancy or active breastfeeding

▦ Sex/Gender

All

▦ Ages

18 Years to N/A

▦ Accepts Healthy Volunteers

No

▦ Contacts

Chris Takimoto, MD PhD   650-352-4150   medical@fortyseveninc.com
Hassan Movahhed   650-352-4150   medical@fortyseveninc.com

Multimodal Narcotic Limited Perioperative Pain Control With Colorectal Surgery

Study ID:

NCT02958566

Sponsor:

University of Illinois College of Medicine at Peoria

Information provided by (Responsible Party):

University of Illinois College of Medicine at Peoria (University of Illinois College of Medicine at Peoria)

Tracking Information

▦ **First Submitted Date**

November 4, 2016

▦ **Start Date**

January 2017

▦ **Current Primary Outcome Measures**

Length of Hospital Stay[Time Frame: 30 days]
    Total time in hospital from admission to discharge

Days to Return of Bowel Function[Time Frame: 30 days]
    Time from operation to first passage of flatus or bowel movement

Medication cost[Time Frame: 30 days]
    Total cost of inpatient medications

Hospital stay cost[Time Frame: 30 days]
    Total cost of hospital stay

▦ **Primary Completion Date**

December 2017

▦ **Last Update Posted Date**

March 20, 2017

▦ **Current Secondary Outcome Measures**

Amount of narcotics used[Time Frame: 30 days]
    Total amount of narcotics patient consumed

Complications[Time Frame: 30 days]
    Death, prolonged ileus (insertion of NG tube or lack of bowel function on POD 3), respiratory failure, renal failure, SSI, leak, pneumonia, UTI, DVT/PE, cardiac event/MI

Descriptive Information

▦ Offical Title

- Multimodal Narcotic Limited Perioperative Pain Control With Colorectal Surgery as Part of an Enhanced Recovery After Surgery Protocol: A Randomized Prospective SingleCenter Trial.

▦ Brief Summary

The General Objective of this study is to investigate the cost and efficacy of treating patients undergoing colorectal surgical resections with an opioid limited pain control regimen as part of an Enhanced Recovery After Surgery (ERAS) Protocol. This group will be compared to a traditional opioid based pain control regimen.

▦ Detailed Description

Postoperative ileus is a well-known problem for patients who have undergone a colorectal procedure. It is manifested as abdominal distension, accumulation of gas and fluid within the bowels and delayed bowel function (flatus or defecation). It is estimated that with traditional perioperative care for open colon resection postoperative ileus can lead to a length of stay (LOS) of 10 days. Such factors include the use of narcotics, immobilization, over-hydration with IV fluid etc. With about 350,000 colon and small bowel resections occurring annually and a bill to the healthcare system greater than US $20 billion, even decreasing LOS by one or two days can result in substantial cost savings.

All patients undergoing colorectal surgery require medications for pain control. The mainstay of current treatment includes narcotics/opioids. The effect of these medicines on mu receptors of the intestine contribute to delayed bowel function. Protocols that limit the use of narcotics/opioids may reduce the risk of ileus, thus reducing length of stay and reducing cost.

A prospective randomized clinical trial at a single tertiary referral academic affiliated medical center (OSF St. Francis Medical Center). Patients undergoing minimally invasive (laparoscopic or robotic) colorectal resection will be considered for inclusion. Surgery will be performed by two surgeons participating in the study protocol. Patient accrual is intended to begin May 1, 2016 and terminate either after 80 patients have been accrued or December 31, 2018, whichever is first. Informed consent will be obtained and preoperative education will be provided (appendix A). Patients will be randomized to one of two groups. The randomization scheme is a random-permuted-block design without stratification. The block size is a random number between 4 and 8. Personnel who are unassociated with patient screening, enrollment, or follow-up will create the allocation sequence and will use a computerized, random number generator. The allocation sequence will be transferred to sequentially numbered, opaque envelopes for purposes of allocation concealment. Clinical trial coordinators/physicians will verify patient eligibility and informed consent before opening the envelope to obtain the treatment assignment. The experimental group will be placed on a narcotic limited protocol as described below. All used medications are FDA approved. No investigational medicines will be used.

▦ Study Type

Interventional

▦ Study Phase

Phase 4

▦ Condition

- Colon Cancer
- Colon Diverticulosis
- Colonic Neoplasms
- Colonic Diverticulitis
- Pain, Postoperative
- Ileus
- Ileus Paralytic
- Ileus; Mechanical
- Constipation Drug Induced
- Constipation
- Rectum Cancer
- Rectum Neoplasm

▦ Intervention

Drug: Acetaminophen

Other Names:

Tylenol

Ofirmev

Drug: Gabapentin

Other Names:

Neurontin

Drug: Orphenadrine

Other Names:

Norflex

Drug: Lidocaine

Drug: Marcaine

Drug: Ketamine

Drug: Methadone

Drug: Tramadol

Other Names:

Ultram

Drug: Ketorolac
Other Names:

Toradol

Drug: Morphine Sulfate

Drug: Fentanyl

Drug: Dilaudid

Drug: Hydrocodone-Acetaminophen Tab 5-325 MG

Other Names:

Norco

Drug: Morphine Sulfate
PCA

Drug: Fentanyl
PCA

Drug: Dilaudid
PCA

Drug: HYDROCODONE/ACETAMINOPHEN 5 Mg-325 Mg ORAL TABLET
Breakthrough

Other Names:
Norco

■ Study Arms

Active Comparator: Narcotic

Morphine, Dilaudid or Fentanyl patient controlled anesthesia (PCA) for the immediate postoperative period, in addition to Norco 5-325 mg 1-2 tabs Q4H PRN, or equivalent medication.

Post-operative day 1: PCA will be discontinued and the patients will have IV narcotics PRN: Morphine 1-2 mg Q2H PRN, fentanyl 50-75 mcg Q2H PRN or Dilaudid 0.5 mg Q2H PRN

Experimental: Non-Narcotic

Gabapentin 300 mg PO, orphenadrine 60 mg IV, acetaminophen 1000 mg PO or IV on Morning of surgery. Lidocaine 100 mg prior to incision, lidocaine 1mg/kg/hour during procedure, marcaine in all incisions. Ketamine and methadone per anesthesia. Acetaminophen 1000 mg PO or IV, gabapentin 300 mg PO, tramadol 50 mg PO in PACU. Acetaminophen 600 mg PO Q 6 hours, tramadol 50 mg PO Q 6 hours, gabapentin 300 mg PO Q 6 hours, orphenadrine 60 mg IV Q 12 hours, ketorolac 15 mg IV Q 6 hours for 48 hours post-operatively.

Recruitment Information

■ **Recruitment Status**

Recruiting

■ **Estimated Enrollment**

80

- ◼ **Completion Date**

  December 2018

- ◼ **Primary Completion Date**

  December 2017

- ◼ **Eligibility Criteria**

  Inclusion Criteria:

  - Males or females above the age of 18
  - Patients undergoing laparoscopic or robotic colorectal resections

  Exclusion Criteria:

  - History of constipation
  - Pre-existing use of narcotics or opioids
  - Pre-existing renal or hepatic failure
  - Mental illness, mental retardation, or inability to participate in informed consent due to mental status
  - Pre-existing dementia
  - Allergy to any protocol medication
  - Emergency operation
  - Subjects who are incarcerated or wards of the state
  - Minors
  - Subjects with inflammatory bowel disease, active colitis, or pre-existing intra-abdominal inflammation. Diverticulitis without active infection/inflammation will not be excluded.

- ◼ **Sex/Gender**

  All

- ◼ **Ages**

  18 Years to N/A

- ◼ **Accepts Healthy Volunteers**

  No

- ◼ **Contacts**

  Mohammed Almzayyen, MD   mohavt@gmail.com

  Marc A Sarran, MD   marc.sarran@gmail.com

Azacitidine Combined With Pembrolizumab and Epacadostat in Subjects With Advanced Solid Tumors (ECHO-206)

Study ID:

NCT02959437

Sponsor:

Incyte Corporation

Information provided by (Responsible Party):

Incyte Corporation (Incyte Corporation)

Tracking Information

- ◼ **First Submitted Date**

  November 7, 2016

- ◼ **Primary Completion Date**

  September 2021

- ◼ **Start Date**

  January 24, 2017

- ◼ **Last Update Posted Date**

  January 12, 2018

- ◼ **Current Primary Outcome Measures**

  Part 1: Frequency, duration, and severity of adverse events[Time Frame: Baseline through 42-49 days after end of treatment, estimated up to 18 months.]

      A treatment-emergent AE was defined as an event occurring after exposure to at least 1 dose of study drug. A treatment-related AE was defined as an event with a definite, probable, or possible causality to study medication. A serious AE is an event resulting in death, hospitalization, persistent or significant disability/incapacity, or is life threatening, a congenital anomaly/birth defect or requires medical or surgical intervention to prevent 1 of the outcomes above. The intensity of an AE was graded according to the National Cancer Institute common terminology criteria for adverse events (NCI-CTCAE) version 4.03: Grade 1 (Mild); Grade 2 (Moderate); Grade 3 (Severe); Grade 4 (life-threatening).

Part 2: Objective response rate based on modified Response Evaluation Criteria in Solid Tumors version 1.1 (mRECIST v1.1)[Time Frame: Every 9 weeks for the duration of study participation; estimated to be 18 months.]

Defined as the percentage of subjects having a complete response or partial response.

Current Secondary Outcome Measures

Part 1: Objective response rate based on mRECIST v1.1[Time Frame: Every 9 weeks for the duration of study participation; estimated to be 18 months]

Defined as the percentage of subjects having a complete response or partial response.

Part 2: Frequency, duration, and severity of adverse events[Time Frame: Baseline through 42-49 days after end of treatment, estimated up to 18 months.]

A treatment-emergent AE was defined as an event occurring after exposure to at least 1 dose of study drug. A treatment-related AE was defined as an event with a definite, probable, or possible causality to study medication. A serious AE is an event resulting in death, hospitalization, persistent or significant disability/incapacity, or is life threatening, a congenital anomaly/birth defect or requires medical or surgical intervention to prevent 1 of the outcomes above. The intensity of an AE was graded according to the National Cancer Institute common terminology criteria for adverse events (NCI-CTCAE) version 4.03: Grade 1 (Mild); Grade 2 (Moderate); Grade 3 (Severe); Grade 4 (life-threatening).

Parts 1 and 2: Percentage of responders determined by immunohistochemistry[Time Frame: Baseline and Week 5 or Week 6.]

Responder is defined as an increase in the number of tumor-infiltrating lymphocytes or the ratio of CD8+ lymphocytes to T regulatory cells infiltrating tumor post-treatment versus pretreatment with pembrolizumab and epacadostat in combination with azacitidine.

Parts 1 and 2: Progression-free survival based on mRECIST v1.1.[Time Frame: Every 9 weeks for the duration of study participation; estimated to be 18 months.]

Defined as the time from date of first dose of study drug until the earliest date of disease progression per mRECIST v1.1, or death due to any cause, if occurring sooner than progression.

Parts 1 and 2: Duration of response based on mRECIST v1.1[Time Frame: Every 9 weeks for the duration of study participation; estimated to be 18 months.]

Defined as the time from earliest date of disease response until the earliest date of disease progression per mRECIST v1.1, or death due to any cause, if occurring sooner than progression.

Descriptive Information

Offical Title

A Phase 1/2 Study Exploring the Safety, Tolerability, Effect on the Tumor Microenvironment, and Efficacy of Azacitidine in Combination With Pembrolizumab and Epacadostat in Subjects With Advanced Solid Tumors and Previously Treated Stage IIIB or Stage IV Non-Small Cell Lung Cancer and Stage IV Microsatellite-Stable Colorectal Cancer (ECHO-206)

Brief Summary

This is an open-label, Phase 1/2 study in subjects with advanced or metastatic solid tumors. The study will be divided into 2 parts (Part 1 and 2). Part 1 is a dose-escalation assessment to evaluate the safety and tolerability of the DNA methyltransferase inhibitor azacitidine in combination with the programmed death receptor-1 (PD-1) inhibitor pembrolizumab and the indoleamine 2,3-dioxygenase (IDO-1) inhibitor epacadostat. Once the recommended doses have been determined, subjects with previously treated NSCLC and microsatellite-stable colorectal cancer (CRC) will be enrolled into expansion cohorts in Part 2.

Study Type

Interventional

Study Phase

Phase 1/Phase 2

Condition

- Solid Tumor
- Advanced Cancer
- Metastatic Cancer

Intervention

Drug: Azacitidine

Five doses of azacitidine will be administered by subcutaneous injection or intravenously (IV) over Days 1 to 7 in Cycles 1 and 2.

Drug: Pembrolizumab

Pembrolizumab will be administered in a 30-minute IV infusion every 3 weeks on Day 1 of each 21-day cycle.

Drug: Epacadostat

Epacadostat tablets will be administered orally twice daily.

Study Arms

Experimental: Azacitidine + Pembrolizumab + Epacadostat

Part 1 is an open-label 3 + 3 + 3 dose-escalation design based on observing each dose level for a period of 21 days. Part 2 will evaluate the recommended dose determined in Part 1.

Recruitment Information

Recruitment Status

Recruiting

Estimated Enrollment

142

Completion Date

October 2021

Primary Completion Date

September 2021

Eligibility Criteria

Inclusion Criteria:

- Willingness to provide written informed consent for the study.
- Part 1: Subjects with histologically or cytologically confirmed advanced or metastatic solid tumors that have failed prior standard therapy (disease progression; subject refusal or intolerance is also allowable).
- Part 2: Subjects with histologically or cytologically confirmed NSCLC:
- Stage IIIB or metastatic (Stage IV) NSCLC (according to American Joint Committee on Cancer 7th edition guidelines) who have had disease progression after available therapies for advanced or metastatic disease that are known to confer clinical benefit, been intolerant to treatment, or refused standard treatment.
- Prior systemic regimens must include previously approved therapies, including a platinum-containing chemotherapy regimen; a tyrosine kinase inhibitor for tumors with driver mutations; and checkpoint inhibitors where approved (except Cohort A1, which must be checkpoint inhibitor-naive).
- Must have disease progression on a prior PD-1-pathway targeted agent (Cohort A2) or must be PD-1 pathway-targeted treatment naive (Cohort A1).
- Subjects with recurrent (unresectable) or metastatic CRC:
- Have histologically confirmed microsatellite stable (MSS) CRC.
- Stage IV MSS CRC (according to American Joint Committee on Cancer 7th edition guidelines) who have had disease progression after available therapies for advanced or metastatic disease that are known to confer clinical benefit, been intolerant to treatment, or refused standard treatment.
- Prior systemic regimens must include previously approved therapies, including fluoropyrimidine-, oxaliplatin-, and irinotecan-based chemotherapy; an anti-VEGF therapy (if no contraindication); and if KRAS wild type and no contraindication, an anti-epidermal growth factor receptor (EGFR) therapy; and progressed after the last administration of approved therapy.
- Has baseline tumor biopsy specimen available or willingness to undergo a pretreatment and on-treatment tumor biopsy to obtain the specimen.
- Eastern Cooperative Oncology Group (ECOG) performance status of 0 or 1.

Exclusion Criteria:

- Laboratory parameters not within the protocol-defined range.
- Receipt of anticancer medications or investigational drugs within a defined interval before the first administration of study drug.
- Has not recovered from toxic effects of prior therapy to ≤ Grade 1.
- Active or inactive autoimmune disease or syndrome.
- Active infection requiring systemic therapy.
- Known active central nervous system (CNS) metastases and/or carcinomatous meningitis.
- History or presence of an abnormal ECG that, in the investigator's opinion, is clinically meaningful.
- Has received a live vaccine within 30 days of planned start of study therapy.
- Prior receipt of an IDO inhibitor.

Sex/Gender

All

Ages

18 Years to N/A

hTERT Immunotherapy Alone or in Combination With IL-12 DNA Followed by Electroporation in Adults With Solid Tumors at High Risk of Relapse

Study ID:

NCT02960594

Sponsor:

Inovio Pharmaceuticals

Information provided by (Responsible Party):

Inovio Pharmaceuticals (Inovio Pharmaceuticals)

Tracking Information

■ **First Submitted Date**

November 4, 2016

■ **Start Date**

December 2014

■ **Current Primary Outcome Measures**

Adverse events graded in accordance with "Common Terminology Criteria for Adverse Events (CTCAE)", NCI version 4.03[Time Frame: Up to 2 years from first study treatment]

Injection site reactions including, but not necessarily limited to, local skin erythema, induration, pain and tenderness at administration site[Time Frame: Up to 14 weeks]

Changes in safety laboratory parameters[Time Frame: Up to 2 years from first study treatment]

■ **Primary Completion Date**

December 2018

■ **Last Update Posted Date**

November 24, 2017

Descriptive Information

■ **Offical Title**

A Study of hTERT Immunotherapy Alone or in Combination With IL-12 DNA Followed by Electroporation in Adults With Solid Tumors at High Risk of Relapse Post Definitive Surgery and Standard Therapy

■ **Brief Summary**

This is a Phase I, open label study to evaluate the safety, tolerability, and immunogenicity of INO-1400 alone or in combination with INO-9012, delivered by electroporation in subjects with high-risk solid tumor cancer with no evidence of disease after surgery and standard therapy. Subjects will be enrolled into one of six treatment arms. Subjects will be assessed according to standard of care. Restaging and imaging studies will be performed to assess disease relapse per NCCN guidelines. RECIST will be used to validate the findings in cases of relapse.

■ **Study Type**

Interventional

■ **Study Phase**

Phase 1

■ **Condition**

- Breast Cancer
- Lung Cancer
- Pancreatic Cancer
- Head and Neck Cancer
- Ovarian Cancer
- ColoRectal Cancer

- Gastric Cancer
- Esophageal Cancer
- HepatoCellular Carcinoma

■ **Intervention**

Biological: INO-1400

    Other Names:

    hTERT

    Biological: INO-9012

    Other Names:

    IL-12

    Biological: INO-1401

    Other Names:

    SynCon TERT

■ **Study Arms**

Experimental: Arm 1
    2 mg INO-1400 delivered intramuscularly followed by electroporation at Day 0, Weeks 4, 8, and 12

Experimental: Arm 2
    8 mg INO-1400 delivered intramuscularly followed by electroporation at Day 0, Weeks 4, 8, and 12

Experimental: Arm 3
    2 mg INO-1400 + 0.5 mg INO-9012 delivered intramuscularly followed by electroporation at Day 0, Weeks 4, 8, and 12

Experimental: Arm 4
    2 mg INO-1400 + 2 mg INO-9012 delivered intramuscularly followed by electroporation at Day 0, Weeks 4, 8, and 12

Experimental: Arm 5
    8 mg INO-1400 + 0.5 mg INO-9012 delivered intramuscularly followed by electroporation at Day 0, Weeks 4, 8, and 12

Experimental: Arm 6
    8 mg INO-1400 + 2 mg INO-9012 delivered intramuscularly followed by electroporation at Day 0, Weeks 4, 8, and 12

Experimental: Arm 7
    2 mg INO-1401 delivered intramuscularly followed by electroporation at Day 0, Weeks 4, 8, and 12

Experimental: Arm 8
    8 mg INO-1401 delivered intramuscularly followed by electroporation at Day 0, Weeks 4, 8, and 12

Experimental: Arm 9
    8 mg INO-1401 + 0.5 mg INO-9012 delivered intramuscularly followed by electroporation at Day 0, Weeks 4, 8, and 12

Experimental: Arm 10
    8 mg INO-1401 + 2 mg INO-9012 delivered intramuscularly followed by electroporation at Day 0, Weeks 4, 8, and 12

Recruitment Information

■ **Recruitment Status**

Recruiting

■ **Estimated Enrollment**

90

■ **Eligibility Criteria**

■ **Completion Date**

December 2018

■ **Primary Completion Date**

December 2018

Inclusion Criteria:

- 1. Signed and dated written IRB approved informed consent;
- 2. Males or females aged ≥18 years;
- 3. Subjects with breast, lung or pancreatic carcinoma who are at high risk of relapse post definitive therapy at least 4 and no more than 24 weeks from completion of definitive therapy at the time of signing informed consent as described below for each indication:
- Breast carcinoma:

- Lung carcinoma:
- Pancreatic carcinoma:
- Head and neck squamous cell carcinoma:
- Ovarian cancer:
- Colorectal cancer
- Gastric and esophageal cancer
- Hepatocellular carcinoma

Exclusion Criteria:
- 1. Previous treatment wth any TERT or IL-12 containing therapy, or any other DNA immunotherapy;
- 2. Any concurrent condition requiring the continued or anticipated use of systemic steroids (excluding non-systemic inhaled, topical skin and/or eye drop-containing corticosteroids) or immunosuppressive therapy (excludes low dose methotrexate). All other systemic corticosteroids must be discontinued at least 4 weeks prior to first Study Treatment;
- 3. Administration of any vaccine within 4 weeks of the first study treatment

Sex/Gender
All

Ages
18 Years to N/A

Accepts Healthy Volunteers
No

Contacts
Inovio Call Center   267-440-4237   clinical.trials@inovio.com

---

Erlotinib Hydrochloride in Reducing Duodenal Polyp Burden in Patients With Familial Adenomatous Polyposis at Risk of Developing Colon Cancer

Study ID:
NCT02961374

Sponsor:
National Cancer Institute (NCI)

Information provided by (Responsible Party):
National Cancer Institute (NCI) (National Cancer Institute (NCI))

Tracking Information

First Submitted Date
November 10, 2016

Primary Completion Date
September 1, 2019

Start Date
October 27, 2017

Last Update Posted Date
December 12, 2017

Current Primary Outcome Measures

Incidence of grade 2/3 adverse event (AE) rate assessed according to National Cancer Institute's (NCI) Common Terminology Criteria for Adverse Events (CTCAE) version 4.0[Time Frame: Up to 2.5 years]

Mean percent change in duodenal polyp burden assessed by esophagogastroduodenoscopy[Time Frame: Baseline to 6 months post-intervention]

For all measurements of response, the 95% confidence intervals will be provided.

Current Secondary Outcome Measures

Absolute and percent change in desmoid tumor size[Time Frame: Baseline to 2.5 years]

Laboratory measures will be correlated with participant outcomes (i.e., polyp burden, adverse events) and with each other as well. Cut-points will be determined based on previously defined and accepted standards. Descriptive statistics and simple scatter plots will be generated to review the tissue-based biomarker data. For continuous variables, the actual and % change in the level of each of the biomarkers from preto post-intervention will be explored using Wilcoxon signed rank tests, and paired sample t-tests. All categorical variables will be analyzed using chi-square tests or Fisher's ex

Absolute and percent change in duodenal polyp number[Time Frame: Baseline to 6 months]

Laboratory measures will be correlated with participant outcomes (i.e., polyp burden, adverse events) and with each other as well. Cut-points will be determined based on previously defined and accepted standards. Descriptive statistics and simple scatter plots will be generated to review the tissue-based biomarker data. For continuous variables, the actual and % change in the level of each of the biomarkers from preto post-intervention will be explored using Wilcoxon signed rank tests, and paired sample t-tests. All categorical variables will be analyzed using chi-square tests or Fisher's ex

Absolute and percent changes in lower gastrointestinal polyp burden[Time Frame: Baseline to 2.5 years]

Laboratory measures will be correlated with participant outcomes (i.e., polyp burden, adverse events) and with each other as well. Cut-points will be determined based on previously defined and accepted standards. Descriptive statistics and simple scatter plots will be generated to review the tissue-based biomarker data. For continuous variables, the actual and % change in the level of each of the biomarkers from preto post-intervention will be explored using Wilcoxon signed rank tests, and paired sample t-tests. All categorical variables will be analyzed using chi-square tests or Fisher's ex

Absolute and percent changes in number for the subset of participants with ileal pouch anal anastomosis or ileo-rectal anastomosis with rectal stump[Time Frame: Baseline to 2.5 years]

Laboratory measures will be correlated with participant outcomes (i.e., polyp burden, adverse events) and with each other as well. Cut-points will be determined based on previously defined and accepted standards. Descriptive statistics and simple scatter plots will be generated to review the tissue-based biomarker data. For continuous variables, the actual and % change in the level of each of the biomarkers from preto post-intervention will be explored using Wilcoxon signed rank tests, and paired sample t-tests. All categorical variables will be analyzed using chi-square tests or Fisher's ex

Change in differentially expressed genes of duodenal polyps and uninvolved tissue[Time Frame: Baseline to 2.5 years]

Laboratory measures will be correlated with participant outcomes (i.e., polyp burden, adverse events) and with each other as well. Cut-points will be determined based on previously defined and accepted standards. Descriptive statistics and simple scatter plots will be generated to review the tissue-based biomarker data. For continuous variables, the actual and % change in the level of each of the biomarkers from preto post-intervention will be explored using Wilcoxon signed rank tests, and paired sample t-tests. All categorical variables will be analyzed using chi-square tests or Fisher's ex

EGFR and Wnt gene expression[Time Frame: Up to 2.5 years]

Laboratory measures will be correlated with participant outcomes (i.e., polyp burden, adverse events) and with each other as well. Cut-points will be determined based on previously defined and accepted standards. Descriptive statistics and simple scatter plots will be generated to review the tissue-based biomarker data. For continuous variables, the actual and % change in the level of each of the biomarkers from preto post-intervention will be explored using Wilcoxon signed rank tests, and paired sample t-tests. All categorical variables will be analyzed using chi-square tests or Fisher's ex

Immune response signaling in duodenal adenomas and uninvolved tissue[Time Frame: Up to 2.5 years]

Laboratory measures will be correlated with participant outcomes (i.e., polyp burden, adverse events) and with each other as well. Cut-points will be determined based on previously defined and accepted standards. Descriptive statistics and simple scatter plots will be generated to review the tissue-based biomarker data. For continuous variables, the actual and % change in the level of each of the biomarkers from preto post-intervention will be explored using Wilcoxon signed rank tests, and paired sample t-tests. All categorical variables will be analyzed using chi-square tests or Fisher's ex

Incidence of all adverse events assessed according to NCI CTCAE version 4.0[Time Frame: Up to 2.5 years]

All registered and treated participants will be evaluable for AEs from the time of their first dose of weekly erlotinib treatment. To evaluate the AE profile for this treatment, the maximum grade for each type of adverse event will be recorded for each participant and frequency tables will be reviewed to determine the overall patterns. The number and severity of adverse events will be tabulated and summarized across all grades. Grade 2+ adverse events will be similarly described and summarized separately. Overall toxicity incidence, as well as toxicity profiles will be explored and summarized.

Descriptive Information

▨ Offical Title

Phase II Trial of Weekly Erlotinib Dosing to Reduce Duodenal Polyp Burden Associated With Familial Adenomatous Polyposis

▨ Brief Summary

This phase II trial studies the side effects of erlotinib hydrochloride and how well it works in reducing duodenal polyp burden in patients with familial adenomatous polyposis at risk of developing colon cancer. Erlotinib hydrochloride may stop the growth of tumor cells by blocking some of the enzymes needed for cell growth.

▨ Detailed Description

PRIMARY OBJECTIVES:

I. To assess the mean percent change in duodenal polyp burden (sum of diameters from all polyps) from baseline to 6 months post-intervention for familial adenomatous polyposis (FAP) subjects receiving weekly erlotinib hydrochloride (erlotinib).

II. To assess the grade 2/3 adverse event rate in this population and compare it to historical data.

SECONDARY OBJECTIVES:

I. To evaluate all adverse events at least possibly attributed to weekly erlotinib.

II. To assess the absolute and percent change in duodenal polyp number from baseline to 6 months.

III. To assess the absolute and percent changes in lower gastrointestinal polyp burden and number for the subset of participants with ileal pouch anal anastomosis (IPAA) or ileo-rectal anastomosis with rectal stump.

IV. To assess the absolute and percent change in desmoid tumor size in participants who have baseline and follow up computed tomography (CT)s performed as part of their standard of care.

V. Gene expression profiles in duodenal adenomas and uninvolved tissue will be compared between baseline and endpoint samples using negative binomial statistics (DESeq2).

VI. Identify differentially expressed genes between duodenal polyps and uninvolved tissue at endpoint compared to baseline.

VII. Evaluate the effect of weekly erlotinib on EGFR and Wnt target gene expression in duodenal adenomas.

VIII. Evaluate the effect of weekly erlotinib on immune response signaling in duodenal adenomas and uninvolved tissue.

OUTLINE:

Patients receive erlotinib hydrochloride orally (PO) once weekly. Treatment continues for up to 6 months in the absence of disease progression or unacceptable toxicity.

After completion of study treatment, patients are followed up at 30 days.

- **Study Type**

  Interventional

- **Study Phase**

  Phase 2

- **Condition**

  - APC Gene Mutation
  - Attenuated Familial Adenomatous Polyposis
  - Familial Adenomatous Polyposis

- **Intervention**

  Drug: Erlotinib Hydrochloride

    Given PO

  Other Names:

    Cp-358,774

    OSI-774

    Tarceva

    Other: Laboratory Biomarker Analysis

    Correlative studies

- **Study Arms**

  Experimental: Treatment (erlotinib hydrochloride)

    Patients receive erlotinib hydrochloride PO once weekly. Treatment continues for up to 6 months in the absence of disease progression or unacceptable toxicity.

Recruitment Information

- **Recruitment Status**

  Recruiting

- **Estimated Enrollment**

  70

- **Completion Date**

  September 1, 2019

- **Primary Completion Date**

  September 1, 2019

- **Eligibility Criteria**

  Inclusion Criteria:

  - PRE-REGISTRATION INCLUSION
  - **Diagnosis of familial adenomatous polyposis (FAP) or attenuated familial adenomatous polyposis (AFAP), defined as at least one of the following:**
  - Genetic diagnosis with confirmed APC mutation (Clinical Laboratory Improvement Act [CLIA] certified lab or research testing)
  - Obligate carrier
  - Clinical diagnosis of classic FAP with >= 100 colorectal adenomas status post colectomy and a family history of FAP

- Ability to understand and the willingness to sign a written informed consent document
- Willing to discontinue taking nonsteroidal anti-inflammatory drugs (NSAIDS) for 30 days prior to initiation of and during intervention; exception: use of =< 81 mg daily or =< 650 mg weekly aspirin is allowed
- Willing to discontinue smoking for the duration of study intervention
- Willing to provide mandatory biospecimens as specified in the protocol
- REGISTRATION INCLUSION
- Eastern Cooperative Oncology Group (ECOG) performance status =< 1
- Leukocytes (white blood cells [WBC]) >= 3,000/uL (>= 2,500/uL for African-American participants)
- Platelet count >= 100 x 10^9/L
- Hemoglobin >= 11.5 g/dL
- Total bilirubin =< 1.5 x institutional upper limit of normal (ULN)
- Alkaline phosphatase =< 1.5 x institutional upper limit of normal (ULN)
- Aspartate aminotransferase (AST)/serum glutamic-oxaloacetic transaminase (SGOT) =< 2 x institutional upper limit of normal (ULN)
- Alanine aminotransferase (ALT)/serum glutamate pyruvate transaminase (SGPT) =< 2 x institutional upper limit of normal (ULN)
- Creatinine =< institutional upper limits of normal (ULN)
- Urinary testing results within institutional limits of normal or deemed clinically insignificant
- Spigelman 2-3
- Not pregnant or breast feeding; women of child-bearing potential and men must agree to use adequate contraception (hormonal or barrier method of birth control; abstinence) prior to study entry and for the duration of study participation; should a woman become pregnant or suspect she is pregnant while participating in this study, she should inform her study physician immediately; breastfeeding should be discontinued if the mother is treated with erlotinib
- Willing to use adequate contraception to avoid pregnancy or impregnation until 2 weeks after discontinuing study agent

Exclusion Criteria:

- PRE-REGISTRATION EXCLUSION
- Any prior treatment with erlotinib or other agent whose primary mechanism of action is known to inhibit EGFR
- History of allergic reactions attributed to compounds of similar chemical or biologic composition to erlotinib
- Use of potent CYP3A4 inhibitors, such as ketoconazole, atazanavir, clarithromycin, indinavir, itraconazole, nefazodone, nelfinavir, ritonavir, saquinavir, telithromycin, troleandomycin, voriconazole, and grapefruit or grapefruit juice
- Use of CYP3A4 inducers such as rifampicin, rifabutin, rifapentine, phenytoin, carbamazepine, phenobarbital, and St. John's wort
- Use of any other investigational agents =< 12 weeks prior to pre-registration
- **Uncontrolled intercurrent illness or recent surgical procedure that in the opinion of the investigative team would limit compliance with study requirements, including, but not limited to:**
- Ongoing or active infection
- Symptomatic congestive heart failure
- Myocardial infarction =< 6 months prior to intervention
- Severely impaired lung function
- Nonmalignant medical illnesses that are uncontrolled or whose control may be jeopardized by the treatment with study intervention
- Diagnosed liver disease, such as cirrhosis, chronic active hepatitis, or chronic persistent hepatitis
- Unstable angina pectoris
- Cardiac arrhythmia
- Psychiatric illness/social situations
- History of invasive malignancy =< 3 years prior to pre-registration; exception: adequately treated carcinoma of the cervix, carcinoma in situ, or basal or squamous cell carcinomas of the skin
- Use of anticoagulation medications, including but not limited to coumadin, warfarin, plavix
- REGISTRATION EXCLUSION
- Histologically-confirmed high grade dysplasia (HGD), cancer, or polyp burden that is not quantifiable
- Regular (>= 2 times per week) use of drugs that alter the pH of the gastrointestinal tract (GI) tract, such as proton pump inhibitors (PPI) and antacids; exceptions: individuals who use prescription PPIs and have approval from their primary health care provider to replace the PPI with an H2 receptor agonist, i.e. ranitidine, for the duration of the trial will be eligible
- Gastrointestinal bleeding; note that the presence of any symptoms (dyspnea, fatigue, angina, weakness, malaise, melena, hematochezia, hematemesis, anemia, abdominal pain) will require clinical assessment to rule out gastrointestinal bleeding

■ Sex/Gender

All

■ **Ages**

18 Years to 69 Years

■ **Accepts Healthy Volunteers**

No

A Phase 1/2 Study to Investigate the Safety, Biologic and Anti-tumor Activity of ONCOS-102 in Combination With Durvalumab in Subjects With Advanced Peritoneal Malignancies

Study ID:

NCT02963831

Sponsor:

Ludwig Institute for Cancer Research

Information provided by (Responsible Party):

Ludwig Institute for Cancer Research (Ludwig Institute for Cancer Research)

Tracking Information

■ **First Submitted Date**

November 10, 2016

■ **Start Date**

September 7, 2017

■ **Primary Completion Date**

July 2020

■ **Last Update Posted Date**

November 29, 2017

■ **Current Primary Outcome Measures**

Number of Adverse Events[Time Frame: up to 24 weeks]

Clinical laboratory tests, vital sign and weight measurements, physical exams, performance status evaluation, imaging scans and any other medically indicated assessments, including subject interviews, will be performed to detect new abnormalities and deteriorations of any pre-existing conditions. The investigator will evaluate any laboratory abnormalities for clinical significance, and clinically significant abnormalities will be recorded as adverse events. All clinically significant abnormalities and deteriorations from time of signing the informed consent to the end of study visit will be recorded in the Case Report Forms as adverse events and graded according to the Common Terminology Criteria for Adverse Events (CTCAE) Version 4.03.

■ **Current Secondary Outcome Measures**

Clinical Benefit (Complete Response, Partial Response and Stable Disease)[Time Frame: up to 24 weeks]

Clinical Benefit is defined as percentage of subjects who are in the study and not in progression at the end of Week 24.

Objective Response Rate[Time Frame: a least 4 weeks]

Progression-free survival[Time Frame: up to 4 years]

Overall Survival[Time Frame: up to 4 years]

Descriptive Information

■ **Offical Title**

A Phase 1/2 Dose Escalation Study With Expansion Cohorts to Investigate the Safety, Biologic and Anti-tumor Activity of ONCOS-102 in Combination With Durvalumab in Subjects With Advanced Peritoneal Malignancies

■ **Brief Summary**

This is a two-part Phase 1/2 dose escalation and dose expansion study of the GMCSFencoding adenovirus, ONCOS-102, in combination with anti-programmed death ligand-1 (PDL1) antibody, durvalumab, in adult subjects with peritoneal disease who have failed prior standard chemotherapy and have histologically confirmed platinum-resistant or refractory epithelial ovarian cancer or colorectal cancer.

Study Type

Interventional

Study Phase

Phase 1/Phase 2

Condition

- ColoRectal Cancer
- Platinum-resistant Ovarian Cancer

Intervention

Biological: ONCOS-102

ONCOS-102 will be administered intraperitoneally via a peritoneal Hickmann catheter (or institutionally preferred alternative) at weekly intervals for 6 weeks.

Drug: Durvalumab

Durvalumab will be administered by IV infusion once every four weeks for a total of 12 four-week cycles.

Other Names:

MEDI4736

Study Arms

Experimental: Dose Escalation

During Phase 1 of the study, subjects will be evaluated for DLTs before proceeding to a subsequent cohort. Dose escalation for the determination of RCD will be performed based on the available dose levels and the respective rules for a standard 3 + 3 dose escalation study design.

For Cohort A, ONCOS-102 (1×10^{11} VP) will be given as monotherapy the first six weeks, and then durvalumab (1500 mg) will be starting on day 71.

For Cohorts B and C, ONCOS-102 will be administered for a total of 6 weeks while durvalumab will be given for a total of 12 four-week cycles.

Experimental: Cohort 1: Platinum-resistant epithelial ovarian cancer

ONCOS-102 will be administered for a total of 6 weeks, while durvalumab will be administered for a total of 12 cycles, starting on Day 15.

Experimental: Cohort 2: Colorectal cancer

ONCOS-102 will be administered for a total of 6 weeks, while durvalumab will be administered for a total of 12 cycles, starting on Day 15.

Recruitment Information

Recruitment Status

Recruiting

Estimated Enrollment

78

Completion Date

October 2022

Primary Completion Date

July 2020

Eligibility Criteria

Inclusion Criteria:

1. Subjects with peritoneal disease who have failed prior standard chemotherapy and have histologic confirmation of platinum-resistant or refractory epithelial ovarian cancer, fallopian tube cancer, primary peritoneal cancer, endometrial cancer, cervical cancer, vaginal and vulvar cancer, uterine sarcomas including leiomyosarcoma, carcinosarcoma or high grade endometrial stromal sarcoma, gastroesophageal cancer, pancreatic cancer, cholangiocarcinoma, colorectal cancer, gastrointestinal neuroendocrine tumors, or mesothelioma will be enrolled.

2. The subject is willing to undergo a core needle biopsy during screening and during Cycle 2, Study Week 5. Archival tumor samples are requested, but are not required for eligibility.

3. Previously treated for advanced cancer with no additional therapy options available known to prolong survival.

4. Laboratory parameters for vital functions should be in the normal range or not clinically significant.

5. Eastern Cooperative Oncology Group (ECOG) performance status ≤ 1

Exclusion Criteria:

1. Treatment with an investigational agent within 4 weeks of starting study treatment or prior treatment with a checkpoint inhibitor (cytotoxic T-lymphocyte-associated protein 4 (CTLA-4), programmed cell death protein 1 (PD-1) or programmed death ligand 1 (PD-L1) antibodies).

2. Subjects with known active central nervous system metastasis, glioma and nervous system malignancies including carcinomatous meningitis or other invasive malignancy within 5 years except for noninvasive malignancies such as cervical carcinoma in situ, non-melanomatous carcinoma of the skin or ductal carcinoma in situ of the breast that has/have been surgically cured.

3. Known immunodeficiency or known to have evidence of acute or chronic or human immunodeficiency virus (HIV), Hepatitis B, or Hepatitis C or other uncontrolled inter-current illnesses.

4. Ongoing bowel perforation or presence of bowel fistula or abscess or history of small or large bowel obstruction within 3 months of registration, including subjects with palliative gastric drainage catheters. Subjects with palliative diverting ileostomy or colostomy are allowed if they have been symptom-free for more than 3 months.

5. Subjects with clinically significant cardiovascular disease, history of organ transplant or allogeneic bone marrow transplant, active known or history of autoimmune disease that might recur or major surgery within 28 days prior to the first dose or still recovering from prior surgery.

■ **Sex/Gender**

All

■ **Ages**

18 Years to N/A

■ **Accepts Healthy Volunteers**

No

■ **Contacts**

Lisa Shohara   212-450-1515   clintrialinformation@licr.org

Danielle McCabe   212-450-1515   clintrialinformation@licr.org

Increasing Uptake of Evidence-Based Screening Services Through CHW-led Multi-modality Intervention

Study ID:

NCT02970136

Sponsor:

University of Miami

Information provided by (Responsible Party):

University of Miami (University of Miami)

Tracking Information

■ **First Submitted Date**

November 18, 2016

■ **Start Date**

April 11, 2017

■ **Current Primary Outcome Measures**

Increased proportion of participants who are screened for all four conditions[Time Frame: 6 months]

■ **Current Secondary Outcome Measures**

Increase in screening for each of the four conditions individually[Time Frame: 6 months]

Testing rates among minority populations in non-clinical settings[Time Frame: 6 months]

■ **Primary Completion Date**

August 30, 2020

■ **Last Update Posted Date**

May 18, 2017

Descriptive Information

■ **Offical Title**

Increasing Uptake of Evidence-Based Screening Services Through CHW-led Multi-modality Intervention: South Florida Center for Reducing Health Disparities

■ **Brief Summary**

The purpose of this research study is to determine the best way to increase screening for cervical cancer, colorectal cancer, HIV, and Hepatitis C among underscreened Hispanic, Haitian and African-American individuals in Hialeah, South Dade, and Little

Haiti. The investigator will compare home testing led by a community health worker (CHW) versus clinic testing guided by a CHW. Community Health Workers are people who have undergone several weeks of community outreach and health education training. During the study period the participant will continue to receive all of their regular medical care from their regular health care providers. If the participant does not have a health care provider, the Community Health Workers would be able to help in referring the participant for care at a local health care clinic located in their community.

Study Type

Interventional

Study Phase

N/A

Condition

- Human Papillomavirus
- Human Immunodeficiency Virus
- Hepatitis C
- ColoRectal Cancer

Intervention

Device: OraQuick Swab

OraQuick for oral fluid HIV antibody testing

Device: Fecal Immunochemical Test

Fecal Immunochemical stool test specific for human hemoglobin

Device: OraQuick Fingerstick

Patients will be tested for Hepatitis C infection using a fingerstick

Other: Standard Screening Tests

Patients will be navigated to a local health center for standard screening tests

Other: HPV Self-Sampling Test

Patients will be using swab to check for HPV infection

Study Arms

Experimental: Home Based Screening

The participant will have the option of choosing between the clinic visit or receiving home-based screening tests (OraQuick Swab, OraQuick Fingerstick, Fecal Immunochemical Test) delivered by the community health worker

Active Comparator: Clinic Based Screening

The participant will meet the Community Health Worker and will be navigated to a clinic appointment for standard screening tests

Recruitment Information

Recruitment Status

Recruiting

Estimated Enrollment

900

Completion Date

February 28, 2022

Primary Completion Date

August 30, 2020

Eligibility Criteria

Inclusion Criteria:

1. live in one of the three target communities

2. self-identify as Haitian, Hispanic and/or Black.

3. be 50-64 years old

4. need at least one of the four recommended screening services as per USPSTF121 guidelines as follows: never having had a HIV test b) never having had a HCV test c) not having a Pap smear in the last three years d) not having had a colonoscopy in last 10 years and/or stool-based test in the last year.

Exclusion Criteria:

1. plan to move out of the community during the next six months;

2. current or prior enrollment (5 five years) in any research study that involved screening for these conditions.

3. Are adults unable to consent

4. Are individuals who are not yet adults (infants, children, teenagers)

5. Pregnant women

6. Prisoners

Sex/Gender

All

Ages

50 Years to 65 Years

Accepts Healthy Volunteers

Accepts Healthy Volunteers

Contacts

Dinah Trevil   3052437283   dtrevil@med.miami.edu

Study of MK-8353 in Combination With Pembrolizumab (MK-3475) in Participants With Advanced Malignancies (MK-8353-013)

Study ID:

NCT02972034

Sponsor:

Merck Sharp & Dohme Corp.

Information provided by (Responsible Party):

Merck Sharp & Dohme Corp. (Merck Sharp & Dohme Corp.)

Tracking Information

First Submitted Date

November 21, 2016

Start Date

January 13, 2017

Primary Completion Date

December 20, 2020

Last Update Posted Date

September 13, 2017

Current Primary Outcome Measures

Percentage of Participants Who Experience an Adverse Event (AE)[Time Frame: Up to 27 months]
Percentage of Participants Who Discontinue Study Drug Due to an AE[Time Frame: Up to 24 months]

Percentage of Participants Who Experience a Dose-limiting Toxicity (DLT)[Time Frame: During Cycle 1 (Up to 21 days)]

Current Secondary Outcome Measures

Objective Response Rate (ORR) Based on Response Evaluation Criteria in Solid Tumors version 1.1 (RECIST 1.1) as Assessed by the Investigator[Time Frame: Up to 24 months]

Descriptive Information

Offical Title

A Phase Ib Study to Evaluate the Safety and Tolerability of MK-8353 in Combination With Pembrolizumab in Patients With Advanced Malignancies

Brief Summary

This study will evaluate the safety, tolerability and preliminary efficacy of MK-8353 when administered in combination with pembrolizumab (MK-3475). There are two parts in this study: Part 1 will be dose escalation and confirmation, and Part 2 will be a cohort expansion. In Part 1, the recommended phase II dose (RP2D) of MK-8353 in combination with a fixed dose of pembrolizumab in participants with advanced malignancies will be identified and confirmed. Participants will be initially enrolled to receive MK-8353 at 350 mg twice a day (BID) in combination with pembrolizumab at a fixed dose of 200 mg on Day 1 of each 3-week cycle (Q3W) for up to 24 months of treatment. In Part 2, participants with advanced colorectal cancer (CRC) who received at least one and up to five prior lines of therapy will be enrolled at the RP2D in the expansion cohort to further evaluate safety and efficacy.

The protocol has been amended to lower the starting doses of MK-8353 in combination with pembrolizumab. In addition,

3 arms have been added: one in which MK-8353 will be administered continuously once a day (QD) in combination with pembrolizumab, one optional arm in which MK-8353 will be administered 1 week on/1 week off QD in combination with pembrolizumab and one optional arm in which participants undergo a MK-8353 QD run-in period prior to starting combination therapy with pembrolizumab.

Study Type

Interventional

Study Phase

Phase 1

Condition

- Neoplasms
- Colorectal Cancer

Intervention

Drug: MK-8353

   PO capsule

   Biological: Pembrolizumab

   IV infusion

Other Names:

   MK-3475

Study Arms

Experimental: MK-8353 BID Continuous+Pembro

   Participants receive MK-8353 orally (PO) two times each day (BID) on Days 1 through 21 of each 21-day cycle PLUS pembrolizumab (pembro) 200 mg intravenously (IV) on Day 1 of each 21-day cycle for up to 35 cycles.

Experimental: MK-8353 QD Continuous+Pembro

   Participants receive MK-8353 PO once each day (QD) on Days 1 through 21 of each 21-day cycle PLUS pembrolizumab 200 mg IV on Day 1 of each 21-day cycle for up to 35 cycles.

Experimental: MK-8353 QD 1 Week On/1 Week Off+Pembro

   Optional Arm: Participants receive MK-8353 PO QD on Days 1 to 7, Days 15 to 21 and Days 29 to 35 PLUS pembrolizumab 200 mg IV on Day 1 and Day 22 of each 42-day period (based on 2 cycles of 21 days) for up to 35 cycles.

Experimental: MK-8353 QD Run-in then MK-8353 QD Continuous+Pembro

   Optional Arm: Participants undergo an MK-8353 PO QD run-in period from Day -14 to Day -1 prior to Cycle 1 during which they receive MK-8353 PO QD. After the run-in period, participants receive MK-8353 PO QD on Days 1 through 21 of each 21-day cycle PLUS pembrolizumab 200 mg IV on Day 1 of each 21-day cycle for up to 35 cycles.

Recruitment Information

Recruitment Status

Recruiting

Estimated Enrollment

96

Completion Date

December 20, 2020

Primary Completion Date

December 20, 2020

Eligibility Criteria

Inclusion Criteria:

- Part 1: Has a histologicallyor cytologically-documented, locally-advanced or metastatic solid malignancy and has received ≥1 and <6 prior line of cancer treatment regimen(s).
- Part 2: Has a histologically-confirmed adenocarcinoma originating from the colon or rectum (Stage 4 American Joint Committee on Cancer [AJCC] 7th edition). Appendiceal cancer is included. AND Has experienced disease progression or was intolerant to at least 1 and up to 5 systemic chemotherapy regimen(s) for metastatic CRC that must have included flururopyrimidines and irinotecan or oxaliplatin, ± anti-vascular endothelial growth factor (VEGF) or anti-epidermal growth factor receptor (EGFR)(if indicated by RAS mutational status).
- Provides an archival or newly obtained tumor tissue sample and blood samples for biomarker analysis.
- Has ≥1 measurable lesion as defined by RECIST 1.1 on imaging studies.
- Has a performance status of 0 or 1 on the Eastern Cooperative Oncology Group (ECOG) Performance Scale.
- Has adequate organ function
- Female participants of childbearing potential who are willing to use either 2 adequate barrier methods, or to abstain from

heterosexual activity throughout the study.

- Male participants of childbearing potential must agree to use an adequate method of contraception.

Exclusion Criteria:

- Has disease that is suitable for local treatment administered with curative intent.
- Part 1: Has received prior therapy with cancer vaccines, or compounds targeting programmed cell death ligand 1 (PD-L1), PD-L2, cytotoxic T-lymphocyte-associated protein 4 (CTLA-4), or Mitogen-activated protein kinase (MAPK)/Extracellular signal-regulated Kinase (MEK).
- Part 2: Has received prior therapy with cancer vaccines, or compounds targeting PD-1 (including Merck pembrolizumab [MK-3475]), PD-L1, PD-L2, CTLA-4, lymphocyte-activation gene 3 (LAG-3), CD-137, OX-40 (tumor necrosis factor receptor superfamily, member 4 [TNFRSF4], also known as CD134), cluster of differentiation 40 (CD-40), glucocorticoid-induced TNFR-related protein (GITR), serine/threonine-protein kinase B-Raf (BRAF), MEK or other molecules in the MAPK pathway.
- Is currently participating in or has participated in a study of an investigational agent or using an investigational device within 4 weeks prior to the first dose of study drug.
- Has a diagnosis of immunodeficiency or is receiving chronic systemic steroid therapy (in doses exceeding 10 mg daily of prednisone equivalent) or any other form of immunosuppressive therapy within 7 days prior to the first dose of study drug.
- Has had a prior anticancer monoclonal antibody (mAb) within 4 weeks prior to study Day 1 or has not recovered (i.e. ≤ Grade 1 or at Baseline) from adverse events (AEs) due to agents administered more than 4 weeks earlier.
- Has had prior chemotherapy, targeted small molecule therapy, or radiation therapy within 14 days prior to study Day 1 or who has not recovered (i.e., ≤Grade 1 or at baseline) from AEs due to a previously administered agent.
- Has received transfusion of blood products (including platelets or red blood cells) or administration of colony stimulating factors within 4 weeks prior to study Day 1.
- Has a known additional malignancy that is progressing or requires active treatment.
- Has known active central nervous system (CNS) metastases and/or carcinomatous meningitis.
- Has active autoimmune disease that has required systemic treatment in past 2 years (i.e. with use of disease modifying agents, corticosteroids or immunosuppressive drugs).
- Has a history of (non-infectious) pneumonitis that required steroids or current pneumonitis.
- Has a history of interstitial lung disease.
- Has an active infection requiring systemic therapy.
- Is pregnant or breastfeeding, or expecting to conceive or father children within the projected duration of the study.
- Has a known history of Human Immunodeficiency Virus (HIV).
- Has known active Hepatitis B or Hepatitis C.
- Has received a live-virus vaccination within 30 days of planned treatment start.

▦ **Sex/Gender**

All

▦ **Ages**

18 Years to N/A

▦ **Accepts Healthy Volunteers**

No

▦ **Contacts**

Toll Free Number   1-888-577-8839

TVB 2640 for Resectable Colon Cancer Other Resectable Cancers; a Window Trial.

Study ID:
NCT02980029

Sponsor:
Mark Evers

Information provided by (Responsible Party):
University of Kentucky (Mark Evers)

Tracking Information

First Submitted Date

October 12, 2016

Start Date

January 2017

Primary Completion Date

August 2018

Last Update Posted Date

January 10, 2018

Current Primary Outcome Measures

Malonyl carnitine and tripalmitin levels will be measured in the preand post-treatment blood samples using mass spectrometry blood samples using mass spectrometry.[Time Frame: Up to 56 Days]

Current Secondary Outcome Measures

- Expression of markers of tumor growth and cell proliferation (Ki67, β-catenin, c-Myc, survivin, p-AKT, etc) in the pretreatment (where available) and post-treatment tumor samples will be evaluated using IHC[Time Frame: Up to 56 Days]

  FASN levels in the pre-treatment and post-treatment tumor samples will be evaluated using IHCsamples will be evaluated using IHC.[Time Frame: Up to 56 Days]

  TIP47 levels in pre-treatment (where available) and post-treatment tumor samples will be evaluated using IHC.[Time Frame: Up to 56 Days]

  Comprehensive profile of cellular metabolites involved in various pathways (glycolysis, PPP, Krebs cycle, glutaminolysis) will be assessed in the post-treatment tumor samples using mass spectrometry analyses.[Time Frame: Up to 56 Days]

  Mutation status of tumors will be evaluated by the Clearseq comprehensive cancer panel, which targets over 145 cancerassociated genes, including APC, CTNNB1, TP53, PIK3CA, BRAF and KRAS.[Time Frame: Up to 56 Days]

  Levels of TVB-2640 will be measured in the post-treatment blood samples using mass spectrometry analysis.[Time Frame: Up to 56 Days]

  Toxicities will be graded as per NCI-CTCAE v4.03, based on recorded adverse events, physical examinations, and clinical laboratory assessments.[Time Frame: Up to 56 Days]

Descriptive Information

Offical Title

Pharmacodynamic Effects of Fatty Acid Synthase (FASN) Inhibition With TVB-2640 in Resectable Colon Cancer and Other Resectable Cancers; a Window Trial.

Brief Summary

Primary Objective

- To evaluate the pharmacodynamic effects on metabolic endpoints (malonyl carnitine and tripalmitin levels) following short-term treatment with TVB-2640 in patients with resectable cancers

Secondary Objectives

- To determine if short-term treatment with TVB-2640 decreases cancer cell proliferation.

- To examine other biological endpoints and determine if TVB-2640 inhibits cell survival signaling and lipid biogenesis.

- To perform comprehensive metabolomic analysis in tumor tissues to identify metabolic alterations induced by TVB-2640 treatment.

- To correlate FASN levels in tumor with metabolic and biological endpoints to determine if FASN inhibition has more pronounced effects in patients with increased expression.

Detailed Description

This study will test the hypothesis that inhibition of FASN activity blocks tumor lipid biosynthesis and alters the cellular metabolism in colon and other resectable cancers.

- The study is a randomized, double-blind, placebo-controlled pharmacodynamic study.

- Potentially eligible patients will be screened in the University of Kentucky Markey Cancer Center clinics. Eligible patients with histologically or cytologically confirmed resectable cancers without any distant metastases will be identified. Upon obtaining informed consent, patients will be enrolled into the study and randomized to TVB-2640 or placebo in a 2:1 fashion. Subjects and clinical investigators will be blinded to treatment group assignment.

- Baseline blood samples will be collected on Day 0 for all patients.

- All enrolled patients will receive the study drug (TVB-2640 or placebo) at a BSA-derived flat dose, orally once daily, starting Day 1. They will receive the study drug for 10-21 days (minimum of 10 days and a maximum of 21 days), i.e. from Day 1 to Day 10-21. The last dose of the study drug will be on the day before the surgical resection.

- For patients in both randomization groups, surgery will be performed anytime during the window of Day 11Day 22. On the day of surgery, surgical resection specimen and blood samples will be collected.

- All patients will be evaluated and graded for adverse events according to the NCI Common Terminology for Adverse Events (CTCAE), version 4.03.

- Patients will be followed for 4 weeks after the last dose of the study drug to monitor for any drug-related adverse events.

Study Type

Interventional

Study Phase

Phase 1

Condition

- Colon Cancer

Intervention

Drug: TVB-2640

TVB-2640 is a potent and reversible inhibitor of the FASN enzyme. TVB-2640 inhibits the β-ketoacyl reductase (KR) enzymatic activity of the FASN enzyme. TVB-2640 is uncompetitive towards both NADPH and acetoacetyl-CoA in inhibiting KR activity.

Other: Placebo

Placebo

Study Arms

Experimental: TVB-2640

TVB-2640 is a potent and reversible inhibitor of the FASN enzyme.

Placebo Comparator: Placebo

Placebo

Recruitment Information

Recruitment Status

Recruiting

Estimated Enrollment

48

Completion Date

August 2018

Primary Completion Date

August 2018

Eligibility Criteria

Inclusion Criteria:

- Histologically or cytologically confirmed, resectable colon cancer without distant metastases, who are candidates for surgical resection of the tumor.
- Willing and able to provide written informed consent prior to initiation of any study procedures.
- Male or female who is ≥ 18 years of age on day of signing informed consent
- Eastern Cooperative Oncology Group (ECOG) performance status of 0 (fully active, able to carry out all pre-disease activities without restriction) or 1 (unable to perform physically strenuous activity but ambulatory and able to carry out work of a light or sedentary nature).
- Adequate bone marrow function as evidenced by:
1. Hemoglobin ≥ 9 g/dL
2. ANC count ≥ 1.5 X 109/L
3. Platelets ≥ 100 X 109/L
- No significant ischemic heart disease or myocardial infarction (MI) within 6 months before the first dose of study drug and currently has adequate cardiac function, as evidenced by a left ventricular ejection fraction (LVEF) of ≥ 50% as assessed by multi-gated acquisition (MUGA) or ultrasound/echocardiography (ECHO); and corrected QT interval (QTc) < 470 msec
- Female subject of childbearing potential should have a negative urine or serum pregnancy within 72 hours prior to receiving the first dose of study medication. If the urine test is positive or cannot be confirmed as negative, a serum pregnancy test will be required.
- Female patients of childbearing potential should be willing to use 2 methods of birth control, be surgically sterile, or abstain from heterosexual activity for the course of the study through 90 days after the last dose of study medication. Subjects of childbearing potential are those who have not been surgically sterilized or have not been free from menses for > 1 year.
- Male patients should agree to use an adequate method of contraception starting with the first dose of study therapy through 90 days after the last dose of study therapy, or documented to be surgically sterile
- Willing to participate in the study and comply with all study requirements.

Exclusion Criteria:

- Inability to swallow oral medications or impairment of GI function or GI disease that may significantly alter drug absorption (including, but not limited to active inflammatory bowel disease, malabsorption syndrome). Concomitant therapy with antacids and anti-emetics is permissible

- History of risk factors for torsades de pointes (e.g., heart failure, hypokalemia, family history of long QT syndrome). Concomitant use of medications with a low risk of QT/QTc prolongation (including, but not limited to diphenhydramine, famotidine, ondansetron) is permissible.
- Known psychiatric or substance abuse disorders that would interfere with cooperation with the requirements of the trial.
- Having received cancer-directed therapy (chemotherapy, radiotherapy, hormonal therapy, biologic or immunotherapy, etc) or an investigational drug within 4 weeks (6 weeks for mitomycin C and nitrosoureas) or 5 half-lives of that agent (whichever is shorter) before the first dose of study drug.
- Pregnant, breastfeeding, or expecting to conceive or father children within the projected duration of the trial, starting with the prescreening or screening visit through 90 days after the last dose of trial treatment
- Inoperable on the basis of co-existent medical problems
- History of clinically significant dry eye (xerophthalmia) or other corneal abnormality or, if a contact lens wearer, does not agree to abstain from contact lens use from Day 1 through the last dose of study drug.
- Other concurrent disease (cardiovascular, renal, hepatic, etc.) or laboratory abnormality that, in the investigator's opinion would increase the risk of participating in the study.

Sex/Gender

All

Ages

18 Years to 99 Years

Accepts Healthy Volunteers

Accepts Healthy Volunteers

Contacts

Mark B Evers, MD   859-257-4500   mark.evers@uky.edu

Phase 2 Study of GVAX (With CY) and Pembrolizumab in MMR-p Advanced Colorectal Cancer

Study ID:

NCT02981524

Sponsor:

Sidney Kimmel Comprehensive Cancer Center

Information provided by (Responsible Party):

Sidney Kimmel Comprehensive Cancer Center (Sidney Kimmel Comprehensive Cancer Center)

Tracking Information

First Submitted Date

December 1, 2016

Start Date

May 26, 2017

Current Primary Outcome Measures

Antitumor activity measured as objective response rate (ORR, assessed by RECIST 1.1)[Time Frame: 4 years]

Current Secondary Outcome Measures

Number of Participants with Adverse Events as a Measure of Safety and Tolerability[Time Frame: 4 years]

Progression Free Survival (PFS)[Time Frame: 4 years]

Overall Survival (OS)[Time Frame: 4 years]

The duration of response among subjects who demonstrate an objective response to treatment with CY/GVAX in combination with pembrolizumab.[Time Frame: 4 years]

Primary Completion Date

March 2021

Last Update Posted Date

July 11, 2017

Descriptive Information

▧ Offical Title

A Phase 2 Study of GVAX Colon Vaccine (With Cyclophosphamide) and Pembrolizumab in Patients With Mismatch Repair-Proficient (MMR-p) Advanced Colorectal Cancer

▧ Brief Summary

This study will be looking at the objective response rate (ORR) as measured by RECIST in in patients with mismatch repair-proficient (MMR-p), advanced colorectal cancer that treated with CY/GVAX in combination with Pembrolizumab.

▧ Study Type

Interventional

▧ Study Phase

Phase 2

▧ Condition

- Metastatic Colorectal Cancer

▧ Intervention

Drug: CY

    CY is administered intravenously at 200 mg/m2

Other Names:

    Cyclophosphamide, Cytoxan

    Biological: GVAX

    GVAX is administered intradermally at 5E8 colon cancer cells + 5E7 GM-CSF secreting

Other Names:

    Colon cancer vaccine

    Drug: Pembrolizumab

    Pembrolizumab is administered intravenously at 200 mg

Other Names:

    KEYTRUDA, MK-3475

▧ Study Arms

Experimental: CY/GVAX with Pembrolizumab

    During each 21 day cycles, Cyclophosphamide (CY) is administered on Day 1 at 200 mg/m2 followed by Pembrolizumab at 200mg, the colon cancer vaccine (GVAX) is administered on Day 2 at 5E8 colon cancer cells + 5E7 GM-CSF secreting cells.

Recruitment Information

▧ Recruitment Status

Recruiting

▧ Estimated Enrollment

30

▧ Completion Date

March 2025

▧ Primary Completion Date

March 2021

▧ Eligibility Criteria

Inclusion Criteria:

1. Documented mismatch repair-proficient cancer of colorectum, who have received at least two prior lines of therapy for metastatic disease
2. ECOG Performance Status of 0 to 1
3. Adequate organ function as defined by study-specified laboratory tests
4. Must use acceptable form of birth control through the study and for 120 days after final dose of study drug
5. Signed informed consent form
6. Willing and able to comply with study procedures

Exclusion Criteria:

1. Currently have or have history of certain study-specified heart, liver, kidney, lung, neurological, immune or other medical conditions
2. Systemically active steroid use

3. Another investigational product within 28 days prior to receiving study drug

4. Major surgery or significant traumatic injury (or unhealed surgical wounds) occurring within 28 days prior to receiving study drug

5. Chemotherapy, radiation, hormonal, or biological cancer therapy within 28 days prior to receiving study drug

6. Pregnant or lactating

7. Unwilling or unable to comply with study procedures

Sex/Gender

All

Ages

18 Years to 100 Years

Accepts Healthy Volunteers

No

Contacts

Anna Ferguson, RN   410-614-7186   afergus1@jhmi.edu
Mark Yarchoan, MD   mark.yarchoan@jhmi.edu

AZD9150 With MEDI4736 in Patients With Advanced Pancreatic, Non-Small Lung and Colorectal Cancer

Study ID:
NCT02983578

Sponsor:
M.D. Anderson Cancer Center

Information provided by (Responsible Party):
M.D. Anderson Cancer Center (M.D. Anderson Cancer Center)

Tracking Information

First Submitted Date
December 1, 2016

Primary Completion Date
March 2021

Start Date
March 2, 2017

Last Update Posted Date
January 31, 2018

Current Primary Outcome Measures

Disease Control Rate[Time Frame: 4 months]

Disease control defined as a Complete Response, Partial Response or Stable Disease, according to RECIST version 1.1 criteria.

Evaluation of Tumor-Based Biomarkers in Paired Pre and Post Treatment Biopsies[Time Frame: Baseline up to 30 days after last study drug dose]

PD-L1 Protein Levels in the Membrane of Circulating Tumor Cells[Time Frame: Baseline up to 30 days after last study drug dose]

Current Secondary Outcome Measures

Objective Response[Time Frame: 2 months]

Objective response defined as Partial Response or Complete Response according to RECIST 1.1 criteria.

Duration of Response[Time Frame: 4 months]

Duration of response according to RECIST version 1.1 criteria (measured from the time measurement criteria are first met for Complete Response or Partial Response, whichever is first recorded, until the first date that recurrent or Progressive Disease is objectively documented (taking as reference for Progressive Disease the smallest measurements recorded on study).

Descriptive Information

Offical Title

Phase II Clinical Trial Evaluating Intravenous AZD9150 (Antisense STAT3) With MEDI4736 (Anti-PD-L1) in Patients With

Advanced Pancreatic, Non-Small Cell Lung Cancer, and Mismatch Repair Deficient Colorectal Cancer

Brief Summary

The goal of this clinical research study is to learn if AZD9150 given in combination with MEDI4736 (durvalumab) can help to control advanced pancreatic, lung, or colorectal cancer.

This is an investigational study. AZD9150 and MEDI4736 are not FDA approved or commercially available. They are currently being used for research purposes only. The study doctor can explain how the study drugs are designed to work.

Up to 75 participants will take part in this study. All will be enrolled at MD Anderson.

Detailed Description

Study Drug Administration:

Every study cycle will be 28 days.

If you are found to be eligible to take part in this study, you will begin study treatment within 28 days after the screening tests are performed. You will receive AZD9150 by vein over 1 hour 3 times before the first dose of MEDI4736 (7, 5, and 3 days beforehand), and then on Days 1, 8, 15, and 22 of every cycle.

You will receive MEDI4736 by vein over about 1 hour on Day 1 of every cycle, about 30 minutes after the AZD9150 infusion.

Length of Treatment:

You may continue receiving the study drugs for as long as the doctor thinks is in your best interest. You will no longer be able to receive the study drugs if the disease gets worse, if intolerable side effects occur, or if you are unable to follow study directions.

Study Visits:

On Day 1 of Cycle 1 and beyond:

- You will have a physical exam.
- Blood (about 4 teaspoons) and urine will be collected for routine tests.
- Blood (about 2 teaspoons) will be drawn to check your thyroid function.
- If you can become pregnant, blood (about 1 teaspoon) or urine will be collected for a pregnancy test.

On Days 8 and 22 of Cycles 1 and beyond:

- You will have a physical exam.
- Blood (about 4 teaspoons) will be drawn for routine tests (Cycle 1 only).

On Day 15 of Cycles 1 and beyond:

- You will have a physical exam.
- Blood (about 4 teaspoons) will be drawn for routine tests.
- Urine will be collected for routine tests (Cycle 1 only).

On Day 22 of Cycles 1 and beyond:

- Blood (about 2½ tablespoons) will be drawn for biomarker testing.
- You will have a core tumor biopsy for biomarker testing.

Every 2 months, you will have a PET/CT scan or MRI to check the status of the disease.

End-of-Treatment Visit:

About 30 days after your last dose of the study drugs:

- You will have a physical exam.
- Blood (about 4 tablespoons) and urine will be collected for routine tests.
- Blood (about 2 teaspoons) will be drawn to check your thyroid function.
- Blood (about 2½ tablespoons) will be drawn for biomarker testing.
- You will have a PET/CT scan or MRI to check the status of the disease.
- If you can become pregnant, urine will be collected for a pregnancy test.

Follow-Up:

About 1-3 months after your last dose of the study drugs, you will have a PET/CT scan or MRI to check the status of the disease.

If you cannot come to MD Anderson for your follow-up visits, you may be called every 12 weeks and asked about how you are doing. These calls will last about 10 minutes each.

Your participation on the study will be over at the end of the follow-up period.

Treatment Beyond Progression:

If the disease appears to be getting worse or the tumors appear to be getting larger, you may still be able to receive the study drugs if you and your doctor decide it is in your best interest. The study doctor will discuss this option with you. If you choose to receive the study drugs after the disease gets worse, you will sign an additional informed consent form.

Study Type

Interventional

Study Phase

Phase 2

Condition

- Malignant Neoplasm of Digestive Organs Intestinal Tract Primary
- Malignant Neoplasm of Respiratory and Intrathoracic Organ Carcinoma

Intervention

Drug: AZD9150

AZD9150 3 mg/kg administered by vein on Days 1, 8, 15, and 22 of every 28 day cycle.

Drug: MEDI4736

MEDI4736 fixed dose of 1500 mg (20 mg/kg Q4W) administered monthly.

Other Names:

Durvalumab

Study Arms

Experimental: Advanced Non-Small Cell Lung Cancer Group

Participants receive AZD9150 every week and MED4736 every 4 weeks.

Participants receive treatment until progression or unacceptable toxicity.

Experimental: Mismatch Repair-Deficient Colorectal Cancer Group

Participants receive AZD9150 every week and MED4736 every 4 weeks.

Participants receive treatment until progression or unacceptable toxicity.

Experimental: Pancreatic Cancer Group

Participants receive AZD9150 every week and MED4736 every 4 weeks.

Participants receive treatment until progression or unacceptable toxicity.

Recruitment Information

Recruitment Status

Recruiting

Estimated Enrollment

75

Completion Date

March 2022

Primary Completion Date

March 2021

Eligibility Criteria

Inclusion Criteria:

1. The patient/legal representative must be able to read and understand the informed consent form (ICF) and must have been willing to give written informed consent and any locally required authorisation (eg, Health Insurance Portability and Accountability Act in the USA; European Union Data Privacy Directive in the EU) before any study-specific procedures, including screening evaluations, sampling, and analyses.

2. Has a histological confirmation of pancreatic cancer, mismatch deficient colorectal cancer, or NSCLC that is refractory to standard therapy or for which no standard of care regimen currently exists.

3. Male and female patients must be at least 18 years of age.

4. Has an Eastern Cooperative Oncology Group (ECOG) PS score of 0 or 1.

5. Has measurable disease, defined as at least 1 lesion that can be accurately measured in at least 1 dimension (longest diameter to be recorded) with a minimum size of 10 mm by computerised tomography (CT) scan, except lymph nodes which must have minimum short axis size of 15 mm (CT scan slice thickness no greater than 5 mm in both cases). Indicator lesions must not have been previously treated with surgery, radiation therapy, or radiofrequency ablation unless there is documented progression after therapy.

6. Has adequate organ and marrow function as defined below. Transfusions intended to elevate any parameters below solely for the intent of meeting study eligibility are not permitted. Leukocytes >/=3000 mcL, Absolute neutrophil count >/=1500 mcL, Platelets >/=100 000 mcL, Hemoglobin >/=9 g/dL, Total bilirubin </=1.5 x ULN; total bilirubin </=3×ULN in patients with documented Gilbert's Syndrome (unconjugated hyperbilirubinaemia) or in the presence of liver metastases, ALT and AST </=2.5×ULN if no demonstrable liver metastases or </=5×ULN in the presence of liver metastases, Creatinine within normal limits OR, for patients with levels above institutional normal: Creatinine clearance measured by 24-hour urine collection >/=60 mL/min, OR Calculated corrected creatinine clearance >/=60 mL/min/1.73 m^2 using the Cockcroft-Gault formula (Cockcroft and Gault 1976) corrected for the body surface area.

7. Women of childbearing potential and men who are sexually active with a female partner of childbearing potential must be surgically sterilised, practicing abstinence, or agree to use 2 birth control methods before study entry, for the duration of study participation, and for 20 weeks after the final dose of study drug; cessation of birth control after this point should be discussed with a responsible physician. Women of childbearing potential are defined as those who are not surgically sterile (ie, bilateral

tubal ligation, bilateral oophorectomy, or complete hysterectomy) or postmenopausal (defined as 12 months with no menses without an alternative medical cause). Two methods of contraception which are considered accurate per protocol must be combined. Periodic abstinence, the rhythm method, and the withdrawal method are not acceptable methods of birth control.

8. Women of childbearing potential also may not be breast feeding and must have a negative serum or urine pregnancy test within 72 hours before the start of study treatment.

9. The patient/legal representative must be willing to provide written consent for collection of formalin fixed paraffin-embedded blocks or slides from archival diagnostic histology samples, where available.

Exclusion Criteria:

1. Has a spinal cord compression unless asymptomatic, radiographically stable over the last 4 weeks, and not requiring steroids for at least 4 weeks before the start of study treatment.

2. Presently has a second malignancy other than SCCHN, or history of treatment for invasive cancer other than SCCHN in the past 3 years. Exceptions are: Previously treated in-situ carcinoma (ie, noninvasive), Cervical carcinoma stage 1B or less, Noninvasive basal cell and squamous cell skin carcinoma, Radically treated prostate cancer (prostatectomy or radiotherapy) with normal prostate-specific antigen, and not requiring ongoing antiandrogen hormonal therapy

3. Patients must have completed previous cancer-related treatments before enrollment. Any concurrent chemotherapy, radiotherapy, immunotherapy, or biologic, or hormonal therapy for cancer excludes the patient (concurrent use of hormones for noncancer-related conditions [eg, insulin for diabetes or hormone replacement therapy] is acceptable). The following intervals between end of the prior treatment and first dose of study drug must be observed: Port-a-cath placement: no waiting required. Minor surgical procedures: >/=7 postoperative days. Major surgery: >/=4 weeks. Radiotherapy: >/=4 weeks. Chemotherapy: >/=4 weeks. Immunotherapy or investigational anticancer therapy with agents other than mAbs: >/=4 weeks. Immunotherapy or investigational anticancer therapy with mAbs: >/=6 weeks. Immunosuppressive medication: >/=4 weeks with the exceptions of intranasal or inhaled corticosteroids or systemic corticosteroids at physiologic doses not to exceed 10mg/day of prednisone or equivalent.

4. Is still experiencing toxicity related to prior treatment and assessed as CTCAE grade >1. Exceptions are alopecia and/or anorexia. The eligibility of patients who are still experiencing irreversible toxicity that is not reasonably expected to be exacerbated by the study drugs in this study (eg, hearing loss) must be reviewed and approved by both the Principal Investigator and Medical Monitor.

5. Has experienced immune-related AEs (irAEs) while receiving prior immunotherapy (including anti-CTLA4 treatment) and assessed as CTCAE grade >/= 3

6. Has active or prior documented autoimmune disease within the past 2 years with the exceptions of vitiligo, Grave's disease, and/or psoriasis not requiring systemic treatment

7. Has active or prior documented inflammatory bowel disease (eg, Crohn's disease, ulcerative colitis)

8. Has a history of primary immunodeficiency

9. Has undergone an organ transplant that requires use of immunosuppressive treatment

10. Has a history of interstitial lung disease or pneumonitis from any cause

11. Has a history of allergic reactions attributed to the study treatments (AZD9150 or MEDI4736), their compounds, or agents of similar chemical or biologic composition (eg, antibody therapeutics)

12. Suffers from a comorbidity that in the opinion of the Investigator renders the patient unsuitable for participation in the study. Such comorbidity may include, but is not limited to, uncontrolled intercurrent illness such as active infection, severe active peptic ulcer disease or gastritis, myocardial infarction within 6 months before entry, congestive heart failure, symptomatic congestive heart failure, active cardiomyopathy, unstable angina pectoris, cardiac arrhythmia, uncontrolled hypertension, or psychiatric illness/social situations that would limit compliance with study requirements.

13. As judged by the Investigator, has any evidence of severe or uncontrolled systemic diseases such as active bleeding diatheses, is positive for human immunodeficiency virus (HIV), or has active hepatitis B virus (HBV) and/or hepatitis C virus (HCV)

14. Has a known history of tuberculosis

15. Has a condition that, in the opinion of the Investigator, would interfere with the evaluation of the study drugs or the interpretation of patient safety or study results

16. Has received a live attenuated vaccine within 28 days before the first dose of study drug

17. Judgment by the Investigator that the patient should not participate in the study if the patient is unlikely to comply with study procedures, restrictions, and requirements

18. Patients with clinically active brain metastases (known or suspected) are excluded unless the brain metastases have been previously treated and are considered stable. Stable brain metastases are defined as no change on CT scan or magnetic resonance imaging (MRI) scan for a minimum of 2 months AND no change in steroid dose for a minimum of 4 weeks, unless change due to intercurrent infection or other acute event.

19. Female subjects who are pregnant, breast-feeding or male or female patients of reproductive potential who are not employing an effective method of birth control

■ Sex/Gender

All

■ Ages

18 Years to N/A

Combination Chemotherapy, Bevacizumab, and/or Atezolizumab in Treating Patients With Deficient DNA Mismatch Repair Metastatic Colorectal Cancer

Study ID:

NCT02997228

Sponsor:

National Cancer Institute (NCI)

Information provided by (Responsible Party):

National Cancer Institute (NCI) (National Cancer Institute (NCI))

Tracking Information

■ **First Submitted Date**

December 19, 2016

■ **Start Date**

November 7, 2017

■ **Primary Completion Date**

April 30, 2022

■ **Last Update Posted Date**

February 6, 2018

■ **Current Primary Outcome Measures**

Progression free survival (PFS)[Time Frame: From the time from randomization until first confirmed progression or death from any cause, assessed up to 5 years]

The experimental arms will be compared to the control arm by the log-rank test stratified by BRAF status, metastatic disease: (liver-only, extra-hepatic), and prior adjuvant therapy for colon cancer (yes, no). Hazard ratios and associated confidence intervals from a stratified Cox regression model will also be reported along with estimates of the distributions of time to PFS event by the method of Kaplan and Meier.

■ **Current Secondary Outcome Measures**

Disease control rate (CR + PR + stable disease [SD]) assessed by RECIST 1.1[Time Frame: At 12 months]

Will be analyzed by a logistic regression models that control for the stratification factors (BRAF status, liver involvement, and adjuvant chemo). Observed proportions along with confidence intervals will be presented by treatment.

Duration of overall response (CR or PR) as assessed by RECIST 1.1[Time Frame: From the time of first response to first confirmed progression by the study investigator or death from any cause, assessed up to 5 years]

Will be analyzed using the stratified log rank test. Kaplan-Meier plots will illustrate the distribution of these endpoints by treatment. Stratified Cox regression models will be used to estimate hazard ratios and associated confidence intervals.

Incidence of adverse events as defined by Common Terminology Criteria for Adverse Events (CTCAE) version 4[Time Frame: Up to 30 days after last course]

Objective response rate (ORR) (complete response [CR] or partial response [PR]) assessed by Response Evaluation Criteria in Solid Tumors (RECIST) 1.1[Time Frame: Up to 5 years]

Will be analyzed by a logistic regression models that control for the stratification factors (BRAF status, liver involvement, and adjuvant chemo). Observed proportions along with confidence intervals will be presented by treatment.

Overall survival (OS)[Time Frame: The time from randomization to death from any cause, assessed up to 5 years]

Will be analyzed using the stratified log rank test. Kaplan-Meier plots will illustrate the distribution of these endpoints by treatment. Stratified Cox regression models will be used to estimate hazard ratios and associated confidence intervals.

PFS[Time Frame: From randomization until first progression by retrospective central independent scan review or death from any cause, assessed up to 5 years]

Surgical conversion rate defined as the proportion of patients that have surgery with curative intent[Time Frame: Up to 5 years]

Will be analyzed by a logistic regression models that control for the stratification factors (BRAF status, liver involvement, and adjuvant chemo). Observed proportions along with confidence intervals will be presented by treatment.

Descriptive Information

Offical Title

Colorectal Cancer Metastatic dMMR Immuno-Therapy (COMMIT) Study: A Randomized Phase III Study of mFOLFOX6/Bevacizumab Combination Chemotherapy With or Without Atezolizumab or Atezolizumab Monotherapy in the First-Line Treatment of Patients With Deficient DNA Mismatch Repair (dMMR) Metastatic Colorectal Cancer

Brief Summary

This randomized phase III trial studies how well combination chemotherapy, bevacizumab, and/or atezolizumab work in treating patients with deficient DNA mismatch repair colorectal cancer that has spread to other places in the body. Drugs used in chemotherapy, such as fluorouracil, oxaliplatin, and leucovorin calcium, work in different ways to stop the growth of tumor cells, either by killing the cells, by stopping them from dividing, or by stopping them from spreading. Monoclonal antibodies, such as bevacizumab and atezolizumab, may interfere with the ability of tumor cells to grow and spread. Giving combination chemotherapy, bevacizumab, and atezolizumab may work better in treating patients with colorectal cancer.

Detailed Description

PRIMARY OBJECTIVES:

I. To determine the efficacy, based on progression-free survival (PFS), of fluorouracil, oxaliplatin, and leucovorin calcium (mFOLFOX6)/bevacizumab plus atezolizumab (combination) and atezolizumab (single agent) as compared to mFOLFOX6/bevacizumab (control).

SECONDARY OBJECTIVES:

I. To compare the overall survival. II. To compare the objective response rates (ORR) per Response Evaluation Criteria in Solid Tumors (RECIST) 1.1.

III. To determine the safety profiles of the combination of mFOLFOX6/bevacizumab/atezolizumab and atezolizumab monotherapy in patients with mismatch-repair deficient (dMMR) metastatic colorectal cancer (mCRC).

IV. To compare the surgical conversion rate. V. To compare disease control rate (complete response [CR] + partial response [PR] + stable disease [SD]) at 12 months.

VI. To determine the duration of response and stable disease. VII. To determine the progression-free survival (PFS) by retrospective central independent scan review.

TERTIARY OBJECTIVES:

I. To compare the health-related quality of life and patient-reported symptoms. II. To bank tissue and blood samples for other future correlative studies from patients enrolled on the study.

OUTLINE: Patients are randomized to 1 of 3 arms.

ARM I: Patients receive bevacizumab intravenously (IV) over 30-90 minutes on day 1, oxaliplatin IV over 2 hours on day 1 of courses 1-10, leucovorin calcium IV over 2 hours on day 1, and fluorouracil IV over 46-48 hours on days 1 and 2. Courses repeat every 2 weeks in the absence of disease progression or unacceptable toxicity.

ARM II: Patients receive atezolizumab IV over 30-60 minutes on day 1. Treatment repeats every 2 weeks for up to 48 courses in the absence of disease progression or unacceptable toxicity.

ARM III: Patients receive atezolizumab IV over 30-60 minutes on day 1. Courses with repeat every 2 weeks for up to 48 courses in the absence of disease progression or unacceptable toxicity. Patients also received bevacizumab IV over 30-90 minutes on day 1, oxaliplatin IV over 2 hours on day 1 courses 1-10, leucovorin calcium IV over 2 hours on day 1, and fluorouracil IV over 46-48 hours on day 1. Courses repeat every 2 weeks in the absence of disease progression or unacceptable toxicity.

After completion of study treatment, patients are followed up every 8 weeks for 18 months, and then every 12 weeks for up to 5 years.

Study Type

Interventional

Study Phase

Phase 3

Condition

- Colorectal Adenocarcinoma
- Mismatch Repair Deficiency
- Stage IV Colorectal Cancer AJCC v7
- Stage IVA Colorectal Cancer AJCC v7
- Stage IVB Colorectal Cancer AJCC v7

Intervention

Drug: Atezolizumab
  Given IV

Other Names:
  MPDL 3280A

MPDL 328OA

MPDL-3280A

MPDL3280A

MPDL328OA

RG7446

RO5541267

Tecentriq

Biological: Bevacizumab

Given IV

Other Names:

Anti-VEGF

Anti-VEGF Humanized Monoclonal Antibody

Anti-VEGF rhuMAb

Avastin

Bevacizumab Biosimilar BEVZ92

Bevacizumab Biosimilar BI 695502

Bevacizumab Biosimilar CBT 124

Bevacizumab Biosimilar FKB238

BEVACIZUMAB, LICENSE HOLDER UNSPECIFIED

Immunoglobulin G1 (Human-Mouse Monoclonal rhuMab-VEGF Gamma-Chain Anti-Human Vascular Endothelial Growth Factor), Disulfide With Human-Mouse Monoclonal rhuMab-VEGF Light Chain, Dimer

Recombinant Humanized Anti-VEGF Monoclonal Antibody

rhuMab-VEGF

Drug: Fluorouracil

Given IV

Other Names:

5-Fluoro-2,4(1H, 3H)-pyrimidinedione

5-Fluorouracil

5-Fluracil

5-FU

AccuSite

Carac

Fluoro Uracil

Fluouracil

Flurablastin

Fluracedyl

Fluracil

Fluril

Fluroblastin

Ribofluor

Ro 2-9757

Ro-2-9757

Other: Laboratory Biomarker Analysis

Correlative studies

Drug: Leucovorin Calcium

Given IV

Other Names:

Adinepar

Calcifolin

Calcium (6S)-Folinate

Calcium Folinate

Calcium Leucovorin

Calfolex

Calinat

Cehafolin

Citofolin

Citrec

citrovorum factor

Cromatonbic Folinico

Dalisol

Disintox

Divical

Ecofol

Emovis

Factor, Citrovorum

Flynoken A

Folaren

Folaxin

FOLI-cell

Foliben

Folidan

Folidar

Folinac

Folinate Calcium

folinic acid

Folinic Acid Calcium Salt Pentahydrate

Folinoral

Folinvit

Foliplus

Folix

Imo

Lederfolat

Lederfolin

Leucosar

leucovorin

Rescufolin

Rescuvolin

Tonofolin

Wellcovorin

Drug: Oxaliplatin
Given IV

Other Names:

1-OHP

Ai Heng

Aiheng

Dacotin

Dacplat

Diaminocyclohexane Oxalatoplatinum

Eloxatin

Eloxatine

JM-83

Oxalatoplatin

Oxalatoplatinum

RP 54780

RP-54780

SR-96669

Other: Quality-of-Life Assessment
Ancillary studies

Other Names:
Quality of Life Assessment

Study Arms

Active Comparator: Arm I (bevacizumab, mFOLFOX6)

Patients receive bevacizumab IV over 30-90 minutes on day 1, oxaliplatin IV over 2 hours on day 1 of courses 1-10, leucovorin calcium IV over 2 hours on day 1, and fluorouracil IV over 46-48 hours on days 1 and 2. Courses repeat every 2 weeks in the absence of disease progression or unacceptable toxicity.

Experimental: Arm II (atezolizumab)

Patients receive atezolizumab IV over 30-60 minutes on day 1. Treatment repeats every 2 weeks for up to 48 courses in the absence of disease progression or unacceptable toxicity.

Experimental: Arm III (atezolizumab, bevacizumab, mFOLFOX6)

Patients receive atezolizumab IV over 30-60 minutes on day 1. Courses with repeat every 2 weeks for up to 48 courses in the absence of disease progression or unacceptable toxicity. Patients also received bevacizumab IV over 30-90 minutes on day 1, oxaliplatin IV over 2 hours on day 1 courses 1-10, leucovorin calcium IV over 2 hours on day 1, and fluorouracil IV over 46-48 hours on day 1. Courses repeat every 2 weeks in the absence of disease progression or unacceptable toxicity.

Recruitment Information

Recruitment Status

Recruiting

Estimated Enrollment

347

Completion Date

April 30, 2022

Primary Completion Date

April 30, 2022

Eligibility Criteria

Inclusion Criteria:

- The patient must have signed and dated an Institutional Review Board (IRB)-approved consent form that conforms to federal and institutional guidelines
- Eastern Cooperative Oncology Group (ECOG) performance status of 0, 1 or 2
- Diagnosis of metastatic adenocarcinoma of colon or rectum without previous chemotherapy or any other systemic therapy for metastatic colorectal cancer
- Tumor determined to be mismatch-repair deficient (dMMR) by Clinical Laboratory Improvement Act (CLIA)-certified immunohistochemical (IHC) assay with a panel of all four IHC markers, including MLH1, MSH2, PMS2, and MSH6; Note: microsatellite instability high (MSI-H) diagnosed by microsatellite instability (MSI) testing (either Bethesda markers or Pentaplex panel) or by next-generation sequencing (NGS) is not eligible unless dMMR is confirmed by CLIA-certified

immunohistochemical (IHC) assay with a panel of all four IHC markers including MLH1, MSH2, PMS2 and MSH6

- An adequate amount of archived tumor tissue, either from primary colorectal cancer site or metastatic lesions, for central confirmation of dMMR status:
- Either whole or part of the formalin-fixed paraffin-embedded (FFPE) block containing tumor tissue; or
- At least 8 unstained slides containing tumor sections
- Documentation by positron emission tomography(PET)/computed tomography (CT) scan, CT scan, or magnetic resonance imaging (MRI) that the patient has untreated measurable metastatic disease per RECIST 1.1
- No immediate need for surgical intervention for the primary tumor or palliative diversion/bypass
- Obtained within 28 days prior randomization: absolute neutrophil count (ANC) must be >= 1500/mm^3
- Obtained within 28 days prior randomization: platelet count must be >= 100,000/mm^3
- Obtained within 28 days prior randomization: hemoglobin must be >= 8 g/dL
- Obtained within 28 days prior randomization: total bilirubin must be =< 1.5 x ULN (upper limit of normal) for the lab unless the patient has a bilirubin elevation > 1.5 x ULN to 3 x ULN due to Gilbert's disease or similar syndrome involving slow conjugation of bilirubin; and
- Obtained within 28 days prior randomization: alkaline phosphatase must be =< 2.5 x ULN for the lab with the following exception: patients with documented liver metastases or bone involvement alkaline phosphatase must be =< 5 x ULN; and
- Obtained within 28 days prior randomization: aspartate aminotransferase (AST) and alanine aminotransferase (ALT) must be =< 3 x ULN for the lab with the following exception: for patients with documented liver metastases, AST and ALT must be =< 5 x ULN
- Obtained within 28 days prior randomization: serum creatinine =< 1.5 x ULN for the lab or measured or calculated creatinine clearance >= 30 mL/min
- A urine sample tested for proteinuria by the dipstick method must indicate 0 -1+ protein; if dipstick reading is >= 2+, a 24-hour urine specimen must demonstrate < 1.0 g of protein per 24 hours
- International normalized ratio of prothrombin time (INR) and prothrombin time (PT) must be =< 1.5 x ULN for the lab within 28 days before randomization; patients who are therapeutically treated with an agent such as warfarin may participate if they are on a stable dose and no underlying abnormality in coagulation parameters exists per medical history
- Pregnancy test done within 14 days prior randomization must be negative (for women of childbearing potential only); pregnancy testing should be performed according to institutional standards; should a woman become pregnant or suspect she is pregnant while she or her partner is participating in this study, she should inform her treating physician immediately
- Women of child-bearing potential must agree to use adequate contraception (hormonal or barrier method of birth control; abstinence) prior to study entry, for the duration of study participation, and for 5 months (150 days) after the last dose of atezolizumab, 6 months after the last dose of bevacizumab, and 6 months after the last dose of mFOLFOX6; Men with female partners of child-bearing potential must agree to use adequate contraception prior to the study, for the duration of study participation, and for 6 months after the last dose of bevacizumab and 6 months after the last dose of mFOLFOX6

Exclusion Criteria:

- **Patients with central nervous system (CNS) metastases are excluded, with the following exceptions:**
- **Patients with asymptomatic untreated CNS metastases may be enrolled, provided all eligibility criteria are met, as well as the following:**
- Evaluable or measurable disease outside the CNS
- No metastases to brain stem, midbrain, pons, medulla, cerebellum, or within 10 mm of the optic apparatus (optic nerves and chiasm)
- No history of intracranial hemorrhage or spinal cord hemorrhage
- No ongoing requirement for dexamethasone for CNS disease; patients on a stable dose of anticonvulsants are permitted.
- No neurosurgical resection or brain biopsy within 28 days prior to randomization
- **Patients with asymptomatic treated CNS metastases may be enrolled, provided all eligibility criteria are met, as well as the following:**
- Radiographic demonstration of improvement upon the completion of CNS-directed therapy and no evidence of interim progression between the completion of CNS-directed therapy and the screening radiographic study
- No stereotactic radiation or whole-brain radiation within 28 days prior to randomization
- Screening CNS radiographic study >= 28 days from completion of radiotherapy and >= 14 days from discontinuation of corticosteroids
- Known hypersensitivity to Chinese hamster ovary cell products or other recombinant human antibodies, fluoropyrimidines, folic acid derivatives or oxaliplatin
- Uncontrolled high blood pressure defined as systolic blood pressure (BP) > 150 mmHg or diastolic BP 90 mmHg with or without anti-hypertensive medication; patients with initial BP elevations are eligible if initiation or adjustment of BP medication lowers pressure to meet entry criteria
- **Any of the following cardiac conditions:**
- Documented New York Heart Association (NYHA) class III or IV congestive heart failure
- Myocardial infarction within 6 months prior to randomization
- Unstable angina within 6 months prior to randomization

- Symptomatic arrhythmia
- Serious or non-healing wound, skin ulcer, or bone fracture
- History of transient ischemic attack (TIA), cerebrovascular accident (CVA), gastrointestinal (GI) perforation or arterial thrombotic event within 6 months prior to randomization or symptomatic peripheral ischemia
- Other malignancies are excluded unless the patient has completed therapy for the malignancy >= 12 months prior to randomization and is considered disease-free; patients with the following cancers are eligible if diagnosed and treated within the past 12 months: in situ carcinomas or basal cell and squamous cell carcinoma of the skin
- Known DPD (dihydro pyrimidine dehydrogenase) deficiency
- Symptomatic peripheral sensory neuropathy >= grade 2 (Common Terminology Criteria for Adverse Events [CTCAE] version [v] 4.0) in patients with no prior oxaliplatin therapy
- Prior treatment with oxaliplatin chemotherapy within 6 months prior to randomization
- **Prior treatment with anti-PD-1, or anti-PD-L1 therapeutic antibody or pathway-targeting agents; patients who have received prior treatment with anti-CTLA-4 may be enrolled provided the following requirements are met:**
- Minimum of 12 weeks from the first dose of anti-CTLA-4 and > 6 weeks from the last dose to randomization
- No history of severe immune-related adverse effects (CTCAE Grade 3 and 4) from anti-CTLA-4
- **Patients who have had chemotherapy or radiotherapy within 4 weeks (6 weeks for nitrosoureas or mitomycin C) prior to entering the study or those who have not recovered from adverse events (other than alopecia) due to agents administered more than 4 weeks earlier are excluded; however, the following therapies are allowed:**
- Hormone-replacement therapy or oral contraception
- Herbal therapy > 7 days prior to randomization (herbal therapy intended as anticancer therapy must be discontinued at least 1 week prior to randomization)
- Palliative radiotherapy for bone metastases > 14 days prior to randomization
- Treatment with systemic immunostimulatory medications (including, but not limited to interferon [IFN]-alpha or interleukin [IL]-2 within 42 days prior to randomization
- Treatment with systemic immunosuppressive medications (including, but not limited to, prednisone, cyclophosphamide, azathioprine, methotrexate, thalidomide, and anti-tumor necrosis factor [anti-TNF] agents) within 14 days prior to randomization; however,
- Patients who have received acute, low dose, systemic immunosuppressant medications (e.g., a one-time dose of dexamethasone for nausea; or chronic daily treatment with corticosteroids with a dose of =< 10 mg/day methylprednisolone equivalent) may be enrolled
- The use of inhaled corticosteroids and mineralocorticoids (e.g., fludrocortisone) for patients with orthostatic hypotension or adrenocortical insufficiency is allowed
- Patients taking bisphosphonate therapy for symptomatic hypercalcemia; use of bisphosphonate therapy for other reasons (e.g., bone metastasis or osteoporosis) is allowed
- Patients requiring treatment with a receptor activator of nuclear factor kappa-B ligand (RANKL) inhibitor (e.g., denosumab) who cannot discontinue it before treatment with atezolizumab
- Treatment with any other investigational agent within 4 weeks prior to randomization
- Known clinically significant liver disease, including active viral, alcoholic, or other hepatitis; cirrhosis; fatty liver; and inherited liver disease; however,
- Patients with past or resolved hepatitis B infection (defined as having a negative hepatitis B surface antigen [HBsAg] test and a positive anti-HBc [antibody to hepatitis B core antigen] antibody test) are eligible
- Patients positive for hepatitis C virus (HCV) antibody are eligible only if polymerase chain reaction (PCR) is negative for HCV ribonucleic acid (RNA)
- History or risk of autoimmune disease, including, but not limited to, systemic lupus erythematosus, rheumatoid arthritis, inflammatory bowel disease, vascular thrombosis associated with antiphospholipid syndrome, Wegener's granulomatosis, Sjogren's syndrome, Bell's palsy, Guillain-Barre syndrome, multiple sclerosis, autoimmune thyroid disease, vasculitis, or glomerulonephritis; however,
- Patients with a history of autoimmune hypothyroidism on a stable dose of thyroid replacement hormone may be eligible
- Patients with controlled type 1 diabetes mellitus on a stable insulin regimen may be eligible
- **Patients with eczema, psoriasis, lichen simplex chronicus or vitiligo with dermatologic manifestations only (e.g., patients with psoriatic arthritis would be excluded) are permitted provided that they meet the following conditions:**
- Patients with psoriasis must have a baseline ophthalmologic exam to rule out ocular manifestations
- Rash must cover less than 10% of body surface area (BSA)
- Disease is well controlled at baseline and only requiring low potency topical steroids (e.g., hydrocortisone 2.5%, hydrocortisone butyrate 0.1%, fluocinolone 0.01%, desonide 0.05%, alclometasone dipropionate 0.05%)
- No acute exacerbations of underlying condition within the last 12 months (not requiring psoralen plus ultraviolet A radiation [PUVA], methotrexate, retinoids, biologic agents, oral calcineurin inhibitors; high potency or oral steroids)
- History of idiopathic pulmonary fibrosis, pneumonitis (including drug induced), organizing pneumonia (i.e., bronchiolitis obliterans, cryptogenic organizing pneumonia, etc.), or evidence of active pneumonitis on screening chest computed tomography (CT) scan; history of radiation pneumonitis in the radiation field (fibrosis) is permitted
- History of severe allergic, anaphylactic, or other hypersensitivity reactions to chimeric or humanized antibodies or fusion

proteins

- Patients with known active tuberculosis (TB) are excluded
- Severe infections within 28 days prior to randomization, including but not limited to, hospitalization for complications of infection, bacteremia, or severe pneumonia
- Signs or symptoms of infection within 14 days prior to randomization
- Received oral or intravenous (IV) antibiotics within 14 days prior to randomization; patients receiving prophylactic antibiotics (e.g., for prevention of a urinary tract infection or chronic obstructive pulmonary disease) are eligible
- Major surgical procedure, open biopsy, or significant traumatic injury within 28 days prior to randomization or anticipation of need for a major surgical procedure during the course of the study
- Administration of a live, attenuated vaccine within 28 days prior to randomization or anticipation that such a live, attenuated vaccine will be required during the study and up to 5 months after the last dose of atezolizumab; Note: influenza vaccination should be given during influenza season only (approximately October to March); patients must not receive live, attenuated influenza vaccine within 28 days prior to randomization or at any time during the study
- Psychiatric illness/social situations that would limit compliance with study requirements
- Pregnant women are excluded from this study; breastfeeding should be discontinued if the mother is treated with atezolizumab; (Note: pregnancy testing should be performed within 14 days prior to randomization according to institutional standards for women of childbearing potential)
- **Patients positive for human immunodeficiency virus (HIV) are NOT excluded from this study, but HIV-positive patients must have:**
- A stable regimen of highly active anti-retroviral therapy (HAART); and
- No requirement for concurrent antibiotics or antifungal agents for the prevention of opportunistic infections; and
- A CD4 count above 250 cells/uL and an undetectable HIV viral load on standard PCR-based tests
- Patients with prior allogeneic bone marrow transplantation or prior solid organ transplantation

Sex/Gender

All

Ages

18 Years to N/A

Accepts Healthy Volunteers

No

Durvalumab and Tremelimumab in Treating Patients With Microsatellite Stable Metastatic Colorectal Cancer to the Liver

Study ID:

NCT03005002

Sponsor:

City of Hope Medical Center

Information provided by (Responsible Party):

City of Hope Medical Center (City of Hope Medical Center)

Tracking Information

First Submitted Date

December 23, 2016

Start Date

June 28, 2017

Primary Completion Date

September 2018

Last Update Posted Date

September 12, 2017

Current Primary Outcome Measures

Hepatic tumor response as assessed by Response Evaluation Criteria in Solid Tumors (RECIST) version 1.1[Time Frame: Up to 1 year]

Will be summarized using a 90% exact Clopper-Pearson confidence interval

Incidence of adverse events assessed by NCI CTCAE version 4.03[Time Frame: Up to 1 year]

Toxicities observed will be summarized in terms of type and severity.

Current Secondary Outcome Measures

Extrahepatic disease response assessed by RECIST 1.1[Time Frame: Up to 1 year]

Hepatic PFS[Time Frame: From study treatment to first progression in the treated liver or death (whichever occurs first), assessed up to 1 year]

This will be reported for the overall population (safety analysis set) and will be described for liver only (time to hepatic progress or death) and for overall disease burden (progression free survival per se). Progression free survival will be estimated using the product-limit (Kaplan-Meier) method, with any loss to follow-up as censoring.

OS[Time Frame: From study treatment to death, assessed up to 1 year]

Overall survival will be estimated using the product-limit (Kaplan-Meier) method, with any loss to follow-up as censoring.

Overall PFS[Time Frame: From study treatment to progressive disease (hepatic and extrahepatic) and death, assessed up to 1 year]

This will be reported for the overall population (safety analysis set) and will be described for liver only (time to hepatic progress or death) and for overall disease burden (progression free survival per se). Progression free survival will be estimated using the product-limit (Kaplan-Meier) method, with any loss to follow-up as censoring.

Overall response rate (both hepatic and extrahepatic disease) assessed by RECIST 1.1[Time Frame: Up to 1 year]

Descriptive Information

Offical Title

A Pilot Feasibility Study of Durvalumab (MEDI4736) and Tremelimumab Following Radioembolization in Patients With Metastatic Microsatellite Stable (MSS) Colorectal Cancer to the Liver

Brief Summary

This pilot clinical trial studies the side effects and how well durvalumab and tremelimumab work in treating patients with microsatellite stable colorectal cancer that has spread to the liver. Monoclonal antibodies, such as durvalumab and tremelimumab, may interfere with the ability of tumor cells to grow and spread.

Detailed Description

PRIMARY OBJECTIVES:

I. Establish the safety of durvalumab and tremelimumab following radioembolization with selective internal radiation (SIR)-Spheres in patients with microsatellite stable (MSS) metastatic colorectal cancer to the liver.

II. Determine the hepatic response rate of SIR-Spheres followed by durvalumab and tremelimumab in patients with MSS metastatic colorectal cancer to the liver.

SECONDARY OBJECTIVES:

I. Estimate the progression free survival (PFS) and overall survival (OS) of the overall treated population.

II. Describe the overall response rate of the treated population. III. Describe the extra-hepatic response in the treated population (abscopal responses).

TERTIARY OBJECTIVES:

I. Describe intra-tumor immune alterations following SIR-Spheres, and following durvalumab plus tremelimumab in comparison to baseline through serial hepatic metastases biopsies.

II. Describe the immune alterations in the blood following SIR-Spheres and following durvalumab plus tremelimumab.

OUTLINE:

Patients receive durvalumab intravenously (IV) over 60 minutes and tremelimumab IV over 60 minutes on day 1. Treatment repeats every 4 weeks for up to 4 courses in the absence of disease progression or unacceptable toxicity. Beginning at week 17, patients receive durvalumab IV over 60 minutes on day 1. Treatment repeats every 4 weeks for up to 9 courses in the absence of disease progression or unacceptable toxicity.

After completion of study treatment, patients are followed up periodically.

Study Type

Interventional

Study Phase

Phase 1

Condition

- Metastatic Carcinoma in the Liver
- MLH1 Gene Mutation
- MSH6 Gene Mutation
- PMS2 Gene Mutation

- Stage IV Colorectal Cancer
- Stage IVA Colorectal Cancer
- Stage IVB Colorectal Cancer

Intervention

Biological: Durvalumab

Given IV

Other Names:

Immunoglobulin G1, Anti-(Human Protein B7-H1) (Human Monoclonal MEDI4736 Heavy Chain), Disulfide with Human Monoclonal MEDI4736 Kappa-chain, Dimer

MEDI-4736

MEDI4736

Other: Laboratory Biomarker Analysis

Correlative studies

Biological: Tremelimumab

Given IV

Other Names:

Anti-CTLA4 Human Monoclonal Antibody CP-675,206

CP-675

CP-675,206

CP-675206

Ticilimumab

Study Arms

Experimental: Treatment (durvalumab, tremelimumab)

Patients receive durvalumab IV over 60 minutes and tremelimumab IV over 60 minutes on day 1. Treatment repeats every 4 weeks for up to 4 courses in the absence of disease progression or unacceptable toxicity. Beginning at week 17, patients receive durvalumab IV over 60 minutes on day 1. Treatment repeats every 4 weeks for up to 9 courses in the absence of disease progression or unacceptable toxicity.

Recruitment Information

Recruitment Status

Recruiting

Estimated Enrollment

18

Completion Date

September 2018

Primary Completion Date

September 2018

Eligibility Criteria

Inclusion Criteria:

- Documented informed consent of the subject and/or legally authorized representative
- Eastern Cooperative Oncology Group (ECOG) performance status of 0 or 1
- Life expectancy of > 12 weeks
- Hemoglobin >= 9.0 g/dL
- Absolute neutrophil count (ANC) >= 1.5 x 10^9/L (>= 1500 per mm^3)
- Platelet count >= 75 x 10^9/L (>= 75,000 per mm^3)
- Serum bilirubin =< 1.5 x institutional upper limit of normal (ULN)
- Aspartate aminotransferase (AST) (serum glutamic-oxaloacetic transaminase [SGOT])/alanine aminotransferase (ALT) (serum glutamate pyruvate transaminase [SGPT]) =< 5 x institutional upper limit of normal given that all patients have liver metastases
- Serum creatinine clearance (CL) > 40 mL/min by the Cockcroft-Gault formula or by 24-hour urine collection for determination of creatinine clearance
- Female subjects must either be of non-reproductive potential (ie, post-menopausal by history: >= 60 years old and no menses for >= 1 year without an alternative medical cause; AND/OR history of hysterectomy, AND/OR history of bilateral tubal ligation, AND/OR history of bilateral oophorectomy) or must have a negative serum pregnancy test upon study entry
- Subject is willing and able to comply with the protocol for the duration of the study including undergoing treatment and scheduled visits and examinations including follow up

- Patients must have received at least one prior line of therapy for the treatment of metastatic disease with a fluoropyrimidine in combination with oxaliplatin and/or irinotecan; patients with prior adjuvant therapy who progressed within 6 months of completion of treatment may be eligible
- Patients must have liver-only metastases or predominant liver metastatic disease
- Patients should have microsatellite stable (MSS) tumor by polymerase chain reaction (PCR) assay or mismatch repair protein proficient (MMRP) tumor by immunohistochemistry as confirmed by the presence of MLH1, MSH2, MSH6, and PMS2; the diagnosis of colorectal cancer should be confirmed by pathology either on the primary tumor or from a prior biopsy of a metastatic disease site
- Patients should have been identified by their respective physicians as candidates for radioembolization and scheduled to undergo such a procedure
- Patients should agree to serial liver metastases biopsy pre-treatment, post-radioembolization, and post-combination immunotherapy
- Patients should have measurable metastatic disease in the liver, defined (for the purpose of this study) as at least 1 measurable lesion more than 2 cm in size and readily accessible to ultrasound (US) or computed tomography (CT)-guided biopsy
- Patients should not be deemed candidate for curative hepatic resection

Exclusion Criteria:

- Involvement in the planning and/or conduct of the study (applies to both AstraZeneca staff and/or staff at the study site) or previous enrollment in the present study
- Participation in another clinical study with an investigational product during the last 4 weeks
- Any previous treatment with a PD1 or PD-L1 inhibitor, including durvalumab or an anti-CTLA4, including tremelimumab
- **History of another primary malignancy except for:**
- Malignancy treated with curative intent and with no known active disease >= 2 years before the first dose of study drug and of low potential risk for recurrence
- Adequately treated non-melanoma skin cancer or lentigo maligns without evidence of disease
- Adequately treated carcinoma in situ without evidence of disease eg, cervical cancer in situ
- Receipt of the last dose of chemotherapy or tyrosine kinase inhibitors should be at least 3 weeks prior to durvalumab and tremelimumab dosing; monoclonal antibodies such as bevacizumab, ziv-aflibercept, ramucirumab, cetuximab, and panitumumab should be at least 6 weeks prior to durvalumab and tremelimumab therapy
- Clinical ascites
- Liver involvement by > 50% with metastatic disease determined by the investigator
- Complete portal vein thrombosis on CT scans
- Failure to satisfy minimum criteria of lung shunting (> 20%) or presence of extrahepatic gastrointestinal activity on microaggregated albumin (MAA) scan or angiogram that preclude SIR-Spheres
- Prior external beam radiation to the liver
- Mean QT interval corrected for heart rate (QTc) >= 470 ms calculated from 3 electrocardiograms (ECGs) using Fridericia's correction
- Current or prior use of immunosuppressive medication within 28 days before the first dose of durvalumab or tremelimumab, with the exceptions of intranasal, topical, and inhaled corticosteroids or systemic corticosteroids at physiological doses, which are not to exceed 10 mg/day of prednisone, or an equivalent corticosteroid
- Any unresolved toxicity (> Common Terminology Criteria for Adverse Events [CTCAE] grade 2) from previous anti-cancer therapy; subjects with irreversible toxicity that is not reasonably expected to be exacerbated by the investigational product may be included (e.g., hearing loss, peripherally neuropathy)
- Any prior systemic anti-cancer immunotherapy treatment
- Active or prior documented autoimmune disease within the past 2 years; NOTE: Subjects with vitiligo, Grave's disease, or psoriasis not requiring systemic treatment (within the past 2 years) are not excluded
- Active or prior documented inflammatory bowel disease (e.g., Crohn's disease, ulcerative colitis)
- History of primary immunodeficiency
- History of allogeneic organ transplant
- Uncontrolled intercurrent illness including, but not limited to, ongoing or active infection, symptomatic congestive heart failure, uncontrolled hypertension, unstable angina pectoris, cardiac arrhythmia, active peptic ulcer disease or gastritis, active bleeding diatheses including any subject known to have evidence of acute or chronic hepatitis B, hepatitis C or human immunodeficiency virus (HIV), or psychiatric illness/social situations that would limit compliance with study requirements or compromise the ability of the subject to give written informed consent
- Known history of previous clinical diagnosis of tuberculosis
- History of leptomeningeal carcinomatosis
- Receipt of live attenuated vaccination within 30 days prior to study entry or within 30 days of receiving durvalumab or tremelimumab
- Any condition that, in the opinion of the investigator, would interfere with evaluation of study treatment or interpretation of patient safety or study results
- Symptomatic or uncontrolled brain metastases requiring concurrent treatment, inclusive of but not limited to surgery, radiation and/or corticosteroids

- Subjects with uncontrolled seizures
- Patients with symptomatic extrahepatic metastases
- Female patients who are pregnant or breastfeeding or male or female patients of reproductive potential who are not willing to employ effective birth control from screening to 180 days after the last dose of durvalumab + tremelimumab combination therapy or 90 days after the last dose of durvalumab monotherapy, whichever is the longer time period
- Known allergy or hypersensitivity to investigational product (IP) or any excipient

Sex/Gender

All

Ages

19 Years to N/A

Accepts Healthy Volunteers

No

Study of Durvalumab and Tremelimumab After Radiation for Microsatellite Stable Metastatic Colorectal Cancer Progressing on Chemotherapy

Study ID:

NCT03007407

Sponsor:

NSABP Foundation Inc

Information provided by (Responsible Party):

NSABP Foundation Inc (NSABP Foundation Inc)

Tracking Information

First Submitted Date

December 7, 2016

Start Date

July 31, 2017

Primary Completion Date

March 2019

Last Update Posted Date

September 12, 2017

Current Primary Outcome Measures

Overall objective response rate of dual immune checkpoint blockade[Time Frame: Through treatment, up to 1.3 years]
Overall objective response rate (ORR) by RECIST 1.1 criteria

Current Secondary Outcome Measures

Proportion of patients who have achieved clinical benefit[Time Frame: Through study completion, up to 2.5 years]
Proportion of patients who have achieved clinical benefit defined as CR and PR and stable disease that lasts at least 4 months

The time during which mCRC responds to study therapy[Time Frame: After cycles 2, 4, 6, 8, 10, and 12 and through study completion, up to 2.5 years]
Time to first progression from study entry per RECIST 1.1 criteria

Frequency of adverse events assessed by CTCAE 4.0, from beginning of treatment to 90 days after last dose[Time Frame: During treatment to 90 days after last dose of study therapy]
Frequency of adverse events categorized using the NCI Common Terminology Criteria for Adverse Events version 4.0

Descriptive Information

Offical Title

A Phase II Study of the Dual Immune Checkpoint Blockade With Durvalumab (MEDI4736) Plus Tremelimumab Following Palliative Hypofractionated Radiation in Patients With Microsatellite Stable (MSS) Metastatic Colorectal Cancer Progressing on Chemotherapy

Brief Summary

This study is being done to look at the safety and response to the combination of two investigational drugs, tremelimumab and durvalumab, when given after radiation therapy for patients with microsatellite stable (MSS) metastatic colorectal cancer. Tremelimumab and durvalumab recognize specific proteins on the surface of cancer cells and trigger the immune system to destroy the cancer cells.

In order to learn more about certain characteristics of colorectal cancer tumors, this study includes special research tests using samples from diagnostic tumors, fresh tumor samples from an area where the cancer has spread, and blood samples.

Detailed Description

The FC-9 study is designed as a phase II, open label, single arm study of the dual immune checkpoint blockade with the combination of durvalumab and tremelimumab following hypofractionated palliative radiation in patients with microsatellite stable (MSS) metastatic colorectal cancer (mCRC) who have progressed on chemotherapy. The primary aim is to determine the anti-tumor efficacy of the dual immune checkpoint blockade with durvalumab plus tremelimumab. The secondary aims are to determine the clinical benefit rate, duration of response, tolerability and correlates of response. Tumor response at unirradiated target lesions will be measured at baseline and every 2 cycles using RECIST 1.1.

Following three doses of hypofractionated palliative radiation (Days −2, −1, and Day 0 prior to Cycle 1), patients will receive the combination of tremelimumab (75 mg IV infusion) and durvalumab (1500 mg IV infusion) on Day 1 for 4 cycles. Beginning with Cycle 5 through Cycle 12, patients will receive durvalumab alone (1500 mg/IV infusion) on Day 1 of each 28 day cycle.

The sample size will be between 12 and 21 evaluable patients. Twelve evaluable patients will be treated in the first stage of the study. If there are no responses among the 12 evaluable patients, the study will be terminated. If the study goes on to the second stage, a total of 21 evaluable patients will be studied.

Submission of tumor tissue and blood samples for FC-9 correlative science studies will be a study requirement for all patients. Requirements will include archived tumor samples from the diagnostic biopsy; additional biopsies of fresh tissue from an accessible lesion prior to radiation therapy and after 2 cycles of study therapy; and blood sample collections.

Study Type

Interventional

Study Phase

Phase 2

Condition

- Colorectal Cancer Metastatic

Intervention

Drug: durvalumab

Following three doses of hypofractionated palliative radiation (Days −2, −1, and Day 0 prior to Cycle 1), patients will receive durvalumab (1500 mg IV infusion) on Day 1 for 4 cycles (in combination with tremelimumab). Beginning with Cycle 5 through Cycle 12, patients will receive durvalumab alone (1500 mg/IV infusion) on Day 1 of each 28 day cycle.

Other Names:

MEDI4736

Drug: Tremelimumab

Following three doses of hypofractionated palliative radiation (Days −2, −1, and Day 0 prior to Cycle 1), patients will receive tremelimumab (75 mg IV infusion) on Day 1 for 4 cycles (in combination with durvalumab).

Study Arms

Experimental: durvalumab and tremelimumab

Recruitment Information

Recruitment Status

Recruiting

Estimated Enrollment

21

Completion Date

March 2019

Primary Completion Date

March 2019

Eligibility Criteria

Inclusion Criteria:

- The ECOG performance status must be 0 or 1.
- There must be histologic confirmation of a diagnosis of colorectal adenocarcinoma.
- The tumor must have been determined to be microsatellite stable (MSS).
- There must be documentation by PET/CT scan, CT scan, or MRI, that the patient has evidence of measurable metastatic disease per RECIST 1.1.

- Patients must have an accessible metastatic lesion for pretreatment core biopsy.
- Unless either drug is medically contraindicated, patients must have received oxaliplatin and irinotecan as part of standard metastatic chemotherapy regimens.
- The patient must have multiple sites of metastatic disease with at least one lesion amenable to treatment with stereotactic radiation therapy (SBRT) in the lung or liver and at least one lesion not being irradiated and meeting RECIST 1.1.
- **At the time of study entry, blood counts performed within 2 weeks prior to study entry must meet the following criteria:**
- ANC must be greater than or equal to 1500/mm3,
- Platelet count must be greater than or equal to 100,000/mm3; and
- Hemoglobin must be greater than or equal to 9 g/dL.
- **The following criteria for evidence of adequate hepatic function performed within 2 weeks prior to study entry must be met:**
- Total bilirubin must be less than or equal to 1.5 x ULN (upper limit of normal) for the lab unless the patient has a bilirubin elevation greater than 1.5 x ULN to 3 x ULN due to Gilbert's disease or similar syndrome involving slow conjugation of bilirubin; and
- AST and ALT must be less than or equal to 2.5 x ULN for the lab with the following exception: for patients with documented liver metastases, AST and ALT must be less than or equal to 5 x ULN.
- Adequate renal function within 4 weeks prior to study entry, defined as serum creatinine less than or equal to 1.5 x ULN for the lab or measured or calculated creatinine clearance greater than 40 mL/min by Cockcroft-Gault formula.
- All hematologic, gastrointestinal, and genitourinary chemotherapy toxicities must be less than Grade 2 at the time study therapy is to begin. (Note: Transfusions may be used to correct hemoglobin for patients experiencing anemia from therapy who otherwise would be eligible for the study.
- Patients with reproductive potential (male/female) must agree to use accepted and highly effective methods of contraception while receiving study therapy and for at least 6 months after the completion of study therapy. The definition of effective method of contraception will be based on the investigator's discretion.
- Female patients must either be of non-reproductive potential (i.e., post-menopausal by history: greater than or equal to 60 years old and no menses for greater than or equal to 1 year without an alternative medical cause; OR history of hysterectomy, OR history of bilateral tubal ligation, OR history of bilateral oophorectomy) or must have a negative serum pregnancy test upon study entry.

Exclusion Criteria:

- Diagnosis of anal or small bowel carcinoma.
- Colorectal cancer other than adenocarcinoma, e.g., sarcoma, lymphoma, carcinoid.
- Previous therapy with any PD-1 or PD-L1 inhibitor including durvalumab or anti-CTLA4 (including tremelimumab) for any malignancy.
- Receipt of live attenuated vaccination within 30 days prior to study entry or within 30 days of receiving study therapy.
- Active or chronic hepatitis B or hepatitis C.
- Symptomatic or uncontrolled brain metastases requiring concurrent treatments, uncontrolled spinal cord compression, carcinomatous meningitis, or new evidence of brain or leptomeningeal disease; uncontrolled seizures.
- Active infection or chronic infection requiring chronic suppressive antibiotics.
- Active or documented inflammatory disease.
- Known history of human immunodeficiency virus (HIV) or acquired immunodeficiency-related (AIDS) illnesses.
- Current or prior use of immunosuppressive medication within 28 days before the first dose of study therapy with the exceptions of intranasal corticosteroids or systemic corticosteroids at physiological doses that do not exceed 10mg/day of prednisone or an equivalent corticosteroid.
- History of allogeneic organ transplantation.
- **Any of the following cardiac conditions:**
- Documented NYHA Class III or IV congestive heart failure,
- Myocardial infarction within 6 months prior to study entry,
- Unstable angina within 6 months prior to study entry,
- Symptomatic arrhythmia. If QTc greater than or equal to 470ms, confirmation of eligible QTc requires mean calculation from 2 additional electrocardiograms (ECGs) 2–5 minutes apart using Fridericia's Correction Formula (mean less than 470 ms).
- Uncontrolled high blood pressure defined as systolic blood pressure (BP) greater than or equal to 150 mmHg or diastolic BP greater than or equal to 100 mmHg with or without anti-hypertensive medication. Patients with initial BP elevations are eligible if initiation or adjustment of BP medication lowers pressure to meet entry criteria.
- Active or prior documented inflammatory bowel disease (e.g., Crohn's disease, ulcerative colitis).
- Ongoing or active gastritis or peptic ulcer disease.
- Active bleeding diatheses.
- Known history of previous diagnosis of tuberculosis.
- History of hypersensitivity to durvalumab or tremelimumab or any excipients of these drugs.

- Known history or confirmation of active pneumonia, pneumonitis, symptomatic interstitial lung disease, or definitive evidence of interstitial lung disease described on CT scan, MRI, or chest x-ray in asymptomatic patients; dyspnea at rest requiring current continuous oxygen therapy.
- Active or prior documented autoimmune disease within the past 2 years. (Note: Patients with vitiligo, Grave disease, or psoriasis not requiring systemic treatment within the past 2 years are eligible.)
- Other malignancies unless the patient is considered to be disease-free and has completed therapy for the malignancy greater than or equal to 12 months prior to study entry. Patients with the following cancers are eligible if diagnosed and treated within the past 12 months: carcinoma in situ of the cervix, and basal cell and squamous cell carcinoma of the skin.
- Psychiatric or addictive disorders or other conditions that, in the opinion of the investigator, would preclude the patient from meeting the study requirements or interfere with interpretation of study results.
- Pregnancy or lactation at the time of study entry. (Note: Pregnancy testing should be performed within 14 days prior to study entry according to institutional standards for women of childbearing potential.)
- Use of any investigational agent. Use and/or receipt of the last dose of anti-cancer therapy (chemotherapy, immunotherapy, endocrine therapy, targeted therapy, biologic therapy, tumor embolization, monoclonal anti-bodies) within 14 days prior to the first dose of study therapy.

Sex/Gender

All

Ages

18 Years to N/A

Accepts Healthy Volunteers

No

Contacts

Diana Gosik, RN, BS   412-339-5333   diana.gosik@nsabp.org

A Dose Escalation Phase I Study to Assess the Safety and Clinical Activity of Multiple Cancer Indications

Study ID:

NCT03018405

Sponsor:

Celyad (formerly named Cardio3 BioSciences)

Information provided by (Responsible Party):

Celyad (formerly named Cardio3 BioSciences) (Celyad (formerly named Cardio3 BioSciences))

Tracking Information

First Submitted Date

January 10, 2017

Start Date

December 2016

Primary Completion Date

May 2020

Last Update Posted Date

January 18, 2018

Current Primary Outcome Measures

Incidence of Treatment-Emergent Adverse Events [Safety and Tolerability] of NKR-2 infusion[Time Frame: 24 months]

Safety defined by Occurrence of adverse events (AEs) and serious adverse events (SAEs) during the study treatment until 30 days after the last study treatment administration.

Current Secondary Outcome Measures

Clinical activity of the treatment in each tumor type[Time Frame: 24 months]

Clinical activity of the treatment in each tumor type

Descriptive Information

Offical Title

- A Multi-national, Open-label, Dose Escalation Phase I Study to Assess the Safety and Clinical Activity of Multiple Administrations of NKR-2 in Patients With Different Metastatic Tumor Types (THINK THerapeutic Immunotherapy With NKR-2)

Brief Summary

THINK (THerapeutic Immunotherapy with NKR-2) is a multinational (EU/US) open-label Phase I study to assess the safety and clinical activity of multiple administrations of autologous NKR-2 cells in seven refractory cancers, including five solid tumors (colorectal, ovarian, bladder, triple-negative breast and pancreatic cancers) and two hematological tumors (acute myeloid leukemia and multiple myeloma).

The trial will test three dose levels. At each dose, the patients will receive three successive administrations, two weeks apart, NKR-2 cells. The dose escalation part of the study will enroll up to 24 patients while the extension phase would enroll 86 additional patients.

Study Type

Interventional

Study Phase

Phase 1/Phase 2

Condition

- Colorectal Cancer (CRC)
- Ovarian Cancer (Epithelial and Fallopian Tube)
- Urothelial Carcinoma
- Triple-negative Breast Cancer (TNBC)
- Pancreatic Cancer
- Acute Myeloid Leukemia/Myelodysplastic Syndrome
- Multiple Myeloma (MM)

Intervention

Biological: NKR-2 cells

The intervention will consist of an infusion of NKR-2 cells administered every 2 weeks (14 days) for a total of 3 infusions within 4 weeks (28 days).

Other Names:

NKG2D CAR-T cells

Study Arms

Experimental: Hematological tumors

The dose escalation arm for hematological tumors will use a 3 +3 design to determine the maximum tolerated dose.

Experimental: Solid Tumors

The dose escalation arm for solid tumors will use a 3 +3 design to determine the maximum tolerated dose.

Recruitment Information

Recruitment Status

Recruiting

Completion Date

August 2020

Estimated Enrollment

122

Primary Completion Date

May 2020

Eligibility Criteria

Inclusion Criteria:

1. Men or women ≥ 18 years old at the time of signing the ICF

2. Patient with Colorectal cancer, epithelial ovarian cell or fallopian tube carcinoma, urothelial carcinoma, Triple Negative Breast cancer, pancreatic cancer, AML/MDS or Multiple Myeloma

3. Disease must be measurable according to the corresponding guidelines

4. Patient with an ECOG performance status 0 or 1

5. Patient with adequate bone marrow reserve, hepatic and renal functions

Detailed disease specific criteria exist and can be discussed with contacts listed below.

Exclusion Criteria:

1. Patient with a tumor metastasis in the central nervous system

2. Patients who have received another cancer therapy within 2 weeks before the planned day for the apheresis

3. Patients who receive or are planned to receive any other investigational product within the 3 weeks before the planned day for the first NKR-2 administration

4. Patients who are planned to receive concurrent growth factor, systemic steroid or other immunosuppressive therapy or

cytotoxic agent

5. Patients who have received other cell therapies

6. Patients who underwent major surgery within 4 weeks before the planned day for the first treatment

▥ Sex/Gender

All

▥ Ages

18 Years to N/A

▥ Accepts Healthy Volunteers

No

▥ Contacts

Jim Kostka   Think   info@celyad.com
Bikash Verma   bverma@celyad.com

A Study of OMP-305B83 in Subjects With Metastatic Colorectal Cancer

Study ID:

NCT03035253

Sponsor:

OncoMed Pharmaceuticals, Inc.

Information provided by (Responsible Party):

OncoMed Pharmaceuticals, Inc. (OncoMed Pharmaceuticals, Inc.)

Tracking Information

▥ First Submitted Date

December 22, 2016

▥ Start Date

December 2016

▥ Primary Completion Date

January 2019

▥ Last Update Posted Date

January 27, 2017

▥ Current Primary Outcome Measures

Incidence of dose limiting toxicities[Time Frame: Subjects will be treated and observed for DLT through the end of the first cycle (Days 0-28).]

The maximum tolerated dose (MTD) or maximum administered dose (MAD) will be determined in patients treated with OMP-305B83 in combination with FOLFIRI

▥ Current Secondary Outcome Measures

Safety of OMP-305B83 in combination with FOLFIRI will be assessed by adverse event monitoring, physical exams, vital signs, clinical laboratory testing, ECGs, echocardiograms, anti-OMP-305B83 testing, and subject interview on an ongoing basis.[Time Frame: Through study completion, an average of 8 months]

Immunogenicity (in terms of formation of anti-drug antibod(ies) against OMP-305B83 in percentage of subjects) of OMP-305B83 in combination with FOLFIRI[Time Frame: Through study completion, an average of 8 months]

Response Rate assessed by RECIST criteria 1.1[Time Frame: At 56 day intervals while on treatment, through study completion, an average of 8 months]

Response Rate assessed by tumor marker CEA[Time Frame: At 28 day intervals while on treatment, through study completion, an average of 8 months]

Progression Free Survival[Time Frame: Up to 5 years]

Descriptive Information

▥ Offical Title

A Phase 1b Study of OMP-305B83 Plus FOLFIRI as Second Line Therapy in Subjects With Metastatic Colorectal Cancer

Brief Summary

The purpose of this study is to test the safety and efficacy of an experimental drug, OMP-305B83, when given in combination with FOLFIRI. OMP-305B83 is a humanized bispecific monoclonal antibody and was developed to target cancer stem cells. Based on preclinical studies, it is believed that OMP-305B83 may block the growth of cancer stem cells and may also impair the productive growth of new blood vessels, which tumors need to grow and spread.

The study is sponsored by OncoMed Pharmaceuticals, which is referred to as OncoMed or the Sponsor.

Detailed Description

This is an open-label, Phase 1b dose escalation and expansion study of OMP-305B83 plus FOLFIRI to evaluate the safety, efficacy, and pharmacokinetics of OMP-305B83 in combination with FOLFIRI in patients with metastatic Colorectal Cancer. This study consists of a screening period, a treatment period, and a post-treatment follow-up period in which patients will be followed for survival for up to 5 years. Patients will be enrolled in two stages: a dose-escalation stage and an expansion phase.

Study Type

Interventional

Study Phase

Phase 1

Condition

- Metastatic Colorectal Cancer

Intervention

Drug: OMP-305B83

Other Names:

bispecific monoclonal antibody

Drug: FOLFIRI

Treatment will consist of OMP-305B83 and the FOLFIRI chemotherapy regimen.

Study Arms

Experimental: OMP-305B83 combined with FOLFIRI

Recruitment Information

Recruitment Status

Recruiting

Estimated Enrollment

30

Completion Date

January 2019

Primary Completion Date

January 2019

Eligibility Criteria

Inclusion Criteria:

- Measurable disease per response evaluation criteria in solid tumors (RECIST) v1.1
- Age >21 years
- Eastern Cooperative Oncology Group (ECOG) performance status of 0 or 1
- Adequate organ and marrow function
- For women of childbearing potential and men with partners of childbearing potential, agreement (by patient and/or partner) to use two effective forms of contraception from study entry through at least 6 months after the termination visit.
- Ability to understand and the willingness to sign a written informed consent document

Exclusion Criteria:

- Receiving any other investigational agents or any other anti-cancer therapy
- Receiving prior hepatic intra-arterial chemotherapy
- Known significant clinically significant gastrointestinal disease
- Patients with brain metastases (treated or untreated) leptomeningeal disease, uncontrolled seizure disorder, or active neurologic disease
- Significant intercurrent illness that will limit the patient's ability to participate in the study or may result in their death over the next 18 months
- Pregnant or nursing women
- Inability to comply with study and follow up procedure

▨ **Sex/Gender**

All

▨ **Ages**

21 Years to N/A

▨ **Accepts Healthy Volunteers**

No

▨ **Contacts**

Robert J Stagg, PharmD   650-995-8289

A Study of SC-006 in Subjects With Advanced Cancer

Study ID:

NCT03035279

Sponsor:

AbbVie

Information provided by (Responsible Party):

AbbVie (AbbVie)

Tracking Information

▨ **First Submitted Date**

January 23, 2017

▨ **Start Date**

March 8, 2017

▨ **Primary Completion Date**

July 1, 2020

▨ **Last Update Posted Date**

February 2, 2018

▨ **Current Primary Outcome Measures**

Number of participants with dose-limiting toxicities (DLT)[Time Frame: Minimum first cycle of dosing (21-day cycles)]

DLTs graded according to the National Cancer Institute's Common Terminology Criteria for Adverse Events (NCI CTCAE) version 4.03.

▨ **Current Secondary Outcome Measures**

Overall Survival (OS)[Time Frame: Approximately 2 years]

OS is defined as the time from the participant's first dose date to death due to any cause.

Progression Free Survival (PFS)[Time Frame: Approximately 2 years]

PFS time is defined as the time from the participant's first dose of study drug (Day 1) to either the participant's disease progression or death due to any cause.

Time to Cmax (Tmax) of SC-006[Time Frame: Approximately 1 year]

Time to Cmax of SC-006

Area under the plasma concentration-time curve within a dosing interval (AUC) of SC-006[Time Frame: Approximately 1 year]

Area under the plasma concentration-time curve within a dosing interval of SC-006

Duration of Clinical Benefit (DOCB)[Time Frame: Approximately 2 years]

DOCB is defined as the time from the initial partial response (PR), complete response (CR), or stable disease to disease progression.

Objective Response Rate (ORR)[Time Frame: Approximately 2 years]

ORR is defined as the percentage of participants whose best overall response is either complete response (CR) or partial response (PR), as determined by Investigator assessment using Response Evaluation Criteria in Solid Tumors (RECIST) version 1.1

Terminal half life (T1/2) of SC-006[Time Frame: Approximately 1 year]

Terminal half life (T1/2) of SC-006

Duration of response (DOR)[Time Frame: Approximately 2 years]

DOR is defined as the time from the participant's initial objective response (CR or PR) to disease progression or death, whichever occurs first.

Observed plasma concentrations at trough (Ctrough) of SC-006[Time Frame: Approximately 1 year]
Observed plasma concentrations at trough of SC-006

Clinical Benefit Rate (CBR) defined as CR, PR, or stable disease (SD)[Time Frame: Approximately 2 years]
CBR is defined as the percentage of participants who achieve a best response of CR, PR, or stable disease (SD).

Maximum observed serum concentration (Cmax) of SC-006[Time Frame: Approximately 1 year]
Maximum observed serum concentration of SC-006

Descriptive Information

▦ Offical Title

An Open Label Study of SC-006 in Subjects With Advanced Cancer

▦ Brief Summary

This is a multicenter, open-label, Phase 1 study in participants with colorectal cancer (CRC), and consists of Part A (dose regimen finding), followed by Part B (dose expansion). Part A (dose regimen finding) will involve dose escalation and possible dose interval modification to define the maximum tolerated dose (MTD) and/or recommended Phase 2 dose (RP2D) and schedule. Part B (dose expansion) will enroll additional participants who will be treated with a study drug dose at or below the MTD determined in Part A.

▦ Study Type

Interventional

▦ Study Phase

Phase 1

▦ Condition

- Colorectal Cancer (CRC)

▦ Intervention

Drug: SC-006
Intravenous

▦ Study Arms

Experimental: SC-006
SC-006 intravenous (IV) (various doses and dose regimens)

Recruitment Information

▦ Recruitment Status

Recruiting

▦ Estimated Enrollment

108

▦ Completion Date

December 22, 2020

▦ Primary Completion Date

July 1, 2020

▦ Eligibility Criteria

Inclusion Criteria:

- Participants with histologically or cytologically confirmed advanced metastatic or unresectable colorectal cancer (CRC) that is relapsed, refractory, or progressive following at least 2 prior systemic regimens in the metastatic setting.
- Participants with an Eastern Cooperative Oncology Group (ECOG) of 0 1.
- Participants with adequate hematologic, hepatic, and renal function.

Exclusion Criteria:

- Participants with prior exposure to a pyrrolobenzodiazepine or indolinobenzodiazepine based drug.

▦ Sex/Gender

All

▦ Ages

18 Years to N/A

▦ Accepts Healthy Volunteers

Accepts Healthy Volunteers

Tucatinib (ONT-380) and Trastuzumab in Treating Patients With HER2+ Metastatic Colorectal Cancer

Study ID:

NCT03043313

Sponsor:

Academic and Community Cancer Research United

Information provided by (Responsible Party):

Academic and Community Cancer Research United (Academic and Community Cancer Research United)

Tracking Information

⬛ **First Submitted Date**

January 31, 2017

⬛ **Start Date**

June 23, 2017

⬛ **Primary Completion Date**

June 30, 2019

⬛ **Last Update Posted Date**

February 12, 2018

⬛ **Current Primary Outcome Measures**

Objective response rate defined as a complete response (CR) or partial response (PR) measured by Response Evaluation Criteria in Solid Tumors 1.1 over the treatment period, with the exception that 4-week confirmatory scans will not be required[Time Frame: Up to 2 years]

> The proportion of unconfirmed tumor responses (successes) will be estimated by the number of successes divided by the total number of evaluable patients. The null hypothesis that the proportion of evaluable patients with CR or PR (p) equals 0.2 (H0: p=0.2) will be tested against the alternative that this proportion equals 0.4 (HA: p=0.4). Confidence intervals for the true success proportion will be calculated using the normal approximation.

⬛ **Current Secondary Outcome Measures**

Clinical best response is defined as the proportion of patients who experience stable disease for >= 6 months, or a best response of complete or Partial response[Time Frame: Up to 2 years]

> Will be estimated by the 95% confidence interval estimates.

Duration of response[Time Frame: Up to 2 years]

> Defined for all evaluable patients who have achieved an objective response as the date at which the patient?s earliest best objective status is first noted to be either a complete or partial response to the earliest date progression is documented. The duration of response will be assessed descriptively.

Incidence of adverse events of grade 2 and above[Time Frame: Up to 2 years]

> Adverse events will be described by grade for grade 2 and above with and without attribution considered. All eligible patients that have initiated treatment will be considered evaluable for assessing adverse event rate(s). The maximum grade for each type of adverse event will be recorded for each patient, and frequency tables will be reviewed to determine patterns. Additionally, the relationship of the adverse event(s) to the study treatment will be taken into consideration.

Overall survival[Time Frame: From registration to death due to any cause, assessed up to 2 years]

> The distribution of overall survival will be estimated using the method of Kaplan-Meier.

Progression free survival[Time Frame: From registration to the earliest date of documented disease progression, assessed up to 2 years]

> The distribution of time to progression will be estimated using the method of Kaplan-Meier.

Descriptive Information

⬛ **Offical Title**

MOUNTAINEER: A Phase II, Open Label Study of Tucatinib Combined With Trastuzumab in Patients With HER2+ Metastatic Colorectal Cancer

⬛ **Brief Summary**

This phase II trial studies how well the HER2 inhibitor tucatinib (ONT-380, ARRY-380) works in combination with trastuzumab in treating patients with HER2-positive (HER2+) metastatic colorectal cancer (CRC). Tucatinib may stop the growth of tumor cells by blocking HER2, a receptor needed for cell growth in patients with HER2+ tumors. Monoclonal antibodies, such as trastuzumab, may interfere with the ability of HER2+ tumor cells to grow and spread. Giving tucatinib and trastuzumab in combination may work better in treating patients with HER2+ metastatic CRC.

Detailed Description

PRIMARY OBJECTIVES:

I. To assess the objective response rate (ORR) of tucatinib in combination with trastuzumab in patients with HER2 positive (+) metastatic CRC.

SECONDARY OBJECTIVES:

I. To assess the clinical benefit rate (CBR) (stable disease [SD] for >= 6 months, or best response of complete response [CR] or partial response [PR]) of tucatinib in combination with trastuzumab.

II. To assess the progression free survival (PFS) of tucatinib in combination with trastuzumab.

III. To assess the duration of response of tucatinib in combination with trastuzumab.

IV. To assess the overall survival (OS) of tucatinib in combination with trastuzumab.

V. To assess the safety and tolerability of tucatinib in combination with trastuzumab.

TERTIARY OBJECTIVES:

I. To determine whether the combination of tucatinib and trastuzumab eliminates HER2 amplified circulating tumor deoxyribonucleic acid (DNA) (ctDNA) from peripheral blood.

II. To explore any correlation between tissue and blood based biomarkers and clinical outcomes.

OUTLINE:

Patients receive tucatinib orally (PO) twice daily (BID) on days 1-21 and trastuzumab intravenously (IV) on day 1. Courses repeat every 21 days in the absence of disease progression or unacceptable toxicity.

After completion of study treatment, patients are followed up at 30 days and then every 12 weeks.

Study Type

Interventional

Study Phase

Phase 2

Condition

- Colorectal Adenocarcinoma
- ERBB2 Gene Amplification
- HER2/Neu Positive
- KRAS wt Allele
- NRAS wt Allele
- Recurrent Colorectal Carcinoma
- Stage III Colorectal Cancer AJCC v7
- Stage IIIA Colorectal Cancer AJCC v7
- Stage IIIB Colorectal Cancer AJCC v7
- Stage IIIC Colorectal Cancer AJCC v7
- Stage IV Colorectal Cancer AJCC v7
- Stage IVA Colorectal Cancer AJCC v7
- Stage IVB Colorectal Cancer AJCC v7

Intervention

Other: Laboratory Biomarker Analysis
    Correlative studies

    Biological: Trastuzumab

    Given IV

Other Names:
    ABP 980

    Anti-c-ERB-2

    Anti-c-erbB2 Monoclonal Antibody

    Anti-ERB-2

    Anti-erbB-2

    Anti-erbB2 Monoclonal Antibody

Anti-HER2/c-erbB2 Monoclonal Antibody

Anti-p185-HER2

c-erb-2 Monoclonal Antibody

HER2 Monoclonal Antibody

Herceptin

Herceptin Biosimilar PF-05280014

Herceptin Trastuzumab Biosimilar PF-05280014

MoAb HER2

Monoclonal Antibody c-erb-2

Monoclonal Antibody HER2

Ogivri

PF-05280014

rhuMAb HER2

RO0452317

Trastuzumab Biosimilar ABP 980

Trastuzumab Biosimilar PF-05280014

Trastuzumab-dkst

Drug: Tucatinib

Given PO

Other Names:

ARRY-380

Irbinitinib

ONT-380

▨ Study Arms

Experimental: Treatment (ErbB-2 inhibitor tucatinib, trastuzumab)

Patients receive ErbB-2 inhibitor tucatinib PO BID on days 1-21 and trastuzumab IV on day 1. Courses repeat every 21 days in the absence of disease progression or unacceptable toxicity.

Recruitment Information

▨ Recruitment Status

Recruiting

▨ Estimated Enrollment

25

▨ Completion Date

June 30, 2020

▨ Primary Completion Date

June 30, 2019

▨ Eligibility Criteria

Inclusion Criteria:

- Histologically and/or cytologically confirmed and radiographically measurable adenocarcinoma of the colon or rectum that is metastatic and/or unresectable; subjects must have been treated with a fluoropyrimidine (e.g., 5-fluorouracil or capecitabine), oxaliplatin, irinotecan, and an anti-VEGF monoclonal antibody (bevacizumab, ramucirumab, or ziv-aflibercept), or have contraindication to such treatment

- **Molecular testing result from Clinical Laboratory Improvement Act (CLIA)-certified laboratory confirming that the tumor tissue has at least one of the following:**

- HER2 overexpression (3+ immunohistochemistry [IHC]); Note: HER2 2+ IHC is eligible if the tumor is amplified by fluorescence in situ hybridization (FISH)

- HER2 amplification by in situ hybridization assay (FISH or chromogenic in situ hybridization [CISH] signal ratio >= 2.0 or gene copy number > 6)

- HER2 amplification by CLIA-certified next generation sequencing (NGS) sequencing assay

- RAS (KRAS and NRAS) wild-type in primary or metastatic tumor tissue

- At least one site of disease that is measurable by Response Evaluation Criteria in Solid Tumors (RECIST) criteria that has not been previously irradiated; if the patient has had previous radiation to the target lesion(s), there must be evidence of progression since the radiation

- Eastern Cooperative Oncology Group (ECOG) performance status (PS) of 0, 1, or 2
- Life expectancy greater than 3 months
- Absolute neutrophil count (ANC) >= 1000/mm^3 obtained =< 7 days prior to registration
- Platelet count >= 75,000/mm^3 obtained =< 7 days prior to registration
- Hemoglobin >= 8.0 g/dL obtained =< 7 days prior to registration
- Total bilirubin =< 1.5 x upper limit of normal (ULN); patients with known history of Gilbert syndrome and total bilirubin < 2 x ULN and normal aspartate aminotransferase (AST)/alanine aminotransferase (ALT) are eligible, obtained =< 7 days prior to registration
- AST and ALT =< 2.5 x ULN (=< 5 x ULN if liver metastases are present) obtained =< 7 days prior to registration
- Calculated creatinine clearance must be >= 50 ml/min using the Cockcroft-Gault formula obtained =< 7 days prior to registration
- International normalized ratio (INR) and activated partial thromboplastin time (aPTT) =< 1.5 X ULN unless on medication known to alter INR and/or aPTT
- Left ventricular ejection fraction (LVEF) >= 50% as assessed by echocardiogram (ECHO) or multiple-gated acquisition scan (MUGA) documented =< 28 days prior to registration
- Women of child bearing potential and male partners of women of child bearing potential must agree to use two medically accepted methods of contraception, one of them being a barrier method during the study and for 7 months after the last study drug administration
- Note: women of childbearing potential include women who have experienced menarche and who have not undergone successful surgical sterilization (hysterectomy, bilateral tubal ligation, or bilateral oophorectomy) or are not postmenopausal; postmenopause is defined as amenorrhea >= 12 consecutive months
- Negative serum pregnancy test done =< 7 days prior to registration for women of childbearing potential only
- Capable of understanding and complying with the protocol requirements and has signed the informed consent document
- Willing to return to enrolling institution for follow-up (during the active monitoring phase of the study)
- Willing to provide mandatory tissue and blood samples for correlative research purposes

Exclusion Criteria:

- Radiation therapy, hormonal therapy, biologic therapy, experimental therapy, or chemotherapy for cancer =< 21 days prior to registration
- Prior anti-HER2 targeting therapy
- Uncontrolled intercurrent illness including, but not limited to, ongoing or active infection, symptomatic congestive heart failure, unstable angina pectoris, cardiac arrhythmia, or psychiatric illness/social situations that would limit compliance with study requirements
- Not recovered to baseline or Common Terminology Criteria for Adverse Events (CTCAE) =< grade 1 from toxicity due to all prior therapies except alopecia and neuropathy; alopecia and neuropathy must have resolved to =< grade 2; congestive heart failure (CHF) must have been =< grade 1 in severity at the time of occurrence and must have resolved completely prior to registration
- Clinically significant cardiac disease such as history of ventricular arrhythmia requiring therapy, currently uncontrolled hypertension (defined as persistent systolic blood pressure > 150 mm Hg and/or diastolic blood pressure > 100 mm Hg on antihypertensive medications), or any history of symptomatic CHF
- Any of the following:
- Pregnant women
- Nursing women
- Men or women of childbearing potential who are unwilling to employ adequate contraception
- Patient with known central nervous system (CNS) metastasis (radiated or resected lesions are permitted, provided the lesions are fully treated and inactive, patient is asymptomatic, and no steroids have been administered for at least 30 days)
- Inability to swallow pills or any significant gastrointestinal disease which would preclude the adequate oral absorption of medications
- Use of a strong CYP3A4 inducer or inhibitor, or strong CYP2C8 inducer or inhibitor within 3 elimination half-lives of the inhibitor or inducer prior to first dose of study treatment
- Major surgical procedure, open biopsy, or significant traumatic injury =< 28 days prior to registration (=< 56 days for hepatectomy, open thoracotomy, major neurosurgery) or anticipation of need for major surgical procedure during the course of the study
- Serious, non-healing wound, ulcer, or bone fracture
- History of myocardial infarction, unstable angina, cardiac or other vascular stenting, angioplasty, or cardiac surgery =< 6 months prior to registration
- Immunocompromised patients and patients known to be human immunodeficiency virus (HIV) positive and currently receiving antiretroviral therapy
- NOTE: patients known to be HIV positive, but without clinical evidence of an immunocompromised state, are eligible for this trial
- Acute or chronic active hepatitis B or C infection, or other serious chronic infection requiring ongoing treatment

- Known chronic liver disease, autoimmune hepatitis, or sclerosing cholangitis
- Receiving any other investigational agent which would be considered as a treatment for the primary neoplasm
- Other active malignancy =< 2 years prior to registration which required systemic treatment
- EXCEPTIONS: non-melanotic skin cancer or carcinoma-in-situ of the cervix
- Co-morbid systemic illnesses or other severe concurrent disease which, in the judgment of the local investigator, would make the patient inappropriate for entry into this study or interfere significantly with the proper assessment of safety and toxicity of the prescribed regimens
- Unable or unwilling to abide by the study protocol or cooperate fully with the investigator or designee

Sex/Gender

All

Ages

18 Years to N/A

Accepts Healthy Volunteers

No

Standard of Care Alone or in Combination With Ad-CEA Vaccine and Avelumab in People With Previously Untreated Metastatic Colorectal Cancer QUILT-2.004

Study ID:

NCT03050814

Sponsor:

National Cancer Institute (NCI)

Information provided by (Responsible Party):

National Institutes of Health Clinical Center (CC) (National Cancer Institute (NCI))

Tracking Information

First Submitted Date

February 10, 2017

Start Date

April 5, 2017

Primary Completion Date

August 1, 2020

Last Update Posted Date

January 23, 2018

Current Primary Outcome Measures

Progression free survival.[Time Frame: 18 months after first dose]
   Proportion of patients that have progressive disease after 18 months

Current Secondary Outcome Measures

Safety[Time Frame: 30 days after treatment discontinuation]
   list of adverse event frequency

Immunologic analysis of samples from peripheral blood[Time Frame: 3-4 years]
   Immunologic analysis of samples from peripheral blood

Immunologic analysis of samples from tumor[Time Frame: 3-4 years]
   Immunologic analysis of samles from tumor

Overall response rate[Time Frame: every 2 months until disease progression]
   Proportion of patients whose tumors shrunk after therapy

Correlative analysis of immune endpoints with clinical outcomes[Time Frame: Progression]
   Correlation between immune endpoints and median amount of time it takes disease to worsen after treatment

Overall survival[Time Frame: death]
   Median amount of time subject survives after therapy.

Descriptive Information

Offical Title

A Randomized Phase II Trial of Standard of Care Alone or in Combination With Ad-CEA Vaccine and Avelumab in Patients With Previously Untreated Metastatic Colorectal Cancer

Brief Summary

Background:

Colorectal cancer is a common cancer in the U.S. It causes the second most cancer-related deaths. The drug avelumab and vaccine Ad-CEA together help the immune system fight cancer.

Objective:

To test if avelumab and Ad-CEA plus standard therapy treats colorectal cancer that has spread to other sites better than standard therapy alone.

Eligibility:

People ages 18 and older with untreated colorectal cancer that has spread in the body

Design:

Participants will be screened with:

Test to see if their cancer has a certain deficiency

Blood, urine, and heart tests

Scans

Medical history

Physical exam

Tumor sample. This can be from a previous procedure.

A small group of participants will get Ad-CEA and avelumab plus standard therapy. This is FOLFOX plus bevacizumab for up to 24 weeks then capecitabine plus bevacizumab.

The others will have treatment in 2-week cycles. They will be Arm A or B:

Arm A: FOLFOX and bevacizumab by IV days 1 and 2 for 12 cycles. After that, capecitabine by mouth twice a day and bevacizumab by IV on day 1.

Arm B: Ad-CEA injection every 2-12 weeks. Avelumab by IV on day 1 of each cycle. FOLFOX and bevacizumab by IV days 2 and 3 for 12 cycles. Then, capecitabine by mouth twice a day and bevacizumab through IV on day 2.

Participants will repeat screening tests during the study.

Participants will be treated until their disease gets worse or they have bad side effects. Arm A participants can join Arm B. They will have a visit 4 5 weeks after they stop therapy.

Detailed Description

Background

- Colorectal cancer (CRC) is the fourth most common cancer diagnosis in the United States and accounts for the second most cancer-related deaths.
- Programmed death ligand 1 (PD-L1) is a transmembrane protein that was first identified for its role in the maintenance of self-tolerance and prevention of autoimmunity. Blockade of the interaction between PD-L1 on tumor cells and PD-1 on T cells is expected to reverse T cell suppression within tumors. These agents are dependent on underlying T cell activation against the tumor cell to be effective.
- Avelumab is a fully human IgG1 anti-PDL1 antibody that selectively binds to PD-L1 and competitively blocks its interaction with PD-1.
- In ongoing phase 1 trials of avelumab, the agent has been well tolerated and has shown clinical activity. Clinical trials with anti-PD-1/L1 agents in colorectal cancer have resulted in minimal activity in patients who do not have mismatch repair deficiency (MMR-D)
- Therapeutic cancer vaccines targeting overexpressed proteins offer a potential method to activate T cells against tumors.
- A novel adenovirus based, CEA-targeting vaccine has demonstrated cytolytic T cell responses in patients with metastatic colorectal cancer.
- Standard of care agents in first line metastatic CRC have properties been associated with improved immune response via immunologic cell death and immunogenic modulation.

Objectives

- -To determine if there is an improvement progression free survival among patients with metastatic colorectal cancer lacking a mismatch repair deficiency who are treated with standard of care + antiPDL1 monoclonal antibody + Ad-CEA therapeutic cancer vaccine compared with standard of care alone.

Eligibility

- Subjects age 18 and older with previously untreated pathologically confirmed colorectal cancer; prior adjuvant therapy is acceptable
- ECOG performance status less than or equal to 1

- Normal organ and bone marrow function
- Subjects with active autoimmune diseases requiring treatment and subjects requiring system steroids (except for physiologic doses for steroid replacement) are not allowed
- Tumor sample and whole blood sample must be available for proteomics, genomics and transcriptomics analyses.
- Subjects with metastatic colorectal cancer with mismatch repair deficiency (MMR-D or MSI-High) will not be eligible

Design

- This is a randomized, multicenter phase II clinical trial designed to evaluate the potential improvement in progression free survival (PFS) when Avelumab and Ad-CEA vaccine are used in combination with standard of care therapy in metastatic colorectal cancer when compared with standard of care alone (FOLFOX-A).
- A lead in cohort, comprising the first 6 evaluable subjects enrolled, will be treated with avelumab + AdCEA vaccine + standard of care in order to assess the safety of the combination.
- If no more than 1 subject in the lead in cohort experiences a dose limiting toxicity attributable to the IND agents, 70 evaluable subjects will be randomized on a 1:1 basis to receive either Avelumab + Ad-CEA vaccine + standard of care (Arm B) or standard of care alone (Arm A).
- Standard of care therapy consists of 6 12 two week cycles of bevacizumab + FOLFOX (5-FU, leucovorin, oxaliplatin) followed by two week cycles of bevacizumab + capecitabine until disease progression.
- Subjects assigned Arm A that have progressive disease will be offered Avelumab + Ad-CEA vaccine in combination with a standard chemotherapy regimen.
- Kaplan-Meier curves and a two-tailed log-rank test will be the primary analysis methods.
- The accrual ceiling for the study is set at 81.

Study Type

Interventional

Study Phase

Phase 2

Condition

- Colorectal Cancer

Intervention

Drug: Avelumab

10 mg/kg IV over 30-60 min on Day 1

Biological: Ad-CEA vaccine

Subcutaneous injection in the thigh prior to Avelumab on Day 1 of cycles 1, 2 3, 5, 7, 9; every 6 cycles thereafter.

Drug: Bevacizumab

5mg/kg IV over 30-90 min on day 1 (Arm A) or 2 (Arm B). Part of the standard of care therapy.

Drug: 5-FU

400mg/m2 (only Arm A) IV bolus on day 1. Part of the standard of care therapy.

Drug: Leucovorin

400mg/m2 IV over 2 hours on day 1 (Arm A) or Day 2 (Arm B). Part of the standard of care therapy.

Drug: Oxaliplatin

85mg/m2 (Arm A) or 68mg/m2 (Arm B) IV over 2 hours on day 1 (Arm A) or Day 2 (Arm B). Part of the standard of care therapy.

Drug: Capecitabine

625 mg/m2 twice a day by mouth. Part of the standard of care therapy.

Drug: 5-FU

2400 mg/m2 (Arm A and B) IV over 46 hours (+/-2 hours) to start on Day 1 (ARM A) or Day 2 (Arm B). Part of the stanard of care therapy.

Study Arms

Experimental: Lead in

The first 6 evaluable subjects will be treated with avelumab + Ad-CEA vaccine + standard of care in order to assess safety

Active Comparator: Arm A

Standard of care alone FOLFOX (5-FU, leucovorin, oxaliplatin) + bevacizumab + for up to 12 2-week cycles followed by maintenance therapy with bevacizumab + capecitabine until disease progression.

Experimental: Arm B

FOLFOX + bevacizumab + avelumab + Ad-CEA vaccine (given weeks 0,2,4,8,12,16 and then every 12 weeks) for up to 12 2-week cycles followed by maintenance therapy with bevacizumab + capecitabine + avelumab + Ad-CEA vaccine (following the every 12 week dosing schedule) until disease progression.

◼ Publications

(Includes publications given by the data provider as well as publications identified by ClinicalTrials.gov Identifier (NCT Number) in Medline.)Morse MA, Chaudhry A, Gabitzsch ES, Hobeika AC, Osada T, Clay TM, Amalfitano A, Burnett BK, Devi GR, Hsu DS, Xu Y, Balcaitis S, Dua R, Nguyen S, Balint JP Jr, Jones FR, Lyerly HK. Novel adenoviral vector induces T-cell responses despite anti-adenoviral neutralizing antibodies in colorectal cancer patients. Cancer Immunol Immunother. 2013 Aug;62(8):1293-301. doi: 10.1007/s00262-013-1400-3. Epub 2013 Apr 30. (https://www.ncbi.nlm.nih.gov/pubmed/23624851)

Herbst RS, Soria JC, Kowanetz M, Fine GD, Hamid O, Gordon MS, Sosman JA, McDermott DF, Powderly JD, Gettinger SN, Kohrt HE, Horn L, Lawrence DP, Rost S, Leabman M, Xiao Y, Mokatrin A, Koeppen H, Hegde PS, Mellman I, Chen DS, Hodi FS. Predictive correlates of response to the anti-PD-L1 antibody MPDL3280A in cancer patients. Nature. 2014 Nov 27;515(7528):563-7. doi: 10.1038/nature14011. (https://www.ncbi.nlm.nih.gov/pubmed/25428504)

Balint JP, Gabitzsch ES, Rice A, Latchman Y, Xu Y, Messerschmidt GL, Chaudhry A, Morse MA, Jones FR. Extended evaluation of a phase 1/2 trial on dosing, safety, immunogenicity, and overall survival after immunizations with an advanced-generation Ad5 [E1-, E2b-]-CEA(6D) vaccine in late-stage colorectal cancer. Cancer Immunol Immunother. 2015 Aug;64(8):977-87. doi: 10.1007/s00262-015-1706-4. Epub 2015 May 9. (https://www.ncbi.nlm.nih.gov/pubmed/25956394)

Recruitment Information

◼ Recruitment Status

Recruiting

◼ Completion Date

August 1, 2021

◼ Estimated Enrollment

81

◼ Primary Completion Date

August 1, 2020

◼ Eligibility Criteria

- INCLUSION CRITERIA:

- Subjects must have previously untreated metastatic colorectal cancer and have no contraindications to treatment with the standard of care regimen as determined by the investigator. Prior adjuvant therapy is acceptable (including immunotherapy), but must have been completed at least 6 months prior to metastatic disease diagnosis.

- Patients should not be eligible for potentially curative surgical intervention in the case of oligometastic disease at the time of enrollment or must have actively refused after explicit discussion of potential benefit of this intervention with multidisciplinary team.

- Histologically confirmed colorectal cancer

- Patients must have measurable disease by RECIST criteria.

- Age greater than or equal to18 years. Because safety data is not known with this agent in patients less than 18 years old, children are excluded from this study.

- ECOG performance status less than or equal to 1.

- Patients must have normal organ and marrow function as defined below:

- Creatinine clearance (Cockroft-Gault calculated or 24-hour urine) greater than or equal to 30 mL/min.

- Adequate hepatic function defined by a total bilirubin level less than or equal to 1.5 (SqrRoot) the upper limit of normal range (ULN), an aspartate aminotransferase (AST), level less than or equal to 2.5 (SqrRoot) ULN, and an alanine aminotransferase (ALT) level less than or equal to 2.5 (SqrRoot) ULN or, for subjects with documented metastatic disease to the liver, AST and ALT levels less than or equal to 5 (SqrRoot) ULN.

- Hematological eligibility parameters (within16 days of enrollment):

- Granulocyte count greater than or equal to 1,500/mm^3

- Platelet count greater than or equal to 100,000/mm^3

- Hemoglobin greater than or equal to 9 g/dL

- The effects of Ad-CEA vaccine and Avelumab on the developing human fetus are unknown. For this reason and because Ad-CEA vaccine and Avelumab as well as other therapeutic agents used in this trial are known to be teratogenic, women of child-bearing potential and men must agree to use adequate contraception (hormonal or barrier method of birth control; abstinence) prior to study entry and for the duration of study participation and for a period of 4 months after the last treatment with avelumab or 6 months after the last administration of bevacizumab, whichever occurs later. Should a woman become pregnant or suspect she is pregnant while she or her partner is participating in this study, she should inform her treating physician immediately.

- Ability of subject to understand and the willingness to sign a written informed consent document.

EXCLUSION CRITERIA:

- Metastatic colorectal cancer with mismatch repair deficiency (MMR-D or MSI-High).

- Concurrent treatment for cancer except agents specified within the treatment protocol.

- Prior surgery or gastrointestinal perforation within 28 days of enrollment.

- Persisting toxicity related to prior therapy (NCI CTCAE v4.03 Grade > 1); however alopecia, sensory neuropathy Grade <=2, or other Grade <=2 AEs not constituting a safety risk based on investigator's judgment are acceptable.
- Known history of testing positive for HIV or known acquired immunodeficiency syndrome.
- Hepatitis B virus (HBV) or hepatitis C virus (HCV) infection at screening (positive HBV surface antigen or HCV RNA if anti-HCV antibody screening test positive)
- Any significant disease that, in the opinion of the investigator, may impair the patient s tolerance of study treatment.
- Active autoimmune disease that might deteriorate when receiving an immuno-stimulatory agent. Patients with diabetes type I, vitiligo, psoriasis, or hypoor hyperthyroid diseases not requiring immunosuppressive treatment are eligible
- Current use of immunosuppressive medication, EXCEPT for the following: a. intranasal, inhaled, topical steroids, or local steroid injection (e.g., intra-articular injection); b. Systemic corticosteroids at physiologic doses less than or equal to 10 mg/day of prednisone or equivalent; c. Steroids as premedication for hypersensitivity reactions (e.g., CT scan premedication).
- Patients who are receiving any other investigational agents within 28 days before start of study treatment.
- Prior organ transplantation including allogenic stem-cell transplantation.
- Subjects with active central nervous system (CNS) metastases causing clinical symptoms or metastases that require therapeutic intervention are excluded. Subjects with a history of treated CNS metastases (by surgery or radiation therapy) are not eligible unless they have fully recovered from treatment, demonstrated no progression for at least 2 months, and do not require continued steroid therapy. Subjects with CNS metastases incidentally detected during Screening which do not cause clinical symptoms and for which standard of care suggests no therapeutic intervention is needed are eligible.
- Active infection, requiring systemic therapy,
- Clinically significant (i.e., active) cardiovascular disease: cerebral vascular accident/stroke (< 6 months prior to enrollment), myocardial infarction (< 6 months prior to enrollment), unstable angina, congestive heart failure (greater than or equal to New York Heart Association Classification Class II), or serious cardiac arrhythmia requiring medication.
- Other severe acute or chronic medical conditions including immune colitis, inflammatory bowel disease, immune pneumonitis, pulmonary fibrosis or psychiatric conditions including recent (within the past year) or active suicidal ideation or behavior; or laboratory abnormalities that may increase the risk associated with study participation or study treatment administration or may interfere with the interpretation of study results and, in the judgment of the investigator, would make the patient inappropriate for entry into this study.
- Pregnant women and breastfeeding mothers are excluded due to unknown impact on embryos or infants.
- Known alcohol or drug abuse.
- Known prior severe hypersensitivity to investigational product or any component in its formulations, including known severe hypersensitivity reactions to monoclonal antibodies (NCI CTCAE v4.03 Grade greater than or equal to 3).
- Patients with a known hypersensitivity/allergy to any of the standard of care agents used in this study or related compounds (e.g. platinum compounds) are excluded
- Prior history of hypertensive crisis or hypertensive encephalopathy.
- Serious, non-healing wound, active ulcer, or untreated bone fracture, including tumorrelated pathological fracture.
- Evidence of bleeding diathesis or significant coagulopathy (in the absence of therapeutic anticoagulation).
- Patients being treated with medications with drug-drug interactions with study agents will require evaluation by to determine if full doses of all study treatments can be given safely. Significant drug-drug interactions will need to be addressed prior to enrollment. Alternatively, the patient will not be eligible.
- Vaccination within 4 weeks of the first dose of avelumab and while on trials is prohibited except for administration of inactivated vaccines

Sex/Gender

All

Ages

18 Years to 100 Years

Accepts Healthy Volunteers

No

Contacts

Diana Martin, R.N.   (240) 760-7969   diana.martin@nih.gov

A Phase 1/2 Safety Study of Intratumorally Dosed INT230-6

Study ID:

NCT03058289

Sponsor:

Intensity Therapeutics, Inc.

Information provided by (Responsible Party):

Intensity Therapeutics, Inc. (Intensity Therapeutics, Inc.)

Tracking Information

▨ **First Submitted Date**

February 10, 2017

▨ **Start Date**

February 9, 2017

▨ **Primary Completion Date**

July 2019

▨ **Last Update Posted Date**

January 30, 2018

▨ **Current Primary Outcome Measures**

Rate and severity of treatment-emergent adverse events ≥ grade 3 attributed to study drug using the NCI Common Terminology Criteria for Adverse Events (CTCAE v.4.03) (Scale 1 to 5)[Time Frame: Up to 3 years]

The primary objective is to assess the safety and tolerability of single and multiple intratumoral doses of INT230-6 in subjects with advanced or recurrent malignancies. This will be assessed by the rate of ≥ grade 3 AE's attributed to INT230-6 and not the underlying disease.

All recorded adverse events will be listed and tabulated by system organ class, preferred term, and dose and coded according to the most current version of MedDRA. The incidence of adverse events will be tabulated and reviewed for potential significance and clinical importance.

Adverse Events will be summarized for all reported data and by study period: a) up to and including 28 days post last dose of initial treatment, and b) from first dose of re-initiation of treatment, for subjects who re-initiate study therapy while in follow-up, up to 28 days post-dose of the last re-treatment dose.

▨ **Current Secondary Outcome Measures**

Preliminary Efficacy: Control or Regression of Injected Tumors by Measurement of Length, Width and Height (in centimeters) Radio-graphically Using Computer Tomography or Magnetic Resonance Imaging to Calculate Tumor Volumes (cubic centimeters) Over Time.[Time Frame: Up to 18 months]

Assess the preliminary efficacy of INT230-6 by measuring the length, width and height (centimeters) of injected tumor during the dosing and afterward.

Determine pharmacokinetic parameter Peak Plasma (Cmax in ng/mL) of each of the 3 main components of INT230-6.[Time Frame: Up to 5 months]

Characterize the peak plasma profile for the three INT230-6 components after single and then multiple IT tumor site injections for safety purposes.

Determine key pharmacokinetic parameter, Area Under the Curve (AUC) (ng

hr/mL) of each of the 3 main components of INT230-6.[Time Frame: Up to 5 months]

Characterize the pharmacokinetic AUC profile of each of the three INT230-6 components for AUC after single IT tumor site injection for safety purposes.

Key pharmacokinetic parameters, half live (hours) of each of the 3 main components of INT230-6.[Time Frame: Up to 5 months.]

Characterize the half life of each of the three INT230-6 components after single and multiple IT tumor site injections for safety purposes.

Descriptive Information

▨ **Offical Title**

A Phase 1/2 Safety Study of Intratumorally Administered INT230-6 in Adult Subjects With Advanced Refractory Cancers

▨ **Brief Summary**

This study evaluates the intratumoral administration of escalating doses of a novel, experimental drug, INT230-6. The study is being conducted in patients with several types of refractory cancers including those at the surface of the skin (melanoma, head and neck, lymphoma, breast) and tumors within the body such (pancreatic, colon, liver, lung, etc.). Sponsor also plans to test INT230-6 in combination with anti-PD-1 antibodies.

▨ **Detailed Description**

- INT230-6 is comprised of a 3 agents in a fixed ratio a cell permeation enhancer and two, potent anti-cancer payloads (cisplatin and vinblastine sulfate). The penetration enhancer facilitates dispersion of the two drugs throughout injected tumors and enables increased diffusion into cancer cells. (Nonclinical safety studies showed no findings following drug injection into healthy tissues.)

Historically physicians administer the two active drugs comprising INT230-6 by intravenous (IV) infusion to achieve a systemic blood level at the limit of tolerability. The objective is destroy both visible tumors and unseen circulating cancer cells (micro-metastases). Unfortunately, dosing drugs IV delivers only a small amount with a low concentration at the tumor site. This approach especially for late stage cancers is not highly effective and often quite toxic to the patient.

Attempts at direct intratumoral injection with chemotherapeutic agents have not shown the ability to treat the injected tumor, non-injected tumors or micro-metastases. This lack of efficacy for local administration is due possibly to poor dispersion and a lack of cell uptake of the agents.

Due to the use of the novel cell penetration enhancing agent INT230-6 treatment demonstrates strong efficacy in animals having large tumors. The Sponsor's in vivo, non-clinical data shows that INT230-6 thoroughly saturates and kills injected tumors. In addition, the drug induces an adaptive (T-cell mediated) immune response that attacks not only the injected tumor, but non-injected tumors and unseen micro-metastases. Cured animals become permanently immunized against the type of cancer that INT230-6 eliminates.

Clinical trial IT-01 will thus seek to determine the safety and potential efficacy of dosing INT230-6 directly into several different types of cancers. In addition animal studies showed a strong synergy of INT230-6 with immune modulation agents. Thus as part of study IT-01 the Sponsor will seek to understand the safety and efficacy of INT230-6 when administered in combination with immuno-therapeutic agents such as antibodies that target Programmed Cell Death (PD-1 or anti-PD-1) receptors.

This study seek to understand whether tumor regression can be achieved and patient outcomes improved.

Study Type

Interventional

Study Phase

Phase 1/Phase 2

Condition

- Melanoma
- Head and Neck Cancer
- Lymphoma
- Breast Cancer
- Pancreatic Cancer
- Liver Cancer
- Colon Cancer
- Lung Cancer
- Glioblastoma

Intervention

Drug: INT230-6

INT230-6 is clear sterile solution administered by injection directly into the tumor to be treated.

The product contains a cell permeation agent with cisplatin and vinblastine sulfate at fixed concentrations.

The drug is stored frozen and must be dosed at room temperature.

Escalation of the drug dose and number of injected tumors is possible in subsequent treatment sessions.

The drug dose to be administered is set by the tumor volume of the target lesions not the subject's body surface area

Biological: anti-PD-1

A concomitant anti-PD-1 will be added in cohort D

Biological: anti-PD-1 antibody

A concomitant anti-PD-1 antibody could be added for cohort E

Study Arms

Experimental: Cohort A

INT230-6 injections every 28 days for 5 sessions into only superficial tumors, low starting dose, low concentration per tumor.

Experimental: Cohort B1

INT230-6 injections every 28 days for 5 sessions into superficial or deep tumors, low starting dose, low drug concentration per tumor

Experimental: Cohort B2

INT230-6 injections every 28 days for 5 sessions into superficial or deep tumors, medium starting dose, low drug concentration per tumor

Experimental: Cohort B3

INT230-6 injections every 28 days for 5 sessions into superficial or deep tumors, high starting dose, low drug concentration per tumor

Experimental: Cohort C1

INT230-6 injections every 28 days for 5 sessions into superficial or deep tumors, low starting dose, high drug concentration per tumor

Experimental: Cohort C2

INT230-6 injections every 28 days for 5 sessions into superficial or deep tumors, medium starting dose, high drug concentration per tumor

Experimental: Cohort C3

INT230-6 injections every 28 days for 5 sessions into superficial or deep tumors, high starting dose, high drug concentration per tumor

Experimental: Cohort D

INT230-6 injections every 28 days for 5 sessions into superficial or deep tumors, dosing per any B or C cohorts (having acceptable tolerability) with addition of anti-PD-1 antibodies

Experimental: Cohort E

INT230-6 injections every 14 days for 5 sessions into superficial or deep tumors treated, dosing per any B, C or D cohorts (having acceptable tolerability) an anti-PD-1 antibody could be added

Recruitment Information

▓ **Recruitment Status**

Recruiting

▓ **Estimated Enrollment**

60

▓ **Completion Date**

August 2020

▓ **Primary Completion Date**

July 2019

▓ **Eligibility Criteria**

Inclusion Criteria:

1. Men and Women > 18 years of age with Eastern Cooperative Oncology Group (ECOG) performance status < 2;

2a. Eligibility: U.S. Sites

Includes subjects with loco-regional disease that have relapsed/recurred within 6 months of chemo-radiation and who have no standard of care.

Includes patients (subjects) with metastatic disease having injections into only superficial lesions that have failed (includes progression, relapse or intolerance) or not be a candidate for approved therapies. Note, patients (subjects) that have approved therapies available, which might confer clinical benefit, may be enrolled as long as the physician properly explains the nature of the treatment, and obtains consent ".

Includes patients (subjects) with metastatic disease having at least one deep tumor injection who have failed (includes progression, relapse or intolerance) all approved lines of therapy prior to enrollment unless they are not an appropriate candidate for a particular approved therapy or no approved therapy exists.

Note: There is no limit on the number of prior therapies that a patient (subject) may have received prior to enrollment in any cohort.

2b. Eligibility: Canadian Sites

Subjects with advanced or metastatic solid tumors that have disease progression after treatment with approved, available therapies (in site's country) for the cancer type or for whom available therapies have limited benefit and the subject refuses the available therapy. Includes subjects with locoregional disease that have relapsed/recurred within 6 months of chemo-radiation; or who have no standard of care or beneficial options. No limit on the number of prior treatments;

3. Subjects must have measurable disease by RECIST 1.1 criteria including one target tumor for injection. Superficial tumors must have one tumor greater than or equal to 1.0 cm, deep tumors greater than or equal to 1.0 cm (as measured by caliper (for non-injected tumors only) or image guidance);

4. Subjects must have a minimum of one injectable lesion as determined by the investigator (for superficial tumors) or radiologist (deep tumors).

5. Prior chemotherapy or immunotherapy (tumor vaccine, cytokine, or growth factor given to control the cancer: systemic or IT) must have been completed at least 4 weeks prior to enrollment and all adverse events have either returned to baseline (or resolved to < grade 1); note: subjects who have received prior platinum therapy are eligible irrespective of their response.

6. Prior systemic radiation therapy (either IV, intrahepatic or oral) completed at least 4 weeks prior to study drug administration.

7. Prior focal radiotherapy completed at least 4 weeks prior to study drug administration.

8. Prior major treatment-related surgery completed at least 4 weeks prior to study drug administration;

9. No prior primary or metastatic brain or meningeal tumors unless clinically and radiographically stable as well as off steroid therapy for at least 2 months;

10a. Life expectancy ≥8 weeks all (US); 10b. Life expectancy ≥12 weeks; ≥ 8 weeks superficial tumors (Canada);

11. Subjects who may become pregnant or who are sexually active with a partner who could become pregnant are to use an effective form of barrier contraception during the study and for at least 60 days for female patients and 180 days for male patients after administration of study drug; and

12. Screening laboratory values must meet the following criteria:

1. White Blood Cell (WBC) ≥2000/µL (≥2 x 10^9/L)

2. Neutrophils ≥1000/µL (≥1 x 10^9/L)

3. Platelets ≥70x103/µL (≥ 70 x 10^9/L) (superficial tumor dosing only)

4. Hemoglobin ≥8 g/dL (≥80 g/L) (superficial tumor dosing only)

5. Creatinine within the institution's laboratory upper limit of normal (ULN) or calculated creatinine clearance >50 ml/min

6. alanine aminotransferase /aspartate aminotransferase (ALT/AST) ≤2.5 x ULN without, and ≤ 5 x ULN with hepatic metastases

7. Bilirubin ≤2 x ULN (except subjects with Gilbert's syndrome, who must have total bilirubin < 3.0 mg/dL (<52 µmol/L))

8. For patients with planned deep tumor injections: prothrombin time (PT), activated partial thromboplastin time (aPPT), and international normalized ratio (INR) within normal limits; Platelet count ≥100,000/µL; hemoglobin ≥ 9 gm/dL.

13. Additional criteria for cohort D (anti-PD1 combo) will be supplied in an appendix at a later date.

Exclusion Criteria:

1. History of severe hypersensitivity reactions to cisplatin or vinblastine or other products of the same class;

2. Other prior malignancy, except for adequately treated basal or squamous cell skin cancer or superficial bladder cancer, or any other cancer from which the subject has been disease-free for at least 5 years;

3. Underlying medical condition that, in the Principal Investigator's opinion, will make the administration of study drug hazardous or obscure the interpretation of toxicity determination or adverse events;

4. Concurrent medical condition requiring the use of immunosuppressive medications, or systemic or topical corticosteroids; systemic or topical corticosteroids must be discontinued at least 4 weeks prior to enrollment. Inhaled or intranasal corticosteroids (with minimal systemic absorption may be continued if the subject is on a stable dose). Non-absorbed intra-articular steroid injections will be permitted; or use of other investigational drugs (drugs not marketed for any indication) within 30 days prior to study drug administration. Use of steroids as prophylactic treatment for subjects with contrast allergies to diagnostic imaging contrast dyes will be permitted;

5. For deep tumor cohorts, patients who require uninterrupted anticoagulants of any type, on daily aspirin therapy, or NSAIAs.

6. U.S. ONLY: For all Cohorts, patients who refuse approved therapy for which they are a suitable candidate are not eligible for enrollment on this trial.

7. Additional criteria for cohort D (anti-PD1 combo) will be supplied in an appendix at a later date.

▨ **Sex/Gender**

All

▨ **Ages**

18 Years to N/A

▨ **Accepts Healthy Volunteers**

No

▨ **Contacts**

Jeanne Lewis   860-815-7185   jlewis@ce3inc.com
Lisa Kamen   203-605-1041   lkamen@intensitytherapeutics.com

Study of Chemotherapy With or Without Hepatic Arterial Infusion for Patients With Unresectable Metastatic Colorectal Cancer to the Liver

Study ID:

NCT03069950

Sponsor:

Memorial Sloan Kettering Cancer Center

Information provided by (Responsible Party):

Memorial Sloan Kettering Cancer Center (Memorial Sloan Kettering Cancer Center)

Tracking Information

▨ **First Submitted Date**

February 28, 2017

▨ **Start Date**

February 28, 2017

Primary Completion Date

February 2020

Last Update Posted Date

November 6, 2017

Current Primary Outcome Measures

Resection rate assessed using RECIST (version 1.1)[Time Frame: 3 months]

Treatment evaluation will be done using RECIST (version 1.1) The patient will be assessed with repeat CT scans as specified. If at any time after 3 cycles (or 3 months) the patient is able to undergo a complete resection of all hepatic metastases they will proceed to operative assessment.

Descriptive Information

Offical Title

A Randomized, Multicenter Phase II Study of Panitumumab Plus FOLFIRI With or Without Hepatic Arterial Infusion as Second-Line Treatment in Patients With Wild Type RAS Who Have Unresectable Hepatic Metastases From Colorectal Cancer

Brief Summary

The purpose of this study is to see if patients treated with both regional chemotherapy using the HAI pump and intravenous chemotherapy are able to have their liver tumors removed surgically (resected), versus treatment with only intravenous chemotherapy.

Study Type

Interventional

Study Phase

Phase 2

Condition

- Colorectal Adenocarcinoma Metastatic to the Liver

Intervention

Drug: Floxuridine (FUDR)

5-Fluouracil (5FU) (1000 mg/m2/day continuous infusion over two days)

Drug: Irinotecan (CPT-11)

Irinotecan (CPT) (150 mg/m2 IV over 30 min to an hour) on Day 1 and Day 15.

Drug: FLUOROURACIL

5-Fluouracil (5FU) (1200 mg/m2/day continuous infusion over two days)

Drug: PANITUMUMAB

Panitumumab (6 mg/kg IV over 60 min)

Drug: DEXAMETHASONE

flat dose of 25 mg on Day 1

Drug: Leucovorin

Leucovorin (LV) (400 mg/m2 IV over 30 min to an hour)

Study Arms

Experimental: HAI FUDR/Dex in addition to Pmab plus FOLFIRI

Panitumumab plus FOLFIRI on Day 1 and Day 15 of each cycle. HAI pump therapy with FUDR and Dex on Day 1 of each cycle. Patients will start protocol therapy approximately 2 weeks after surgery. All patients will receive Panitumumab (6 mg/kg IV over 60 min). The HAI FUDR group will receive FOLFIRI in the following dosing; 5-Fluouracil (5FU) (1000 mg/m2/day continuous infusion over two days), Leucovorin (LV) (400 mg/m2 IV over 30 min to an hour), and Irinotecan (CPT) (150 mg/m2 IV over 30 min to an hour) on Day 1 and Day 15.

Experimental: Pmab plus FOLFIRI alone

The dosing of FOLFIRI in the systemic arm will be 5-Fluouracil (5FU) (1200 mg/m2/day continuous infusion over two days), Leucovorin (LV) (400 mg/m2 IV over 30 min to an hour), bolus 5FU 400mg/ m2 and Irinotecan (CPT) (150 mg/m2 IV over 30 min to an hour) on Day 1 and 15.

Recruitment Information

Recruitment Status

Recruiting

Estimated Enrollment

80

Completion Date

February 2020

Primary Completion Date

February 2020

Eligibility Criteria

Inclusion Criteria:

- History of histologically confirmed colorectal adenocarcinoma metastatic to the liver with no clinical or radiographic evidence of extrahepatic disease. Confirmation of diagnosis must be performed by the enrolling institution.
- Patients must have a primary L sided colorectal cancer, (at or distal to the splenic flexure)
- Confirmed RAS/RAF wild type tumor. Paraffin-embedded tumor tissue obtained from the primary tumor or metastasis
- Have received prior treatment for metastatic disease with oxaliplatin-based regimen and either
- Had disease progression OR
- Had stable disease OR
- Discontinued oxaliplatin due to neuropathy
- **Patients must meet the following criteria for unresectability as determined by two hepatobiliary surgeons and one radiologist:**
- When a margin negative resection would require resection of all three hepatic veins, both portal veins, or the retrohepatic vena cava.
- Requiring a resection that leaves less than 2 hepatic segments (not including the caudate lobe) behind with adequate arterial/portal inflow, venous outflow and biliary drainage.

A patient is considered resectable if the procedure includes a minor wedge or thermo-ablation encompassing 10% or less of the volume of the remaining 2 segments.

- Patient⊠s liver metastases must comprise <70% of the liver parenchyma. All patients must be clinically fit to undergo surgery as determined by the pre-operative evaluation
- **Lab values within 14 days prior to enrollment/randomization:**
- WBC ≥ 3.0 K/uL
- ANC > 1.5 K/uL
- Platelets ≥ 100,000/uL
- **Renal function (≤ 10 days prior to enrollment/randomization) °Creatinine ≤ 1.5 mg/dL or creatinine clearance ≥ 50 mL/min calculated by the Cockcroft-Gault method as follows:**

Cockcroft-Gault method as follows:

- Male creatinine clearance = (140 -age in years) x (weight in Kg) / (serum Cr in mg/dl x 72)
- Female creatinine clearance = (140 age in years) x (weight in Kg) x 0.85 / (serum Cr in mg/dl x 72) (use of creatinine clearance per protocol based on chemotherapy regimen)
- Hepatic function, as follows: (≤ 10 days prior to enrollment/randomization)
- Total Bilirubin ≤ 1.5 mg/dl
- Calcium ≥ lower limit of normal (≤ 48 hours prior to enrollment/randomization)
- KPS ≥ 60% (ECOG (or Karnofsky) performance status (preferably 0 or 1/≥ 60% for Karnofsky))

Exclusion Criteria:

- Patients < 18 years of age
- Patients who have received more than one chemotherapy regimen for metastatic disease
- Patients who are chemotherapy naïve
- Prior radiation to the liver (Prior radiation therapy to the pelvis is acceptable if completed at least 4 weeks prior to registration)
- Active infection

°Active infection includes patients with positive blood cultures

- Prior treatment with HAI FUDR
- Prior TACE
- Female patients who are pregnant or lactating or planning to become pregnant within 6 months after the end of the treatment (female patients of child-bearing potential must have negative pregnancy test ≤ 72 hours before enrollment and randomization, and must have a negative pregnancy test ≤ 72 hours prior to treatment start)
- If a patient has any serious medical problems which may preclude receiving this type of treatment
- Patients with history or known presence of primary CNS tumors, seizures not well-controlled with standard medical therapy, or history of stroke will also be excluded.
- Serious or non-healing active wound, ulcer, or bone fracture
- History of interstitial lung disease e.g. pneumonitis or pulmonary fibrosis or evidence of interstitial lung disease on baseline chest CT scan
- Patients who have a diagnosis of Gilbert⊠s disease
- **History of other malignancy, except:**

1. Malignancy treated with curative intent and with no known active disease present for ≥ 3 years prior to randomization and felt to be at low risk for recurrence by the treating physician

2. Adequately treated non-melanomatous skin cancer or lentigo maligna without evidence of disease

3. Adequately treated cervical carcinoma in situ without evidence of disease

▪ Sex/Gender

All

▪ Ages

18 Years to N/A

▪ Accepts Healthy Volunteers

No

▪ Contacts

Andrea Cercek, MD   646-888-4189   cerceka@mskcc.org

Michael D'Angelica, MD   212-639-3226

A Study of the Safety and Tolerability of ABBV-621 in Participants With Previously Treated Solid Tumors and Hematologic Malignancies

Study ID:

NCT03082209

Sponsor:

AbbVie

Information provided by (Responsible Party):

AbbVie (AbbVie)

Tracking Information

▪ First Submitted Date

March 14, 2017

▪ Start Date

April 3, 2017

▪ Primary Completion Date

November 16, 2018

▪ Last Update Posted Date

February 2, 2018

▪ Current Primary Outcome Measures

Segment 1: Area under the serum concentration time curve (AUC) of ABBV-621[Time Frame: Up to 64 days]
  Area under the serum concentration time curve (AUC) of ABBV-621.

Segment 1: Maximum observed serum concentration (Cmax) of ABBV-621[Time Frame: Up to 64 days]
  Maximum observed serum concentration (Cmax) of ABBV-621.

Segment 1: Terminal phase elimination rate constant (β)[Time Frame: Up to 64 days]
  Terminal phase elimination rate constant (β).

Segment 2: Objective response rate (ORR)[Time Frame: Approximately 6 months]
  ORR is defined as the proportion of participants with a response of partial response (PR) or better per Response Evaluation Criteria In Solid Tumors (RECIST) 1.1 for colorectal cancer (CRC) and other solid tumor participants, or per the International Working Group (IWG) criteria for Acute Myeloid Leukemia (AML) participants, or per the Lugano response criteria for Non-Hodgkin Lymphoma (NHL) participants.

Segment 1: Maximum Tolerated Dose (MTD) and/or Recommended Phase 2 Dose (RP2D) for ABBV-621[Time Frame: Up to 21 days]
  The MTD and/or RP2D of ABBV-621 will be determined during the dose escalation phase (Segment I) of the study.

Segment 1: Time to Cmax (Tmax) of ABBV-621[Time Frame: Up to 64 days]
  Time to Cmax (Tmax) of ABBV-621.

▪ Current Secondary Outcome Measures

QTcF Change from Baseline[Time Frame: Up to 64 days]

QT interval measurement corrected by Fridericia's formula (QTcF) mean change from baseline by dose level

Segment 2: Dose limiting toxicity (DLT)[Time Frame: Up to 21 days after first day of study drug administration]

A drug-related toxicity is an adverse event or laboratory value outside of the reference range that is judged by the Investigator and/or AbbVie as a "reasonable possibility" of being related to the study drug.

Descriptive Information

▦ Offical Title

An Open-Label, Phase 1, First-In-Human Study of Safety and Tolerability of TRAIL Receptor Agonist ABBV-621 in Subjects With Previously Treated Solid Tumors and Hematologic Malignancies

▦ Brief Summary

This is an open-label, Phase I, dose-escalation study to determine the maximum tolerated dose (MTD) and/or recommended phase two dose (RPTD), and evaluate the safety, efficacy, and pharmacokinetic (PK) profile of ABBV-621 for participants with previously treated solid tumors or hematologic malignancies. The study will consist of 2 segments: Segment I (Dose Escalation) and Segment II (Dose Expansion).

▦ Study Type

Interventional

▦ Study Phase

Phase 1

▦ Condition

- Solid Tumors
- Hematologic Malignancies

▦ Intervention

Drug: ABBV-621

Intravenous

▦ Study Arms

Experimental: Escalating Arm 1

ABBV-621 via intravenous administration at escalating dose levels in participants with solid tumors.

Experimental: Escalating Arm 2

ABBV-621 via intravenous administration at escalating dose levels in participants with acute myeloid leukemia (AML).

Experimental: Expansion Arm 1

Additional participants with solid tumors will be enrolled in a dose expansion cohort that will further evaluate ABBV-621.

Experimental: Expansion Arm 2

Additional participants with colorectal cancer (CRC) will be enrolled in a dose expansion cohort that will further evaluate ABBV-621.

Experimental: Expansion Arm 3

Additional participants with AML will be enrolled in a dose expansion cohort that will further evaluate ABBV-621.

Recruitment Information

▦ Recruitment Status

Recruiting

▦ Estimated Enrollment

92

▦ Completion Date

April 29, 2020

▦ Primary Completion Date

November 16, 2018

▦ Eligibility Criteria

Inclusion Criteria:

- Must have a diagnosis of a solid tumor, AML or non-Hodgkin lymphoma (NHL).
- Must have received at least one prior systemic therapy, and must have relapsed or progressed after, or failed to respond to any/all available effective therapy or therapies.
- Must have measurable disease (by RECIST 1.1 for those with solid tumors; by Lugano classification for those with NHL), except those with AML, who must have histologically confirmed relapsed or refractory disease.

- Must have an Eastern Cooperative Oncology Group (ECOG) Performance Score of 0 2.
- Must have adequate hematologic, renal and hepatic function.

Exclusion Criteria:

- Participants with history of brain metastases who have not shown clinical and radiographic stable disease for at least 28 days after definitive therapy.
- Receipt of any systemic anti-cancer agent, including investigational anti-cancer products, within 21 days prior to study drug administration or 5 half-lives, whichever is longer.
- Participant with a history of cirrhosis or other indication of significant hepatic function compromise including primary hepatobiliary malignancy (cholangiocarcinoma or hepatocellular carcinoma).
- Participant with a positive diagnosis of hepatitis A, B, or C.

Sex/Gender

All

Ages

18 Years to 100 Years

Accepts Healthy Volunteers

No

Contacts

ABBVIE CALL CENTER   847.283.8955   abbvieclinicaltrials@abbvie.com

A Study of Epacadostat in Combination With Pembrolizumab and Chemotherapy in Subjects With Advanced or Metastatic Solid Tumors (ECHO-207/KEYNOTE-723)

Study ID:

NCT03085914

Sponsor:

Incyte Corporation

Information provided by (Responsible Party):

Incyte Corporation (Incyte Corporation)

Tracking Information

First Submitted Date

February 28, 2017

Start Date

May 2, 2017

Primary Completion Date

April 2021

Last Update Posted Date

December 18, 2017

Current Primary Outcome Measures

Phase 1: Safety and tolerability assessed by frequency, duration, and severity of adverse events (AEs)[Time Frame: Through 90 days after end of treatment, estimated to be up to 27 months per subject]

A treatment-emergent AE is defined as an event occurring after exposure to at least 1 dose of study drug. A treatment-related AE is defined as an event with a definite, probable, or possible causality to study medication. A serious AE is an event resulting in death, hospitalization, persistent or significant disability/incapacity, or is life threatening, a congenital anomaly/birth defect or requires medical or surgical intervention to prevent 1 of the outcomes above. The intensity of an AE is graded according to the National Cancer Institute common terminology criteria for adverse events (NCI-CTCAE) version 4.03: Grade 1 (Mild); Grade 2 (Moderate); Grade 3 (Severe); Grade 4 (life-threatening).

Phase 2: Objective response rate (ORR) based on Response Evaluation Criteria in Solid Tumors v1.1 (RECIST v1.1)[Time Frame: Every 9 weeks through duration of treatment, estimated to be up to 24 months per subject]

Defined as percentage of subjects with a complete response (CR) or partial response (PR)

Current Secondary Outcome Measures

Phase 1: ORR based on RECIST v1.1[Time Frame: Every 9 weeks through duration of treatment, estimated to be up to 24 months per subject]

Defined as percentage of subjects with a CR or PR

Phase 2: Safety and tolerability assessed by frequency, duration, and severity of AEs[Time Frame: Through 90 days after end of treatment, estimated to be up to 27 months per subject]

A treatment-emergent AE is defined as an event occurring after exposure to at least 1 dose of study drug. A treatment-related AE is defined as an event with a definite, probable, or possible causality to study medication. A serious AE is an event resulting in death, hospitalization, persistent or significant disability/incapacity, or is life threatening, a congenital anomaly/birth defect or requires medical or surgical intervention to prevent 1 of the outcomes above. The intensity of an AE is graded according to the National Cancer Institute common terminology criteria for adverse events (NCI-CTCAE) version 4.03: Grade 1 (Mild); Grade 2 (Moderate); Grade 3 (Severe); Grade 4 (life-threatening).

Phases 1 and 2: Duration of response (DOR) per RECIST v1.1[Time Frame: Every 9 weeks through duration of treatment, estimated to be up to 24 months per subject]

DOR defined as time from earliest date of CR or PR until the earliest date of disease progression or death due to any cause, if occurring sooner than disease progression.

Phases 1 and 2: Progression-free survival RECIST v1.1[Time Frame: Every 9 weeks through duration of treatment, estimated to be up to 24 months per subject]

Defined as time from date of first dose of study medication until the earliest date of disease progression or death due to any cause, if occurring sooner than progression.

Descriptive Information

Offical Title

A Phase 1/2, Open-Label, Safety, Tolerability, and Efficacy Study of Epacadostat in Combination With Pembrolizumab and Chemotherapy in Subjects With Advanced or Metastatic Solid Tumors (ECHO-207/KEYNOTE-723)

Brief Summary

This is an open-label, nonrandomized, Phase 1/2 study in subjects with advanced or metastatic solid tumors. Phase 1 is an assessment to evaluate the safety and tolerability of epacadostat when given in combination with pembrolizumab and chemotherapy. Once the recommended doses have been confirmed, subjects with advanced or metastatic CRC, PDAC, NSCLC (squamous or nonsquamous), UC, SCCHN or any advanced or metastatic solid tumor who progressed on previous therapy with a PD-1 or PD-L1 inhibitor will be enrolled in Phase 2.

Study Type

Interventional

Study Phase

Phase 1/Phase 2

Condition

- Advanced or Metastatic Solid Tumors
- Advanced or Metastatic Colorectal Cancer (CRC)
- Pancreatic Ductal Adenocarcinoma (PDAC)
- Non-Small Cell Lung Cancer (NSCLC; Squamous or Nonsquamous)
- Advanced or Metastatic Solid Tumor That Progressed on Previous Therapy With a Programmed Cell Death Protein 1 (PD-1) Inhibitor
- Advanced or Metastatic Solid Tumor That Progressed on Previous Therapy With a Programmed Cell Death Ligand 1 (PD-L1) Inhibitor
- Advanced or Metastatic Urothelial Carcinoma (UC)
- Advanced or Metastatic Squamous Cell Carcinoma of the Head and Neck (SCCHN)

Intervention

Drug: Epacadostat

Epacadostat oral twice-daily continuous daily dosing at the protocol-defined dose

Other Names:

INCB024360

Drug: Pembrolizumab

Pembrolizumab 200 mg IV every 3 weeks

Drug: Oxaliplatin

Oxaliplatin 85 mg/m^2 IV on Days 1 and 15

Drug: Leucovorin

Leucovorin 400 mg/m^2 IV on Days 1 and 15

Drug: 5-Fluorouracil

5-Fluorouracil total dose of 2400 mg/m^2 on Days 1 and 15

Drug: Gemcitabine

Gemcitabine 1000 mg/m^2 IV on Days 1, 8, and 15

Drug: nab-Paclitaxel

nab-Paclitaxel 125 mg/m^2 IV on Days 1, 8, and 15

Drug: Carboplatin

Carboplatin AUC 6 IV on Day 1 every 3 weeks

Drug: Paclitaxel

Paclitaxel 200 mg/m^2 IV on Day 1 every 3 weeks

Drug: Pemetrexed

Pemetrexed 500 mg/m^2 IV on Day 1 every 3 weeks

Drug: Cyclophosphamide

Cyclophosphamide 50 mg orally once daily

Drug: Carboplatin

Carboplatin AUC 5 IV on Day 1 every 3 weeks

Drug: Cisplatin

Cisplatin 75 mg/m^2 on Day 1 every 3 weeks

- Study Arms

Experimental: Treatment Group A

Epacadostat + pembrolizumab + mFOLFOX6 (oxaliplatin, leucovorin, 5-fluorouracil)

Experimental: Treatment Group B

Epacadostat + pembrolizumab + gemcitabine and nab-paclitaxel

Experimental: Treatment Group C

Epacadostat + pembrolizumab + carboplatin and paclitaxel

Experimental: Treatment Group D

Epacadostat + pembrolizumab + pemetrexed and investigators choice of platinum agent

Experimental: Treatment Group E

Epacadostat + pembrolizumab + cyclophosphamide

Experimental: Treatment Group F

Epacadostat + pembrolizumab + gemcitabine and investigators choice of platinum agent

Experimental: Treatment Group G

Epacadostat + pembrolizumab + investigators choice of platinum agent and 5-fluorouracil

Recruitment Information

- **Recruitment Status**

Recruiting

- **Estimated Enrollment**

421

- **Completion Date**

October 2022

- **Primary Completion Date**

April 2021

- **Eligibility Criteria**

Inclusion Criteria:

- Histologically or cytologically confirmed diagnosis of selected advanced or metastatic solid tumors.
- Presence of measurable disease per RECIST v1.1.
- Eastern Cooperative Oncology Group (ECOG) performance status of 0 or 1.

Exclusion Criteria:

- Laboratory and medical history parameters not within the Protocol-defined range.
- Receipt of anticancer medications or investigational drugs within the Protocol-defined intervals before the first administration of study drug.
- Previous radiotherapy within 2 weeks of starting study therapy.
- Known active central nervous system (CNS) metastases and/or carcinomatous meningitis.
- Has not recovered to ≤ Grade 1 from toxic effects of previous therapy and/or complications from previous surgical intervention before starting study therapy.
- Receipt of a live vaccine within 30 days of planned start of study therapy.
- Active infection requiring systemic therapy.
- Subjects who have any active or inactive autoimmune disease or syndrome.
- Women who are pregnant or breastfeeding.

Sex/Gender

All

Ages

18 Years to N/A

Accepts Healthy Volunteers

No

Contacts

Incyte Corporation Call Center   1.855.463.3463   medinfo@incyte.com

Incyte Corporation Call Center (ex-US)   +800 00027423   globalmedinfo@incyte.com

Panitumumab in Combination With Trametinib in Cetuximab-Refractory Stage IV Colorectal Cancer

Study ID:

NCT03087071

Sponsor:

M.D. Anderson Cancer Center

Information provided by (Responsible Party):

M.D. Anderson Cancer Center (M.D. Anderson Cancer Center)

Tracking Information

First Submitted Date

March 10, 2017

Primary Completion Date

December 2021

Start Date

December 29, 2017

Last Update Posted Date

January 23, 2018

Current Primary Outcome Measures

Response Rate (RR)[Time Frame: Day 10 of Cycle 4 (14 day cycles) and every 4 cycles until 28-35 days after last dose of study drug]

Response rate (RR) defined Complete Response (CR): Disappearance of all target lesions. Any pathological lymph nodes (whether target or non-target) must have reduction in short axis to <10 mm.

Response Rate (RR)[Time Frame: Day 10 of Cycle 4 (14 day cycles) and every 4 cycles until 28-35 days after last dose of study drug]

Response rate (RR) defined as Partial Response (PR): At least a 30% decrease in the sum of the diameters of target lesions, taking as reference the baseline sum diameters.

Measurable lesions defined as in RECIST version 1.1.

Descriptive Information

Offical Title

A Phase II Enrichment Study of Panitumumab as a Single Agent or in Combination With Trametinib in Cetuximab-Refractory

Stage IV Colorectal Cancer Patients

Brief Summary

The goal of this clinical research study is to learn if panitumumab alone or in combination with trametinib can help to control advanced colorectal cancer. The safety of these drugs will also be studied.

Detailed Description

Study Groups:

If participant is found to be eligible to take part in this study, participant will be assigned to 1 of 3 groups based on the results of the genetic testing done at screening.

- If participant is in Group 1 or 3, participant will receive panitumumab alone.
- If participant is in Group 2, participant will receive will receive panitumumab and trametinib.

If participant is in Group 1 or 3 and the disease appears to get worse, participant may be able to cross-over to group 2 and begin to receive the panitumumab and trametinib combination therapy.

Study Drug Administration:

Each study cycle is 14 days.

Participant will receive panitumumab by vein over about 60-90 minutes on Day 1 of each cycle. After the first dose, participant will be checked for side effects for about 60 minutes after the dose. If no intolerable side effects occur, participant's next dose will last about 30 minutes and participant will be checked for side effects for 30 minutes afterward.

If participant is in Group 2, participant will take trametinib by mouth 1 time every day.

Participant should take the trametinib tablets in the morning at about the same time each day, at least 1 hour before or 2 hours after a meal. Participant should swallow the capsules with about 1 cup (8 ounces) of water. Participant should swallow each capsule whole (without chewing), one right after the other.

At the end of each study cycle or if participant stops taking the study drug, participant should return any unused trametinib capsules to the study nurse.

Length of Study:

Participant may continue receiving the study drug(s) for as long as the doctor thinks it is in participant's best interest. Participant will no longer be able to receive the study drug(s) if the disease gets worse, if intolerable side effects occur, or if participant is unable to follow study directions.

Study Visits:

On Day 1 of every cycle:

- Blood (about 6 tablespoons) will be drawn for routine and biomarker testing.
- If the doctor thinks it is needed, participant will have an eye exam.
- Participant will have a physical exam (Cycles 1-4, and every even-numbered cycle after that)
- Participant will have an EKG (Cycles 1-4, and every even-numbered cycle after that).
- Participant will have either an ECHO or MUGA scan (Cycles 2, 4, and 10, and then every 6 cycles after that)

On Day 10 of Cycle 2, if the doctor thinks it is needed, participant will have an eye exam.

On Day 10 of Cycle 4 and every 4 cycles after that (Cycles 8, 12, 16, and so on):

- Participant will have a CT of participant's chest and CT/MRI of participant's abdomen and pelvis.
- If the doctor thinks it is needed, participant will have an eye exam.

End of Treatment Visit:

Within 28-35 days after participant's last dose of study drug, participant will have an end-of-treatment visit. The following tests and procedures will be performed:

- Participant will have a physical exam.
- Blood (about 5 tablespoons) will be drawn for routine and biomarker testing.
- Participant will have an EKG and either an ECHO or MUGA scan.
- Participant will have a CT scan of participant's chest and a CT scan or MRI of participant's abdomen and pelvis.
- If the doctor thinks it is needed, participant will have an eye exam.
- If participant can become pregnant, blood (about 1 teaspoon) will be collected for a pregnancy test.

Long-Term Follow-Up:

Every 3 months after the end of treatment visit, a member of the study staff will contact participant to ask how participant is doing. This contact will take place either during a regularly scheduled clinic visit or by phone. Each phone call should last about 10 minutes.

This is an investigational study. Panitumumab is FDA approved and commercially available for the treatment of colorectal cancer. Trametinib is FDA approved and commercially available for the treatment of melanoma. The combination of these drugs is considered investigational in the treatment of advanced colorectal cancer.The study doctor can explain how the study drugs are designed to work.

Up to 84 participants will be enrolled in this study. All will take part at MD Anderson.

Study Type

Interventional

Study Phase

Phase 2

Condition

- Colorectal Cancer

Intervention

Drug: Panitumumab

Cohort 1 and 3: Panitumumab 6 mg/kg by vein on Day 1 of a 14 Day cycle.

Cohort 2: Panitumumab 4.8 mg/kg by vein on Day 1 of a 14 Day cycle.

Other Names:

Vectibix

Drug: Trametinib

2 mg by mouth once a day.

Other Names:

GSK1120212

Study Arms

Experimental: Cohort 1

Cohort 1 comprised of patients with detectable EGFR S492R or other ectodomain mutations in circulating free tumor DNA.

Participants receive Panitumumab until disease progression.

If the disease appears to get worse, participants may be able to cross-over to group 2 and begin to receive the panitumumab and trametinib combination therapy.

Experimental: Cohort 2

Cohort 2 comprised of patients with detectable KRAS or NRAS mutations in exons 2, 3, or 4; or BRAF codon 600 mutations in circulating free tumor DNA.

Participants receive Panitumumab and Trametinib combination therapy until disease progression.

Experimental: Cohort 3

Cohort 3 comprised of patients who do not have any of the detectable mutations listed in Cohort 1 or 2.

Participants receive Panitumumab until disease progression.

If the disease appears to get worse, participants may be able to cross-over to group 2 and begin to receive the Panitumumab and Trametinib combination therapy.

Recruitment Information

Recruitment Status

Recruiting

Estimated Enrollment

84

Completion Date

December 2021

Primary Completion Date

December 2021

Eligibility Criteria

Inclusion Criteria:

1. Histologically or cytologically confirmed colorectal adenocarcinoma, with metastatic disease documented on diagnostic imaging studies

2. Progression during or within 6 months after fluoropyrimidine, irinotecan, and oxaliplatin. For oxaliplatin-based therapy, failure of therapy will also include patients who progressed within 12 months of adjuvant therapy and patients who had oxaliplatin discontinued secondary to toxicity or allergic reaction. Patients with a known history of Gilbert's disease who cannot receive irinotecan or patients who are intolerant of irinotecan or fluoropyrimidine are eligible.

3. Confirmed wild-type status in KRAS exons 2, 3, and 4; NRAS exons 2, 3, and 4; and BRAF, by standard of care testing of tumor specimen. Tissue used for testing may have been collected prior to treatment with cetuximab.

4. Patient must have been already tested and have available results of the mutations status of KRAS/NRAS/BRAF and EGFR from the circulating tumor DNA within 10 weeks prior to starting study therapy.

5. Previous treatment with cetuximab with evidence of clinical benefit, as defined by complete response, partial response, or

prolonged stable disease with 16 or more weeks of treatment without radiographic progression, as assessed by the treating physician and documented in the medical record. This treatment may have occurred at any point in the patient's clinical course for treatment of metastatic colorectal cancer.

6. Ultimate progression through previous treatment with cetuximab, with documented clinical progression. Patients who discontinued cetuximab for any other reason, such as decline in performance status, hypersensitivity, or other adverse effects of therapy, are not eligible.

- 7. All prior treatmentrelated toxicities must be CTCAE (Version 4.0) </= Grade 1 (except </= Grade 2 for alopecia or peripheral neuropathy).

8. Radiographically measurable disease present per RECIST 1.1

9. Age >/= 18 years

10. Eastern Cooperative Oncology Group (ECOG) performance status 0 or 1

11. Blood counts performed within 3 weeks prior to starting study therapy must have absolute neutrophil count >/= 1,500/mm3, platelets >/= 100,000/mm3, and hemoglobin >/= 9 g/dL

12. Liver function tests performed within 3 weeks prior to starting study therapy must have total bilirubin </= 1.5 x upper limit of normal (ULN), alanine aminotransferase and aspartate aminotransferase </= 2.5 x ULN (or </= 5 x ULN if liver metastases are present), and albumin >/= 2.5 g/dL

13. Serum creatinine performed within 3 weeks prior to starting study therapy must be </= 1.5 x ULN, or have calculated creatinine clearance (using Cockcroft-Gault formula) of >/= 50 mL/minute.

14. PT/INR and PTT performed within 3 weeks prior to starting study therapy must be </= 1.5 x ULN

15. Left Ventricular Ejection fraction (LVEF) >/= LLN by ECHO or MUGA within 3 weeks prior to starting study therapy.

16. Women of childbearing potential must have a negative serum pregnancy test within 14 days prior to randomization and must agree to use effective contraception throughout the treatment period and for 4 months after the last dose of study treatment.

17. Ability to sign informed consent form. Informed consent form for this study must be signed prior to the performance of any study-specific procedures and initiation of any study therapy.

18. Ability to swallow and retain oral medication, with no clinically significant gastrointestinal abnormalities that may alter absorption such as malabsorption syndrome or major resection of the stomach or bowels.

19. In cohort 1, must have EGFR S492R or other ectodomain mutation detected from circulating tumor DNA from plasma collected after progression to prior cetuximab. May have a concomitant mutation in KRAS, NRAS, or BRAF, if there is at least a 5-fold higher allele frequency of the most prevalent EGFR mutation than the most prevalent KRAS/NRAS/BRAF mutation.

20. In cohort 2, must have one or more mutations found in KRAS exon 2, 3, or 4; NRAS exon 2, 3, or 4; BRAF codon 600. May have a concomitant EGFR ectodomain mutation, if the most prevalent EGFR ectodomain mutation does not have over a 5-fold higher allele frequency than the most prevalent KRAS/NRAS/BRAF mutation.

21. In cohort 3, must not have EGFR ectodomain mutation or any mutations in KRAS, NRAS, or BRAF.

22. Patients must have consented to the MD Anderson ATTACC protocol prior to inclusion.

Exclusion Criteria:

1. Past treatment with any MEK or ERK inhibitor or with panitumumab

2. Previous retreatment with cetuximab following progression on initial course of cetuximab therapy

3. Known untreated brain metastasis or brain metastasis treated within 3 months prior to enrollment in this trial

4. Symptomatic or untreated leptomeningeal or brain metastases or spinal cord compression.

5. History of interstitial lung disease or pneumonitis

6. History of any other malignancy within 3 years, except for adequately treated carcinoma in situ of the cervix or non-melanoma skin cancer and/or subjects with indolent second malignancies are eligible.

7. Prior treatment within 21 days of the first dose of study drug with any other chemotherapy, immunotherapy, biologic therapy, vaccine therapy, or investigational treatment, or failure to recover from adverse effects of prior therapies administered over 4 weeks prior to Study Day 1. All toxicities from prior therapies must be </= Grade 1 (or </= Grade 2 for alopecia or peripheral neuropathy). Prior systemic treatment in the adjuvant setting is allowed.

8. Any major surgery, extensive radiotherapy, chemotherapy with delayed toxicity, biologic therapy, or immunotherapy within 21 days prior to randomization and/or daily chemotherapy without the potential for delayed toxicity within 14 days prior to randomization.

9. Impaired cardiac function or clinically significant cardiac disease, as defined: a) Left ventricular ejection fraction < lower limit of normal (LLN) on multiple gated acquisition scan (MUGA) or echocardiogram; b) Congenital long QT syndrome or family history of unexpected sudden cardiac death; c) QTc corrected with Bazett's formula (QTcB) >/= 480 ms.; d) History or evidence of current clinically significant uncontrolled arrhythmias. Note subjects with atrial fibrillation controlled for >30 days prior to dosing are eligible;

10. Continuation of criteria above: e) History of acute coronary syndromes (including myocardial infarction and unstable angina), coronary angioplasty, or stenting within 6 months prior to randomization; f) History or evidence of current >/= Class II congestive heart failure as defined by New York Heart Association (NYHA); g) Treatment refractory hypertension defined as a blood pressure of systolic> 140 mmHg and/or diastolic > 90 mm Hg which cannot be controlled by anti-hypertensive therapy; h) Patients with intra-cardiac defibrillators.

11. Any serious and/or unstable pre-existing medical disorder (aside from malignancy exception above), psychiatric disorder, or other conditions that could interfere with subject's safety, obtaining informed consent, or compliance to the study procedures.

12. History of retinal vein occlusion (RVO)

13. Pregnant or breastfeeding, or planning to become pregnant within 6 months after the end of treatment.

14. History of organ allograft or other history of immunodeficiency.

15. Inability or unwillingness to comply with study and/or follow-up requirements

16. Known immediate or delayed hypersensitivity reaction or idiosyncrasy to drugs chemically related to study drug, or excipients or to dimethyl sulfoxide (DMSO).

17. Known Human Immunodeficiency Virus (HIV), Hepatitis B virus (HBV), or Hepatitis C virus (HCV) infection. Subjects with laboratory evidence of cleared HBV and HCV infection will be permitted.

18. Current use of a prohibited medication.

Sex/Gender

All

Ages

18 Years to N/A

Accepts Healthy Volunteers

No

Contacts

Eduardo Vilar Sanchez, MD, PHD   713-563-4743   CR   Study   Registration@mdanderson.org

APN401 in Treating Patients With Recurrent or Metastatic Pancreatic Cancer, Colorectal Cancer, or Other Solid Tumors That Cannot Be Removed by Surgery

Study ID:

NCT03087591

Sponsor:

Wake Forest University Health Sciences

Information provided by (Responsible Party):

Wake Forest University Health Sciences (Wake Forest University Health Sciences)

Tracking Information

First Submitted Date

January 13, 2017

Start Date

April 28, 2017

Primary Completion Date

April 2018

Last Update Posted Date

May 5, 2017

Current Primary Outcome Measures

Incidence of adverse events Common Terminology Criteria for Adverse Events version 4.0[Time Frame: Up to 1 year]

Will be categorized by organ system and severity, graded according to the National Cancer Institute Common Terminology Criteria for Adverse Events

Current Secondary Outcome Measures

Clinical response as assessed by RECIST[Time Frame: Up to 5 years]

Will be summarized as frequency counts and percentages.

Immune response as measured by frequency of immune cells[Time Frame: Up to 1 year]

Will be summarized as medians and ranges. The effects of treatment will be analyzed using paired t-tests or the non-parametric counterpart.

Immune response as measured by interferon production[Time Frame: Up to 1 year]

Will be summarized as medians and ranges. The effects of treatment will be analyzed using paired t-tests or the non-parametric counterpart.

Immune response as measured by neutrophil to lymphocyte ratio[Time Frame: Up to 1 year]

Will be summarized as medians and ranges. The effects of treatment will be analyzed using paired t-tests or the non-parametric counterpart.

Overall survival (OS)[Time Frame: From the initial infusion to confirmation of progression or death, assessed up to 5 years]

Exploratory survival plots will be estimated using the Kaplan Meier approach and median OS will be estimated if enough events occur.

Progression-free survival (PFS)[Time Frame: From the initial infusion to confirmation of progression or death, assessed up to 5 years]

Exploratory survival plots will be estimated using the Kaplan Meier approach and median PFS will be estimated if enough events occur.

Survival as assessed by RECIST[Time Frame: Up to 5 years]

Will be summarized as frequency counts and percentages.

Descriptive Information

▧ Offical Title

Safety and Immunologic Activity of Multiple Infusions of APN401

▧ Brief Summary

This phase I trial studies the side effects and best dose of APN401 in treating patients with pancreatic cancer, colorectal cancer, or other solid tumors that have spread to other places in the body or have come back. APN401 may stop the growth of tumor cells by blocking some of the enzymes needed for cell growth.

▧ Detailed Description

PRIMARY OBJECTIVES:

I. To determine the toxicities and establish the safety of multiple infusions of small interfering ribonucleic acid (siRNA)-transfected peripheral blood mononuclear cells APN401 (APN401).

SECONDARY OBJECTIVES:

I. To determine the immunologic effects of multiple infusions of APN401. II. To document clinical response and survival.

OUTLINE:

Patients receive siRNA-transfected peripheral blood mononuclear cells APN401 intravenously (IV) over 30 minutes on days 1, 29, and 57 in the absence of disease progression or unacceptable toxicity.

After completion of study treatment, patients are followed up for 5 years.

▧ Study Type

Interventional

▧ Study Phase

Phase 1

▧ Condition

- Metastatic Malignant Neoplasm in the Brain
- Metastatic Solid Neoplasm
- Recurrent Colorectal Carcinoma
- Recurrent Pancreatic Carcinoma
- Recurrent Solid Neoplasm
- Stage IV Colorectal Cancer
- Stage IV Pancreatic Cancer
- Stage IVA Colorectal Cancer
- Stage IVA Pancreatic Cancer
- Stage IVB Colorectal Cancer
- Stage IVB Pancreatic Cancer
- Unresectable Solid Neoplasm

▧ Intervention

Other: Laboratory Biomarker Analysis

Correlative studies

Biological: siRNA-transfected Peripheral Blood Mononuclear Cells APN401

Given IV

Other Names:

APN401

siRNA-transfected PBMC APN401

Study Arms

Experimental: Treatment (APN401)

Patients receive siRNA-transfected peripheral blood mononuclear cells APN401 IV over 30 minutes on days 1, 29, and 57 in the absence of disease progression or unacceptable toxicity.

Recruitment Information

Recruitment Status

Recruiting

Estimated Enrollment

10

Completion Date

April 2018

Primary Completion Date

April 2018

Eligibility Criteria

Inclusion Criteria:

- Patients with histologically confirmed inoperable, recurrent or metastatic malignant solid tumors, deemed incurable, and who have either:
- Failed to respond to standard therapy or
- For whom no standard therapy is available or
- Refuse to receive standard therapies
- The study is intended to enroll patients with pancreatic and colorectal cancer; patients with other types of solid tumors will require approval by the principal investigator
- Measurable disease as defined by Response Evaluation Criteria in Solid Tumors (RECIST)
- Patients with treated, stable, and asymptomatic brain metastases are eligible
- Patients on every 3 or every 4 week systemic therapy programs must be at least 4 weeks since treatment and recovered from any clinically significant toxicity experienced; patients on weekly or daily systemic therapy programs and patients receiving radiation must be at least 1 week since treatment and recovered from any clinically significant toxicity experienced; must be at least 4 weeks and have recovered from major surgery
- Eastern Cooperative Oncology Group (ECOG) performance status 0 or 1
- White blood cells >= 3000/uL
- Platelets >= 100,000/uL
- Hematocrit >= 28%
- Creatinine =< 1.6 mg/dL
- Aspartate aminotransferase (AST) and alanine aminotransferase (ALT) < 2.5 x upper limit of normal
- Bilirubin =< 1.6 mg/dL (except patients with Gilbert's syndrome, who must have a total bilirubin less than 3.0 mg/dL)
- Albumin >= 3.0 g/dL
- International normalized ratio (INR) =< 1.5

Exclusion Criteria:

- Women must not be pregnant or breastfeeding; all women of childbearing potential must have a blood test within 72 hours to rule out pregnancy; women of childbearing potential and sexually active males must be strongly advised to use an accepted and effective method of contraception; women of childbearing potential (WOCBP) must be using an adequate method of contraception to avoid pregnancy throughout the study and for 26 weeks after the last dose of investigational product, in such a manner that the risk of pregnancy is minimized; sexually mature females who have not undergone a hysterectomy or who have not been postmenopausal naturally for at least 24 consecutive months (i.e., who have had menses at some time in the preceding 24 consecutive months) are considered to be of childbearing potential; women who are using oral contraceptives, other hormonal contraceptives (vaginal products, skin patches, or implanted or injectable products), or mechanical products such as an intrauterine device or barrier methods (diaphragm, condoms, spermicides) to prevent pregnancy, or are practicing abstinence or where their partner is sterile (e.g., vasectomy) should be considered to be of childbearing potential
- Untreated, progressing, or symptomatic brain metastases
- Autoimmune disease, as follows: patients with a history of inflammatory bowel disease are excluded as are patients with a history of symptomatic disease (e.g., rheumatoid arthritis, systemic progressive sclerosis [scleroderma], systemic lupus erythematosus, autoimmune vasculitis [e.g., Wegener's granulomatosis]); patients with motor neuropathy considered of autoimmune origin (e.g., Guillain-Barre syndrome and myasthenia gravis) are excluded; patients with a history of autoimmune thyroiditis are eligible if their current thyroid disorder is treated and stable with replacement or other medical therapy
- Any other malignancy from which the patient has been disease-free for less than 2 years, with the exception of adequately treated and cured basal or squamous cell skin cancer, superficial bladder cancer or carcinoma in situ of the cervix
- Other ongoing systemic therapy for cancer, including any other experimental treatment; these include concomitant therapy with any of the following: IL-2, interferon, ipilimumab, pembrolizumab, nivolumab, or other immunotherapy; cytotoxic

chemotherapy; and targeted therapies

- Ongoing requirement for an immunosuppressive treatment, including the use of glucocorticoids or cyclosporine, or with a history of chronic use of any such medication within the last 4 weeks before enrollment; patients are excluded if they have any concurrent medical condition that requires the use of systemic steroids (the use of inhaled or topical steroids is permitted)

- Infection with human immunodeficiency virus (HIV)

- Active infection with hepatitis B; active or chronic infection with hepatitis C

- Clinically significant pulmonary dysfunction, as determined by medical history and physical examination; patients with a history of pulmonary dysfunction must have pulmonary function tests with a forced expiratory volume in 1 second (FEV1) >= 60% of predicted and a diffusing capacity of the lung for carbon monoxide (DLCO) >= 55% (corrected for hemoglobin)

- Clinically significant cardiovascular abnormalities (e.g., congestive heart failure or symptoms of coronary artery disease), as determined by medical history and physical examination; patients with a history of cardiac disease must have a normal cardiac stress test (treadmill, echocardiogram, or myocardial perfusion scan) within the past 6 months of study entry

- Active infections or oral temperature > 38.2 degrees Celsius (C) within 48 hours of study entry

- Systemic infection requiring chronic maintenance or suppressive therapy

- Patients are excluded for any underlying medical or psychiatric condition, which in the opinion of the investigator, will make treatment hazardous or obscure the interpretation of adverse events, such as a condition associated with frequent rashes or diarrhea

Sex/Gender

All

Ages

18 Years to N/A

Accepts Healthy Volunteers

No

Pembrolizumab and XL888 in Patients With Advanced Gastrointestinal Cancer

Study ID:

NCT03095781

Sponsor:

Emory University

Information provided by (Responsible Party):

Emory University (Emory University)

Tracking Information

First Submitted Date

March 22, 2017

Start Date

June 28, 2017

Primary Completion Date

June 2021

Last Update Posted Date

July 7, 2017

Current Primary Outcome Measures

Recommended phase II dose of the combination of XL888 and pembrolizumab as assessed by National Cancer Institute Common Terminology Criteria for Adverse Events version 4.0[Time Frame: Cycle length 21 days. Outcome determined on day 22 (after completion of cycle 1)]

Summary statistics will be presented. Toxicities will be presented as worst toxicity per patient and will be reported as percent toxicity.

Current Secondary Outcome Measures

Overall response rate as assessed by Response Evaluation Criteria in Solid Tumors (RECIST) 1.1[Time Frame: Up to 2 years after cycle 1, day 1. Cycle length is 21 days.]

RECIST version 1.1 will be used in this study for assessment of tumor response. While either CT or MRI may be utilized, as per RECIST 1.1, CT is the preferred imaging technique in this study.

Overall survival[Time Frame: Up to 1 year after cycle 1, day 1. Each cycle is 21 days.]

Once a subject experiences confirmed disease progression or starts a new anti-cancer therapy, the subject moves into the survival follow-up phase and should be contacted by telephone every 12 weeks to assess for survival status until death, withdrawal of consent, or the end of the study, whichever occurs first.

Progression free survival[Time Frame: Up to 6 months after cycle 1, day 1. Each cycle is 21 days]
Summary statistics will be presented.

Response duration as assessed by RECIST 1.1[Time Frame: Up to 2 years after cycle 1, day 1. Each cycle is 21 days.]
Summary statistics will be presented.

Descriptive Information

Offical Title

Phase Ib Trial of Pembrolizumab and XL888 in Patients With Advanced Gastrointestinal Malignancies

Brief Summary

This phase Ib trial studies the side effects and best dose of Hsp90 inhibitor XL888 when given together with pembrolizumab in treating patients with advanced gastrointestinal cancer that has spread to other places in the body. XL888 may stop the growth of tumor cells by blocking some of the enzymes needed for cell growth. Monoclonal antibodies, such as pembrolizumab, may block tumor growth in different ways by targeting certain cells. Giving XL888 with pembrolizumab may work better in treating patients with gastrointestinal cancer.

Detailed Description

PRIMARY OBJECTIVES:

I. Determine the recommended phase II dose for the combination of XL888 and pembrolizumab.

SECONDARY OBJECTIVES:

I. Define the toxicity profile of the combination of XL888 and pembrolizumab.

II. Evaluate the activity of the combination of XL888 and pembrolizumab in previously treated patients with gastrointestinal tumors.

TERTIARY OBJECTIVES:

I. Evaluate the effect of the combination on the immune profile in the serum and in tumor biopsies.

OUTLINE: This is a dose-escalation study of Hsp90 inhibitor XL888.

Patients receive pembrolizumab intravenously (IV) over 30 minutes on day 1 and XL888 orally (PO) on day 1, 4, 8, 11, 15, and 18. Courses repeat every 21 days in the absence of disease progression or unacceptable toxicity.

After completion of study treatment, patients are followed up at 30 days and periodically thereafter.

Study Type

Interventional

Study Phase

Phase 1

Condition

- Adenocarcinoma of the Gastroesophageal Junction
- Colorectal Adenocarcinoma
- Metastatic Pancreatic Adenocarcinoma
- Non-Resectable Cholangiocarcinoma
- Non-Resectable Hepatocellular Carcinoma
- Recurrent Cholangiocarcinoma
- Recurrent Colorectal Carcinoma
- Recurrent Gastric Carcinoma
- Recurrent Hepatocellular Carcinoma
- Recurrent Pancreatic Carcinoma
- Recurrent Small Intestinal Carcinoma
- Small Intestinal Adenocarcinoma
- Stage III Colorectal Cancer
- Stage III Gastric Cancer
- Stage III Hepatocellular Carcinoma
- Stage III Pancreatic Cancer
- Stage III Small Intestinal Cancer
- Stage IIIA Colorectal Cancer
- Stage IIIA Gastric Cancer

- Stage IIIA Hepatocellular Carcinoma
- Stage IIIA Small Intestinal Cancer
- Stage IIIB Colorectal Cancer
- Stage IIIB Gastric Cancer
- Stage IIIB Hepatocellular Carcinoma
- Stage IIIB Small Intestinal Cancer
- Stage IIIC Gastric Cancer
- Stage IV Colorectal Cancer
- Stage IV Gastric Cancer
- Stage IV Hepatocellular Carcinoma
- Stage IV Pancreatic Cancer
- Stage IV Small Intestinal Cancer
- Stage IVA Colorectal Cancer
- Stage IVA Hepatocellular Carcinoma
- Stage IVA Pancreatic Cancer
- Stage IVB Colorectal Cancer
- Stage IVB Hepatocellular Carcinoma
- Stage IVB Pancreatic Cancer
- Unresectable Pancreatic Carcinoma
- Unresectable Small Intestinal Carcinoma

Intervention

Drug: XL888

  Given PO

Other Names:

  Heat Shock Protein 90 Inhibitor XL888

  Hsp90 Inhibitor XL888

  Biological: Pembrolizumab

  Given IV

Other Names:

  Keytruda

  Lambrolizumab

  MK-3475

  SCH 900475

Study Arms

Experimental: Treatment (pembrolizumab, XL888)

  Patients receive pembrolizumab IV over 30 minutes on day 1 and XL888 PO on days 1, 4, 8, 11, 15, and 18. Courses repeat every 21 days in the absence of disease progression or unacceptable toxicity.

Recruitment Information

Recruitment Status

Recruiting

Estimated Enrollment

50

Completion Date

June 2023

Primary Completion Date

June 2021

Eligibility Criteria

Inclusion Criteria:

- Patients with stage IV or locally advanced unresectable gastrointestinal adenocarcinomas (gastric, gastroesophageal junction [GEJ], cholangiocarcinoma, hepatocellular, pancreas, colorectal, small intestinal tumors) who have failed at least one prior therapy (dose escalation phase)
- Patients with pancreatic adenocarcinoma; patients must have histologic diagnosis and either locally advanced unresectable or metastatic disease that has failed at least one standard regimen; eight patients must have tumors that are accessible for biopsy and sign the informed consent for paired biopsy study (dose escalation phase, arm A)

- Patients with colorectal adenocarcinoma; patients must have histologic diagnosis and either locally advanced unresectable or metastatic disease and have previously received oxaliplatin, irinotecan, and fluoropyrimidine; eight patients must have tumors that are accessible for biopsy and sign the informed consent for paired biopsy study (dose escalation phase, arm B)
- Be willing and able to provide written informed consent/assent for the trial
- Have measurable disease based on Response Evaluation Criteria in Solid Tumors (RECIST) 1.1
- Have a performance status of 0 or 1 on the Eastern Cooperative Oncology Group (ECOG) performance scale
- Absolute neutrophil count (ANC) ≥ 1,500 cells/μL
- Platelets ≥ 100,000 cells/μL
- Hemoglobin ≥ 9 g/dL or ≥ 5.6 mmol/L without transfusion or erythropoietin (EPO) dependency (within 7 days of assessment)
- Serum creatinine ≤ 1.5 x upper limit of normal (ULN) OR measured or calculated creatinine clearance (glomerular filtration rate [GFR] can also be used in place of creatinine or creatinine clearance [CrCl]) ≥ 60 mL/min for subject with creatinine levels > 1.5 x institutional ULN
- Creatinine clearance should be calculated per institutional standard
- Serum total bilirubin ≤ 1.5 x ULN OR direct bilirubin ≤ ULN for subjects with total bilirubin levels > 1.5 ULN
- Aspartate aminotransferase (AST) (serum glutamic oxaloacetic transaminase [SGOT]) and alanine aminotransferase (ALT) (serum glutamic pyruvic transaminase [SGPT]) ≤ 2.5 x ULN OR ≤ 5 x ULN for subjects with liver metastases
- Albumin ≥ 2.5 mg/dL
- International normalized ratio (INR) or prothrombin time (PT) ≤ 1.5 x ULN unless subject is receiving anticoagulant therapy as long as PT or partial thromboplastin time (PTT) is within therapeutic range of intended use of anticoagulants
- Activated partial thromboplastin time (aPTT) ≤ 1.5 x ULN unless subject is receiving anticoagulant therapy as long as PT or PTT is within therapeutic range of intended use of anticoagulants
- Female subject of childbearing potential should have a negative urine or serum pregnancy within 72 hours prior to receiving the first dose of study medication; if the urine test is positive or cannot be confirmed as negative, a serum pregnancy test will be required
- Male subjects of childbearing potential must agree to use an adequate method of contraception, starting with the first dose of study therapy through 120 days after the last dose of study therapy.
- Note: Abstinence is acceptable if this is the usual lifestyle and preferred contraception for the subject
- Female subjects of childbearing potential must be willing to use an adequate method of contraception for the course of the study through 120 days after the last dose of study medication
- Note: Abstinence is acceptable if this is the usual lifestyle and preferred contraception for the subject

Exclusion Criteria:

- Is currently participating and receiving study therapy or has participated in a study of an investigational agent and received study therapy or used an investigational device within 4 weeks of the first dose of treatment
- Has a diagnosis of immunodeficiency or is receiving systemic steroid therapy or any other form of immunosuppressive therapy within 7 days prior to the first dose of trial treatment
- Has a known history of active tuberculosis (TB) (Bacillus tuberculosis)
- Hypersensitivity to pembrolizumab or history of severe allergic or hypersensitivity reactions to excipients (e.g., polyethylene glycol [PEG] 300 and polysorbate 80)
- Clinically significant cardiovascular disease or peripheral vascular (e.g. myocardial infarction, unstable angina within 6 months of study entry), symptomatic congestive heart failure, serious uncontrolled cardiac arrhythmia requiring medications, baseline corrected QT (QTc) > 450 msec or previous history of QT prolongation while taking other medications
- Other medications, or severe acute/chronic medical or psychiatric condition, or laboratory abnormality that may increase the risk associated with study participation or study drug administration, or may interfere with the interpretation of study results, and in the judgment of the investigator would make the subject inappropriate for entry into this study
- Has had a prior anti-cancer monoclonal antibody (mAb) within 4 weeks prior to study day 1 or who has not recovered (i.e., ≤ grade 1 or at baseline) from adverse events due to agents administered more than 4 weeks earlier
- Has had prior chemotherapy, targeted small molecule therapy, or radiation therapy within 2 weeks prior to study day 1 or who has not recovered (i.e., ≤ grade 1 or at baseline) from adverse events due to a previously administered agent
- Note: Subjects with ≤ grade 2 neuropathy are an exception to this criterion and may qualify for the study
- Note: If subject received major surgery, they must have recovered adequately from the toxicity and/or complications from the intervention prior to starting therapy
- Has a known additional malignancy that is progressing or requires active treatment; exceptions include basal cell carcinoma of the skin or squamous cell carcinoma of the skin that has undergone potentially curative therapy or in situ cervical cancer
- Has known active central nervous system (CNS) metastases and/or carcinomatous meningitis; subjects with previously treated brain metastases may participate provided they are stable (without evidence of progression by imaging for at least four weeks prior to the first dose of trial treatment and any neurologic symptoms have returned to baseline), have no evidence of new or enlarging brain metastases, and are not using steroids for at least 7 days prior to trial treatment; this exception does not include carcinomatous meningitis which is excluded regardless of clinical stability
- Has active autoimmune disease that has required systemic treatment in the past 2 years (i.e. with use of disease modifying agents, corticosteroids or immunosuppressive drugs); replacement therapy (eg., thyroxine, insulin, or physiologic corticosteroid replacement therapy for adrenal or pituitary insufficiency, etc.) is not considered a form of systemic treatment

- Has known history of, or any evidence of active, non-infectious pneumonitis
- Has an active infection requiring systemic therapy
- Has known substance abuse disorders that would interfere with cooperation with the requirements of the trial
- Is pregnant or breastfeeding, or expecting to conceive or father children within the projected duration of the trial, starting with the pre-screening or screening visit through 120 days after the last dose of trial treatment
- Has received prior therapy with an anti-programmed death (PD)-1, anti-PD-L1, or anti-PD-L2 agent
- Has a known history of human immunodeficiency virus (HIV) (HIV 1/2 antibodies)
- Has known active hepatitis B (e.g., hepatitis surface antigen [HBsAg] reactive) or hepatitis C (e.g., hepatitis C virus [HCV] ribonucleic acid [RNA] [qualitative] is detected)
- Has received a live vaccine within 30 days of planned start of study therapy
- Note: Seasonal influenza vaccines for injection are generally inactivated flu vaccines and are allowed; however intranasal influenza vaccines (e.g., Flu-Mist) are live attenuated vaccines, and are not allowed

■ **Sex/Gender**

All

■ **Ages**

18 Years to N/A

■ **Accepts Healthy Volunteers**

No

■ **Contacts**

Bassel El-Rayes, MD   404-778-2670   bassel.el-rayes@emoryhealthcare.org

Regorafenib Plus 5-Fluorouracil/Leucovorin Beyond Progression in mCRC

Study ID:

NCT03099486

Sponsor:

Fox Chase Cancer Center

Information provided by (Responsible Party):

Fox Chase Cancer Center (Fox Chase Cancer Center)

Tracking Information

■ **First Submitted Date**

March 23, 2017

■ **Start Date**

October 6, 2017

■ **Current Primary Outcome Measures**

Progression free survival (PFS) at 2 months[Time Frame: 2 months]

PFS at 2 months in mCRC patients who progress on regorafenib monotherapy and are treated with regorafenib and 5-FU/LV combination therapy.

■ **Current Secondary Outcome Measures**

Overall survival rate[Time Frame: 1 years]

Overall survival will be calculated from the day of first treatment until death

Best overall response[Time Frame: 1-2 years]

This will be calculated from the day of first treatment dose until disease progression or death, whichever occurs earlier

Number of toxicities due to regorafenib and 5-FU/LV combination therapy[Time Frame: 1-2 years]

Number of toxicities due to combination therapy will be summarized by frequencies and grades of toxicities due to the combination therapy according to CTCAE 4.03 criteria

■ **Primary Completion Date**

October 22, 2019

■ **Last Update Posted Date**

November 20, 2017

Descriptive Information

Offical Title

A Pilot Phase II, Single Arm, Open Label, Investigator-initiated Clinical Trial of Regorafenib Plus 5-Fluorouracil/Leucovorin (5FU/LV) Beyond Progression on Regorafenib Monotherapy in Metastatic Colorectal Cancer (mCRC)

Brief Summary

This is a single arm open label pilot phase II trial of Regorafenib PO plus 5-FU/LV infusion in 15 mCRC patients who progressed on prior Regorafenib monotherapy as well as 5-FU containing chemotherapy combinations.The study will enroll mCRC patients with prior progression on standard multi-agent combination chemotherapy and progression on regorafenib monotherapy.

Study Type

Interventional

Study Phase

Phase 2

Condition

- Colorectal Cancer

Intervention

Drug: Regorafenib

The dose of Regorafenib is 160 mg PO daily D1-D21 of 28-day cycle or last tolerated dose while on Regorafenib monotherapy.

Drug: 5-FU

5-FU dose D1 and D15 of 28 day cycle i400 mg/m2 bolus over 10 mins followed by 2400 mg/m2 continuous infusion over 46 hours

Drug: Leucovorin

D1 and D15 of 28 day cycle Leucovorin 400 mg/m2 over 2 hours,

Study Arms

Experimental: Regorafenib + 5FU/LV Treatment Arm

Recruitment Information

Recruitment Status

Recruiting

Estimated Enrollment

15

Completion Date

October 22, 2020

Primary Completion Date

October 22, 2019

Eligibility Criteria

Inclusion Criteria:

1. mCRC with prior progression on standard multi-agent combination chemotherapy and regorafenib as a standard approved monotherapy. Progression on prior regorafenib is required for inclusion in this clinical study. Prior regimens may include FOLFOX -/+ bevacizumab, FOLFIRI -/+ bevacizumab or -/+ cetuximab (if KRAS wild-type) or panitumumab (if KRAS wilt-type). Other prior regimens may include 5-FU or capecitabine -/+ bevacizumab, irinotecan -/+ cetuximab or panitumumab, FOLFIRI -/+ ziv-aflibercept or ramucirumab.

2. Patients treated with oxaliplatin in an adjuvant setting should have progressed during or within 6 months of completion of adjuvant therapy. Patients who progress more than 6 months after completion of oxaliplatin containing adjuvant treatment must be retreated. Patients who have withdrawn from standard treatment due to unacceptable toxicity warranting discontinuation of treatment and precluding retreatment with the same agent prior to progression of disease will also be allowed in the study.

3. Patients previously treated with chemotherapy must have at least 4 weeks period between the last dose of previous chemotherapy and the first dose in this clinical study. Patients previously treated with biologics such as Avastin, Zaltrap, Erbitux, and Vectibix must have at least 6 weeks period between the last dose of previous chemotherapy and the first dose in this clinical study.

4. Measurable metastatic disease that is refractory.

5. Eastern Cooperative Oncology Group (ECOG) performance status 0 or 1.

6. Patients are included regardless of KRAS/NRAS, BRAF, p53, or microsatellite instability (MSI) status

7. Age ≥ 18 years.

8. Life expectancy of at least 8 weeks (2 months).

9. Subjects must be able to understand and be willing to sign the written informed consent form. A signed informed consent form must be appropriately obtained prior to the conduct of any trial-specific procedure.

10. Adequate bone marrow, liver and renal function as assessed by the following laboratory requirements:

- Total bilirubin ≤ 1.5 x the upper limits of normal (ULN)
- Alanine aminotransferase (ALT) and aspartate amino-transferase (AST) ≤ 2.5 x ULN (≤ 5 x ULN for subjects with liver involvement of their cancer)
- Alkaline phosphatase limit ≤ 2.5 x ULN (≤ 5 x ULN for subjects with liver involvement of their cancer)
- Serum creatinine ≤ 1.5 x the ULN
- International normalized ratio (INR)/ Partial thromboplastin time (PTT) ≤ 1.5 x ULN.
- Platelet count > 100000 /mm3, hemoglobin (Hb) > 9 g/dL, absolute neutrophil count (ANC) ≥ 1500/mm3. Blood transfusion to meet the inclusion criteria will not be allowed.

11. Subject must be able to swallow and retain oral medication.

12. Up to 5 of the 15 patients will be allowed to have had other approved or investigational drugs after prior progression of Regorafenib monotherapy. (all patients enrolled in this trial must have had prior progression on regorafenib therapy). This may include TAS102, off-label therapy that may have been prescribed based on tumor genomic profiling or any investigational agents on a clinical trial.

13. No more than grade 2 toxicity with last previous cycle of regorafenib mono therapy.

Exclusion Criteria:

1. Patients receiving any concurrent investigational agents

2. Previous assignment to treatment during this study. Subjects permanently withdrawn from study participation will not be allowed to re-enter study.

3. Uncontrolled hypertension (systolic pressure >140 mm Hg or diastolic pressure > 90 mm Hg [NCI-CTCAE v4.0] on repeated measurement) despite optimal medical management.

4. Active or clinically significant cardiac disease including:

- Congestive heart failure New York Heart Association (NYHA) > Class II.
- Active coronary artery disease.
- Suspected Long QT syndrome defined as QTc interval > 500 milliseconds at baseline.
- Cardiac arrhythmias requiring anti-arrhythmic therapy other than beta blockers or digoxin.
- Unstable angina (anginal symptoms at rest), new-onset angina within 3 months before randomization, or myocardial infarction within 6 months before randomization.

5. Evidence or history of bleeding diathesis or coagulopathy.

6. Any hemorrhage or bleeding event ≥ NCI CTCAE Grade 3 within 4 weeks prior to start of study medication.

7. Subjects diagnosed with thrombotic, embolic, venous, or arterial events, such as cerebrovascular accident (including transient ischemic attacks) deep vein thrombosis or pulmonary embolism within 3 months of start of study treatment.

8. Patients with any previously untreated or concurrent cancer that is distinct in primary site or histology except cervical cancer in-situ, treated ductal carcinoma in situ of the breast, curatively treated nonmelanoma skin carcinoma, noninvasive aerodigestive neoplasms, or superficial bladder tumor. Subjects surviving a cancer that was curatively treated and without evidence of disease for more than 3 years before registration are allowed; all cancer treatments must be completed at least 3 years prior to registration.

9. Patients with phaeochromocytoma.

10. Known history of human immunodeficiency virus (HIV) infection or current chronic or active hepatitis B or C infection requiring treatment with antiviral therapy.

11. Ongoing infection > Grade 2 NCI-CTCAE v4.0.

12. Symptomatic metastatic brain or meningeal tumors.

13. Presence of a non-healing wound, non-healing ulcer, or bone fracture.

14. Major surgical procedure or significant traumatic injury within 28 days before start of study medication

15. Renal failure requiring hemo-or peritoneal dialysis.

16. Dehydration Grade ≥1 NCI-CTCAE v4.0.

17. Patients with seizure disorder requiring medication.

18. Persistent proteinuria ≥ Grade 3 per NCI-CTCAE v4.0 (> 3.5 g/24 hrs, measured by urine protein: creatinine ratio on a random urine sample).

19. Interstitial lung disease with ongoing signs and symptoms at the time of informed consent.

20. Pleural effusion or ascites that causes respiratory compromise (≥ NCI-CTCAE version 4.0 Grade 2 dyspnea).

21. History of organ allograft (including corneal transplant).

22. Known or suspected allergy or hypersensitivity to any of the study drugs, study drug classes, or excipients of the formulations given during the course of this trial.

23. Any malabsorption condition.

24. Women who are pregnant or breast-feeding.

25. Any condition which, in the investigator's opinion, makes the subject unsuitable for trial participation.

26. Substance abuse, medical, psychological or social conditions that may interfere with the subject's participation in the study or evaluation of the study results.

27. Therapeutic anticoagulation with Vitamin-K antagonists (e.g., warfarin) or with heparins and heparinoids.

a. However, prophylactic anticoagulation as described below is allowed: i. Low dose warfarin (1 mg orally, once daily) with PT-INR ≤ 1.5 x ULN is permitted.

ii. Low dose aspirin (≤ 100 mg daily). iii. Prophylactic doses of heparin. iv. Low molecular weight heparin Subjects who are prophylactically treated with an agent such as warfarin or heparin require close monitoring (day5 of cycle 1 and day 1 of each cycle) of their INR/PTT. If either of these values are above the therapeutic range, the doses should be modified and the assessments should be repeated weekly until they are stable.

▨ Sex/Gender

All

▨ Ages

18 Years to N/A

▨ Accepts Healthy Volunteers

No

▨ Contacts

Wafik S El-Deiry, MD   215-214-4233   wafik.eldeiry@fccc.edu

Nivolumab and Ipilimumab and Radiation Therapy in MSS and MSI High Colorectal and Pancreatic Cancer

Study ID:

NCT03104439

Sponsor:

Massachusetts General Hospital

Information provided by (Responsible Party):

Massachusetts General Hospital (Massachusetts General Hospital)

Tracking Information

▨ First Submitted Date

April 3, 2017

▨ Start Date

May 10, 2017

▨ Primary Completion Date

October 31, 2020

▨ Last Update Posted Date

November 27, 2017

▨ Current Primary Outcome Measures

Disease Control Rate[Time Frame: 2 years]

The percentage of participants with disease control following treatment with nivolumab/ipilimumab/radiation. Disease control is defined as the percentage of participants who have achieved complete response (CR), partial response (PR), or stable disease (SD) as defined by Response Evaluation Criteria In Solid Tumors (RECIST). Tumors may be evaluated for response with X-ray, computerized tomography (CT) scan, Magnetic resonance imaging (MRI), FDG (fluorodeoxyglucose) positron emission tomography (PET) scan, PET-CT, or cytology/histology.

▨ Current Secondary Outcome Measures

Median Progression free Survival[Time Frame: 2 years]

Progression-Free Survival (PFS) is defined as the time from the first treatment date to the earlier of progression or death due to any cause. Participants alive without disease progression are censored at date of last disease evaluation.

Median Overall Survival[Time Frame: 2 years]

Overall Survival (OS) is defined as the time from the first treatment date to death due to any cause, or censored at date last known alive.

Descriptive Information

▨ Offical Title

Nivolumab and Ipilimumab and Radiation Therapy in Microsatellite Stable (MSS) and Microsatellite Instability (MSI) High Colorectal and Pancreatic Cancer

▣ Brief Summary

This research study is studying a combination of drugs with radiation therapy as a possible treatment for Microsatellite Stable Colorectal Cancer, Pancreatic Cancer, or MSI High Colorectal Cancer.

The interventions involved in this study are:

- Nivolumab
- Ipilimumab
- Radiation Therapy

▣ Detailed Description

This research study is a Phase II clinical trial. Phase II clinical trials test the safety and effectiveness of an investigational intervention to learn whether the intervention works in treating a specific disease. "Investigational" means that the intervention is being studied.

The FDA (the U.S. Food and Drug Administration) has not approved nivolumab for this specific disease but it has been approved for other uses.

The FDA (the U.S. Food and Drug Administration) has not approved ipilimumab for this specific disease but it has been approved for other uses.

Researchers hope to study the effects of the combination of Nivolumab and Ipilimumab. Many cancers use specific pathways (such as PD-1/PD-L1 and CTLA-4) to evade the body's immune system. Nivolumab and ipilimumab work by blocking the PD-1/PD-L1 and CTLA-4 pathways and thus releasing the brakes on the immune system so it can stop or slow cancer.

Ipilimumab and Nivolumab are both antibodies. An antibody is a cell that attaches to other cells to fight off infection. The antibodies in ipilimumab work by not allowing cancer cell growth. The antibodies in nivolumab work by causing programmed cell death of the cancer cells. Radiation therapy is believed to increase the likelihood of response of immunotherapy (the prevention/treatment of a disease through an immune response).

In this research study, the investigators are studying the combination of nivolumab, ipilimumab and radiation therapy on participants with microsatellite stable colorectal cancer, pancreatic cancer, or MSI high colorectal cancer. The combination of these study drugs have been tested and optimized for safety and is currently being tested in multiple disease types. The study drugs have not been tested and optimized in combination with radiation therapy. The investigators believe that through the combination of the study drugs and radiation therapy the body may produce an immune response to stop the cancer cells from growing.

▣ Study Type

Interventional

▣ Study Phase

Phase 2

▣ Condition

- Microsatellite Stable Colorectal Cancer
- Pancreatic Cancer
- MSI High Colorectal Cancer

▣ Intervention

Drug: Nivolumab

The antibodies in nivolumab work by causing programmed cell death of the cancer cells

Other Names:

Opdivo

Drug: Ipilimumab

The antibodies in ipilimumab work by not allowing cancer cell growth

Other Names:

Yervoy

Radiation: Radiation Therapy

Radiation therapy is believed to increase the likelihood of response of immunotherapy

▣ Study Arms

Experimental: Nivolumab+Ipilimumab

Nivolumab will be administered intravenously 3 times per cycle

Ipilimumab will be administered intravenously once per cycle

Radiation Therapy will be administered per hospital standard

Recruitment Information

Recruitment Status

Recruiting

Estimated Enrollment

80

Completion Date

October 31, 2024

Primary Completion Date

October 31, 2020

Eligibility Criteria

Inclusion Criteria:

- Participants must have histologically or cytologically confirmed adenocarcinoma of colorectal or pancreatic origin
- Age >18 years.
- Eastern Cooperative Oncology Group (ECOG) performance status ≤1
- Life expectancy of greater than 3 months
- Participants must have normal organ and marrow function as defined in Table 1, all screening labs should be performed within 14 days of protocol registration.

Table 1 Adequate Organ Function Laboratory Values

System Laboratory Value

- Hematological
- Absolute neutrophil count (ANC) ≥1500 /mcL
- White blood count (WBC) ≥2000 /mcL
- Platelets ≥100,000 / mcL
- Hemoglobin ≥9 g/dL
- Renal
- **Serum creatinine OR Measured or calculated creatinine clearance (GFR can also be used in place of creatinine or CrCl) ≤ Serum creatinine ≤ 1.5 x ULN or creatinine clearance (CrCl) ≥ 40 mL/min (if using the Cockcroft-Gault formula below):**
- Female CrCl = (140 age in years) x weight in kg x 0.85 72 x serum creatinine in mg/dL
- Male CrCl = (140 age in years) x weight in kg x 1.00 72 x serum creatinine in mg/dL
- Hepatic
- Serum total bilirubin ≤ 1.5 X ULN (upper limit of normal) (subjects with Gilbert Syndrome can have a total bilirubin <3 mg/dL
- aspartate aminotransferase (AST) serum glutamic oxaloacetic transaminase (SGOT) and Alanine Aminotransferase ALT (SGPT) ≤ 3 X ULN OR ≤ 5 X ULN for subjects with liver metastases
- Coagulation
- International Normalized Ratio (INR) or Prothrombin Time (PT)
- Activated Partial Thromboplastin Time (aPTT) ≤1.5 X ULN unless subject is receiving anticoagulant therapy
- as long as PT or PTT is within therapeutic range of intended use of anticoagulants

≤1.5 X ULN unless subject is receiving anticoagulant therapy

- as long as PT or PTT is within therapeutic range of intended use of anticoagulants
- Creatinine clearance should be calculated per institutional standard.
- Women of childbearing potential (WOCBP) must use appropriate method(s) of contraception. WOCBP should use an adequate method to avoid pregnancy for 5 months (30 days plus the time required for nivolumab to undergo five half-lives) after the last dose of investigational drug.
- Women of childbearing potential must have a negative serum or urine pregnancy test (minimum sensitivity 25 IU/L or equivalent units of HCG)
- Women must not be breastfeeding
- Men who are sexually active with WOCBP must use any contraceptive method with a failure rate of less than 1% per year. Men receiving nivolumab and who are sexually active with WOCBP will be instructed to adhere to contraception for a period of 7 months after the last dose of investigational product. Women who are not of childbearing potential, ie, who are postmenopausal or surgically sterile as well as azoospermic men do not require contraception
- Ability to understand and the willingness to sign a written informed consent document.
- Stable dose of dexamethasone 2 mg or less for 7 days prior to initiation of treatment
- One previously unirradiated lesion amenable to radiotherapy 8 Gy x 3 and can meet dose constraints, and another unirradiated measurable lesion > 1 cm in size outside the radiation field that can be used as measurable disease
- Colorectal patients must have documentation of microsatellite status. Immunohistochemistry (IHC) is acceptable.
- Colorectal patients must have received prior Fluorouracil (5FU), Irinotecan and Oxaliplatin (any combination) or have a contraindication to receiving these agents.
- Pancreas patients must have progressed on at least 1 prior line of chemotherapy

Exclusion Criteria:

- Participants who have had chemotherapy, targeted small molecule therapy or study therapy within 14 days of protocol treatment, or those who have not recovered (i.e., ≤ Grade 1 or at baseline) from adverse events due to agents administered more than 2 weeks earlier. Subjects with ≤ Grade 2 neuropathy are an exception to this criterion and may qualify for the study. If subject received major surgery, they must have recovered adequately from the toxicity and/or complications from the intervention prior to starting therapy.
- Participants who are receiving any other investigational agents.
- Patients are excluded if they have an active, known or suspected autoimmune disease other than those listed below. Subjects are permitted to enroll if they have vitiligo, type I diabetes mellitus, residual hypothyroidism due to autoimmune condition only requiring hormone replacement, psoriasis not requiring systemic treatment, or conditions not expected to recur in the absence of an external trigger
- Patients are excluded if they have a condition requiring systemic treatment with either corticosteroids (> 10 mg daily prednisone equivalents) or other immunosuppressive medications within 14 days of study drug administration. Inhaled or topical steroids and adrenal replacement doses > 10 mg daily prednisone equivalents are permitted in the absence of active autoimmune disease. Subjects are permitted to use topical, ocular, intra-articular, intranasal, and inhalational corticosteroids (with minimal systemic absorption). Physiologic replacement doses of systemic corticosteroids are permitted, even if > 10 mg/day prednisone equivalents. A brief course of corticosteroids for prophylaxis (eg, contrast dye allergy) or for treatment of non-autoimmune conditions (eg, delayed-type hypersensitivity reaction caused by contact allergen) is permitted.
- Colorectal patients are excluded if they have had prior systemic treatment with an anti-CTLA4, anti-PD1 (Programmed cell death protein 1) or PDL1 (Programmed death-ligand 1) antibody. Pancreatic patients are excluded if they have previously received anti-CTLA-4 therapy. Prior PD-1 or PDL1 therapy will be permitted for pancreas patients
- Has a known history of active TB (Bacillus Tuberculosis)
- Patients are excluded if they are positive test for hepatitis B virus surface antigen (HBV sAg) or hepatitis C virus ribonucleic acid (HCV antibody) indicating acute or chronic infection
- Patients are excluded if they have known history of testing positive for human immunodeficiency virus (HIV) or known acquired immunodeficiency syndrome (AIDS). These participants are at increased risk of lethal infections when treated with marrow-suppressive therapy. Appropriate studies will be undertaken in participants receiving combination antiretroviral therapy when indicated.
- Uncontrolled intercurrent illness including, but not limited to, ongoing or active infection, symptomatic congestive heart failure, unstable angina pectoris, cardiac arrhythmia, or psychiatric illness/social situations that would limit compliance with study requirements.
- Has known psychiatric or substance abuse disorders that would interfere with cooperation with the requirements of the trial.
- Is pregnant or breastfeeding, or expecting to conceive or father children within the projected duration of the trial, starting with the pre-screening or screening visit through 5 months for woman and 7 months for men, after the last dose of trial treatment.
- Has a known additional malignancy that is progressing or requires active treatment. Exceptions include basal cell carcinoma of the skin and squamous cell carcinoma of the skin that has undergone potentially curative therapy or in situ cervical cancer.
- Has known history of, or any evidence of active, non-infectious pneumonitis.
- Has an active infection requiring systemic therapy.
- Has received a live vaccine within 30 days of planned start of study therapy. Note: Seasonal influenza vaccines for injection are generally inactivated flu vaccines and are allowed; however intranasal influenza vaccines (e.g., Flu-Mist®) are live attenuated vaccines, and are not allowed.
- History of allergy to study drug components
- History of severe hypersensitivity reaction to any monoclonal antibody
- Uncontrolled brain metastases. Patients treated with radiation > 4 weeks prior with follow up imaging showing control are eligible

Sex/Gender

All

Ages

18 Years to N/A

Accepts Healthy Volunteers

No

Contacts

Theodore Hong   617-724-8770   tshong1@partners.org
Tarin Grillo   tgrillo@partners.org

A Clinical Trial of Durvalumab and Tremelimumab, Administered With Radiation Therapy or Ablation in Patients With Colorectal Cancer

Study ID:

NCT03122509

Sponsor:

Memorial Sloan Kettering Cancer Center

Information provided by (Responsible Party):

Memorial Sloan Kettering Cancer Center (Memorial Sloan Kettering Cancer Center)

Tracking Information

▓ **First Submitted Date**

April 18, 2017

▓ **Start Date**

April 24, 2017

▓ **Current Primary Outcome Measures**

Overall Response Rate[Time Frame: 2 years]
based on RECIST criteria

▓ **Primary Completion Date**

April 2019

▓ **Last Update Posted Date**

May 2, 2017

Descriptive Information

▓ **Offical Title**

Phase II Study to Assess the Efficacy of Durvalumab (MEDI4736) and Tremelimumab Plus Radiotherapy or Ablation in Patients With Metastatic Colorectal Cancer

▓ **Brief Summary**

The purpose of this study is to test the safety and effectiveness of two investigational drugs (drugs that are not currently approved by the FDA) given in combination with radiation therapy or ablation.

▓ **Study Type**

Interventional

▓ **Study Phase**

Phase 2

▓ **Condition**

- Metastatic Colorectal Cancer

▓ **Intervention**

Drug: durvalumab

1500 mg durvalumab via IV infusion

Other Names:

(MEDI4736)

Drug: tremelimumab

75 mg tremelimumab via IV infusion

Radiation: Radiotherapy (RT)

Radiotherapy (RT) will be performed using external beam ionizing radiation as standard therapy in accordance with institutional standard practice.

Procedure: ablation

Ablation will be performed percutaneously under image guidance as standard therapy at the discretion of the interventional radiologist in accordance with institutional standard practice.

▓ **Study Arms**

Experimental: durvalumab and tremelimumab plus Radiotherapy (RT)

Patients will receive 1500 mg durvalumab via IV infusion q4w for up to 4 doses/cycles and 75 mg tremelimumab via IV infusion q4w for up to 4 doses/cycles, and then continue 1500 mg durvalumab q4w starting on Week 16. Tremelimumab will be administered first. Durvalumab infusion will start approximately 1 hour after the end of tremelimumab infusion. The duration will be approximately 1 hour for each infusion. Radiotherapy (RT) will be performed using external beam ionizing radiation as standard therapy in accordance with institutional standard practice. RT will be initiated within 7 days after the first of durvalumab and tremelimumab.

Experimental: durvalumab and tremelimumab plus ablation

Patients will receive 1500 mg durvalumab via IV infusion q4w for up to 4 doses/cycles and 75 mg tremelimumab via IV infusion q4w for up to 4 doses/cycles, and then continue 1500 mg durvalumab q4w starting on Week 16. Tremelimumab will be administered first. Durvalumab infusion will start approximately 1 hour after the end of tremelimumab infusion. The duration will be approximately 1 hour for each infusion. The ablation will be performed percutaneously under image guidance as standard therapy at the discretion of the interventional radiologist in accordance with institutional standard practice. Ablation will be performed within 7 days after the first of durvalumab and tremelimumab.

Recruitment Information

Recruitment Status

Recruiting

Estimated Enrollment

33

Completion Date

April 2019

Primary Completion Date

April 2019

Eligibility Criteria

Inclusion Criteria:

- Be willing and able to provide written informed consent for the trial.
- Histologicallyor cytologicallyconfirmed CRC.
- Metastatic CRC.
- Subjects have received at least two standard chemotherapy regimens for which they would be considered eligible (at least one containing a 5-fluoropyrimidine), or systemic chemotherapy is not indicated in the setting of low volume metastatic disease.
- At least one tumor for which palliative RT is considered appropriate standard therapy (cohort 1); or, at least one tumor for which palliative ablation is considered appropriate standard therapy (cohort 2).
- At least one index lesion that will not undergo RT or ablation, and which is measurable based on RECIST 1.1.
- Be ≥ 18 years of age on day of signing informed consent.
- Consent for tumor biopsies (for patients enrolled in stage 1 only) and blood draws for research purposes (for all patients).
- Consent for use of available archived tissue and tumor obtained during a standard procedure, for research purposes.
- Have a performance status of 0 or 1 on the ECOG Performance Scale.
- Female subjects must either be of non-reproductive potential (i.e., post-menopausal by history: ≥60 years old and no menses for ≥ 1 year without an alternative medical cause; OR history of hysterectomy, OR history of bilateral tubal ligation, OR history of bilateral oophorectomy) or must have a negative serum pregnancy test within 2 weeks prior to starting treatment.
- Demonstrate adequate organ function as defined all screening labs should be performed within 4 weeks prior to treatment initiation.
- Hemoglobin ≥ 8.0 g/dL
- Absolute neutrophil count (ANC) ≥1,500 /mcL
- Platelets ≥100,000 / mcL
- Serum creatinine ≤1.5 X upper limit of normal (ULN) OR
- Measured or calculated creatinine clearance (GFR can also be used in place of creatinine or CrCl) OR
- Serum creatinine CL>40 mL/min by the Cockcroft-Gault formula (Cockcroft and Gault 1976) or by 24-hour urine collection for determination of creatinine clearance.
- Serum total bilirubin ≤ 1.5 X ULN OR Direct bilirubin ≤ ULN for subjects with total bilirubin levels > 1.5 ULN
- AST (SGOT) and ALT (SGPT) ≤ 2.5 X ULN OR ≤ 5 X ULN for subjects with liver metastases.

aCreatinine clearance should be calculated per institutional standard.

Exclusion Criteria:

- Is currently participating in or has participated in a study of an investigational agent or using an investigational device within 4 weeks of the first dose of treatment.
- Chemotherapy, monoclonal antibody, targeted small molecule therapy, within 4 weeks prior to dose #1 or who has not recovered (i.e., ≤ Grade 1 or at baseline) from adverse events due to a previously administered agent (excluding alopecia or toxicity not anticipated to interfere with planned treatment on study).
- Known or suspected MSI-H CRC.
- Any prior Grade ≥3 immune-related adverse event (irAE) while receiving any previous immunotherapy agent, or any unresolved irAE >Grade 1, including anti-PD-1, anti-PD-L1, anti-CD137, anti-CTLA-4 antibody or any other antibody or drug specifically targeting T-cell co-stimulation or checkpoint pathways, except for endocrinopathies and asymptomatic amylase/

lipase.

- If subject received major surgery, they must have recovered adequately from the toxicity and/or complications from the intervention per clinical discretion of the investigator prior to starting therapy.
- Concurrent active malignancy that requires systemic treatment.
- Known CNS metastases and/or carcinomatous meningitis. Subjects with previously treated brain metastases may participate provided they are stable without evidence of new or enlarging brain metastases, and are not using steroids for at least 7 days prior to trial treatment.
- Active autoimmune disease requiring systemic immune suppressive treatment within the past 2 years. NOTE: Subjects with vitiligo, Grave's disease, or psoriasis not requiring systemic treatment (within the past 2 years) are not excluded.
- Has active, non-infectious pneumonitis.
- Active or prior documented inflammatory bowel disease.
- History of allogeneic organ transplant.
- Has an active infection requiring systemic therapy.
- Has known psychiatric or substance abuse disorders that would interfere with cooperation with the requirements of the trial.
- Has a known history of Human Immunodeficiency Virus (HIV) (HIV 1/2 antibodies).
- Has known active and untreated Hepatitis B (e.g., HBsAg reactive) or active Hepatitis C (e.g., HCV RNA [qualitative] is detected).
- Has received a live vaccine within 30 days prior to the first dose of trial treatment.
- Current or prior use of immunosuppressive medication within 14 days before the first dose of durvalumab or tremelimumab with the exceptions of premedication and intranasal and inhaled corticosteroids or systemic corticosteroids at physiological doses, which are not to exceed 10mg/day of prednisone, or an equivalent corticosteroid.
- Hypersensitivity to durvalumab or tremelimumab, or any excipients on the formulation.
- Any condition that, in the opinion of the investigator, would interfere with evaluation of study treatment or interpretation of patient safety or study results.
- Female patients who are pregnant or breastfeeding or male or female patients of reproductive potential who are not willing to employ effective birth control from screening to 180 days after the last dose of durvalumab + tremelimumab combination therapy or 90 days after the last dose of durvalumab monotherapy, whichever is the longer time period.
- QT interval corrected for heart rate (QTc) ≥ 470ms calculated from 1 electrocardiogram (ECG) using Fridericia's Correction.
- History of primary immunodeficiency.
- Known history of previous clinical diagnosis of tuberculosis.
- Subjects with uncontrolled seizures.

■ **Sex/Gender**

All

■ **Ages**

18 Years to N/A

■ **Accepts Healthy Volunteers**

No

■ **Contacts**

Neil Segal, MD, PhD   646-888-4187   segaln@mskcc.org
Leonard Saltz, MD   646-888-4286

Phase 1/2 Study Exploring the Safety, Tolerability, and Efficacy of INCAGN01876 Combined With Immune Therapies in Advanced or Metastatic Malignancies

Study ID:
NCT03126110

Sponsor:
Incyte Biosciences International Sàrl

Information provided by (Responsible Party):
Incyte Corporation (Incyte Biosciences International Sàrl)

Tracking Information

First Submitted Date

April 19, 2017

Start Date

April 13, 2017

Primary Completion Date

January 2020

Last Update Posted Date

February 1, 2018

Current Primary Outcome Measures

Phase 1: Safety and tolerability assessed by monitoring frequency, duration, and severity of adverse events (AEs)[Time Frame: Screening through 60 days after end of treatment, up to 18 months]

An AE is defined as any untoward medical occurrence associated with the use of a drug in humans, whether or not considered drug related, that occurs after a subject provides informed consent.

Phase 2: Objective response rate (ORR) based on Response Evaluation Criteria in Solid Tumors (RECIST) v1.1.[Time Frame: Every 8 weeks for 12 months, then every 12 weeks, up to 18 months]

Defined as the percentage of subjects having complete response (CR) or partial response (PR)

Current Secondary Outcome Measures

Phase 1 & Phase 2: ORR based on RECIST v1.1 and modified RECIST v1.1 (mRECIST v1.1)[Time Frame: Assessed every 8 weeks for 12 months, then every 12 weeks, up to 18 months]

Defined as the percentage of subjects having CR or PR

Phase 1 & Phase 2: Duration of response based on RECIST v1.1 and mRECIST v1.1[Time Frame: Assessed every 8 weeks for 12 months, then every 12 weeks, up to 18 months]

Defined as the time from the earliest date of disease response (CR or PR) until earliest date of disease progression or death due to any cause, if occurring sooner than progression.

Phase 1 & Phase 2: Duration of disease control based on RECIST v1.1 and mRECIST v1.1[Time Frame: Assessed every 8 weeks for 12 months, then every 12 weeks, up to 18 months]

Defined as CR, PR, and stable disease (SD) as measured from first report of SD or better until disease progression or death from any cause, if occurring sooner than progression.

Phase 1 & Phase 2: Progression-free survival based on RECIST v1.1 and mRECIST v1.1[Time Frame: Assessed every 8 weeks for 12 months, then every 12 weeks, up to 18 months]

Defined as the time from the start of combination therapy until the earliest date of disease progression or death due to any cause, if occurring sooner than progression.

Phase 1 & Phase 2: Overall survival[Time Frame: 1 year, 2 years, and end of study, up to 24 months]

Determined from the start of combination therapy until death due to any cause.

Phase 1 & Phase 2: Safety and tolerability assessed by monitoring frequency, duration, and severity of adverse events[Time Frame: Screening through 60 days after end of treatment, up to 18 months]

An AE is defined as any untoward medical occurrence associated with the use of a drug in humans, whether or not considered drug related, that occurs after a subject provides informed consent.

Descriptive Information

Offical Title

A Phase 1/2 Study Exploring the Safety, Tolerability, and Efficacy of INCAGN01876 in Combination With Immune Therapies in Subjects With Advanced or Metastatic Malignancies

Brief Summary

The purpose of this study is to determine the safety, tolerability, and efficacy of INCAGN01876 when given in combination with immune therapies in subjects with advanced or metastatic malignancies.

Study Type

Interventional

Study Phase

Phase 1/Phase 2

Condition

- Advanced Malignancies
- Metastatic Malignancies

474

Intervention

Drug: INCAGN01876

In Phase 1 subjects will receive INCAGN01876 administered intravenously (IV) at the protocol-defined dose according to cohort enrollment. In Phase 2, subjects will be administered IV study drug at the recommended dose from Phase 1.

Drug: Nivolumab

Nivolumab will be administered IV at the protocol-defined dose according to assigned treatment group.

Drug: Ipilimumab

Ipilimumab will be administered IV at the protocol-defined dose according to assigned treatment group.

Study Arms

Experimental: INCAGN01876 + Nivolumab
INCAGN01876 combined with nivolumab.

Experimental: INCAGN01876 + Ipilimumab
INCAGN01876 combined with ipilimumab.

Experimental: INCAGN01876 + Nivolumab + Ipilimumab
INCAGN01876 combined with nivolumab and ipilimumab.

Recruitment Information

Recruitment Status

Recruiting

Estimated Enrollment

450

Completion Date

March 2020

Primary Completion Date

January 2020

Eligibility Criteria

Inclusion Criteria:

- Locally advanced or metastatic disease; locally advanced disease must not be amenable to resection with curative intent.
- Phase 1: Subjects with advanced or metastatic solid tumors.
- Phase 1: Subjects who have disease progression after treatment with available therapies.
- Phase 2: Subjects with advanced or metastatic endometrial cancer, gastric cancer (including stomach, esophageal, and GEJ), and SCCHN.
- Presence of measurable disease based on RECIST v1.1.
- Eastern Cooperative Oncology Group (ECOG) performance status 0 to 1.

Exclusion Criteria:

- Laboratory and medical history parameters not within the Protocol-defined range
- Prior treatment with an immune-therapy.
- Receipt of anticancer medications or investigational drugs within protocol-defined intervals before the first administration of study drug.
- Has not recovered to ≤ Grade 1 from toxic effects of prior therapy.
- Active autoimmune disease.
- Known active central nervous system metastases and/or carcinomatous meningitis.
- Evidence of active, noninfectious pneumonitis or history of interstitial lung disease.
- Evidence of hepatitis B virus or hepatitis C virus infection or risk of reactivation.
- Known history of human immunodeficiency virus (HIV; HIV 1/2 antibodies).

Sex/Gender

All

Ages

18 Years to N/A

Accepts Healthy Volunteers

No

Contacts

Incyte Corporation Call Center (US)   1.855.463.3463   medinfo@incyte.com
Incyte Corporation Call Center (ex-US)   +800 00027423   globalmedinfo@incyte.com

A Phase 2 Study of Lamivudine in Patients With p53 Mutant Metastatic Colorectal Cancer

Study ID:

NCT03144804

Sponsor:

Massachusetts General Hospital

Information provided by (Responsible Party):

Massachusetts General Hospital (Massachusetts General Hospital)

Tracking Information

▓ **First Submitted Date**

May 5, 2017

▓ **Start Date**

October 31, 2017

▓ **Current Primary Outcome Measures**

Overall Response Rate[Time Frame: 2 years]

▓ **Current Secondary Outcome Measures**

Progression Free Survival[Time Frame: 2 years]

Overall Survival[Time Frame: 2 years]

Overall Disease Control Rate[Time Frame: 2 years]

▓ **Primary Completion Date**

November 30, 2020

▓ **Last Update Posted Date**

November 6, 2017

Descriptive Information

▓ **Offical Title**

A Phase 2 Study of Lamivudine in Patients With p53 Mutant Metastatic Colorectal Cancer

▓ **Brief Summary**

This research study is studying a drug as a possible treatment for p53 mutant metastatic colorectal cancer.

The drug involved in this study is:

-Lamivudine

▓ **Detailed Description**

This research study is a Phase II clinical trial. Phase II clinical trials test the safety and effectiveness of an investigational drug to learn whether the drug works in treating a specific disease. "Investigational" means that the drug is being studied.

The FDA (the U.S. Food and Drug Administration) has not approved lamivudine for this specific disease but it has been approved for other uses.

In this research study, the investigators are studying the effects of lamivudine on this type of cancer. This drug may help prevent the growth and spread of the cancer cells to other parts of the body. The investigators have discovered that this particular type of colon cancer, which has a p53 mutation may be sensitive to treatment with lamivudine by impairing the ability of the cancer cells to grow.

▓ **Study Type**

Interventional

▓ **Study Phase**

Phase 2

▓ **Condition**

- Colorectal Cancer Metastatic

▓ **Intervention**

Drug: Lamivudine

This drug may help prevent the growth and spread of the cancer cells to other parts of the body.

Other Names:

Combivir

Study Arms

Experimental: Lamivudine

    Lamivudine administered orally every 4 weeks

    Treatment cycles will last 28 consecutive days

    The dosage will be determine by the PI

Recruitment Information

■ **Recruitment Status**

Recruiting

■ **Estimated Enrollment**

32

■ **Completion Date**

November 30, 2024

■ **Primary Completion Date**

November 30, 2020

■ **Eligibility Criteria**

Inclusion Criteria:

- Patients must have histologically confirmed adenocarcinoma of the colon that has metastasized (stage 4) and is TP53 mutant/deleted by a CLIA approved genetic test. Only known loss of function TP53 mutation/deletion will be eligible for this study.
- Participants must have measureable disease, defined as at least on lesion that can be accurately measured in at least one dimension (longest diameter to be recorded for non-nodal lesions and short axis for nodal lesions) as > 20mm with conventional techniques or > 10 mm with spiral CT scan, MRI or calipers by clinical exam. See section 11 for evaluation of measurable disease
- Patients must be resistant to or intolerant of 5FU, oxaliplatin, irinotecan, bevacizumab and cetuximab/panitumumab (if RAS wild type)
- Age 18 or older.
- ECOG performance status ≤2 (Karnofsky ≥60%, see Appendix A)
- Life expectancy of greater than 8 weeks.
- **Participants must have normal organ and marrow function as defined below:**
- absolute neutrophil count ≥1,200/mcL
- platelets ≥75,000/mcL
- total bilirubin ≤1.5 × institutional upper limit of normal within normal
- AST(SGOT)/ALT(SGPT) ≤5 × institutional upper limit of normal
- creatinine within normal institutional limits OR
- creatinine clearance ≥60 mL/min/1.73 m2 for participants with creatinine levels above institutional normal.
- The effects of lamivudine on the developing human fetus are known to be teratogenic. For this reason, women of child-bearing potential and men must agree to use adequate contraception (hormonal or barrier method of birth control; abstinence) prior to study entry and for the duration of study participation. Should a woman become pregnant or suspect she is pregnant while she or her partner is participating in this study, she should inform her treating physician immediately. Men treated or enrolled on this protocol must also agree to use adequate contraception prior to the study, for the duration of study participation, and 4 months after completion of lamivudine administration.
- Ability to understand and the willingness to sign a written informed consent document.

Exclusion Criteria:

- Participants who have had chemotherapy or radiotherapy within 4 weeks (6 weeks for nitrosourea or mitomycin C) prior to entering the study or those who have not recovered from adverse events due to agents administered more than 4 weeks earlier.
- Participants who are receiving any other investigational agents.
- Participants with known brain metastases should be excluded from this clinical trial because of their poor prognosis and because they often develop progressive neurologic dysfunction that would confound the evaluation of neurologic and other adverse events.
- History of allergic reactions attributed to compounds of similar chemical or biologic composition to lamivudine.
- Uncontrolled intercurrent illness including, but not limited to, ongoing or active infection, symptomatic congestive heart failure, unstable angina pectoris, cardiac arrhythmia, or psychiatric illness/social situations that would limit compliance with study requirements.
- Pregnant women are excluded from this study because lamivudine is an agent with the potential for teratogenic or abortifacient effects. Because there is an unknown but potential risk for adverse events in nursing infants secondary to treatment of the mother with lamivudine, breastfeeding should be discontinued if the mother is treated with lamivudine.
- HIV-positive participants on combination antiretroviral therapy are ineligible because of the potential for pharmacokinetic interactions with lamivudine
- HBV positive participants will be excluded given the known effects of lamivudine on HBV.

■ **Sex/Gender**

All

■ **Ages**

18 Years to N/A

■ **Accepts Healthy Volunteers**

No

■ **Contacts**

Aparna R Parikh, MD   617-724-4000   Aparna.Parikh@mgh.harvard.edu

A Study Evaluating the Safety, Pharmacokinetics and Anti-Tumor Activity of ABBV-176 in Subjects With Advanced Solid Tumors Likely to Express Prolactin Receptor (PRLR)

Study ID: **Sponsor:**

NCT03145909   AbbVie

Information provided by (Responsible Party):

AbbVie (AbbVie)

Tracking Information

■ **First Submitted Date**   ■ **Primary Completion Date**

May 5, 2017   June 25, 2019

■ **Start Date**   ■ **Last Update Posted Date**

July 3, 2017   February 2, 2018

■ **Current Primary Outcome Measures**

Dose Escalation Cohort: Tmax of ABBV-176[Time Frame: Up to approximately 57 days]
    Time to Cmax (Tmax) of ABBV-176

Dose Escalation Cohort: AUC∞ for ABBV-176[Time Frame: Up to approximately 57 days]
    AUC∞ is the area under the plasma concentration-time curve from Time 0 to infinite time.

Dose Escalation Cohort: Terminal phase elimination rate constant (β) for ABBV-176[Time Frame: Up to approximately 57 days]
    Terminal phase elimination rate constant (β)

Dose Escalation Cohort: Recommended Phase 2 dose (RPTD) for ABBV-176[Time Frame: Minimum first cycle of dosing (up to 21 days)]
    The RPTD will be determined using available safety and pharmacokinetics data upon completion of the Dose Escalation Cohort.

Dose Escalation Cohort: Cmax of ABBV-176[Time Frame: Up to approximately 57 days]
    Maximum observed plasma concentration (Cmax) of ABBV-176.

Dose Escalation Cohort: Maximum tolerated dose (MTD) of ABBV-176[Time Frame: Minimum first cycle of dosing (up to 21 days)]
    MTD will be defined as the highest dose level at which less than or equal to 33% of participants experience a dose limiting toxicity.

Expanded Recommended Phase Two Dose (RPTD) Cohort: Objective Response Rate (ORR)[Time Frame: Up to approximately 2 years]
    ORR is defined as the proportion of participants with a response of partial response (PR) or better per Response Evaluation Criteria In Solid Tumors (RECIST) 1.1.

Dose Escalation Cohort: AUCt for ABBV-176[Time Frame: Up to approximately 57 days]
    Area Under the Plasma Concentration-time Curve from Time 0 to the Time of the Last Measurable Concentration (AUCt) for ABBV-176.

Dose Escalation Cohort: t1/2 for ABBV-176[Time Frame: Up to approximately 57 days]
Terminal elimination half-life (t1/2)

▨ Current Secondary Outcome Measures

Expanded RPTD Cohort: AUCt for ABBV-176[Time Frame: Up to approximately 15 days]
Area Under the Plasma Concentration-time Curve from Time 0 to the Time of the Last Measurable Concentration (AUCt)

Expanded RPTD Cohort: Tmax of ABBV-176[Time Frame: Up to approximately 15 days]
Time to Cmax (Tmax) of ABBV-176

Expanded RPTD Cohort: Overall Survival (OS)[Time Frame: Up to 2 years after the last dose of study drug]
OS is defined as number of days from the date of the first dose to the date of death for all dosed subjects. For subjects who are not deceased, the data will be censored at the date of the last study visit, or the last know date to be alive, whichever is later.

Expanded RPTD Cohort: Cmax of ABBV-176[Time Frame: Up to approximately 15 days]
Maximum observed plasma concentration (Cmax) of ABBV-176.

Expanded RPTD Cohort: Duration of Response (DOR)[Time Frame: Up to approximately 2 years]
DOR is defined as the time from the date of the participant's documented first response of PR or better to the date of documented disease progression or death due to the disease, whichever occurs first.

Expanded RPTD Cohort: Terminal phase elimination rate constant (β) for ABBV-176[Time Frame: Up to approximately 15 days]
Terminal phase elimination rate constant (β) for ABBV-176

Expanded Recommended Phase Two Dose (RPTD) Cohort: Progression-Free Survival (PFS)[Time Frame: Up to approximately 2 years]
PFS is defined as the time from the participant's first dose of study drug (Day 1) to the date of documented disease progression (per RECIST 1.1), or death due to any cause, whichever occurs first.

Expanded RPTD Cohort: Change in ECOG Performance Status[Time Frame: Up to approximately 2 years]
Change from baseline in Eastern Cooperative Oncology Group (ECOG) Performance Status

Expanded RPTD Cohort: AUC∞ for ABBV-176[Time Frame: Up to approximately 15 days]
Area Under the Plasma Concentration-time Curve from Time 0 to infinite time (AUC∞)

Expanded RPTD Cohort: t1/2 for ABBV-176[Time Frame: Up to approximately 15 days]
Terminal elimination half-life (t1/2) for ABBV-176

Dose Escalation Cohort: Change from Baseline in QTcF[Time Frame: Up to approximately 47 days]
QT interval measurement corrected by Fridericia's formula (QTcF) mean change from baseline

Descriptive Information

▨ Offical Title

A Phase 1 Study Evaluating the Safety, Pharmacokinetics and Anti-Tumor Activity of ABBV-176 in Subjects With Advanced Solid Tumors Likely to Express Prolactin Receptor (PRLR)

▨ Brief Summary

This is an open-label, Phase I, dose-escalation study to determine the maximum tolerated dose (MTD) and the recommended phase two dose (RPTD), and to assess the safety, preliminary efficacy, and pharmacokinetic (PK) profile of ABBV-176 for participants with advanced solid tumors likely to express Prolactin Receptor (PRLR). The study will consist of 2 cohorts: Dose Escalation and Expanded Recommended Phase 2 Dose.

▨ Study Type

Interventional

▨ Study Phase

Phase 1

▨ Condition

- Advanced Solid Tumors Likely to Express Prolactin Receptor (PRLR)

▨ Intervention

Drug: ABBV-176
Intravenous infusion

▨ Study Arms

Experimental: Dose Escalation Cohort

ABBV-176 will be administered via intravenous infusion at escalating dose levels until the maximum tolerated dose is reached.

Experimental: Expanded RPTD Cohort

ABBV-176 via intravenous administration in participants with breast cancer at the Recommended Phase Two Dose (RPTD) determined during the Dose Escalation Cohort

Recruitment Information

■ **Recruitment Status**

Recruiting

■ **Estimated Enrollment**

100

■ **Eligibility Criteria**

Inclusion Criteria:

- Participant has histological confirmation of a locally advanced or metastatic solid tumor of a type associated with Prolactin Receptor (PRLR) expression that has progressed on prior treatment, is not amenable to treatment with curative intent, and has no other therapy options known to provide clinical benefit or the subject is ineligible for such therapies.
- Dose Escalation Cohort: must have breast cancer, colorectal cancer, adrenocortical carcinoma, chromophobe renal cell carcinoma, or hepatocellular carcinoma.
- Expanded Cohort: must have breast cancer.
- **Participant must consent to provide the following for biomarker analyses:**
- Dose Escalation Cohort: archived tumor tissue or fresh tumor biopsy.
- Expanded Cohort: archived tumor tissue and fresh tumor biopsy.
- Participant has Eastern Cooperative Oncology Group (ECOG) performance status 0-1.
- Participant has adequate bone marrow, renal, and hepatic function.

Exclusion Criteria:

- Participant received anticancer therapy including chemotherapy, immunotherapy, radiotherapy, biologic, or any investigational therapy within 21 days before Study Day 1; participant received palliative radiotherapy or small molecule targeted anti-cancer agents within 14 days of Study Day 1.
- Participant has prior exposure to any pyrrolobenzodiazopine-containing agent
- Participant has unresolved, clinically significant toxicities from prior anticancer therapy, defined as greater than Grade 1 on Common Terminology for adverse events.
- Participant has clinically significant uncontrolled conditions.
- Participant has a history of major immunologic reaction to any Immunoglobulin G (IgG).

■ **Sex/Gender**

All

■ **Ages**

18 Years to N/A

■ **Accepts Healthy Volunteers**

No

■ **Contacts**

ABBVIE CALL CENTER   847.283.8955   abbvieclinicaltrials@abbvie.com

■ **Completion Date**

September 3, 2019

■ **Primary Completion Date**

June 25, 2019

High Dose Vitamin C Intravenous Infusion in Patients With Resectable or Metastatic Solid Tumor Malignancies

Study ID:

NCT03146962

Sponsor:

Weill Medical College of Cornell University

Information provided by (Responsible Party):

Weill Medical College of Cornell University (Weill Medical College of Cornell University)

Tracking Information

■ **First Submitted Date**

April 27, 2017

■ **Start Date**

March 29, 2017

■ **Primary Completion Date**

December 2019

■ **Last Update Posted Date**

July 19, 2017

■ **Current Primary Outcome Measures**

- Preliminary antitumor activity measured by pathologic response based on tumor regression grading in cohort A patients. 3-month disease control rate (DCR) will be evaluated using RECIST v 1.1 in cohort B patients.[Time Frame: cohort A 8 weeks, cohort B up to 6 months]

■ **Current Secondary Outcome Measures**

- Progression-free survival (PFS) in cohort B.[Time Frame: cohort A 8 weeks, cohort B up to 6 months]
- Objective response rate (ORR) in cohort B.[Time Frame: cohort A 8 weeks, cohort B up to 6 months]
- Assessment of pharmacokinetics of high dose vitamin C plasma levels concentrations[Time Frame: cohort A 8 weeks, cohort B up to 6 months]
- Safety of high dose vitamin C administration using CTCAE 4.03.[Time Frame: cohort A 8 weeks, cohort B up to 6 months]

Descriptive Information

■ **Offical Title**

A Phase II Study of High Dose Vitamin C Intravenous Infusion in Patients With Resectable or Metastatic Solid Tumor Malignancies

■ **Brief Summary**

This is a single arm, 2-cohort, open-label trial of high dose Vitamin C intravenous infusion in subjects with solid tumor malignancies who are eligible for resection (cohort A) or with KRAS or BRAF mutant metastatic cancer who have received prior systemic treatment (cohort B).

■ **Detailed Description**

This clinical trial is for men and women with resectable or metastatic solid tumor malignancies. The objective of the study is to investigate whether high dose vitamin C infusion leads to pathological tumor response in resectable colorectal, pancreatic, and lung cancer (cohort A) or objective tumor response in KRAS or BRAF mutant solid tumors (cohort B).

Patients enrolled in cohort A will receive high dose Vitamin C infusion for 4 days per week for 2-4 consecutive weeks prior to surgery. Patients enrolled in cohort B will receive high dose Vitamin C infusion for 4 days per week up to 6 months. A tumor sample will be resected after completion of study drug (high dose vitamin C infusion) treatment to examine the effects of study drug (Cohort A only). In addition, organoids will be grown in vitro and continue to be treated with vitamin C added in culture medium to examine tumor response. The resected tumor in this study will

Key eligibility:

- Men and women age 18 and older
- Patients with histologically proven early stage or locally advanced colorectal adenocarcinoma, lung cancer or pancreatic cancer, who are eligible for resection, and have not received chemotherapy or radiotherapy (cohort A) Patients with inoperable, metastatic, KRAS or BRAF mutant colorectal adenocarcinoma, lung cancer and pancreatic cancer, who have received at least 1 line of treatment for metastatic disease (cohort B)

■ **Study Type**

Interventional

■ **Study Phase**

Phase 2

■ **Condition**

- Colorectal Cancer
- Pancreatic Cancer
- Lung Cancer

■ **Intervention**

Drug: Vitamin C

Vitamin C infusion will be administered intravenously at 1.25 g/kg for 4 days per week for 2-4 consecutive weeks (cohort A) or up to 6 months (cohort B).

Other Names:

Ascorbic Acid

▣ Study Arms

Experimental: All Subjects

Vitamin C infusion will be administered intravenously at 1.25 g/kg for 4 days per week for 2-4 consecutive weeks (cohort A) or up to 6 months (cohort B).

Recruitment Information

▣ Recruitment Status

Recruiting

▣ Estimated Enrollment

50

▣ Completion Date

December 2021

▣ Primary Completion Date

December 2019

▣ Eligibility Criteria

Inclusion Criteria:

1. Male or female ≥ 18 years of age.

2. Patients with histologically proven early stage or locally advanced colorectal adenocarcinoma, lung cancer or pancreatic cancer, who are eligible for resection, and have not received chemotherapy or radiotherapy (cohort A)

3. Patients with inoperable, metastatic, KRAS or BRAF mutant colorectal adenocarcinoma, lung cancer and pancreatic cancer, who have received at least 1 line of treatment for metastatic disease (cohort B).

4. ECOG performance status 0-1.

5. Life expectancy of at least 6 months.

6. All women of child-bearing potential and all sexually active male patients must agree to use effective contraception.

7. Patient with adequate organ and marrow function as follows:

- ANC ≥ 1500 mm3, platelets ≥ 100,000/mm3, hemoglobin ≥ 9 g/dL,

- serum creatinine ≤1.8 mg/dL or creatinine clearance > 50 mL/min (Appendix C: Estimating Creatinine Clearance);

- bilirubin ≤ 1.5 mg/dL; alanine aminotransferase (ALT), aspartate transaminase (AST) ≤ 2.5 times the upper limit of normal if no liver involvement or ≤ 5 times the upper limit of normal with liver involvement.

8. Patients with serum electrolytes (including calcium, magnesium, phosphorous, sodium and potassium) within normal limits (supplementation to maintain normal electrolytes is allowed).

10. Patients capable of understanding and complying with the protocol and who have signed the informed consent document.

Exclusion Criteria:

1. Patients with uncontrolled intercurrent illness including, but not limited to uncontrolled infection, symptomatic congestive heart failure (NYHA class III and IV), uncontrolled cardiac arrhythmia, or psychiatric illness/social situations that would limit compliance with study requirements (Appendix B: New York Heart Association (NYHA) Classifications).

2. Patients with active heart disease including myocardial infarction within previous 3 months, symptomatic coronary artery disease, arrhythmias not controlled by medication, unstable angina pectoris, or uncontrolled congestive heart failure (NYHA class III and IV) (Appendix B: New York Heart Association (NYHA) Classifications).

3. Patients who have received systemic chemotherapy or targeted therapy for metastatic disease within 2 weeks from start of study drug treatment (cohort B).

4. Patients who have received an investigational drug within 21 days of the first dose of study drug.

5. Patient who have not recovered to grade ≤ 1 from adverse events (AEs) due to investigational drugs or other medications, which were administered more than 4 weeks prior to the first dose of study drug.

6. Patients who are pregnant or lactating.

7. Patients who are known to be positive for the human immunodeficiency virus (HIV). The effect of Vitamin C on HIV medications is unknown. Note: HIV testing is not required for eligibility, but if performed previously and was positive, the patient is ineligible for the study.

8. Patients who have the inability or unwillingness to abide by the study protocol or cooperate fully with the investigator or designee.

9. Patient who are receiving drugs which are known to interact with Vitamin C, potential risk and eligibility will be evaluated individually by the investigator.

10. Patients who have uncontrolled or severe hyponatremia, hypernatremia, SIADH, hypokalemia, hyperkalemia, hypomagnesemia, or hypermagnesemia

11. Patients who have uncontrolled or severe coagulopathies or a history of clinically significant bleeding within the past 6 months, such as hemoptysis, epistaxis, hematochezia, hematuria, or gastrointestinal bleeding.

12. Patients who have a known predisposition for bleeding such as von Willebrand's disease or other such condition.

13. Patients who require therapeutic doses of any anticoagulant, including low molecular weight heparin (LMWH). Concomitant use of warfarin, even at prophylactic doses, is prohibited.

14. Patients who have uncontrolled seizure disorder, ascites, iron overload, edema, or dehydration.

15. Patients who have glucose-6-phosphate dehydrogenase (G6PD) deficiency, hereditary spherocytosis, or other conditions predisposing patient to hemolysis.

16. Patients who have a history of oxalate renal calculi.

Sex/Gender

All

Ages

18 Years to N/A

Accepts Healthy Volunteers

No

Contacts

Alice Mercado, RN   646-962-3080   alm2051@med.cornell.edu
Scott Sherrin, RN   646-962-3378   sts2039@med.cornell.edu

Study of QRH-882260 Heptapeptide Application in the Colon

Study ID:

NCT03148119

Sponsor:

Danielle Kim Turgeon

Information provided by (Responsible Party):

University of Michigan (Danielle Kim Turgeon)

Tracking Information

First Submitted Date

April 12, 2017

Start Date

March 31, 2017

Primary Completion Date

March 2018

Last Update Posted Date

May 10, 2017

Current Primary Outcome Measures

Incidence of QRH-882260 Heptapeptide administration-related adverse events[Time Frame: 1 year]

Continued monitoring of safety in subjects as measured by the number of Adverse Event (AE) assessments, severity (grade), and relationship to the study drug (any that could be related).

Current Secondary Outcome Measures

Efficacy of QRH-882260 Heptapeptide administration for detection of polypoid and non-polypoid colonic neoplasia[Time Frame: 1 year]

The test product efficacy will be assessed by evaluating the fluorescence intensified measured from suspicious regions of colonic mucosa where the fluorescently-labeled peptide (QRH-882260) is administered. Measurement of peptide binding will be evaluated by the fluorescence intensity measured from the suspicious (target) region and normal tissues (background) to produce a target-to-background ratio.

Descriptive Information

Offical Title

Phase IB Study of QRH-882260 Heptapeptide Application in the Colon

Brief Summary

A Phase 1B study of the efficacy of a topically-administered 7-amino acid peptide labeled with a near-infrared fluorophore Cy5 for detecting neoplastic areas of the colon is proposed. The study will test the efficacy of administering this agent (QRH-882260 Heptapeptide) to human subjects undergoing clinically-indicated colonoscopy for endoscopic resection of known colonic adenomas or for surveillance biopsies of known dysplasia in the setting of irritable bowel disease (IBD). Up to 120 evaluable subjects will be enrolled.

Subjects will be recruited around scheduled standard of care procedures. The endoscopists performing the procedures are all endoscopists credentialed at the University of Michigan to do these procedures. Urine for dipstick pregnancy testing (if applicable) will be collected before the procedure, along with medical information. Vital signs are routinely monitored throughout the clinical procedure and are available in the electronic medical record. The endoscopy will proceed per the University of Michigan Health System (UMHS) standard of care. The endoscopist performing the clinical procedure will evaluate the potential risk (if any) for the subject to continue with the procedure or study. Five mL of the reconstituted QRH-882260 Heptapeptide (~100 µM) will be sprayed onto the site of interest through a catheter in the endoscope. Five minutes after QRH-882260 Heptapeptide application, the unbound peptide will be washed off using the endogator irrigator and the residual liquid will be suctioned. Pictures with white-light and fluorescence will be taken with the scanning fiber based molecular imaging endoscopic probe inserted via the instrument channel of the standard endoscope before the QRH-882260 Heptapeptide application, immediately after application and then again after the QRH-882260 Heptapeptide will be washed off. The area of interest identified will be resected/biopsied per discretion of the endoscopist per clinical care. All specimens taken are for clinical care only (not research use) and will be sent for routine histology per UMHS standard of care.

Study Type

Interventional

Study Phase

Phase 1

Condition

- Colon Cancer Prevention

Intervention

Drug: QRH-882260 Heptapeptide

topical spray; fluorescently-labeled peptide composed of a 7-amino acid sequence [Gln-Arg-His-Lys-Pro-Arg-Glu] attached via a 5 amino acid linker [Gly-Gly-Gly-Ser-Lys] to a near-infrared fluorophore, Cy5. The complete peptide sequence is written as: Gln-Arg-His-Lys-Pro-Arg-Glu-Gly-Gly-Gly-Ser-Lys(Cy5)-NH2, and is abbreviated as: QRHKPRE-GGGSK-(Cy5)-NH2.

Other Names:

QRH

Device: Scanning Fiber Endoscope

Endoscope used for providing the light via laser to image the area of interest in the colon after the QRH has been sprayed and rinsed.

Study Arms

Experimental: Topical QRH Heptapeptide Administration

Recruitment Information

Recruitment Status

Recruiting

Estimated Enrollment

120

Completion Date

March 2018

Primary Completion Date

March 2018

Eligibility Criteria

Inclusion Criteria:

Subject meets at least one of the following criteria:

- At increased risk for colorectal cancer (CRC) and colonic polyps
- Known colonic adenomas scheduled for colonic resection
- Scheduled for outpatient colonoscopy for follow up surveillance of IBD with known dysplasia or who are at high risk for high grade dysplasia
- Subject is scheduled for outpatient colonoscopy in the Medical Procedures Unit at UMHS
- Subject is medically cleared for the procedure (e.g. washout for anticoagulants, co-morbidities) Standard practice guidelines for safely proceeding with the procedure will be sufficient for the study
- Age 18 to 100 years
- Willing and able to sign informed consent

Exclusion Criteria:

Subjects with known allergy or negative reaction to Cy5 (a near-infrared fluorophore) or derivatives

- Subjects on active chemotherapy or radiation treatment
- Pregnant or trying to conceive

■ **Sex/Gender**

All

■ **Ages**

18 Years to 100 Years

■ **Accepts Healthy Volunteers**

No

■ **Contacts**

D K Turgeon, MD   (734)764-6860   kturgeon@med.umich.edu

Elaine M Brady, MBA   (734)647-4794   embrady@med.umich.edu

Lesion Detection Assessment in the Liver: Standard vs Low Radiation Dose Using Varied Post-Processing Techniques

Study ID:

NCT03151564

Sponsor:

M.D. Anderson Cancer Center

Information provided by (Responsible Party):

M.D. Anderson Cancer Center (M.D. Anderson Cancer Center)

Tracking Information

■ **First Submitted Date**

May 9, 2017

■ **Start Date**

May 9, 2017

■ **Primary Completion Date**

May 2020

■ **Last Update Posted Date**

May 12, 2017

■ **Current Primary Outcome Measures**

Metastasis Detection Accuracy[Time Frame: 1 day]

Primary endpoint is metastasis detection accuracy status of each patient, where the standard of care scan reviewed by "truth readers" (independent to the blinded radiologists) serve as the gold standard. If any lesion of a patient is diagnosed as metastasis by "truth readers" or blinded readers' consensus, that patient will be considered true positive and diagnosis positive, respectively. The expected accuracy of standard CT is 95%, and a low dose CT detection be considered non-inferior if its accuracy is 85% or higher.

Descriptive Information

■ **Offical Title**

Lesion Detection Assessment in the Liver: Standard vs Low Radiation Dose Using Varied Post-Processing Techniques

■ **Brief Summary**

The goal of this clinical research study is to compare imaging software and 2 different radiation doses during a standard CT scan in order to "see" problems in the liver and still produce a good image quality.

■ **Detailed Description**

If participant agrees to take part in this study, participant will have a CT scan that is done as part of participant's routine care. This CT scan will be done at the normal radiation dose.

During this scan, participant will also have a scan of the liver at a lower radiation dose, which is part of the research in this study. This will add about a minute to participant's normal scan time.

Information will also be collected from participant's medical record.

After participant's scan, participation in this study will be over.

This is an investigational study. The CT scans in this study are performed using an FDA-approved and commercially available method. The comparison of software used in this study at 2 different radiation doses is considered research.

Up to 104 participants will be enrolled in the study. All will take part at MD Anderson.

Study Type

Interventional

Study Phase

N/A

Condition

- Diseases of Liver
- Colon Carcinoma
- Colorectal Carcinoma
- Liver Metastases

Intervention

- Diagnostic Test: Computed Tomography Scan 50% Dose Reduction

  Participants undergo routine standard of care CT examination for colon carcinoma restaging, then have an additional scan of the liver at 50% dose reduction.

  Other Names:

  CT scan

- Diagnostic Test: Computed Tomography Scan 70% Dose Reduction

  Participants undergo routine standard of care CT examination for colon carcinoma restaging, then have an additional scan of the liver at 70% dose reduction.

  Other Names:

  CT scan

Study Arms

- Experimental: Computed Tomography Scan 50% Dose Reduction

  Participants undergo routine standard of care CT examination for colon carcinoma restaging, then have an additional scan of the liver at 50% dose reduction.

- Experimental: Computed tomography Scan 70% Dose Reduction

  Participants undergo routine standard of care CT examination for colon carcinoma restaging, then have an additional scan of the liver at 70% dose reduction.

Recruitment Information

Recruitment Status

Recruiting

Estimated Enrollment

104

Completion Date

May 2020

Primary Completion Date

May 2020

Eligibility Criteria

Inclusion Criteria:

1. Patient must be >/= 18 years of age and </=90 years of age

2. Men and non-pregnant women

3. Pathology proven diagnosis of colon or colorectal carcinoma

4. Liver metastases on most recent prior M.D. Anderson CT examination

5. Standard of care CT abdomen examination planned WITH IV contrast

Exclusion Criteria:

1. Patients cannot give informed consent

2. Patients cannot undergo CT examination

Sex/Gender

All

Ages

18 Years to 90 Years

Phase 1 Study of LOXO-292 in Patients With Advanced Solid Tumors, RET-Fusion Lung Cancer and Medullary Thyroid Cancer

Study ID:

NCT03157128

Sponsor:

Loxo Oncology, Inc.

Information provided by (Responsible Party):

Loxo Oncology, Inc. (Loxo Oncology, Inc.)

Tracking Information

■ **First Submitted Date**

May 9, 2017

■ **Start Date**

May 9, 2017

■ **Primary Completion Date**

August 2019

■ **Last Update Posted Date**

November 29, 2017

■ **Current Primary Outcome Measures**

Maximum tolerated dose (MTD)[Time Frame: The first 28 days of treatment (Cycle 1)]

Recommended dose for further study[Time Frame: The first 28 days of treatment (Cycle 1) and every cycle (28 days) for approximately 12 months (or earlier if the patient discontinues from the study)]

■ **Current Secondary Outcome Measures**

Number of participants with adverse events as assessed by CTCAE v4.03[Time Frame: From the time of informed consent, for approximately 24 months (or earlier if the patient discontinues from the study), and through Safety Follow-up (28 days after the last dose)]

Number of participants with serious adverse events[Time Frame: From the time of informed consent, for approximately 24 months (or earlier if the patient discontinues from the study), and through Safety Follow-up (28 days after the last dose)]

Number of patients with changes in clinical laboratory results compared to baseline[Time Frame: Day 1 (baseline) , Day 8 and Day 15 of Cycle 1 and every cycle (28 days) beginning with Cycle 2, for approximately 24 months (or earlier if the patient discontinues from the study), and through Safety Follow-up (28 days after the last dose)]

Number of patients with changes upon physical examination compared to baseline[Time Frame: Day 1 (baseline) , Day 8 and Day 15 of Cycle 1 and every cycle (28 days) beginning with Cycle 2, for approximately 24 months (or earlier if the patient discontinues from the study), and through Safety Follow-up (28 days after the last dose)]

Number of patients with changes in vital signs compared to baseline[Time Frame: Day 1 (baseline) , Day 8 and Day 15 of Cycle 1 and every cycle (28 days) beginning with Cycle 2, for approximately 24 months (or earlier if the patient discontinues from the study), and through Safety Follow-up (28 days after the last dose)]

Number of patients with changes in ECGs compared to baseline[Time Frame: Day 1 (baseline) and Day 8 of Cycle 1 and every cycle (28 days) beginning with Cycle 2, for approximately 24 months (or earlier if the patient discontinues from the study), and through Safety Follow-up (28 days after the last dose)]

Area under the plasma concentration time curve from 0 to 24 hours (AUC0-24) of LOXO-292[Time Frame: Days 1 and 8 of Cycle 1 and Day 1 of Cycles 3 and 5]

Maximum plasma concentration (Cmax) of LOXO-292[Time Frame: Days 1 and 8 of Cycle 1 and Day 1 of Cycles 3 and 5]

Time to maximum plasma concentration (Tmax) of LOXO-292[Time Frame: Days 1 and 8 of Cycle 1 and Day 1 of Cycles 3 and 5]

Terminal half-life (t1/2) of LOXO-292[Time Frame: Days 1 and 8 of Cycle 1 and Day 1 of Cycles 3 and 5]

Degree of Accumulation of LOXO-292[Time Frame: Days 1 and 8 of Cycle 1 and Day 1 of Cycles 3 and 5]

Overall response rate[Time Frame: Approximately every 8 weeks for one year, then every 12 weeks, 7 days after the last dose, and every 12 weeks after the last dose (for up to 2 years) in patients who have not progressed.]

As assessed by RECIST v1.1 or RANO, as appropriate to tumor type

Duration of reponse[Time Frame: Approximately every 8 weeks for one year, then every 12 weeks, 7 days after the last dose, and every 12 weeks after the last dose (for up to 2 years) in patients who have not progressed]

In patients with best overall response of complete response or partial response, as assessed by RECIST v1.1 or RANO, as appropriate to tumor type

Best change in tumor size from baseline[Time Frame: Approximately every 8 weeks for one year, then every 12 weeks, 7 days after the last dose, and every 12 weeks after the last dose (for up to 2 years) in patients who have not progressed]

Clinical benefit rate[Time Frame: Approximately every 8 weeks for one year, then every 12 weeks, 7 days after the last dose, and every 12 weeks after the last dose (for up to 2 years) in patients who have not progressed]

Proportion of patients with complete response, partial response, or stable disease for at least 6 months while on LOXO-292, as assessed by RECIST v1.1 or RANO, as appropriate to tumor type

Median duration of progression-free survival following initiation of LOXO-292[Time Frame: Up to 2 years]

Median overall survival following initiation of LOXO-292[Time Frame: Up to 2 years]

Descriptive Information

▣ Offical Title

A Phase 1 Study of Oral LOXO-292 in Patients With Advanced Solid Tumors, Including RET-Fusion Non-Small Cell Lung Cancer, Medullary Thyroid Cancer, and Other Tumors With Increased RET Activity

▣ Brief Summary

This is a Phase 1, open-label, first-in-human study designed to evaluate the safety, tolerability, pharmacokinetics (PK) and preliminary anti-tumor activity of LOXO-292 administered orally to patients with advanced solid tumors, including RET-fusion non-small cell lung cancer (NSCLC), medullary thyroid cancer (MTC) and other tumors with increased RET activity.

▣ Detailed Description

The trial will be conducted in 2 parts: dose escalation (Part 1) and dose expansion (Part 2). During Part 1, patients with advanced NSCLC, advanced MTC or other advanced solid tumors are initially eligible if the tumor has progressed following or has not adequately responded to standard therapy, or if the patient is intolerant of, unlikely to benefit from or refuses standard therapy. During Part 2, patients with NSCLC, MTC or other advanced solid tumor that harbors a RET gene alteration or other evidence of increased RET activity are eligible.

▣ Study Type

Interventional

▣ Study Phase

Phase 1

▣ Condition

- Non-Small Cell Lung Cancer
- Medullary Thyroid Cancer
- Colon Cancer
- Solid Tumor

▣ Intervention

Drug: LOXO-292

Oral LOXO-292

▣ Study Arms

Experimental: LOXO-292

Dose Escalation Multiple doses of LOXO-292 Dose Expansion The maximum tolerated dose (MTD)/recommended dose for further study of LOXO-292 as determined during Dose Escalation

Recruitment Information

▣ Recruitment Status

Recruiting

▣ Estimated Enrollment

180

▣ Completion Date

December 2019

▣ Primary Completion Date

August 2019

Eligibility Criteria

Key Inclusion Criteria:

- Diagnosis during Dose Escalation (Part 1) Patients with a locally advanced or metastatic solid tumor that progressed following standard therapy, or for whom no standard therapy is exists, or who decline standard therapy, or who in the opinion of the Investigator, is not a candidate for, or would be unlikely to tolerate or derive significant clinical benefit from standard therapy.

- Once a safe dose level is achieved that is consistent with inhibiting RET, patients must have advanced NSCLC, MTC or other advanced solid tumor with evidence of RET alteration or other evidence of increased RET activity in tumor tissue and/or blood.

- Any number of prior TKIs.

- Measurable or non-measurable disease as determined by RECIST 1.1 or RANO as appropriate to tumor type.

- Eastern Cooperative Oncology Group (ECOG) score of 0, 1, or 2.

- Adequate hematologic, hepatic and renal function.

- Life expectancy of at least 3 months.

Inclusion Criteria:

- Diagnosis during Dose Expansion (Part 2)

- Group 1: Advanced RET-fusion NSCLC with ≥ 1 prior tyrosine kinase inhibitor (TKI) that inhibit RET

- Group 2: Advanced RET-fusion NSCLC with no prior TKI that inhibits RET

- Group 3: Advanced RET-mutant MTC with ≥ 1 prior TKI that inhibit RET

- Group 4: Advanced RET-mutant MTC with no prior TKI that inhibits RET

- Group 5: Disease not measurable, other RET-altered tumors, other RET alterations, cfDNA positive for RET alteration with tumor discordant or negative, RET mutation-negative MTC with any number of prior TKIs that inhibit RET

- For MTC: PD within the previous 14 months as defined by RECIST 1.1.

- Any number of prior TKIs.

- At least one measurable lesion as defined by RECIST 1.1 or RANO, as appropriate to tumor type, not previously irradiated and not chosen for biopsy during the screening period. Patients without RECIST 1.1 or RANO measurable disease may be eligible for enrollment to Group 5.

- ECOG score of 0, 1, or 2.

- Adequate hematologic, hepatic and renal function.

- Life expectancy of at least 3 months.

Key Exclusion Criteria (Dose Escalation and Dose Expansion):

- For NSCLC patients, a targetable mutation in EGFR, or targetable rearrangement involving ALK or ROS1.

- Investigational agent or anticancer therapy within 5 half-lives or 2 weeks (14 days) prior to planned start of LOXO-292.

- Major surgery (excluding placement of vascular access) within 4 weeks prior to planned start of LOXO-292.

- Radiotherapy with a limited field of radiation for palliation within 1 week of planned start of LOXO-292, with the exception of patients receiving radiation to more than 30% of the bone marrow or with a wide field of radiation, which must be completed at least 4 weeks prior to the first dose of study treatment.

- Symptomatic primary CNS tumor or metastases (stable CNS tumor/metastases is allowed).

- Clinically significant active cardiovascular disease or history of myocardial infarction within 6 months prior to planned start of LOXO-292 or prolongation of the QT interval corrected (QTcF) > 470 msec.

- Required treatment with certain strong CYP3A4 inhibitors or inducers.

Sex/Gender

All

Ages

12 Years to N/A

Accepts Healthy Volunteers

No

Contacts

Patient Advocacy   855-RET-4-292 (855-738-4292)   clinicaltrials@loxoncology.com

Small Media Interventions to Increase Colorectal Cancer Screening Among Chinese Americans

Study ID:

NCT03174444

Sponsor:

University of California, San Francisco

Information provided by (Responsible Party):

University of California, San Francisco (University of California, San Francisco)

Tracking Information

▦ **First Submitted Date**

May 30, 2017

▦ **Start Date**

August 15, 2017

▦ **Primary Completion Date**

November 30, 2017

▦ **Last Update Posted Date**

October 6, 2017

▦ **Current Primary Outcome Measures**

Colorectal Cancer Screening[Time Frame: 9 months]
    Up-to-date receipt of any colorectal cancer screening

Descriptive Information

▦ **Offical Title**

Small Media Interventions to Increase Colorectal Cancer Screening Among Chinese Americans

▦ **Brief Summary**

There have been few studies of small media interventions to promote colorectal cancer screening among Chinese Americans. Based on the results of strong preliminary studies on the promotion of colorectal cancer screening among Asian American populations, this community-academic research team propose to develop a culturally and linguistically appropriate traditional small media print brochure and a novel small media electronic audio-visual application accessible through mobile applications and through a website to promote CRC screening in English, Cantonese, and Mandarin. The team will test in a randomized controlled trial in 3 healthcare systems the efficacy of a combination of these small media interventions and a mailed patient reminder compared to usual care on increasing CRC screening among Chinese American patients.

▦ **Detailed Description**

Chinese Americans are the largest group of Asian Americans, the fastest growing racial population in the U.S. Colorectal cancer is the second most common cancer among Chinese Americans. Screening reduces colorectal cancer mortality and is cost-effective but remains underutilized. Asian Americans and Chinese Americans are less likely than non-Hispanic whites to be screened for colorectal cancer. Factors associated with lack of screening among Asian Americans include recent immigration, lower education, lower English fluency, lack of knowledge, patient-physician language discordance, and lack of physician recommendation.

Although small media and client-reminders are effective in increasing colorectal cancer screening in the general population, no randomized controlled trial has assessed the effect of such interventions on Chinese Americans, particularly those who are limited English proficient. Building on an established community-based participatory research network and strong preliminary studies, the team propose to develop a culturally and linguistically appropriate booklet (small print media) and an audio-visual application accessible through mobile devices and a website (small electronic media) to promote screening. Through an innovative approach that links community organizations that have cultural and linguistic expertise to healthcare systems that have many Chinese American patients, the investigators will test the effect of combining these small media materials and a mailed patient reminder on the rate of screening for colorectal cancer screening among Chinese Americans in this Small Media Interventions for Limited English Speakers (SMILES). The investigators have developed English and Chinese (Cantonese and Mandarin) small print and electronic media materials to promote colorectal cancer screening among Chinese Americans. This RCT will compare the efficacy of a combination of mailed patient reminder and small print and electronic media versus usual care among Chinese American patients who are not up-to-date for colorectal cancer screening recruited from 3 healthcare systems in a randomized controlled trial.

▦ **Study Type**

Interventional

▦ **Study Phase**

N/A

- Condition
  - Colorectal Cancer
  - Cancer Screening
- Intervention

  Behavioral: Small Media

  Bilingual brochures and access to bilingual website

- Study Arms

  Experimental: Small Media

  Participants receive bilingual brochures and access to bilingual website about colorectal cancer screening.

  No Intervention: Control

  Participants receive no information about colorectal cancer screening from the study during the intervention period, but may receive usual care from health care provider.

Recruitment Information

- Recruitment Status

  Recruiting

- Estimated Enrollment

  2000

- Eligibility Criteria

  Inclusion Criteria:
  - Not up-to-date for colorectal cancer screening; self-identified as Chinese or Chinese American, or Asian who speak Chinese, or Asian born in China.

  Exclusion Criteria:
  - Not eligible for colorectal cancer screening for any reason.

- Sex/Gender

  All

- Ages

  50 Years to 75 Years

- Accepts Healthy Volunteers

  Accepts Healthy Volunteers

- Contacts

  Tung Nguyen, MD   415-514-8659   Tung.Nguyen@ucsf.edu

- Completion Date

  September 30, 2018

- Primary Completion Date

  November 30, 2017

Evaluation of Pathway Modulation by Raf, MEK, & Kinase Inhibitors

Study ID:

NCT03176485

Information provided by (Responsible Party):

University of Arizona (University of Arizona)

Sponsor:

University of Arizona

Tracking Information

- First Submitted Date

  June 1, 2017

- Start Date

  October 17, 2014

Primary Completion Date

October 15, 2017

Last Update Posted Date

June 5, 2017

Current Primary Outcome Measures

Modulatory effect of systemic Raf inhibition in the MEK/Erk and PI3 /AKT/mTOR pathways in patients undergoing targeted therapy for metastatic disease[Time Frame: 2 months]

> The primary endpoint of the study is to evaluate the modulatory effect of systemic Raf inhibition in the MEK/Erk and PI3 / AKT/mTOR pathways in patients undergoing targeted therapy for metastatic disease. Changes in relevant proteins will be evaluated using a combined protein expression methodology that in includes immunohistochemistry (IHC) and reverse phase protein microarray (RPPA) technology. The primary endpoint of this study will be assessed in normal skin and skin acutely exposed to solar simulated light.

Current Secondary Outcome Measures

Downstream modulation of direct Ras and MEK inhibition in human keratinocytes and melanocytes following acute solar simulated light exposure in the presence of metastatic disease treatment with Tyrosine kinase and MEK inhibitors.[Time Frame: 2 months]

> The modulatory effect will be evaluated using IHC and RPPA technology.

Modulatory effect of systemic Raf inhibition in the MEK/Erk and PI3 /AKT/mTOR pathways in eligible melanocytic nevi.[Time Frame: 2 months]

> Correlate the type and severity of cutaneous squamous cell carcinoma development in patients treated with BRaf inhibitors and the modulatory profile identified in the proposed primary endpoint.[Time Frame: 2 months]

> Safety of performing solar simulated light studies in patients undergoing Ras inhibition for metastatic disease.[Time Frame: 2 months]

> Modulatory effect of Ras inhibition in Epidermal Growth Factor Receptor (EGFR) and Activating Protein-1 (AP1) signaling pathways (IHC and RPPA).[Time Frame: 2 months]

Descriptive Information

Offical Title

Pilot Study to Evaluate the Signaling Pathway Modulation Demonstrated by Raf, MEK, and Kinase Inhibitors In Human Skin With or Without Solar Simulated Light

Brief Summary

This is a pilot study designed to evaluate the cutaneous effect of systemic inhibition of the tyrosine kinase pathway in the presence or absence of solar simulated light exposure.

A maximum of 45 subjects will be accrued into the overall study we anticipate approximately 25 patients in the Raf inhibitor group and 10 patients each into the Tyrosine Kinase and MEK inhibitor arms of the study.

Detailed Description

The study will evaluate the modulatory effect of systemic Raf inhibition in the MEK/ERK and PI3 /Akt/mTOR pathways in patients undergoing targeted therapy for metastatic disease.

Changes in relevant proteins will be evaluated using a combined protein expression methodology that in includes immunohistochemistry (IHC) and reverse phase protein microarray (RPPA) technology.

The primary endpoint of this study will be assessed in normal skin and skin acutely exposed to solar simulated light

Study Type

Interventional

Study Phase

N/A

Condition

- Metastatic Cancer
- Melanoma
- Colon Cancer
- Differentiated Thyroid Cancer
- Hepatocellular Carcinoma
- Renal Cell Carcinoma
- Metastatic Melanoma
- HCC
- Metastatic Colon Cancer

■ **Intervention**

Other: Solar Simulator

A Multiport UV Solar Simulator Model 600 (Solar Light Co., Inc., Philadelphia, PA) will be used to administer Solar Simulated Light (SSL) exposures to formerly unexposed buttock skin.The device is equipped with six 8mm liquid light guides (LLG), allowing for 6 simultaneously conducted exposures.A large 3x2 endplate places the LLGs several centimeters apart and is specifically designed for Sun Protection Factor (SPF) and photo patch testing. The dose of emission from each LLG can be precisely regulated and the spectrum of emission can be limited to UVA (320-390 nm) or UVB+UVA (290-390 nm). The operator can select between UVA only and a combined Ultraviolet-A (UVA)/ Ultraviolet-B (UVB) spectrum by placement of an optical filter. The spectral output (indicated below) follows the distribution of sunlight from 290 to 390 nm.

Other Names:

Multiport UV Solar Simulator Model 60

■ **Study Arms**

Experimental: ArmA: With Solar Simulated Light Exposure

Experimental: ArmB: With Solar Simulated Light Exposure (Vemurafenib/Dabraf)

Subjects in this study arm undergo the same procedures as Arm A, with the addition of a blood test for the presence of porphyrins

No Intervention: ArmC: Without Solar Simulated Light Exposure

Recruitment Information

■ **Recruitment Status**

Recruiting

■ **Estimated Enrollment**

45

■ **Completion Date**

April 15, 2018

■ **Primary Completion Date**

October 15, 2017

■ **Eligibility Criteria**

Inclusion Criteria:

- Subjects who have not yet initiated but plan to undergo dosing with a Tyrosine Kinase inhibitor (TKI) or Raf inhibitor, either alone or with a MEK inhibitor, for treatment of metastatic melanoma, colon cancer, hepatic cell carcinoma, or thyroid cancer.
- Individuals with normal skin and Fitzpatrick skin type II, III or IV.
- Individuals who are willing to limit sun exposure to the body during the study period, and who agree to wear protective clothing and SPF 50 broad spectrum sunscreen or sunblock on exposed skin when they are outdoors.
- Individuals who have the ability to understand and willingness to sign an informed consent before initiation of study procedures, after the nature of the study is explained to them and they have asked any questions.
- Individuals with a Karnofsky Performance Status of at least 80%.

Exclusion Criteria:

- Individuals with any inflammation or irritation of the skin at the test area (buttocks), or any skin conditions felt by the study physician to contraindicate enrollment.
- Individuals with a history of any skin cancer, melanocytic lesions, actinic keratoses or actinic damage in the test area are ineligible. History of such conditions at a body site other than the test area is not exclusionary if in the opinion of the study physician it will not pose a risk to the subject.
- Individuals who are immunosuppressed by virtue of medication or disease, as determined by the examining study physician. This includes AIDS patients and subjects taking oral steroids.
- Individuals with active infection, psychiatric illness, or other situations that in the opinion of the study physician limit compliance or interfere with the study regimen.
- Individuals with a history of photosensitive diseases including, but not limited to, Lupus Erythematosus, pseudoporphyria, or other diseases that in the opinion of the study physician would pose a risk to the subject or interfere with the study.
- Individuals who have used photosensitizing drugs within the last 30 days prior to study enrollment, or who will be using a photosensitizing drug during the time of the study.
- Individuals who have used any topical medication other than emollients on the test area within 30 days prior to study enrollment.
- Individuals who have used retinoids, steroids, 5-fluorouracil, Levulan, Vaniqua (eflornithine), Solaraze, or Imiquimod (Aldara®) anywhere on the body within 30 days prior to enrollment.
- Individuals must not take mega-doses of vitamins. Mega-doses are defined as more than 5 capsules of standard multivitamins daily or more than the Tolerable Upper Intake Levels of Vitamins, as defined by the Institute of Medicine, National Academy of Sciences. Such vitamin therapy must be discontinued at least 30 days prior to study entry.
- Individuals with a history of natural or artificial sun exposure to the buttocks within 30 days of study participation.
- Individuals with Fitzpatrick skin type I
- Individuals with Fitzpatrick skin type V or VI

- Individuals enrolled in or who plan to enroll in a clinical intervention trial. There must be a 30-day period between completing a previous study and enrolling in this study. The Principal Investigator will have the option to consider an exception for patients on drugs of interest for the purpose of this study.
- Individuals with a known allergy to lidocaine.

Sex/Gender

All

Ages

18 Years to N/A

Accepts Healthy Volunteers

No

Contacts

Clara Curiel-Lewandroski   ccuriel@email.arizona.edu

A Study of BMS-813160 in Combination With Chemotherapy or Nivolumab in Patients With Advanced Solid Tumors

Study ID:

NCT03184870

Sponsor:

Bristol-Myers Squibb

Information provided by (Responsible Party):

Bristol-Myers Squibb (Bristol-Myers Squibb)

Tracking Information

First Submitted Date

June 9, 2017

Start Date

August 4, 2017

Primary Completion Date

March 8, 2021

Last Update Posted Date

January 23, 2018

Current Primary Outcome Measures

Adverse events (AEs)[Time Frame: Approximately 4 years]
    Measured by incidence of AEs

Serious adverse events (SAEs)[Time Frame: Approximately 4 years]
    Measured by incidence of SAEs

AEs meeting protocol-defined dose limiting toxicity criteria[Time Frame: Approximately 6 months]
    Measured by incidence of AEs that meet the protocol-defined dose limiting toxicity criteria

AEs leading to discontinuation[Time Frame: Approximately 4 years]
    Measured by incidence of AEs leading to discontinuation

Death[Time Frame: Approximately 4 years]
    Measured by incidence of deaths

Incidence of laboratory abnormalities[Time Frame: Approximately 4 years]
    Measured by any laboratory test result that is clinically significant or meets the definition of an SAE, any laboratory test result abnormality that required the patient to have study treatment discontinued or interrupted, or any laboratory test result abnormality that required the participant to receive specific corrective therapy

Electrocardiogram (ECG)[Time Frame: Approximately 4 years]
    ECGs will be evaluated by the investigator for any clinically significant changes or for changes meeting dose modifying criteria.

Summary measures of vital signs[Time Frame: Approximately 4 years]

Including weight, body temperature, respiratory rate, pulse oximetry, seated blood pressure and heart rate.

Objective response rate (ORR)[Time Frame: Approximately 4 years]

ORR is defined as the proportion of all treated participants whose Best overall response (BOR) is either complete response or partial response. BOR for a participant will be assessed per Response Evaluation Criteria in Solid Tumors (RECIST) v1.1 by investigator

Median duration of response (DOR)[Time Frame: Approximately 4 years]

DOR for a participant with a BOR of CR or PR, is defined as the time between the date of first response and the date of the first objectively documented tumor progression per RECIST v1.1 or death, whichever occurs first

Progression free survival (PFS) rate[Time Frame: At 24 weeks]

PFS for a participant is defined as the time from the first dosing date to the date of first objectively documented disease progression or death due to any cause, whichever occurs first

Current Secondary Outcome Measures

Maximum observed plasma concentration (Cmax)[Time Frame: Approximately 4 years]
Summary statistics: geometric means and coefficients of variation

Time of maximum observed plasma concentration (Tmax)[Time Frame: Approximately 4 years]
Summary statistics: medians and ranges

Trough observed plasma concentration (Ctrough)[Time Frame: Approximately 4 years]
Summary statistics to assess attainment of steady state: geometric means and coefficients of variation; plots vs time by dose

Observed plasma concentration at the end of the dosing interval (Ctau)[Time Frame: Approximately 4 years]
Summary statistics: geometric means and coefficients of variation

Area under the concentration-time curve from time 0 to 8 hours postdose [AUC(0-8)][Time Frame: Approximately 4 years]
Summary statistics: geometric means and coefficients of variation

Area under the concentration-time curve in one dosing interval [AUC(TAU)][Time Frame: Approximately 4 years]
Summary statistics: geometric means and coefficients of variation

Apparent total body clearance (CLT/F)[Time Frame: Approximately 4 years]
Summary statistics: geometric means and coefficients of variation

Accumulation index, calculated based on ratio of AUC(TAU) and Cmax at steady state to after the first dose (AI)[Time Frame: Approximately 4 years]
Summary statistics: geometric means and coefficients of variation

Renal clearance (CLR)[Time Frame: Approximately 4 years]
Summary statistics: geometric means and coefficients of variation

Percent urinary recovery over 24 hours corrected for molecular weight (%UR)[Time Frame: Approximately 4 years]
Summary statistics: geometric means and coefficients of variation

Ratio of metabolite Cmax to parent Cmax, corrected for molecular (MR   Cmax)[Time Frame: Approximately 4 years]
Summary statistics: geometric means and coefficients of variation

Ratio of metabolite AUC(TAU) to parent AUC(TAU), corrected for molecular weight [MR   AUC(TAU)][Time Frame: Approximately 4 years]
Summary statistics: geometric means and coefficients of variation

Frequency of positive anti-drug antibody (ADA) to nivolumab during combination therapy[Time Frame: Approximately 4 years]
Frequency distribution of baseline ADA-positive participants and ADA-positive participants after initiation of the treatment

Decrease in regulatory T cells (Treg) & tumor-associated macrophages (TAM) in tumor samples[Time Frame: Approximately 4 years]
Examination of tumor-associated immune cells and microenvironment, through proteomics

Descriptive Information

Offical Title

A Phase 1b/2 Study of BMS-813160 in Combination With Chemotherapy or Nivolumab in Patients With Advanced Solid Tumors

Brief Summary

This study will evaluate the safety profile, tolerability, PK, PD, and preliminary efficacy of BMS-813160 in combination with either chemotherapy or nivolumab in participants with metastatic colorectal and pancreatic cancers.

- **Study Type**

  Interventional
- **Study Phase**

  Phase 1/Phase 2
- **Condition**
  - Colorectal Cancer
  - Pancreatic Cancer
- **Intervention**

  Drug: BMS-813160

    specified dose on specified days

    Biological: Nivolumab

  specified dose on specified days

  Other Names:

    Opdivo

    BMS-936558

    Drug: Nab-paclitaxel

    chemotherapy regimen

  Drug: Gemcitabine
    chemotherapy regimen

  Drug: 5-fluorouracil (5-FU)
    chemotherapy regimen

  Drug: Leucovorin
    chemotherapy regimen

  Drug: Irinotecan
    chemotherapy regimen
- **Study Arms**

  Experimental: Combination Therapy 1
    BMS-813160 with 5-fluorouracil (5-FU), leucovorin containing regimens in combination with irinotecan

  Experimental: Combination Therapy 2
    BMS-813160, nab/paclitaxel and gemcitabine

  Experimental: Combination Therapy 3
    BMS-813160 and Nivolumab

  Experimental: Monotherapy
    BMS-813160 Monotherapy

Recruitment Information

- **Recruitment Status**

  Recruiting
- **Estimated Enrollment**

  260
- **Completion Date**

  March 8, 2021
- **Primary Completion Date**

  March 8, 2021
- **Eligibility Criteria**

  For more information regarding Bristol-Myers Squibb Clinical Trial participation, please visit www.BMSStudyConnect.com
  Inclusion Criteria:
  - Participants must have metastatic colorectal or pancreatic cancer
  - Eastern Cooperative Oncology Group (ECOG) performance status of ≤1
  - Ability to swallow pills or capsules
  - All participants will be required to undergo mandatory pre and on-treatment biopsies
  - Adequate marrow function

- Adequate other organ functions
- Ability to comply with study visits, treatment, procedures, PK and PD sample collection, and required study follow-up

Exclusion Criteria:

- Histology other than adenocarcinoma (neuroendocrine or acinar cell)
- Suspected, known, or progressive CNS metastases (Imaging required only if participants are symptomatic)
- Participants with active, known or suspected autoimmune disease
- Participants with a condition requiring systemic treatment with either corticosteroids (> 10 mg daily prednisone equivalents) or other immunosuppressive medications within 14 days of study treatment administration
- Interstitial lung disease that is symptomatic or may interfere with the detection or management of suspected treatment-related pulmonary toxicity
- Prior treatment with CCR2 and/or CCR5 inhibitors
- History of allergy to study treatments or any of its components of the study arm that participant is enrolling

Other protocol defined inclusion/exclusion criteria could apply

▨ **Sex/Gender**

All

▨ **Ages**

18 Years to N/A

▨ **Accepts Healthy Volunteers**

No

▨ **Contacts**

Recruiting sites have contact information. Please contact the sites directly. If there is no contact information.   please email: Clinical.Trials@bms.com

First line of the email MUST contain NCT # and Site #.

Diet and Exercise After Pancreatic Cancer

Study ID:

NCT03187028

Sponsor:

University of Alabama at Birmingham

Information provided by (Responsible Party):

University of Alabama at Birmingham (University of Alabama at Birmingham)

Tracking Information

▨ **First Submitted Date**

May 24, 2017

▨ **Start Date**

August 3, 2017

▨ **Primary Completion Date**

August 31, 2018

▨ **Last Update Posted Date**

January 3, 2018

▨ **Current Primary Outcome Measures**

- Feasibility Recruitment[Time Frame: Baseline]
  Number of participants excluded or not agreeing to participate

- Feasibility Adherence to study protocol activities[Time Frame: Throughout 6 month study period]
  Feasibility measure (e.g. percent of assessments completed, percent of counseling sessions completed, etc.)

- Feasibility Attrition rates[Time Frame: Throughout 6 month study period]
  Number of participants who dropout or are withdrawn

- Feasibility Adverse events[Time Frame: Throughout 6 month study period]
  Recorded by staff

- Feasibility Participant satisfaction[Time Frame: At conclusion of 6 month study period]
  Survey

Current Secondary Outcome Measures

Eastern Cooperative Oncology Group (ECOG) performance status[Time Frame: At 4 timepoints during the 6 month study (pre-surgery if applicable, post-surgery/prior to starting the intervention, 3 months and 6 months)]

Preliminary effect size

Quality of life (assessed using the Functional Assessment of Cancer Therapy index)[Time Frame: At 4 timepoints during the 6 month study (pre-surgery if applicable, post-surgery/prior to starting the intervention, 3 months and 6 months)]

Preliminary effect size

Objective physical functioning[Time Frame: At 4 timepoints during the 6 month study (pre-surgery if applicable, post-surgery/prior to starting the intervention, 3 months and 6 months)]

Preliminary effect size

CA 19-9 (tumor markers)[Time Frame: At 4 timepoints during the 6 month study (pre-surgery if applicable, post-surgery/prior to starting the intervention, 3 months and 6 months)]

Exploratory data related to within and between group (diet and diet+exercise) differences

Completion of pancreatic cancer treatment[Time Frame: At conclusion of 6 month study]

Exploratory data related to within and between group (diet and diet+exercise) differences

Survival rates[Time Frame: At conclusion of 6 month study]

Exploratory data related to within and between group (diet and diet+exercise) differences

Pancreatic cancer recurrence rates[Time Frame: At conclusion of 6 month study]

Exploratory data related to within and between group (diet and diet+exercise) differences

Prognostic blood cytokine biomarkers[Time Frame: At 4 timepoints during the 6 month study (pre-surgery if applicable, post-surgery/prior to starting the intervention, 3 months and 6 months)]

Exploratory data related to within and between group (diet and diet+exercise) differences

Prognostic blood tumor immunity biomarkers[Time Frame: At 4 timepoints during the 6 month study (pre-surgery if applicable, post-surgery/prior to starting the intervention, 3 months and 6 months)]

Exploratory data related to within and between group (diet and diet+exercise) differences

Wearable activity monitor (weekly minutes of physical activity)[Time Frame: At 4 timepoints during the 6 month study (pre-surgery if applicable, post-surgery/prior to starting the intervention, 3 months and 6 months)]

Exploratory data related to within and between group (diet and diet+exercise) differences

Descriptive Information

Offical Title

Diet and Exercise After Pancreatic Cancer: Clinical and Functional Outcomes (Non Canonical WNT Signaling in Colorectal Cancer)

Brief Summary

Determine feasibility of a randomized controlled trial (RCT) in pancreatic cancer patients comparing the effects of diet alone vs. diet+exercise on functional and clinical outcomes.

Detailed Description

Pancreatic cancer causes significant side effects and poorer health-related quality of life (QOL), as well as a 5-year survival rate of only 6%. Importantly, the reduction in physical functioning caused by this cancer and its therapies is associated with higher mortality risk. Although multiple studies in more prevalent cancer types support exercise benefits (e.g., improved physical functioning), data cannot be generalized from one cancer type to another. Little is known about exercise feasibility and benefits in pancreatic cancer patients, and no data regarding potential mechanistic outcomes that may explain the link between poor physical performance status and cancer survival have been reported. We will enroll 20 patients with pancreatic adenocarcinoma who are expected to undergo surgical resection or who are within 3 years of surgical resection, in a pilot project involving a 6-month home-based lifestyle intervention (diet along versus diet+exercise). Research assessments will be done pre-surgery (if applicable), post-surgery (and prior to starting the intervention), 3 months, and 6 months post-surgery. Intervention counseling will be delivered using visual communication (e.g., Skype). Participants will be provided a computer tablet for the intervention with participants randomized to receive exercise counseling also receiving a fitness bracelet to facilitate counseling by the certified Cancer Exercise Trainer. Our primary study aim is to determine feasibility of a randomized controlled trial (RCT) in pancreatic cancer patients comparing the effects of diet alone with diet+exercise on pancreatic cancer-related functional and disease outcomes; feasibility measures include recruitment, retention, intervention adherence, assessment completion, adverse events, and participant satisfaction. Our secondary study aim is to determine the effect of diet+exercise compared with diet alone on physical functioning and QOL. Also, we will draw and store blood samples so that additional funds can be requested to test intervention effects on biomarkers of cancer risk (e.g., tumor immunity, inflammatory cytokines, etc.). The goal of the study is to advance the exercise oncology field into an understudied cancer type and develop an intervention that will improve the survivorship care of pancreatic cancer patients through distance-delivered counseling methods.

Study Type

Interventional

Study Phase

N/A

Condition

- Pancreatic Cancer

Intervention

Behavioral: Diet Only

Diet counseling will be delivered using visual communication (e.g., Skype). Participants will be provided a computer tablet for the intervention with participants randomized to receive diet counseling.

Behavioral: Diet + Exercise

Diet and exercise counseling will be delivered using visual communication (e.g., Skype). Participants will be provided a computer tablet for the intervention with participants randomized to receive diet and exercise counseling.

Study Arms

Active Comparator: Diet only

Diet counseling will be delivered using visual communication (e.g., Skype). Participants will be provided a computer tablet for the intervention with participants randomized to receive diet counseling.

Experimental: Diet + Exercise

Diet and exercise counseling will be delivered using visual communication (e.g., Skype). Participants will be provided a computer tablet for the intervention with participants randomized to receive diet and exercise counseling also receiving a fitness bracelet to facilitate counseling by the certified Cancer Exercise Trainer.

Recruitment Information

Recruitment Status

Recruiting

Estimated Enrollment

50

Completion Date

August 31, 2019

Primary Completion Date

August 31, 2018

Eligibility Criteria

Inclusion Criteria:

- adult 18 years of age or older with resectable pancreatic adenocarcinoma for whom surgery is planned (includes "borderline resectable" if deemed appropriate by surgical investigators) or has occurred within the past 3 years
- English speaking
- Eastern Cooperative Technology Group (ECOG) performance status of 0,1 or 2.
- able to ambulate without assistance
- able to obtain medical clearance

Exclusion Criteria:

- pancreatic cancer recurrence
- dementia or organic brain syndrome
- severe emotional distress
- medical, psychological or social characteristic that would interfere with the ability to fully participate in program activities and assessments
- another diagnosis of cancer in the past 5 years (not including skin or cervical cancer in situ).
- oncologist refuses to allow screening for possible study participation
- current participation in another exercise trial

Sex/Gender

All

Ages

18 Years to N/A

Accepts Healthy Volunteers

No

■ Contacts

Laura Q Rogers, MD, MPH   205-975-1667   rogersl@uab.edu

David Bryan, MS   205-975-1247   dbryan@uab.edu

Implementing Preemptive Pharmacogenomic Testing for Colorectal Cancer Patients in a Community Oncology Clinic

Study ID:

NCT03187184

Sponsor:

Essentia Health

Information provided by (Responsible Party):

Essentia Health (Essentia Health)

Tracking Information

■ **First Submitted Date**

June 12, 2017

■ **Start Date**

May 20, 2017

■ **Primary Completion Date**

May 20, 2018

■ **Last Update Posted Date**

October 10, 2017

■ **Current Primary Outcome Measures**

PGx Test Interpretation[Time Frame: 10 days]

Proportion of patients with pharmacogenomic testing completed and interpreted prior to starting chemotherapy.

■ **Current Secondary Outcome Measures**

Allele Frequency[Time Frame: 10 days]

The proportion of Essentia Health patients with metabolic enzyme alleles that could impact chemotherapy dosing will be reported. Descriptive statistics, proportion and 95% confidence interval (95% CI), will be reported.

Chemotherapy Toxicity[Time Frame: 3 months]

Toxicity will be reported for all patients and the sub-groups of patients with and without the metabolic enzyme alleles that could impact chemotherapy. Descriptive statistics, proportion and 95% confidence interval (95% CI), will be reported. Depending upon the sample sizes involved, either the chi-square test or Fisher's exact test will be used to compare the sub-groups.

Descriptive Information

■ **Offical Title**

Implementing Preemptive Pharmacogenomic Testing for Colorectal Cancer Patients in a Community Oncology Clinic

■ **Brief Summary**

Pharmacogenomics (PGx) studies the interactions between an individuals genes and medications. PGx testing identifies genes within an individual that may affect treatment, efficacy, and toxicity of drugs. With improvements in testing speed, accuracy and cost, it is now possible to perform PGx testing in cancer patients prior to starting chemotherapy. The test results may help a physician personalize chemotherapy dosing. The goal of this study is to determine if PGx testing using the OneOme® Rightmed test is feasible in a community oncology clinic to guide treatment prior to starting chemotherapy. The study will also gather data regarding the frequency of genes within the local population as well as the impact of testing on chemotherapy doses.

■ **Detailed Description**

The goal of personalized medicine is to tailor therapies to an individual patient with a goal of maximizing benefit and minimizing treatment related side effects. Inter-individual variability in metabolic enzymes can have a significant impact on cancer therapies. Pharmacogenomics (PGx) studies the interactions between drugs and genes, and pharmacogenomic screening tests can assess for genetic variations among individuals to personalize medicine. PGx testing identifies genes within an individual that may affect treatment, efficacy, and toxicity of drugs. PGx screening prior to chemotherapy would help identify patients with genetic polymorphisms that are at increased risk for drug toxicity and would benefit from genetic-guided dosing, resulting in decreased risk of adverse events (AEs) related to the chemotherapy. PGx testing is not routinely used in community-based oncology practices. The cost of testing as well as lengthy waits for results have limited routine use of this testing. Advances in testing have reached the point where routine preemptive testing could benefit patients with newly diagnosed cancer.

PGx testing evaluating a large number of metabolic enzymes is now commercially available. OneOme RightMed® is a privately owned company developed by doctors and scientists at Mayo Clinic with a mission "to provide the most cost-effective, comprehensive, personalized, pharmacogenomics analysis integrated into everyday clinical care." OneOme RightMed® currently tests for 22 genes that impact over 340 drugs used in multiple fields of medicine, including oncology. The drugs tested for by OneOme RightMed® were generated from practice guidelines and the FDA's guidelines for genotyping, and drugs with published, clinical evidence supporting genotyping. With developments in sequencing technology, comprehensive PGx testing can now be completed for a modest cost. Testing is done using a prepackaged OneOme RightMed® kit to collect a buccal swab. OneOme RightMed® PGx test uses a DNA Genotek ORAcollect OC-100 buccal swab kit to extract DNA, which is then analyzed through polymerase chain reaction (PCR). The results are available in 10 or less calendar days to the provider and/or pharmacist. The report provides "genotype-derived recommendations" with additional quick references for medication dosing guidance.

Despite clear clinical implications, incorporation of PGx testing has historically been challenging due to potential delay in initiation of therapy and uncertainty of clinical and economic benefits. However, in the past decades, clinically actionable gene-drug interactions, such as the polymorphisms discussed above, have been identified. Additionally, the availability of high-quality genotyping in a timely manner with lower costs makes PGx testing feasible. Pilot studies implementing PGx testing have been conducted at academic centers.10,13-15 Though the knowledge gained from those studies enhanced their ability to implement PGx testing, pilot studies implementing PGx testing in a community-based health care setting in oncology treatment have not been conducted, to the best of our knowledge. Therefore, our pilot study would evaluate the feasibility of implementing PGx testing in routine oncology treatment at a community-based health care center. CRC is a common cancer and the drugs used in treating CRC are affected by PGx. Thus, CRC represents an ideal situation to evaluate the feasibility of routine preemptive PGx testing. While this study represents an initial pilot feasibility study, our ultimate goal is to evaluate the benefits of PGx in the community setting in regards to reduction of toxicity, improved cancer outcomes, and cost savings.

Primary Objective

1. To determine if preemptive PGx testing is feasible in a community oncology clinic.

Secondary Objective

1. To gather pilot data on the proportion of Essentia Health patients with metabolic enzyme alleles that could impact chemotherapy dosing.

2. To evaluate the impact of PGx guided chemotherapy dosing on toxicity.

3. To evaluate the cost-effectiveness of PGx testing in Essentia Health patients with colorectal cancer.

Eligible patients will have a histological diagnosis of colorectal cancer. The intent of the study is to enroll patients as quickly as possible once a decision has been made that a patient is a candidate for chemotherapy for stage 2-4 colorectal cancer. While many patients will be eligible for study participation at their initial consultation with medical oncology, it is also anticipated that some patients may need additional testing prior to eligibility. This would also include patients who have been followed in the medical oncology department that develop a new malignancy or have a recurrence. Patients must be enrolled to the study within 7 days of their initial consultation, or within 7 days of a physician visit, after any additional tests or biopsies have been completed, when the patient is felt to be a suitable candidate for chemotherapy. After obtaining informed consent from eligible patients, a commercially available pharmacogenomics panel, the OneOme RightMed® pharmacogenomic test, will be ordered. Patients will not be responsible for the cost of PGx testing. The study will not prescribe any specific chemotherapy regimens. All decisions regarding the clinical care of the patient will be made by the treating physician. Treatment will not be delayed to wait for PGx results per study protocol, however the treating physician may elect to do so. When PGx test results are available, results will be interpreted by the Oncology Lead Pharmacist at Essentia Health, and recommendations will be made to the treating physician regarding potential chemotherapy does adjustments. The treating physician will have the ultimate decision as to whether chemotherapy dose adjustments are done as a result of PGx testing. Patients will be seen by study staff prior to initiating chemotherapy, and after chemotherapy cycles 1-3 to assess for toxicity and to determine if any dose modifications were done by the treating physician.

Patient demographic data will be collected at baseline. Once patients start chemotherapy, treatment toxicity data will be collected prior to chemotherapy and after cycles 1-3. For patients receiving continuous chemotherapy such as infusional 5-FU or capecitabine concurrent with radiation, a cycle will be defined as 2 weeks. Toxicity data will be collected following Common Terminology Criteria for Adverse Events (CTCAE) v4.0. Data will be collected for common side effects associated with typical colorectal cancer chemotherapy regimens including, leukopenia, neutropenia, anemia, thrombocytopenia, fatigue, nausea/vomiting, diarrhea, mucositis, hand-foot syndrome, peripheral neuropathy, and abdominal pain. Other toxicities identified by study staff will be collected as well. Chemotherapy dose modifications made by the treating physician will be collected for chemotherapy cycles 1-3.

When PGx results are available, study staff will alert the Oncology Lead Pharmacist who will evaluate the results and make recommendations to the treating physician regarding suggested dose modification to the planned chemotherapy regimen. The primary assessment of the analysis will focus on UGT1A1 and DPD.

In cases where the suggested dose modifications are unclear or the results are atypical, the Lead Pharmacist will consult with OneOme RightMed® staff to determine appropriate recommendations. The Lead Pharmacist will also review each patient's current medication list and identify if there are any additional medication concerns related to evaluated genes other than UGT1A1 and DPYD. Any identified additional concerns will be noted on the Results Interpretation and Impact form. Once the form is complete, a copy will be forwarded to the treating physician who will then complete the form to indicate whether any changes to the planned chemotherapy regimen will be made.

Study Type

Interventional

Study Phase

N/A

- Condition
  - Colorectal Cancer
- Intervention

  Device: OneOme RightMed®

  OneOme RightMed® currently tests for 22 genes that impact over 340 drugs used in multiple fields of medicine, including oncology. The drugs tested for by OneOme RightMed® were generated from practice guidelines and the FDA's guidelines for genotyping, and drugs with published, clinical evidence supporting genotyping. Testing is done using a prepackaged OneOme RightMed® kit to collect a buccal swab. OneOme RightMed® PGx test uses a DNA Genotek ORAcollect OC-100 buccal swab kit to extract DNA, which is then analyzed through polymerase chain reaction (PCR).

- Study Arms

  Experimental: OneOme RightMed® Test

  OneOme RightMed® currently tests for 22 genes that impact over 340 drugs used in multiple fields of medicine, including oncology. The drugs tested for by OneOme RightMed® were generated from practice guidelines and the FDA's guidelines for genotyping, and drugs with published, clinical evidence supporting genotyping. Testing is done using a prepackaged OneOme RightMed® kit to collect a buccal swab. OneOme RightMed® PGx test uses a DNA Genotek ORAcollect OC-100 buccal swab kit to extract DNA, which is then analyzed through polymerase chain reaction (PCR).

Recruitment Information

- Recruitment Status

  Recruiting

- Estimated Enrollment

  40

- Completion Date

  December 30, 2018

- Primary Completion Date

  May 20, 2018

- Eligibility Criteria

  Inclusion Criteria:

  1. Histologically proven Stage 2-4 colon or rectal adenocarcinoma with an anticipated need for chemotherapy, which may include neoadjuvant, adjuvant or palliative treatment, and may include oral or intravenous chemotherapy.

  2. Adequate organ function and performance status to receive chemotherapy as determined by the treating physician.

  3. Age ≥ 18 years.

  4. Ability to understand and the willingness to sign a written informed consent documented.

  5. Patients must sign consent within 7 days of the physician visit for newly diagnosed or recurrent colorectal cancer when a patient is initially felt to be a candidate for chemotherapy.

  Exclusion Criteria:

  1. Patients received prior chemotherapy for colorectal cancer in the last 12 months.

  2. Patients received prior OneOme RightMed® pharmacogenomic testing.

- Sex/Gender

  All

- Ages

  18 Years to N/A

- Accepts Healthy Volunteers

  No

- Contacts

  Clinical Research Manager   218-786-1018   mlodozyniec.tammie@essentiahealth.org
  Bret Friday, MD   218-686-3625   bret.friday@essentiahealth.org

Study of Personalized Immunotherapy in Adults With Metastatic Colorectal Cancer

Study ID:

NCT03189030

Sponsor:

Aduro Biotech, Inc.

Information provided by (Responsible Party):

Aduro Biotech, Inc. (Aduro Biotech, Inc.)

Tracking Information

First Submitted Date

June 14, 2017

Start Date

May 2, 2017

Primary Completion Date

December 2020

Last Update Posted Date

January 18, 2018

Current Primary Outcome Measures

Incidence of Treatment-Emergent Adverse Events (Safety and Tolerability)[Time Frame: Through study completion, an average of 12 months]

Number of patients with treatment-related adverse events as assessed by CTCAE v 4.0

Descriptive Information

Offical Title

A Phase 1 Safety and Tolerability Study of Personalized Live, Attenuated, Double-Deleted Listeria Monocytogenes (pLADD) Immunotherapy in Adults With Metastatic Colorectal Cancer

Brief Summary

This study will evaluate the safety and tolerability of a personalized live, attenuated, double-deleted Listeria monocytogenes (pLADD) treatment in adults with metastatic colorectal cancer.

Detailed Description

This single arm study is designed to evaluate the safety and tolerability of a personalized treatment in adults with metastatic colorectal cancer by first analyzing the expression of tumor-associated antigens and then treating the patients with a personalized live, attenuated, double-deleted Listeria monocytogenes (pLADD)-based immunotherapy. pLADD is based on the attenuated form of Listeria monocytogenes that has been genetically modified to reduce its ability to cause disease, while maintaining its ability to stimulate a potent immune response. pLADD is manufactured using patient-specific antigens and is therefore individualized to each patient.

Study Type

Interventional

Study Phase

Phase 1

Condition

- Colorectal Neoplasms

Intervention

Biological: pLADD
   via IV infusion

Study Arms

Experimental: Treatment arm

pLADD treatment cycle is once every 3 weeks; starting dose 1×10^8 colony-forming units (CFU) administered IV over 1 hour, and if tolerated increasing to 1×10^9 CFU

Recruitment Information

Recruitment Status

Recruiting

Estimated Enrollment

15

Eligibility Criteria

Inclusion Criteria:

- metastatic colorectal cancer (mCRC) that is microsatellite stable (MSS)

Completion Date

December 2020

Primary Completion Date

December 2020

- able to provide adequate tumor tissue from at least 1 accessible tumor site
- completed or have developed intolerance to a course of oxaliplatinor irinotecan-based frontline therapy at Screening
- on maintenance standard-of-care chemotherapies or on treatment holiday
- Eastern Cooperative Oncology Group (ECOG) 0 or 1
- adequate organ function
- progression of disease at the time of Enrollment

Exclusion Criteria:

- BRAF V600E mutation
- known allergy to both penicillin and sulfa drugs
- implanted devices that cannot be easily removed
- immunodeficiency, immune compromised state or receiving immunosuppressive therapy

Sex/Gender

All

Ages

18 Years to N/A

Accepts Healthy Volunteers

No

Contacts

Flordeliza J Mendoza, CCRC   650-724-2056   flormend@stanford.edu

Administering Peripheral Blood Lymphocytes Transduced With a Murine T-Cell Receptor Recognizing the G12V Variant of Mutated RAS in HLA-A

Study ID:

NCT03190941

Sponsor:

National Cancer Institute (NCI)

Information provided by (Responsible Party):

National Institutes of Health Clinical Center (CC) (National Cancer Institute (NCI))

Tracking Information

First Submitted Date

June 16, 2017

Start Date

September 21, 2017

Primary Completion Date

December 1, 2022

Last Update Posted Date

February 2, 2018

Current Primary Outcome Measures

- Response rate[Time Frame: 6 weeks (+/2 weeks) after cell infusion, then at week 12, every 3 months x3, every 6 months x2 years.]

    Maximum Tolerated Dose[Time Frame: End of treatment]

Current Secondary Outcome Measures

Survival and persistence of mTCR gene-engineered cells.[Time Frame: approximately 4-5 years]

Descriptive Information

Offical Title

Phase I/II Study Administering Peripheral Blood Lymphocytes Transduced With a Murine T-Cell Receptor Recognizing the G12V Variant of Mutated RAS in HLA-A 1101 Patients

Brief Summary

Background:

A new cancer therapy involves taking white blood cells from a person, growing them in the lab, genetically modifying them, then giving them back to the person. This therapy is called gene transfer using anti-KRAS G12V mTCR cells.

Objective:

To see if anti-KRAS G12 V mTCR cells are safe and can shrink tumors.

Eligibility:

Adults at least 18 years old with cancer that has the KRAS G12V molecule on the surface of tumors.

Design:

In another protocol, participants will:

Be screened

Have cells harvested and grown

Have leukapheresis

In this protocol, participants will have the procedures below.

Participants will be admitted to the hospital.

Over 5 days, participants will get 2 chemotherapy medicines as an infusion via catheter in the upper chest.

A few days later, participants will get the anti-KRAS G12V mTCR cells via catheter.

For up to 3 days, participants will get a drug to make the cells active.

A day after getting the cells, participants will get a drug to increase their white blood cell count. This will be a shot or injection under the skin.

Participants will recover in the hospital for 1 2 weeks. They will have lab and blood tests.

Participants will take an antibiotic for at least 6 months.

Participants will have visits every few months for 2 years, and then as determined by their doctor.

Visits will be 1 2 days. They will include lab tests, imaging studies, and physical exam. Some visits may include leukapheresis or blood drawn.

Participants will have blood collected over several years.

Detailed Description

Background:

- We generated an HLA-A1101-restricted murine T-cell receptor (mTCR) that specifically recognizes the G12V-mutated variant of KRAS (and other RAS family genes), expressed by many human cancers and constructed a single retroviral vector that contains its alpha and beta chains that confers recognition of this antigen when transduced into PBL.
- In co-cultures with HLA-A1101+ target cells expressing this mutated oncogene, mTCR transduced T cells lyse target cells and secrete IFN-gamma with high specificity.

Objectives:

Primary objectives:

- Phase I: determine the safety of administering PBL transduced with anti-KRAS G12V mTCR in concert with preparative lymphodepletion and high dose interleukin-2 (IL-2; aldesleukin).
- Phase II:To determine if anti-KRAS G12V mTCR-transduced PBL can mediate the regression of tumors harboring the RAS G12V mutation.

Eligibility:

Patients must be HLA-A 1101 positive and 18 years of age or older and must have:

-A metastatic or unresectable RAS G12V-expressing cancer which has progressed after standard therapy (if available).

Patients may not have:

-Allergies or hypersensitivities to high dose aldesleukin, cyclophosphamide or fludarabine.

Design:

- This is a Phase I/II, single center study of PBL transduced with anti-KRAS G12D mTCR in HLA-A

11:01 positive patients with advanced solid tumors expressing G12D mutated RAS.

- PBMC obtained by leukapheresis will be cultured in the presence of anti-CD3 (OKT3) and aldesleukin in order to stimulate T-cell growth.
- Transduction is initiated by exposure of these cells to retroviral vector supernatant containing replication-incompetent virus encoding the anti-KRAS G12V mTCR.

- All patients will receive a non-myeloablative lymphocyte depleting preparative regimen of cyclophosphamide and fludarabine.
- On day 0 patients will receive their PBL transduced with the anti-KRAS G12V mTCR and will then begin high dose aldesleukin.
- A complete evaluation of lesions will be conducted approximately 6 weeks (+/2 weeks) after treatment.
- The study will be conducted using a Phase I/II Simon minimax design, with two separate cohorts for the phase II component: Cohort 1pancreatic cancers; Cohort 2: all other RAS G12V cancers.
- A total of 110 patients may be required; approximately 24 patients in the phase I portion of the study and 86 (41, plus an allowance of up to 2 non-evaluable per phase II cohort) patients in the phase II portion of the study.

Study Type

Interventional

Study Phase

Phase 1/Phase 2

Condition

- Pancreatic Cancer
- Gastric Cancer
- Gastrointestinal Cancer
- Colon Cancer
- Rectal Cancer

Intervention

Drug: Cyclophosphamide

Days -7 and -6: Cyclophosphamide 60 mg/kg/day X 2 days IV in 250 mlD5W.

Drug: Fludarabine

Days -7 to -3: Fludarabine 25 mg/m2/day IVPB daily over 30 minutes for 5 days.

Biological: anti-KRAS G12V mTCR

Day 0: Cells will be infused intravenously (IV) on the Patient Care Unit over 20 to 30 minutes.

Drug: Aldesleukin

Aldesleukin will be administered at a dose of 720,000 IU/kg (based on total body weight) as an intravenous bolus over a 15-minute period beginning within 24 hrs of cell infusion and continuing for up to 3 days (maximum 9 doses).

Study Arms

Experimental: Phase I

Non-myeloablative lymphocyte delpleting regimen followed by anti-KRAS G12V mTCR and high dose aldesleukin.

Experimental: Phase II

Non-myeloablative lymphocyte delpleting regimen followed by anti-KRAS G12V mTCR and high dose aldesleukin.

Publications

(Includes publications given by the data provider as well as publications identified by ClinicalTrials.gov Identifier (NCT Number) in Medline.)Dudley ME, Yang JC, Sherry R, Hughes MS, Royal R, Kammula U, Robbins PF, Huang J, Citrin DE, Leitman SF, Wunderlich J, Restifo NP, Thomasian A, Downey SG, Smith FO, Klapper J, Morton K, Laurencot C, White DE, Rosenberg SA. Adoptive cell therapy for patients with metastatic melanoma: evaluation of intensive myeloablative chemoradiation preparative regimens. J Clin Oncol. 2008 Nov 10;26(32):5233-9. doi: 10.1200/JCO.2008.16.5449. Epub 2008 Sep 22. (https://www.ncbi.nlm.nih.gov/pubmed/18809613)

Morgan RA, Dudley ME, Wunderlich JR, Hughes MS, Yang JC, Sherry RM, Royal RE, Topalian SL, Kammula US, Restifo NP, Zheng Z, Nahvi A, de Vries CR, Rogers-Freezer LJ, Mavroukakis SA, Rosenberg SA. Cancer regression in patients after transfer of genetically engineered lymphocytes. Science. 2006 Oct 6;314(5796):126-9. Epub 2006 Aug 31. (https://www.ncbi.nlm.nih.gov/pubmed/16946036)

Robbins PF, Morgan RA, Feldman SA, Yang JC, Sherry RM, Dudley ME, Wunderlich JR, Nahvi AV, Helman LJ, Mackall CL, Kammula US, Hughes MS, Restifo NP, Raffeld M, Lee CC, Levy CL, Li YF, El-Gamil M, Schwarz SL, Laurencot C, Rosenberg SA. Tumor regression in patients with metastatic synovial cell sarcoma and melanoma using genetically engineered lymphocytes reactive with NY-ESO-1. J Clin Oncol. 2011 Mar 1;29(7):917-24. doi: 10.1200/JCO.2010.32.2537. Epub 2011 Jan 31. (https://www.ncbi.nlm.nih.gov/pubmed/21282551)

Recruitment Information

Recruitment Status

Recruiting

Estimated Enrollment

110

Completion Date

December 29, 2023

Primary Completion Date

December 1, 2022

Eligibility Criteria

-INCLUSION CRITERIA:

1. Measurable metatstatic unresectable malignancy expressing G12V mutated KRAS as assessed by one of the following methods: RT-PCR on tumor tissue, tumor DNA sequencing or any other CLIA certified laboratory test on resected tissue. Patients shown to have tumors expressing G12V mutated NRAS and HRAS will also be eligible as these oncogenes share complete amino acid homology with G12V mutated KRAS for their first 80 N-terminal amino acids, completely encompassing the target epitope.

2. Confirmation of G12V mutated KRAS, NRAS or HRAS by the Laboratory of Pathology of the NCI.

3. Patients must be HLA-A 1101 positive.

4. Confirmation of the diagnosis of cancer by the Laboratory of Pathology of the NCI.

5. Patients must have previously received standard systemic therapy for their advanced cancer and have been either non-responders (progressive disease) or have recurred. Specifically;

- For patients with metastatic colorectal cancer, they must have had at least two systemic chemotherapy regimens that include 5FU, leucovorin, bevacizumab, oxaliplatin and irinotecan or have contraindications to receiving those medications.
- For pancreatic cancer, they must have received gemcitabine, 5FU and oxaliplatin or have contraindications to receiving those medications.
- Patients with non-small cell lung cancer (NSCLC) must have had appropriate targeted therapy as indicated by abnormalities in ALK, EGFR or expression of PDL1. Other patients must have had platinum-based chemotherapy.
- Patients with ovarian cancer or prostate cancer must have had approved first line chemotherapy.

6. Patients with 3 or fewer brain metastases that are less than 1 cm in diameter and asymptomatic are eligible. Lesions that have been treated with stereotactic radiosurgery must be clinically stable for 1 month after treatment for the patient to be eligible. Patients

with surgically resected brain metastases are eligible.

7. Greater than or equal to 18 years of age and less than or equal to 70 years of age.

8. Willing to sign a durable power of attorney

9. Able to understand and sign the Informed Consent Document

10. Clinical performance status of ECOG 0 or 1

11. Patients of both genders must be willing to practice birth control from the time of enrollment on this study and for up to four months after treatment.

12. Serology:

- Seronegative for HIV antibody. (The experimental treatment being evaluated in this protocol depends on an intact immune system. Patients who are HIV seropositive can have decreased immune-competence and thus be less responsive to the experimental treatment and more susceptible to its toxicities.)
- Seronegative for hepatitis B antigen, and seronegative for hepatitis C antibody. If hepatitis C antibody test is positive, then patient must be tested for the presence of antigen by RT-PCR and be HCV RNA negative.

13. Women of child-bearing potential must have a negative pregnancy test because of the potentially dangerous effects of the treatment on the fetus.

14. Hematology

- Absolute neutrophil count greater than 1000/mm3 without the support of filgrastim
- WBC greater than or equal to 3000/mm3
- Platelet count greater than or equal to 100,000/mm3
- Hemoglobin > 8.0 g/dL

15. Chemistry:

- Serum ALT/ASTless than or equal to to 2.5 times the upper limit of normal
- Serum creatinine less than or equal to to 1.6 mg/dL
- Total bilirubin less tha or equal to to 1.5 mg/dL, except in patients with Gilbert s Syndrome who must have a total bilirubin less than 3.0 mg/dL.

16. More than four weeks must have elapsed since any prior systemic therapy at the time the patient receives the preparative regimen, and patients toxicities must have recovered to a grade 1 or less (except for toxicities such as alopecia or vitiligo).

17. More than 3 weeks must have elapsed since minor surgical procedures or limited field radiotherapy at the time the patient receives the preparative regimen, and patients toxicities must have recovered to grade 1 or less.

18. Subjects must be co-enrolled in protocol 03-C-0277.

EXCLUSION CRITERIA:

1. Women of child-bearing potential who are pregnant or breastfeeding because of the potentially dangerous effects of the treatment on the fetus or infant.

2. Any form of primary immunodeficiency (such as Severe Combined Immunodeficiency Disease).

3. Active systemic infections (e.g.: requiring anti-infective treatment), coagulation disorders or any other major medical illnesses.

4. Concurrent opportunistic infections (The experimental treatment being evaluated in this protocol depends on an intact immune system. Patients who have decreased immune competence may be less responsive to the experimental treatment and more susceptible to its toxicities).

5. Concurrent systemic steroid therapy.

6. History of severe immediate hypersensitivity reaction to cyclophosphamide, aldesleukin, or fludarabine.

7. History of coronary revascularization or ischemic symptoms

8. Documented LVEF of less than or equal to 45%. Testing is required in patients with:

- Clinically significant atrial and/or ventricular arrhythmias including but not limited to: atrial fibrillation, ventricular tachycardia, second or third degree heart block or have a history of ischemic heart disease or chest pain

- Age greater than or equal to 65 years old

9. Documented FEV1 less than or equal to 50% predicted tested in patients with:

- A prolonged history of cigarette smoking (20 pk/year of smoking within the past 2 years).

- Symptoms of respiratory dysfunction

10. Patients who are receiving any other investigational agents

■ **Sex/Gender**

All

■ **Ages**

18 Years to 70 Years

■ **Accepts Healthy Volunteers**

No

■ **Contacts**

Ellen Bodurian   (866) 820-4505   ncisbirc@mail.nih.gov

Oral STAT3 Inhibitor, C188-9, in Patients With Advanced Cancers

Study ID:

NCT03195699

Sponsor:

StemMed, Ltd., USA

Information provided by (Responsible Party):

StemMed, Ltd., USA (StemMed, Ltd., USA)

Tracking Information

■ **First Submitted Date**

June 9, 2017

■ **Primary Completion Date**

July 2020

■ **Start Date**

November 15, 2017

■ **Last Update Posted Date**

December 27, 2017

■ **Current Primary Outcome Measures**

Maximum Tolerated Dose of C188-9[Time Frame: 6 months]

The maximum tolerated dose of C188-9 will be determined using the dose-limiting toxicity is observed. Dose-limiting toxicity is defined using the CTCAE v5.0. The number of patients with dose-limiting toxicities will be evaluated.

- Pharmacokinetics Cmax[Time Frame: 6 months]

Cmax(obs) will be determined by direct inspection of the plasma drug concentration versus time data point values.

- Pharmacokinetics Tmax[Time Frame: 6 months]

Tmax(obs) will also be determined by direct inspection of the plasma drug concentration versus time data point values.

- Pharmacokinetics AUC(0-t)[Time Frame: 6 months]

AUC(0-t) (where t = the time point for the last sample on the pharmacokinetic profile in which quantifiable drug was detected) will be estimated using linear or linear/log trapezoidal calculation.

Pharmacodynamics of C188-9 in peripheral blood mononuclear cells (PBMC) of patients[Time Frame: 6 months]

Levels of pY-STAT3 measured using Luminex bead-based assays, without and with cytokine stimulation both before and after receiving C188-9 will be measured. Changes in pY-STAT1 and pY-STAT3 over time will be assessed.

Pharmacodynamics of C188-9 in tumors of patients[Time Frame: 6 months]

Levels of pY-STAT3 will be scored by percentage of positive cells and intensity of staining. Analyses will be at only two time points: before and after 28-day cycle.

- Complete Response (CR) Target Lesions[Time Frame: 6 months]

  Complete Response (CR): Disappearance of all target lesions. Any pathological lymph nodes (whether target or non-target) must have reduction in short axis to <10 mm.

- Partial Response (PR) Target Lesions[Time Frame: 6 months]

  Partial Response (PR): At least a 30% decrease in the sum of diameters of target lesions, taking as reference the baseline sum diameters.

- Progressive Disease (PD) Target Lesions[Time Frame: 6 months]

  Progressive Disease (PD): At least a 20% increase in the sum of diameters of target lesions, taking as reference the smallest sum on study (this includes the baseline sum if that is the smallest on study). In addition to the relative increase of 20%, the sum must also demonstrate an absolute increase of at least 5 mm. (Note: the appearance of one or more new lesions is also considered progression).

- Stable Disease (SD) Target Lesions[Time Frame: 6 months]

  Stable Disease (SD): Neither sufficient shrinkage to qualify for PR nor sufficient increase to qualify for PD, taking as reference the smallest sum diameters while on study.

- Complete Response (CR) Non-target Lesions[Time Frame: 6 months]

  Complete Response (CR): Disappearance of all non-target lesions and normalization of tumor marker level. All lymph nodes must be non-pathological in size (<10 mm short axis).

- Non-CR/Non-PD Non-target Lesions[Time Frame: 6 months]

  Non-CR/Non-PD: Persistence of one or more non-target lesion(s) and/or maintenance of tumor marker level above the normal limits.

- Progressive Disease (PD) Non-target Lesions[Time Frame: 6 months]

  Progressive Disease (PD): Unequivocal progression of existing non-target lesions. (Note: the appearance of one or more new lesions is also considered progression).

Best Overall Response[Time Frame: 6 months]

The best overall response is the best response recorded from the start of the study treatment until the end of treatment, taking into account any requirement for confirmation. The patient's best overall response assignment will depend on the findings of both target and non-target disease and will also take into consideration the appearance of new lesions.

Descriptive Information

■ Offical Title

Phase I Study of C188-9, an Oral Inhibitor of Signal Transducer and Activator of Transcription (STAT) 3, in Patients With Advanced Cancers

■ Brief Summary

Many patients have cancers that have increased activity of a protein called STAT3 that contributes critically to the development and growth of their cancer. Despite our knowledge of STAT3's importance to cancer, scientists and doctors have not developed a drug that targets it and that patients can take to treat their cancer more effectively than treatments that are now available. StemMed, Ltd. has developed a compound, C188-9, which can be given by mouth and acts as a direct inhibitor of STAT3. Administration of C188-9 to mice demonstrated that it blocked growth of cancers of the breast, head and neck, lung, and liver and it was safe when administered at high doses to mice, rats, and dogs. In this application, StemMed is proposing to further develop C188-9 for treatment of solid tumors for which the prognosis is dismal. The investigators will determine how safe it is when administered to patients with cancer, determine whether an adequate dose can be administered to patients with cancer that will block STAT3 in their cancer, and determine whether treatment with C188-9 leads to reduced growth of their cancer.

■ Detailed Description

Signal transducer and activator of transcription 3 (STAT3) is a member of a family of seven closely related proteins responsible for transmission of peptide hormone signals from the extracellular surface of cells to the nucleus. STAT3 is a master regulator of most key hallmarks and enablers of cancer, including cell proliferation, resistance to apoptosis, metastasis, immune evasion, tumor angiogenesis, epithelial mesenchymal transition (EMT), response to DNA damage, and the Warburg effect. STAT3 also is a key mediator of oncogene addiction and supports the self-renewal of tumor-initiating cancer stem cells that contribute to cancer initiation, cancer maintenance, and relapse in several types of tumors. STAT3 activity is increased in ~50% of all cancers, due either to naturally occurring STAT3 mutations, as have been demonstrated in human inflammatory hepatocellular adenomas and large granular lymphocytic leukemia, or, more commonly as a result of activation of signaling molecules upstream of STAT3, including receptor tyrosine kinases (RTK; e.g. epidermal growth factor receptor, EGFR), tyrosine kinase-associated receptors (e.g. the family of IL-6 cytokine receptors or G-protein coupled receptors, GPCR), and Src kinases (e.g. Src, Lck, Hck, Lyn, Fyn, or Fgr). Thus, STAT3 is an attractive target for drug development to treat many types of cancer including breast cancer, head and neck squamous cell carcinoma (HNSCC), non-small cell lung cancer (NSCLC), hepatocellular carcinoma (HCC), colorectal cancer (CRC), gastric adenocarcinoma and melanoma.

▨ Study Type

Interventional

▨ Study Phase

Phase 1

▨ Condition

- Breast Cancer
- Head and Neck Squamous Cell Carcinoma
- Non Small Cell Lung Cancer
- Hepatocellular Cancer
- Colorectal Cancer
- Gastric Adenocarcinoma
- Melanoma
- Advanced Cancer

▨ Intervention

Drug: C188-9

Dose level 1. 3.2 mg/kg/day administered in divided doses every 12 hours Dose level 2. 6.4 mg/kg/day administered in divided doses every 12 hours Dose level 3. 12.8 mg/kg/day administered in divided doses every 12 hours Dose level 4. 25.6 mg/kg/day administered in divided doses every 12 hours

▨ Study Arms

Experimental: Dose escalation study

Oral administration of C188-9 for up to 6 28-day cycles

Recruitment Information

▨ Recruitment Status

Recruiting

▨ Estimated Enrollment

30

▨ Completion Date

July 2020

▨ Primary Completion Date

July 2020

▨ Eligibility Criteria

Inclusion Criteria

All of the following inclusion criteria must be fulfilled for eligibility:

1. Age ≥18 years;

2. Patients with histologically confirmed diagnosis of locally-advanced, inoperable, metastatic and/or treatment refractory solid tumors for whom there are no available therapies that will confer clinical benefit;

3. Eastern Cooperative Oncology Group Performance status 0-1;

4. Hemoglobin ≥9.0 g/dL, neutrophil count ≥1.0 x 109/l, platelets ≥100 x 109/L;

5. Adequate renal function capability, as calculated by creatinine clearance >60 ml/min using the Cockroft-Gault formula;

6. Adequate liver function defined as total bilirubin <1.5 x ULN, and aspartate aminotransferase (AST)/alanine aminotransferase (ALT) <3 x ULN. For subjects with liver involvement, AST/ALT <5 x ULN;

7. Measurable disease using clinically appropriate criteria for the type of malignancy, RECIST v 1.1 for solid tumors;

8. Negative blood pregnancy test at the screening visit for women of childbearing potential, defined as: female subjects after puberty unless they have been postmenopausal for at least two years, are surgically sterile, or are sexually inactive and will remain so for the course of the trial;

9. Willingness to avoid pregnancy and breast feeding beginning two weeks before the first C188-9 dose and ending three months after the last trial treatment. Male subjects with female partners of childbearing potential and female subjects of childbearing potential must use adequate contraception in the judgment of the Investigator, such as a two—barrier method or a one—barrier method with spermicide or intrauterine device during trial treatment dosing and for 3 months after the last dose of the study; and

10. Ability to read and understand the informed consent form and willingness and ability to give informed consent and demonstrate comprehension of the trial before undergoing any trial activities.

Exclusion Criteria

Subjects are ineligible to enroll in this trial if they fulfill any of the following exclusion criteria:

1. Previous therapy with:

1. Standard therapy including chemotherapy, immunotherapy, biologic therapy, or any other anticancer therapy within 28 days (or five elimination half-lives for non-cytotoxics, whichever is shorter) of Day 1 of trial drug treatment (6 weeks for nitrosureas or mitomycin);

2. Any investigational agent within 28 days of Day 1 of trial drug treatment or 5 half-lives for a small molecule/targeted therapy;

2. Extensive prior radiotherapy on more than 30% of bone marrow reserves, or prior bone marrow/stem cell transplantation within 5 years from enrollment; Ongoing toxicity (except alopecia) due to a prior therapy, unless returned to baseline or Grade 1 or less;

3. Major surgical intervention or participation in a therapeutic clinical trial within 28 days from Day 1 of the first dose of C188-9;

4. Significantly impaired cardiac function such as unstable angina pectoris, congestive heart failure with New York Heart Association (NYHA) class III or IV, myocardial infarction within the last 12 months prior to trial entry; signs of pericardial effusion, serious arrhythmia (including QTc prolongation of >470 ms and/or pacemaker) or prior diagnosis of congenital long QT syndrome or left ventricular ejection fraction <50% on screening echocardiogram;

5. History of cerebral vascular accident or stroke within the previous 2 years;

6. Uncontrolled hypertension (>160/100mm Hg);

7. History of Grade 3 or 4 allergic reactions attributed to compounds of similar chemical or biologic composition as C188-9 (hydroxyl-naphthalene sulfonamides);

8. Known active metastases in the central nervous system (unless stable by brain imaging studies for at least 1 month without evidence of cerebral edema and no requirements for corticosteroids or anticonvulsants);

9. History of difficulty swallowing, malabsorption, or other chronic gastrointestinal disease or conditions that may hamper compliance and/or absorption of the investigational product;

10. Known human immunodeficiency virus or viral hepatitis;

11. Legal incapacity or limited legal capacity;

12. Pregnant or lactating women;

13. Any other condition, which in the opinion of the investigator, might impair the subject's tolerance of trial treatment, the safety of the individual subject, or the outcome of the trial;

14. Previous treatment of the current malignancy with a STAT inhibitor.

Sex/Gender

All

Ages

18 Years to 65 Years

Accepts Healthy Volunteers

No

Contacts

David J Tweardy, MD   832-413-1362   davidt@stemmedcancer.com

Phase 1 Clinical Trial of Metastasis Inhibitor NP-G2-044 in Patients With Advanced or Metastatic Solid Tumors (Including Lymphoma)

Study ID:

NCT03199586

Sponsor:

Novita Pharmaceuticals, Inc.

Information provided by (Responsible Party):

Novita Pharmaceuticals, Inc. (Novita Pharmaceuticals, Inc.)

Tracking Information

First Submitted Date

June 23, 2017

Start Date

November 3, 2017

■ **Primary Completion Date**	■ **Last Update Posted Date**
September 1, 2019	November 17, 2017

■ **Current Primary Outcome Measures**

Number of participants with treatment related adverse events[Time Frame: 24 months] as assessed by CTCAE V4.03

■ **Current Secondary Outcome Measures**

Anti tumor activity[Time Frame: 24 months.]
Resist 1.1

Descriptive Information

■ **Offical Title**

First-in-Human, Dose Finding, Open Label Phase 1 Clinical Trial of Metastasis Inhibitor NP-G2-044 in Patients With Advanced or Metastatic Solid Tumors (Including Lymphoma)

■ **Brief Summary**

First-in-human phase 1 study to determine safety of NP-G2-044 when given orally on a daily X 28 days followed by a 14 day rest period.

■ **Study Type**

Interventional

■ **Study Phase**

Phase 1

■ **Condition**

- Breast Cancer
- Pancreas Cancer
- Prostate Cancer
- Lung Cancer
- Colon Cancer
- Esophagus Cancer
- Liver Cancer
- Ovary Cancer
- Lymphoma

■ **Intervention**

Drug: NP-G2-044
capsule

■ **Study Arms**

Experimental: NP-G2-044
capsule

Recruitment Information

■ **Recruitment Status**	■ **Completion Date**
Recruiting	December 1, 2019
■ **Estimated Enrollment**	■ **Primary Completion Date**
60	September 1, 2019

■ **Eligibility Criteria**

Inclusion Criteria:

- Disease Related
- Patients must have documented history of histologically confirmed solid tumors (as defined by ASCO/CAP guidelines) originating in breast, pancreas, prostate, lung, colon, esophagus, liver, or ovary, and lymphomas, which are locally advanced or metastatic and who are refractory or intolerant beyond primary treatment for their malignancy, or for lymphoma patients who are not eligible for or who have refused autologous or allogenic hematopoietic stem cell transplant

- Measurable or evaluable disease documented within one month of the planned protocol treatment (Treatment Period Cycle 1, Day 1)first dose of study drug (PK Period Day 1)
- ECOG performance score of 0 and 1
- Able to swallow capsules/tablets

Demographic • Male and females who are 18 years or older

Laboratory Values

- Hemoglobin ≥ 9.0 g/dL
- Absolute neutrophil count ≥ 1500/uL
- Platelet count ≥ 100,000/uL
- Serum creatinine ≤ 1.5 mg/dL or a 24-hour calculated estimated creatinine clearance of ≥ 60 mL/min
- Serum bilirubin ≤ 1.5 mg/dL
- Serum albumin ≥ 3g/dL
- AST (SGOT), ALP and ALT (SGPT) ≤ 2.5 times upper limit of normal (OR ≤ 5 times ULN in the presence of known liver metastases)
- Prothrombin time (PT)/International Normalized Ratio (INR) and partial thromboplastin time (PPT) ≤ 1.5 times the upper limit of normal
- Serum sodium, potassium, magnesium, calcium and phosphorous levels within institutional normal limits; supplements required to maintain normal electrolyte levels will be permitted

Ethical

- Before any study-specific procedure, the appropriate written informed consent must be obtained

Exclusion Criteria:

Disease Related

- Clinical or radiographical evidence of active brain metastasis
- Patients who have not recovered to ≤ grade 1 toxicities except grade 2 alopecia or neuropathy associated with previous chemotherapy, radiotherapy, biologic, hormone or prior investigational therapies.

Medications:

- Chemotherapy or other cancer, radiation or surgical treatments within 2 weeks or five half-lives (whichever is shorter) of the first dose of study drug (PK Period Day 1) planned first protocol treatment (i.e., cycle 1 day 1) or not yet recovered from respective treatments
- Patients who have had allogenic hematopoietic stem cell transplant or allogenic bone marrow transplant
- Patients who have had prior solid organ transplant
- Patients who are on immune suppression drugs or anti-transplant rejection drugs

General:

- History of any medical or psychiatric condition or addictive disorder, or laboratory abnormality that in the opinion of the investigator, may increase the risks associated with study participation or treatments that may interfere with the conduct of the study or the interpretation of study results
- Prior history of clinically significant gastrointestinal bleeding, intestinal obstruction or gastrointestinal perforation within 6 months before planned initiation of study treatment
- Uncontrolled diabetes
- History of long QT syndrome or clinically significant cardiac arrhythmia, other than stable atrial fibrillation
- Mean QTcF > 450 msec in men and mean QTcF > 470 msec in women at screening
- Myocardial infarction within the previous 6 months before planned initiation of study treatment
- Active infection requiring intravenous antibiotics within 2 weeks of the first dose of study drug (PK Period Day 1) before planned initiation of study treatment
- Prior history or current positive tests for hepatitis B, hepatitis C or human immunodeficiency virus
- Currently enrolled in or has not yet completed at least 30 days since ending other investigational device or drug study before planned date of first dose, or the patient is currently receiving other investigational agent(s)
- Pregnant, planning a pregnancy or breast feeding during the study
- Male or female not willing to use adequate contraceptive precautions during the study period
- Unwilling or unable to comply with study requirements or not available for follow-up assessments
- Any disorder that compromises the ability of the patient to give written informed consent and/or to comply with study procedures.

▪ **Sex/Gender**

All

▪ **Ages**

18 Years to N/A

A Phase I/II Study of Pexa-Vec Oncolytic Virus in Combination With Immune Checkpoint Inhibition in Refractory Colorectal Cancer

Study ID:

NCT03206073

Sponsor:

National Cancer Institute (NCI)

Information provided by (Responsible Party):

National Institutes of Health Clinical Center (CC) (National Cancer Institute (NCI))

Tracking Information

▨ **First Submitted Date**

June 30, 2017

▨ **Start Date**

December 7, 2017

▨ **Primary Completion Date**

December 31, 2020

▨ **Last Update Posted Date**

January 5, 2018

▨ **Current Primary Outcome Measures**

List of adverse event frequency[Time Frame: 30 days after last treatment]

▨ **Current Secondary Outcome Measures**

Median amount of time subject survives without disease progression after treatment[Time Frame: 5 month]

Median amount of time subject survives without disease progression after treatment[Time Frame: at progression]

Median amount of time subject survives after therapy[Time Frame: death]

Changes in tumor size and occurrence of metastases[Time Frame: every 2 months until disease progression or intolerable toxicity]

Descriptive Information

▨ **Offical Title**

A Phase I/II Study of Pexa-Vec Oncolytic Virus in Combination With Immune Checkpoint Inhibition in Refractory Colorectal Cancer

▨ **Brief Summary**

Background:

- Immune-based approaches in colorectal cancer have unfortunately with the notable exception of immune checkpoint inhibition in microsatellite instable (MSI-hi) disease been largely unsuccessful. The reasons for this are unclear but no doubt relate to the fact that in advanced disease colorectal cancer appears to be less immunogenic, as evidenced by the lack of infiltrating lymphocytes with advancing T stage
- Pexa-Vec (JX-594) is a thymidine kinase gene-inactivated oncolytic vaccinia virus engineered for the expression of transgenes encoding human granulocytemacrophage colony-stimulating factor (GM-CSF) and beta-galactosidase. Apart from the direct oncolytic activity, oncolytic viruses such as Pexa-Vec have been shown to mediate tumor cell death via the induction of innate and adaptive immune responses
- Tremelimumab is a fully human monoclonal antibody that binds to CTLA-4 expressed on the surface of activated T lymphocytes and causes inhibition of B7-CTLA-4-mediated downregulation of T-cell activation. Durvalumab is a human monoclonal antibody directed against PD-L1.
- The aim of the study is to evaluate whether the anti-tumor immunity induced by Pexa-Vec oncolytic viral therapy can be enhanced by immune checkpoint inhibition.

Objective:

514

-To determine the safety, tolerability and feasibility of Pexa-Vec oncolytic virus in combination with immune checkpoint inhibition in patients with refractory metastatic colorectal cancer.

Eligibility:

- Histologically confirmed metastatic colorectal cancer.
- Patients must have progressed on, been intolerant of or refused prior oxaliplatinand irinotecan-containing, fluorouracil-based, chemotherapeutic regimen and have disease that is not amenable to potentially curative resection. Patients who have a known KRAS wild type tumor must have progressed, been intolerant of or refused cetuximab or panitumumabbased chemotherapy.
- Patients tumors must be documented to be microsatellite-stable (MSS) either by genetic analysis or immunohistochemistry OR microsatellite-high with documented disease progression following anti-PD1/PDL1 therapy.
- Patients must have at least one focus of metastatic disease that is amenable to preand ontreatment biopsy.
- Willingness to undergo mandatory tumor biopsy.

Design:

-The proposed study is Phase I/II study of Pexa-Vec oncolytic virus at two dose levels in combination with immune checkpoint inhibition in patients with metastatic colorectal cancer.

Detailed Description

Background:

- Immune-based approaches in colorectal cancer have unfortunately with the notable exception of immune checkpoint inhibition in microsatellite instable (MSI-hi) disease been largely unsuccessful. The reasons for this are unclear but no doubt relate to the fact that in advanced disease colorectal cancer appears to be less immunogenic, as evidenced by the lack of infiltrating lymphocytes with advancing T stage
- Pexa-Vec (JX-594) is a thymidine kinase gene-inactivated oncolytic vaccinia virus engineered for the expression of transgenes encoding human granulocytemacrophage colony-stimulating factor (GM-CSF) and beta-galactosidase. Apart from the direct oncolytic activity, oncolytic viruses such as Pexa-Vec have been shown to mediate tumor cell death via the induction of innate and adaptive immune responses
- Tremelimumab is a fully human monoclonal antibody that binds to CTLA-4 expressed on the surface of activated T lymphocytes and causes inhibition of B7-CTLA-4-mediated downregulation of T-cell activation. Durvalumab is a human monoclonal antibody directed against PD-L1.
- The aim of the study is to evaluate whether the anti-tumor immunity induced by Pexa-Vec oncolytic viral therapy can be enhanced by immune checkpoint inhibition.

Objective:

-To determine the safety, tolerability and feasibility of Pexa-Vec oncolytic virus in combination with immune checkpoint inhibition in patients with refractory metastatic colorectal cancer.

Eligibility:

- Histologically confirmed metastatic colorectal cancer.
- Patients must have progressed on, been intolerant of or refused prior oxaliplatinand irinotecan-containing, fluorouracil-based, chemotherapeutic regimen and have disease that is not amenable to potentially curative resection. Patients who have a known KRAS wild type tumor must have progressed, been intolerant of or refused cetuximab or panitumumabbased chemotherapy.
- Patients tumors must be documented to be microsatellite-stable (MSS) either by genetic analysis or immunohistochemistry OR microsatellite-high with documented disease progression following anti-PD1/PDL1 therapy.
- Patients must have at least one focus of metastatic disease that is amenable to preand ontreatment biopsy.
- Willingness to undergo mandatory tumor biopsy.

Design:

- The proposed study is Phase I/II study of Pexa-Vec oncolytic virus at two dose levels in combination with immune checkpoint inhibition in patients with metastatic colorectal cancer.
- Patients with advanced microsatellite-stable colorectal cancer (or MSI-hi disease that is refractory to PD-1 monotherapy) will receive Pexa-Vec, administered IV at a dose of either 3×10^{8} plaque forming units (pfu) (DL1) or 10^{9} pfu (DL2) every 2 weeks for 4 doses, in 2 separate cohorts A and B. The first administration will be on Day (minus) 12, followed by administration on Days 2, 16 and 30 (i.e. 4 doses in total).
- Cohort A: In addition to the oncolytic virus patients will also receive durvalumab at a flat dose of 1500 mg as an intravenous infusion beginning on Day 1 followed by q28days until off-treatment criteria are met.
- Cohort B: In addition to the oncolytic virus patients will also receive tremelimumab 75 mg and durvalumab 1500 mg as intravenous infusions beginning on Day 1 followed by q28days for 4 doses with subsequent continuation of the durvalumab alone until off-treatment criteria are met.
- Pexa-Vec will commence on Day (minus) 12 to facilitate tumor biopsies following oncolytic virus alone. All patients will undergo a baseline tumor biopsy and a post treatment biopsy. The timing of the post-treatment biopsy will depend on randomization. The randomization will be balanced with an equal number randomized to each timing group. Patients will be randomized to receive the second biopsy on Day 1 (i.e. after one dose of Pexa-Vec alone) or Day 29 (i.e. after the combination of immune checkpoint inhibition and Pexa-Vec). (Specific dates of biopsy will have a window of 72 hrs to allow for logistical issues; however, the biopsy will not be performed within 48 hrs after PexaVec administration).
- Accrual ceiling will be set at 35 to allow for patients replaceable for reasons other than toxicity.
- Patients will be restaged every 8 weeks +/3 days

Study Type

Interventional

Study Phase

Phase 1/Phase 2

Condition

- Colorectal Cancer
- Colorectal Carcinoma
- Colorectal Adenocarcinoma
- Refractory Cancer
- Colorectal Neoplasms

Intervention

Drug: Durvalumab

  1500 mg of durvalumab via IV infusion on Day 1 of each cycle until patients meet off treatment criteria

  Drug: Tremelimumab

  75 mg of tremelimumab via IV infusion on Day 1 of cycles 1-4

Biological: Pexa-Vec

  3 x 10E8 pfu (DL 1) or 1 x 10E9 pfu (DL 2) via IV infusion for 4 doses: Day 12, Day 2, Day 16 of Cycle 1 and Day 2 of Cycle 2.

Study Arms

Experimental: Cohort A
  Immune checkpoint inhibition Durvalumab

Experimental: Cohort B
  Immune checkpoint inhibition Durvalumab + Tremelimumab

Publications

(Includes publications given by the data provider as well as publications identified by ClinicalTrials.gov Identifier (NCT Number) in Medline.)Rajani KR, Vile RG. Harnessing the Power of Onco-Immunotherapy with Checkpoint Inhibitors. Viruses. 2015 Nov 13;7(11):5889-901. doi: 10.3390/v7112914. Review. (https://www.ncbi.nlm.nih.gov/pubmed/26580645)

Kohlhapp FJ, Kaufman HL. Molecular Pathways: Mechanism of Action for Talimogene Laherparepvec, a New Oncolytic Virus Immunotherapy. Clin Cancer Res. 2016 Mar 1;22(5):1048-54. doi: 10.1158/1078-0432.CCR-15-2667. Epub 2015 Dec 30. Review. (https://www.ncbi.nlm.nih.gov/pubmed/26719429)

Heo J, Reid T, Ruo L, Breitbach CJ, Rose S, Bloomston M, Cho M, Lim HY, Chung HC, Kim CW, Burke J, Lencioni R, Hickman T, Moon A, Lee YS, Kim MK, Daneshmand M, Dubois K, Longpre L, Ngo M, Rooney C, Bell JC, Rhee BG, Patt R, Hwang TH, Kirn DH. Randomized dose-finding clinical trial of oncolytic immunotherapeutic vaccinia JX-594 in liver cancer. Nat Med. 2013 Mar;19(3):329-36. doi: 10.1038/nm.3089. Epub 2013 Feb 10. (https://www.ncbi.nlm.nih.gov/pubmed/23396206)

Recruitment Information

Recruitment Status

Recruiting

Estimated Enrollment

35

Completion Date

December 31, 2021

Primary Completion Date

December 31, 2020

Eligibility Criteria

- INCLUSION CRITERIA:
- Patients must have histopathological confirmation of Colorectal Carcinoma (CRC) by the Laboratory of Pathology of the NCI prior to entering this study.
- Patients must have progressed on, been intolerant of or refused prior oxaliplatinand irinotecan-containing, fluorouracil-based, chemotherapeutic regimen and have disease that is not amenable to potentially curative resection. Patients who have a known KRAS wild type tumor must have progressed, been intolerant of or refused cetuximab or panitumumab-based chemotherapy.
- Patients tumors must be documented to be microsatellite-stable (MSS) either by genetic analysis or immunohistochemistry OR microsatellite-high with documented disease progression following anti-PD1/PDL1 therapy.
- Patients must have at least one focus of metastatic disease that is amenable to preand on-treatment biopsy and be willing to undergo this. Ideally the biopsied lesion should not be one of the target measurable lesions, although this can be up to the discretion of the investigators.
- All patients enrolled will be required to have measurable disease by RECIST 1.1 criteria.

- Age greater than or equal to 18 years. Because no dosing or adverse event data are currently available on the use of Pexa-Vec in combination with tremelimumab and/or durvalumab in patients <18 years of age, children are excluded from this study, but will be eligible for future pediatric trials.
- ECOG performance status 0-1
- **Patients must have acceptable organ and marrow function as defined below:**
- Leukocytes greater than or equal to 3,000/mcL
- absolute neutrophil count greater than or equal to 1,500/mcL
- Platelets greater than or equal to 100,000/mcL
- total bilirubin less than or equal to 1.5X institution upper limit of normal
- Hb > 9g/dl
- AST (SGOT)/ALT (SGPT) less than or equal to 2.5 x institutional upper limit of normal unless liver metastases are present, in which case it must be less than or equal to 5x ULN
- Creatinine <1.5X institution upper limit of normal, OR
- creatinine clearance greater than or equal to 45 mL/min/1.73 m(2), as calculated below, for patients with creatinine levels above institutional normal
- Patient must be able to understand and willing to sign a written informed consent document
- The effects of Pexa-Vec, durvalumab and tremelimumab on the developing human fetus are unknown. For this reason, women of child-bearing potential and men must agree to use adequate contraception (hormonal or barrier method of birth control; abstinence) prior to study entry, for the duration of study participation and up to 180 days after the last dose of durvalumab + tremelimumab combination therapy or 90 days after the last dose of durvalumab monotherapy, whichever is the longer time period. Should a woman become pregnant or suspect she is pregnant while she or her partner is participating in this study, she should inform her treating physician immediately.
- **Evidence of post-menopausal status or negative urinary or serum pregnancy test for female pre-menopausal patients. Women will be considered post-menopausal if they have been amenorrheic for 12 months without an alternative medical cause. The following age-specific requirements apply:**
- Women <50 years of age would be considered post-menopausal if they have been amenorrheic for 12 months or more following cessation of exogenous hormonal treatments and if they have luteinizing hormone and follicle-stimulating hormone levels in the post-menopausal range for the institution or underwent surgical sterilization (bilateral oophorectomy or hysterectomy).
- Women greater than or equal to 50 years of age would be considered post-menopausal if they have been amenorrheic for 12 months or more following cessation of all exogenous hormonal treatments, had radiation-induced menopause with last menses >1 year ago, had chemotherapy-induced menopause with last menses >1 year ago, or underwent surgical sterilization (bilateral oophorectomy, bilateral salpingectomy or hysterectomy. Subject is willing and able to comply with the protocol for the duration of the study including undergoing treatment and scheduled visits and examinations including follow up.
- Body weight >35kg

EXCLUSION CRITERIA:

- Patients who have had anti-cancer therapy (chemotherapy, immunotherapy, endocrine therapy, targeted therapy, biologic therapy, tumor embolization, monoclonal antibodies or other investigation agents), large field radiotherapy, or major surgery must wait 4 weeks after completing treatment prior to entering the study.
- No prior exposure to immune-mediated therapy including, but not limited to, other anti CTLA-4, anti-PD-1, anti-PD-L1, and anti-programmed cell death ligand 2 (anti-PD-L2) antibodies, including therapeutic anticancer vaccines. The exception to this is those whose tumors are MSI-hi and are refractory to anti-PD1 monotherapy.
- Involvement in the planning and/or conduct of the study
- Previous IP assignment in the present study
- Patients who are receiving any other investigational agents.
- Inability to suspend treatment with anti-hypertensive medication (including but not limited to: diuretics, beta-blockers, angiotensin converting enzyme [ACE] inhibitors, aldosterone antagonists, etc.) for 48 hours pre and post each Pexa-Vec administration.
- Patients with severe hypertension who in the opinion of the investigator cannot withhold antihypertensive medication for 48 hours pre and post Pexa-Vec administration.
- Any unresolved toxicity NCI CTCAE Grade greater than or equal to 2 from previous anticancer therapy with the exception of alopecia, vitiligo, and the laboratory values defined in the inclusion criteria
- Patients with Grade greater than or equal to 2 neuropathy will be evaluated on a case-by-case basis
- Patients with known brain metastases will be excluded from this clinical trial because of their poor prognosis and because they often develop progressive neurologic dysfunction that would confound the evaluation of neurologic and other adverse events.
- Uncontrolled intercurrent illness including, but not limited to, hypertension (systolic BP > 160, diastolic BP > 100), ongoing or active systemic infection, symptomatic congestive heart failure, unstable angina pectoris, cardiac arrhythmia, uncontrolled diabetes or psychiatric illness/social situations that would limit compliance with study requirements. For patients with a history of cardiovascular disease, cardiology consultation. Echocardiogram, troponin and creatinine clearance must be obtained prior to enrollment. NOTE: Patients with active cardiac disease (e.g. myocarditis and myocardial infarction) within 12 months of study entry are excluded from study participation.
- HIV-positive patients receiving anti-retroviral therapy are excluded from this study due to the possibility of pharmacokinetic interactions between antiretroviral medications and the investigational agent. HIV positive patients not receiving

antiretroviral therapy are excluded due to the possibility that Durvalumab or Tremelimumab may worsen their condition and the likelihood that the underlying condition may obscure the attribution of adverse events.

- Known significant immunodeficiency due to underlying illness (e.g. HIV/AIDS) and/or immune-suppressive medication including high-dose corticosteroids (defined as greater than or equal to 20 mg/day prednisone or equivalent which is ongoing at the time of randomization and/or was taken for more than 4 weeks within the preceding 2 months of study treatment)

- History of chronic autoimmune disease (e.g. systemic lupus erythematosus or Wegener s granulomatosis, Addison s disease, multiple sclerosis, Graves disease, Hashimoto s thyroiditis, hypophysitis, etc.) with symptomatic disease within the 3 years before enrollment. Note: Active vitiligo or a history of vitiligo will not be a basis for exclusion. In addition, a past history of certain autoimmunity e.g. rheumatoid arthritis or thyroiditis may be allowed per PI discretion provided it has been quiescent for a minimum of three years. The following are exceptions to this criterion:

1. Patients with vitiligo or alopecia

2. Patients with hypothyroidism (e.g. following Hashimoto syndrome) stable on hormone replacement

3. Any chronic skin condition that does not require systemic therapy

4. Patients without active disease in the last 5 years may be included

5. Patients with celiac disease controlled by diet alone

6. Active or history of inflammatory bowel disease (colitis, Crohn s), irritable bowel disease, celiac disease, or other serious, chronic, gastrointestinal conditions associated with diarrhea.

- History of active primary immunodeficiency

- Active infection including tuberculosis (clinical evaluation that includes clinical history, physical examination and radiographic findings, and TB testing (if clinically indicated), hepatitis B (known positive HBV surface antigen (HBsAg) result), hepatitis C. Patients with a past or resolved HBV infection (defined as the presence of hepatitis B core antibody [anti-HBc] and absence of HBsAg) are eligible. Patients positive for hepatitis C (HCV) antibody are eligible only if polymerase chain reaction is negative for HCV RNA.

- Current or prior use of immunosuppressive medication within 14 days before the first dose of durvalumab or tremelimumab. The following are exceptions to this criterion:

- Intranasal, inhaled, topical steroids, or local steroid injections (e.g. intra articular injection)

- Systemic corticosteroids at physiologic doses not to exceed <<10 mg/day>> of prednisone or its equivalent

- Steroids as premedication for hypersensitivity reactions (e.g. CT scan premedication)

- Receipt of live attenuated vaccine within 30 days prior to the first dose of IP. Note:

Patients, if enrolled, should not receive live vaccine whilst receiving IP and up to 30 days after the last dose of IP.

- Female patients who are breastfeeding. Because there is an unknown but potential risk for adverse events in nursing infants secondary to treatment of the mother with Pexa-Vec, breastfeeding should be discontinued if the mother is treated with Pexa-Vec. These potential risks may also apply to other agents used in this study.

- Known allergy or hypersensitivity to IP

- Prior randomization or treatment in a previous durvalumab and/or tremelimumab clinical study regardless of treatment arm assignment.

- History of sarcoidosis syndrome

- Mean QT interval corrected for heart rate (QTc) greater than or equal to 470 ms calculated from 3 electrocardiograms (ECGs) using Fredericia s Correction

- Patients with a history of Interstitial lung disease or pneumonitis

- Subjects with uncontrolled seizures

- History of leptomeningeal carcinomatosis

- History of hypersensitivity reaction to human or mouse antibody products.

- Patients with unhealed surgical wounds for more than 30 days

- Ongoing severe inflammatory skin condition (as determined by the Investigator) requiring medical treatment

- History of severe eczema (as determined by the Investigator) requiring medical treatment

- Patients with tumor(s) invading a major vascular structure (e.g. carotid artery) or other key anatomical structure (e.g. pulmonary airway) in the event of post treatment tumor swelling and/or necrosis (hepatic and portal vein involvement allowed)

- Patients with liver tumors in a location that would potentially result in significant clinical adverse effects in the opinion of investigator if post-treatment tumor swelling were to occur, including at the site of the common bile duct

- Clinically significant and/or rapidly accumulating ascites, pericardial and/or pleural effusions. Mild ascites that does not preclude safe tumor biopsy as protocol specified is allowed at the discretion of the treating physician.

- Medical conditions, per the investigator s judgment, that predispose the patient to untoward medical risk in the event of volume loading (e.g. intravenous [IV] fluid bolus infusion), tachycardia, or hypotension during or following treatment with Pexa-Vec

- Any prior or planned organ transplant (e.g. liver transplant)

- Patients who experienced a severe systemic reaction or side-effect as a result of a previous vaccination with vaccinia

- Pulse oximetry O2 saturation <90% at rest on room air

- **Sex/Gender**

  All

- **Ages**

  18 Years to 99 Years

- **Accepts Healthy Volunteers**

  No

- **Contacts**

  Donna M Hrones, C.R.N.P.   (301) 451-4864   donna.mabry@nih.gov

Investigation of Cecal Intubation Rates and Pain Levels Between Water Exchange and Air Insufflation Flexible Sigmoidoscopy

Study ID:
NCT03209349

Sponsor:
Kelowna Gastroenterology Associates

Information provided by (Responsible Party):
Kelowna Gastroenterology Associates (Kelowna Gastroenterology Associates)

Tracking Information

- **First Submitted Date**

  June 14, 2017

- **Start Date**

  June 14, 2017

- **Primary Completion Date**

  December 8, 2017

- **Last Update Posted Date**

  July 6, 2017

- **Current Primary Outcome Measures**

  Full colon exam[Time Frame: Immediately following the procedure]

  Ability for patient to receive full exam of the colon with minimal discomfort

- **Current Secondary Outcome Measures**

  Recalled Discomfort[Time Frame: Immediately following the procedure]

  Patient will be contacted at 24 hours following the procedure and in order to document whether the scope was more uncomfortable than expected and if the patient would be willing to receive the test again at their next screening interval.

  Adenoma detection rates[Time Frame: Immediately following the procedure]

  Histopathological testing and reporting will follow standard practices and adenoma detection rates will be documented and compared between study arms.

Descriptive Information

- **Offical Title**

  Investigation of Cecal Intubation Rates and Pain Levels Between Water Exchange and Air Insufflation Flexible Sigmoidoscopy: A Randomized Controlled StudyExercise and Low-Dose Ibuprofen for Cognitive Impairment in Colorectal Cancer Patients Receiving Chemotherapy

- **Brief Summary**

  This study evaluates how often patients without sedation that receive screening sigmoidoscopy are able to have their full colon examined without significant discomfort by comparing a new colonoscopy technique known as the water exchange technique to the traditional air insufflation technique. It compares the differences between complete colon exam rates for water exchange when compared to the traditional air technique. Patients will be randomised and blinded to the procedure type.

  Previous studies have shown that the water exchange method is associated with a significant reduction in discomfort and often allows patients to receive colonoscopy without sedation or with only minimal sedation. However, the potential for water exchange to be used in the screening setting has yet to be evaluated. As per standard practices in sigmoidoscopy screening, patients will not be sedated. However, unlike standard practices in sigmoidoscopy screening, while maintaining minimal levels of discomfort, the investigators will attempt to scope beyond the distal colon.

Detailed Description

Purpose:

This study is being conducted to evaluate whether a new technique, known as the water exchange technique can more frequently allow for the full colon to be examined in patients undergoing screening sigmoidoscopy.

Hypothesis & Goals & Objectives:

It is hypothesised that there will be a 20% or greater difference in cecal intubation rate (ability for the colonoscope to reach the Ileocecal juncture, and thereby provide full examination of the colon) at a minimal and acceptable level of discomfort in non-sedated colon screening patients receiving a scope using the water-exchange method, when compared to the air insufflation method.

Justification:

Previous studies have shown that the water exchange method is associated with a significant reduction in discomfort and often allows patients to receive colonoscopy without sedation or with only minimal sedation. The ability to increase the likelihood of full colon examination at minimal discomfort has the opportunity to improve upon screening practices and increase the likelihood of patient participation as discomfort and fear of discomfort is a major factor that limits uptake of sigmoidoscopy and colonoscopy screening.

Research Design:

This study takes a patient and interviewer blinded and randomised study design. Patients will be randomly assigned to receive either the water exchange method or the air insufflation method. Rates of cecal intubation are compared across study arms.

Statistical Analysis Plan:

Effect differences in cecal intubation rates, and responses to whether the scope that they received was more uncomfortable than they expected, and whether they would be willing to receive the test again at their next screening interval will be compared using the Chi-Squared or, when the data necessitates, Fisher's Exact Test. Assuming a non-normal distribution in reported pain scores, the Mann Whitney U test will be used to assess the differences in maximum reported pain according to the Wong Baker Faces Pain Rating Scale between study arms.

The term sigmoidoscopy is used here as patients are prepared for the procedure using a standard sigmoidoscopy protocol, rather than colonoscopy. That is, sedation is not administered; this is a standard practice for sigmoidoscopy procedures but not for colonoscopy.

Study Type

Interventional

Study Phase

N/A

Condition

- Colorectal Cancer

Intervention

Procedure: Water Exchange Sigmoidoscopy

See arm description.

Procedure: Air Insufflation Sigmoidoscopy

See arm description.

Study Arms

Experimental: Water Exchange Sigmoidoscopy

As per standard practices, the patient will be walked to the procedure room and positioned in the left lateral position on the procedure bed, without pre-operative anesthesia. The procedures will be completed within the ambulatory endoscopy clinic at Kelowna General Hospital. The study will use the same colonoscopes that are already being used at KGH for colonoscopy. These are the Olympus 190 series colonoscopes. They can and will be fitted to support both water and air exchange.

For patients assigned the water exchange intervention arm, the insertion of the scope will be followed by infusion and suction of water to minimally distend the lumen. If the lumen does not open, the instrument will be retracted slightly and the infusion started again. As the scope is inserted and progressed through the intestinal lumen some of the infused water will be suctioned back constantly, exchanging clean for opaque water.

Active Comparator: Air Insufflation Sigmoidoscopy

As per standard practices, the patient will be walked to the procedure room and positioned in the left lateral position on the procedure bed, without pre-operative anesthesia. The procedures will be completed within the ambulatory endoscopy clinic at Kelowna General Hospital. The study will use the same colonoscopes that are already being used at KGH for colonoscopy. These are the Olympus 190 series colonoscopes. They can and will be fitted to support both water and air exchange.

For patients assigned to the air insufflation intervention arm, extended sigmoidoscopy will be performed with the minimum insufflation required to reach the cecum.

Recruitment Information

Recruitment Status

Recruiting

Estimated Enrollment

200

Eligibility Criteria

Inclusion Criteria:

- Asymptomatic average risk (as per BC colon screening guidelines) individuals
- Ages 50-74 years of age

Exclusion Criteria:

- A sigmoidoscopy or colonoscopy within 10 years,
- A FIT within 2 years,
- Individuals classified with any high-risk screening criteria in accordance to the

BC colon screening guidelines including:

- a personal history of adenoma,
- a first degree relative that was diagnosed with colorectal cancer or multiple adenomas under the age of 60,
- two or more first degree relatives with colorectal cancer at any age, longstanding inflammatory bowel diseases,
- a family history of familial adenomatous polyposis or hereditary nonpolyposis colorectal cancer, Individuals presenting with rectal pain, rectal bleeding, abdominal pain, or unintentional weight loss at the time of the examination.

Sex/Gender

All

Ages

50 Years to 74 Years

Accepts Healthy Volunteers

Accepts Healthy Volunteers

Contacts

Brent Parker, M.Sc   250-469-4881   brent.parker2@interiorhealth.ca
Adrian Bak, MD   250-763-6433   adrianbak@mac.com

Completion Date

December 8, 2017

Primary Completion Date

December 8, 2017

Study of TAS-102 Plus Radiation Therapy for the Treatment of the Liver in Patients With Hepatic Metastases From Colorectal Cancer

Study ID:

NCT03223779

Sponsor:

Massachusetts General Hospital

Information provided by (Responsible Party):

Massachusetts General Hospital (Massachusetts General Hospital)

Tracking Information

First Submitted Date

July 12, 2017

Start Date

October 13, 2017

Primary Completion Date

January 31, 2021

Last Update Posted Date

January 4, 2018

Current Primary Outcome Measures

Maximum Tolerated Dose (MTD)[Time Frame: From start of treatment until 4 weeks after the end of treatment]

MTD will be determined using a 3 + 3 dose escalation. 3 participants enrolled at the starting dose of 20 mg/m2 BID (Bis in die, Latin for twice daily). Based on the number of dose limiting toxicities (DLT), the dose can be either be increased to 25 mg/m2 BID then 30 mg/m2 BID or it could be reduced to 15 mg/m2 BID.

If 0 out of 3 have DLT, enroll 3 participants at next dose level

If ≥ 2 DLT out of 3 or 6 participants in a dose cohort have DLT, this will be the MTD and 3 additional participants are enrolled at next lowest dose if only 3 were treated at that level so far.

If 1 out of 3 have DLT, 3 more enrolled at current dose level. If no DLT in those 3, move to next dose level. If ≥ 1 DLT, declare this the MTD and enroll 3 additional at next lowest dose if only 3 treated so far.

If ≤ 1 out of 6 DLT at highest dose level below maximally administered dose, MTD is generally the rerecorded phase 2 dose (RP2D). Dose level 3 is RP2D if MTD not reached.

The Duration of Local Control[Time Frame: Baseline, 1 month post treatment, every 6 months for two years or until death]

Local control is the absence of local failure defined as evidence of tumor growth/regrowth that meets Response Evaluation Criteria In Solid Tumors (RECIST) criteria for progressive disease in any direction beyond that present in pre-treatment imaging studies of the treated lesion(s). The duration of local control will be measured from the start date of protocol treatment until the date of local failure.

Marginal failure is defined as appearance of tumor growth at the margin of the target volume.

Nodal failure is defined as failure in regional lymph nodes (i.e. porta-hepatis, para-aortic, diaphragmatic).

Distant failure is defined as appearance of tumor at sites beyond marginal and regional nodal sites.

Intrahepatic recurrence is defined as any new lesion elsewhere in the liver and separate from local failure.

Current Secondary Outcome Measures

Toxicity associated with TAS-102 combined with SBRT[Time Frame: From start of treatment until 4 weeks after the end of treatment]

Summary of the Adverse events experienced during treatment. Adverse events are assessed with Common Terminology Criteria for Adverse Events (CTCAE) 4.0.

Progression Free Survival[Time Frame: from the start of treatment until 2 years, or until time of progression/death]

Progression-free survival (PFS) will be measured from the start date of protocol treatment (first TAS-102 dose and/or first SBRT fraction) to the earlier date of first failure at any pre-treatment or new site (defined in 'Duration of Local Control' section) or death. PFS will be censored at the date of last follow-up for participants still alive who have not failed.

Overall Survival[Time Frame: from the start of treatment until 2 years, or until time of death]

Overall survival (OS) will be measured from the start date of protocol treatment (first TAS-102 dose and/or first SBRT fraction) to the date of death. OS will be censored at the date of last follow-up for participants who are still alive.

Association between KRAS or BRAF mutation status with local control[Time Frame: Baseline, 1 month post treatment, every 6 months for two years or until death]

Association between KRAS or BRAF mutation status with local control will be assessed using Gray's test with death as a competing risk in the absence of local failure. Local control is defined in the 'Duration of Local Control' description.

Serial ctDNA[Time Frame: Baseline, week 1, week 2, 1 month post treatment, at the time of progression]

Serial ctDNA will be analyzed by descriptive methods to identify potential trends and correlations with synchronous radiologic endpoints (baseline, one month post-treatment). ctDNA level (detectable versus negative) at early (week 1, week 2) and post-treatment (one month) assessments will be analyzed for differences in local control

Descriptive Information

Offical Title

Phase Ib/II Study of TAS-102 Plus Radiation Therapy for the Treatment of the Liver in Patients With Hepatic Metastases From Colorectal Cancer

Brief Summary

This research study is studying a drug in combination with radiation therapy as a possible treatment for hepatic metastases from colorectal cancer.

The interventions involved in this study are:

- Trifluridine (TAS-102)
- Radiation Therapy

Detailed Description

This is a Phase I/II clinical trial. Patients are being asked to participate in the Phase I portion of the study. A Phase I clinical trial tests the safety of an investigational intervention and also tries to define the appropriate dose of the investigational drug to use for further studies. "Investigational" means that the intervention is being studied.

The FDA (the U.S. Food and Drug Administration) has approved Trifluridine as a treatment option for this disease.

The FDA has not approved Trifluridine in combination with radiation therapy as a treatment option for this disease.

In this research study, the investigators are determining the safest and most effective dose of Trifluridine in combination with radiation therapy in participants with hepatic metastases from colorectal cancer.

Trifluridine stops DNA replication which may prevent the cancer cells from growing. Radiation may help to kill the cancer cells while protecting normal tissue cells. Studies have shown Trifluridine may make radiation more effective.

Study Type

Interventional

Study Phase

Phase 1/Phase 2

Condition

- Colorectal Cancer

Intervention

Drug: TAS-102

   Trifluridine stops DNA replication which may prevent the cancer cells from growing

Other Names:

   Lonsurf

   Trifluridine

Radiation: Photon SBRT

   SBRT stands for Stereotactic Body Radiation Therapy. Radiation may help to kill the cancer cells while protecting your normal tissue cells

Study Arms

Experimental: TAS-102

   Photon treatments will be performed on a linear accelerator

   Photon SBRT will be given during TAS-102 dosing

   TAS-102 dosing occurs on days 1 through 5 and 8 through 12

   TAS-102 tablets should be taken twice a day orally

Recruitment Information

Recruitment Status

Recruiting

Estimated Enrollment

56

Completion Date

January 31, 2025

Primary Completion Date

January 31, 2021

Eligibility Criteria

Inclusion Criteria:

- Participants must have biopsy-proven diagnosis of a colorectal cancer with 1-4 liver metastases. There is no upper size limit and participants must have at least 800 mL of uninvolved liver. Liver metastases may be diagnosed by imaging alone, no liver biopsy is required. Extrahepatic disease is allowed if 1) it has been stable for 3 months prior to study entry, 2) the dominant disease burden is intrahepatic and 3) the patient is referred for definitive radiation therapy to the disease in the liver.
- Participants must have measurable disease, defined as at least one lesion that can be accurately measured in at least one dimension (longest diameter to be recorded) as ≥ 10 mm with spiral CT scan. See Section 13 for the evaluation of measurable disease.
- Participants may have had prior chemotherapy, targeted biological therapy (i.e. sorafenib), surgery, transarterial chemoembolization (TACE), radiofrequency ablation, or cryosurgery for their disease as long as the prior therapy occurred more than 3 weeks before the first radiation treatment. Patients may not have had prior liver directed radiation, including radioembolization.
- Participants must be 18 years of age or older.
- Because no dosing or adverse event data are currently available on the use of high dose liver radiation in participants <18 years

of age, children are excluded from this study.

- Expected survival must be greater than three months.
- ECOG Performance Status 0 or 1..
- Participants must have liver metastases deemed unresectable due to anatomy, medical fitness, or presence of extrahepatic disease.
- Participants must have normal organ and marrow function as defined below. History of transfusion is acceptable and transfusions may be given to meet eligibility requirements.
- Hgb ≥ 9g/dL
- Absolute neutrophil count ≥ 1,500/mm3
- Platelets ≥ 75,000/mm3
- Total bilirubin ≤ 1.5 X institutional upper limit of normal
- AST (SGOT) and ALT (SGPT) ≤ 1.5 X institutional upper limit of normal
- Creatinine ≤ 1.5 mg/dl or creatinine clearance ≥ 60 mL/min/1.73 m2 (Calculated per Cockroft & Gault formula) for subjects with creatinine levels above institutional normal.
- If patient has underlying cirrhosis, only Child-Pugh classification Group A patients should be included in this study. Clinical assessment of ascites and encephalopathy is required. Child-Pugh classification must be determined for all study participants at the time of eligibility analysis. As albumin and PT/INR are required for Child-Pugh classification; these labs should be drawn with other labs required for eligibility analysis. See Appendix B for Child-Pugh classification table.
- The effects of radiation on the developing human fetus are known to be teratogenic and the safety of TAS-102 in pregnant women and their fetuses has not been established. Therefore, women of child-bearing potential and men must agree to use adequate contraception (hormonal or barrier method of birth control; abstinence) prior to study entry, for the duration of study participation, and for 6 months after stopping study treatment. Should a woman become pregnant or suspect she is pregnant while participating in this study, she should inform her treating physician immediately.
- Ability to understand and the willingness to sign a written informed consent document.
- Ability to take oral medications (i.e. no feeding tube and able to swallow whole)

Exclusion Criteria:

- Women who are pregnant or lactating. Patients must be either surgically sterile (via hysterectomy or bilateral tubal ligation), post menopausal or using acceptable methods of contraception if they are of child bearing potential. Female patients of child bearing potential must have a negative serum or urine pregnancy test within 7 days prior to starting drug. Because there is an unknown but potential risk of adverse events in nursing infants secondary to treatment of the mother with radiation, breastfeeding should be discontinued if the mother is treated with radiation.
- Participants with gross ascites or encephalopathy
- Participants with local conditions or systemic illnesses that would reduce the local tolerance to radiation treatment, such as serious local injuries, active collagen vascular disease, etc.
- Participants who have had prior liver directed radiation treatment, including selective internal radiation (SIRspheres or Theraspheres)
- Participants with a serious medical illness that may limit survival to less than 3 months
- Participants who have had chemotherapy or radiotherapy within 3 weeks (6 weeks for nitrosoureas or mitomycin C) prior to starting study treatment or those who have not recovered from adverse events due to agents administered more than 3 weeks earlier.
- Participants who are receiving any other investigational agents, or any other anti-cancer therapy during study treatment.
- Participants with any uncontrolled intercurrent illness including, but not limited to ongoing or active infection, symptomatic congestive heart failure, unstable angina pectoris, cardiac arrhythmia, or serious psychiatric illness/social situations that would limit compliance with study requirements.
- Participants who have previously received TAS-102

Sex/Gender

All

Ages

18 Years to N/A

Accepts Healthy Volunteers

No

Contacts

Theodore S Hong, MD   617-724-8770   tshong1@mgh.harvard.edu
Tarin Grillo   617-724-3661   tgrillo@mgh.harvard.edu

Pembrolizumab (Anti-PD-1) and AMG386 (Angiopoietin-2 (Ang-2) in Patients With Advanced Solid Tumor

Study ID:

NCT03239145

Sponsor:

Dana-Farber Cancer Institute

Information provided by (Responsible Party):

Dana-Farber Cancer Institute (Dana-Farber Cancer Institute)

Tracking Information

▦ **First Submitted Date**

August 1, 2017

▦ **Start Date**

August 31, 2017

▦ **Current Primary Outcome Measures**

Dose Limiting Toxicity[Time Frame: 2 years]

▦ **Current Secondary Outcome Measures**

Objective Response Rate[Time Frame: 2 years]

Progression Free Survival[Time Frame: 2 years]

Overall Survival[Time Frame: 2 years]

▦ **Primary Completion Date**

August 31, 2020

▦ **Last Update Posted Date**

February 1, 2018

Descriptive Information

▦ **Offical Title**

Phase Ib Study to Test the Safety and Potential Synergy of Pembrolizumab (Anti-PD-1) and AMG386 (Angiopoietin-2 (Ang-2) in Patients With Advanced Solid Tumor

▦ **Brief Summary**

This research study is studying an investigational combination of drugs as a possible treatment for advanced solid tumors: melanoma, ovarian, renal, or colorectal cancer.

The drugs involved in this study are:

- Pembrolizumab
- AMG386

▦ **Detailed Description**

This research study is a Phase Ib clinical trial, which tests the safety of an investigational combination of drugs and also tries to define the appropriate dose of the investigational drugs to use for further studies. "Investigational" means that the drug is being studied.

FDA (the U.S. Food and Drug Administration) has not approved of the combination of the study drugs pembrolizumab and AMG386 as a treatment for any disease. However, the FDA has approved pembrolizumab by itself for melanoma and non-small cell lung cancer.

Pembrolizumab is a humanized monoclonal antibody, or specialized type of protein, produced in the laboratory for use in treating patients with the participant disease. Pembrolizumab is designed to augment the natural ability of the immune system to recognize and target cancer cells.

AMG386 is a drug that may kill tumor cells and blocks blood vessels that supply the tumor with nutrients and oxygen. Drugs that block blood vessel formation are called "anti-angiogenic" therapies. AMG386 has been used and is currently being used in other clinical trials treating different types of cancer. Information from these other clinical trials suggests that this drug may help stop tumor growth.

In this research study, the investigators are interested in looking at the combination of AMG386 with pembrolizumab because research done in the laboratory has suggested that the immunotherapy effect could be limited by the presence of tumor vessels in a process called angiogenesis. Adding AMG386 to pembrolizumab may help overcome this limitation and augment the effect of pembrolizumab.

This combination of study drugs is being researched to:

- Determine the safety and tolerability of pembrolizumab and AMG386 at different dose levels.
- Determine the side effects of pembrolizumab and AMG386 when they are given in combination
- Determine if pembrolizumab in combination with AMG386 is a possible treatment for cancer

- Determine if pembrolizumab in combination with AMG386 changes immune cells in the blood or tumor

■ **Study Type**

Interventional

■ **Study Phase**

Phase 1

■ **Condition**

- Advanced Solid Tumor

■ **Intervention**

Drug: Pembrolizumab

Pembrolizumab is designed to augment the natural ability of the immune system to recognize and target cancer cells

Other Names:

Keytruda

Drug: Trebananib

AMG386 is a drug that may kill tumor cells and blocks blood vessels that supply the tumor with nutrients and oxygen

Other Names:

AMG 386

■ **Study Arms**

Experimental: Pembrolizumab + Trebananib
Part 1 Standard 3+3 Dose Escalation

Experimental: Pembrolizumab + Trebananib (Melanoma)
Part 2 Dose Expansion

Experimental: Pembrolizumab + Trebananib (Ovarian)
Part 2 Dose Expansion

Experimental: Pembrolizumab + Trebananib (Colorectal)
Part 2 Dose Expansion

Experimental: Pembrolizumab + Trebananib (Renal Cell Carcinoma)
Part 2 Dose Expansion

Recruitment Information

■ **Recruitment Status**

Recruiting

■ **Estimated Enrollment**

60

■ **Completion Date**

August 31, 2024

■ **Primary Completion Date**

August 31, 2020

■ **Eligibility Criteria**

Inclusion Criteria:

- Be willing and able to provide written informed consent for the trial.
- Be ≥ 18 years of age on day of signing informed consent.
- Have measurable disease based on RECIST 1.1.
- In dose escalation (Phase I), patients must have histologically or cytologically confirmed metastatic disease from any solid tumor that is incurable and fulfills one of the following criteria:
- Has demonstrated progression of disease following at least one line of effective systemic therapy. Prior treatment with anti-CTLA-4 antibody (including ipilimumab) is allowable OR
- For which effective therapy does not exist
- In dose expansion (part 2), patients must have histologically or cytologically confirmed unresectable or metastatic melanoma, renal cell carcinoma, ovarian cancer, or colorectal cancer.
- Renal cell patients must have had at least one prior VEGF TKI.
- Ovarian cancer patients must be resistant to platinum therapy (i.e. within 6 months of last platinum therapy).
- Patients with colorectal cancer should have progressed on at least one fluorouracil plus irinotecan or oxaliplatin containing regimen.

- Patients with melanoma should have unresectable or metastatic disease. Melanoma patients with BRAF V600E or V600K mutation-positive melanoma who have previously received a BRAF inhibitor with or without a MEK inhibitor) are eligible.
- In the dose expansion cohort patients should be willing to provide tissue from a newly obtained core or excisional biopsy of a tumor lesion (pre-treatment) and post-treatment biopsy. Newly-obtained is defined as a specimen obtained up to 6 weeks (42 days) prior to initiation of treatment on Day 1. Subjects for whom newly-obtained samples cannot be provided (e.g., inaccessible, subject safety concern, or unwilling to undergo biopsy) may submit an archived specimen only upon agreement from the Sponsor. Paired biopsies will be needed from 20 patients in the dose expansion cohort, ideally 5 per disease indication
- Have a performance status of 0 or 1 on the ECOG Performance Scale (see Appendix A)
- Demonstrate adequate organ function as defined in Table 1, all screening labs should be performed up to 14 days before treatment initiation.
- System Laboratory Value
- Hematological
- Absolute neutrophil count (ANC) ≥1,500 /mcL
- Platelets ≥100,000 / mcL
- Hemoglobin ≥9 g/dL or ≥5.6 mmol/L without transfusion or EPO dependency (within 7 days of assessment)
- Renal

--Serum creatinine OR Measured or ≤1.5 X upper limit of normal (ULN) OR calculateda creatinine clearance ≥60 mL/min for subject with creatinine levels (GFR can also be used in place of > 1.5 X institutional ULN creatinine or CrCl)

- Hepatic
- Serum total bilirubin ≤ 1.5 X ULN OR Direct bilirubin ≤ ULN for subjects with total bilirubin levels > 1.5 ULN AST (SGOT) and ALT (SGPT) ≤ 2.5 X ULN OR ≤ 5 X ULN for subjects with liver metastases
- Albumin >2.5 mg/dL
- Coagulation
- International Normalized Ratio (INR) ≤1.5 X ULN unless subject is receiving therapy as or Prothrombin Time (PT) long as PT or PTT is within therapeutic range of intended use of anticoagulants
- Activated Partial Thromboplastin Time ≤1.5 X ULN unless subject is receiving (aPTT) anticoagulant therapy as long as PT or PTT is within therapeutic range of intended use of anticoagulants
- Creatinine clearance should be calculated per institutional standard.
- Urine protein-creatinine ratio (UPCR) ≤ 1 on spot urinalysis or protein ≤ 500 mg/24 hour urine
- Female subject of childbearing potential should have a negative serum pregnancy test within 24 hours prior to receiving the first dose of study medication.
- Female subjects of childbearing potential (Section 5.11.2) must be willing to use an adequate method of contraception as outlined in Section 5.11.2 Contraception, for the course of the study through 120 days after the last dose of study medication. Should a woman become pregnant or suspect she is pregnant while she is participating in this study, she should inform her treating physician immediately.
- Abstinence is acceptable if this is the usual lifestyle and preferred contraception
- Male subjects of reproductive potential (Section 5.11.2) must agree to use an adequate method of contraception as outlined in Section 5.11.2Contraception, starting with the first dose of study therapy through 120 days after the last dose of study therapy.
- Abstinence is acceptable if this is the usual lifestyle and preferred contraception for the subject.

Exclusion Criteria:

- Is currently participating and receiving study therapy or has participated in a study of an investigational agent and received study therapy or used an investigational device within 4 weeks of the first dose of treatment.
- Has a diagnosis of immunodeficiency including subjects infected with Human Immunodeficiency Virus (HIV).
- Is receiving systemic steroid therapy or any other form of immunosuppressive therapy within 7 days prior to the first dose of trial treatment.
- Has a known history of active TB (Bacillus Tuberculosis).
- Has had a prior anti-cancer monoclonal antibody (mAb) within 4 weeks prior to study Day 1 or who has not recovered (i.e., ≤ Grade 1 or at baseline) from adverse events due to agents administered more than 4 weeks earlier.
- Has had prior chemotherapy, targeted small molecule therapy, or radiation therapy within 2 weeks prior to study Day 1 or who has not recovered (i.e., ≤ Grade 1 or at baseline) from adverse events due to a previously administered agent.
- Subjects with ≤ Grade 2 neuropathy are an exception to this criterion and may qualify for the study.
- If subject received major surgery, they must have recovered adequately from the toxicity and/or complications from the intervention prior to starting therapy.
- Has a known additional malignancy that is progressing or requires active treatment. -Exceptions include basal cell carcinoma of the skin or squamous cell carcinoma of the skin that has undergone potentially curative therapy or in situ cervical cancer.
- Lesions suspected to be at higher-risk for bleeding such as bowel involvement with tumor that invades into the bowel wall or involves the intraluminal component of bowel by imaging or direct visualization or central pulmonary lesions.
- Ulcerated skin lesions
- Full anti-coagulant therapy coumadin. Patients may be receiving therapeutic lovenox, fragmin, or other heparin product that does not require laboratory monitoring.

- Poorly-controlled hypertension as defined BP > 150/100 mmHg, or SBP > 180 mmHg when DBP < 90 mmHg, on at least 2 repeated determinations on separate days within 3 months prior to study enrollment.
- History within 6 months prior to treatment of myocardial infarction, severe/unstable angina pectoris, CABG, NYHA class III or IV CHF, stroke or TIA.
- History within 3 months prior to treatment of Grade 3-4 GI bleeding/hemorrhage, treatment resistant peptic ulcer disease, erosive esophagitis or gastritis, infectious or inflammatory bowel disease, diverticulitis, pulmonary embolus, or other uncontrolled thromboembolic event.
- Patients who are less than 4 weeks post-op after major surgery.
- History of allergic reactions attributed to compounds of similar chemical or biologic composition to pembrolizumab and trebananib including history of allergic reactions to bacterially produced proteins.
- Has known active central nervous system (CNS) metastases and/or carcinomatous meningitis. Subjects with previously treated brain metastases may participate provided they are stable (without evidence of progression by imaging for at least four weeks prior to the first dose of trial treatment and any neurologic symptoms have returned to baseline), have no evidence of new or enlarging brain metastases, and are not using steroids for at least 7 days prior to trial treatment. This exception does not include carcinomatous meningitis which is excluded regardless of clinical stability.
- Has active autoimmune disease that has required systemic treatment in the past 2 years (i.e. with use of disease modifying agents, corticosteroids or immunosuppressive drugs). Replacement therapy (eg., thyroxine, insulin, or physiologic corticosteroid replacement therapy for adrenal or pituitary insufficiency, etc.) is not considered a form of systemic treatment.
- Treatment within 30 days prior to enrollment/randomization with strong immune modulators including but not limited to systemic cyclosporine, tacrolimus, sirolimus, mycophenolate mofetil, methotrexate, azathioprine, rapamycin, thalidomide, and lenalidomide.
- Uncontrolled intercurrent illness including, but not limited to, ongoing or active infection, interstitial lung disease or active, non-infectious pneumonitis, nephritis, pancreatitis, symptomatic congestive heart failure, unstable angina pectoris, cardiac arrhythmia, or psychiatric illness/social situations that would limit compliance with study requirements.
- Has a history of (non-infectious) pneumonitis that required steroids or current pneumonitis.
- Has proteinuria
- Has an active infection requiring systemic therapy.
- Has a history or current evidence of any condition, therapy, or laboratory abnormality that might confound the results of the trial, interfere with the subject's participation for the full duration of the trial, or is not in the best interest of the subject to participate, in the opinion of the treating investigator.
- Has known psychiatric or substance abuse disorders that would interfere with cooperation with the requirements of the trial.
- Is pregnant or breastfeeding, or expecting to conceive or father children within the projected duration of the trial, starting with the pre-screening or screening visit through 120 days after the last dose of trial treatment.
- Patient with melanoma, ovarian cancer, renal cell carcinoma, colorectal cancer, and other solid tumors who have received prior therapy with an anti-PD-1, anti-PD-L1, or anti-PD-L2 antibody.
- Has received trebananib or another angiopoietin-2 directed therapy (prior treatment with bevacizumab is not an exclusion criteria)
- Has active Hepatitis B (e.g., HBsAg reactive) or Hepatitis C (e.g., HCV RNA [qualitative] is detected).
- Has received a live vaccine within 30 days of planned start of study therapy.

Sex/Gender

All

Ages

18 Years to N/A

Accepts Healthy Volunteers

No

Contacts

Janice Russell   617-632-5458   janice   russell@dfci.harvard.edu

A Study Exploring the Safety and Efficacy of INCAGN01949 in Combination With Immune Therapies in Advanced or Metastatic Malignancies

Study ID:

NCT03241173

Sponsor:

Incyte Biosciences International Sàrl

Information provided by (Responsible Party):

Incyte Corporation (Incyte Biosciences International Sàrl)

Tracking Information

▧ **First Submitted Date**

August 2, 2017

▧ **Start Date**

October 2, 2017

▧ **Primary Completion Date**

May 2021

▧ **Last Update Posted Date**

January 18, 2018

▧ **Current Primary Outcome Measures**

Phase 1: Participants With Treatment-Emergent Adverse Events (TEAEs) [Safety and Tolerability][Time Frame: Screening through 60 days after end of treatment, up to 18 months]

> TEAEs defined as any untoward medical occurrence associated with the use of a drug in humans, whether or not considered drug related, that occurs after a subject provides informed consent.

Phase 2: Objective response rate (ORR) based on Response Evaluation Criteria in Solid Tumors (RECIST) v1.1[Time Frame: Assessed every 8 weeks for 12 months, then every 12 weeks, up to 18 months]

> Defined as the percentage of subjects having a complete response (CR) or partial response (PR).

▧ **Current Secondary Outcome Measures**

Phase 1 & Phase 2: ORR based on RECIST v1.1 and modified RECIST (mRECIST) v1.1[Time Frame: Assessed every 8 weeks for 12 months, then every 12 weeks, up to 18 months]

> Defined as the percentage of subjects having a CR or PR.

Phase 1 & Phase 2: Duration of response based on RECIST v1.1 and mRECIST v1.1[Time Frame: Assessed every 8 weeks for 12 months, then every 12 weeks, up to 18 months]

> Defined as the time from the earliest date of disease response (CR or PR) until earliest date of disease progression or death due to any cause, if occurring sooner than progression.

Phase 1 & Phase 2: Disease control rate based on RECIST v1.1 and mRECIST v1.1[Time Frame: Assessed every 8 weeks for 12 months, then every 12 weeks, up to 18 months]

> Defined as the percentage of subjects having a CR, PR, or stable disease (SD).

Phase 1 & Phase 2: Duration of disease control based on RECIST v1.1 and mRECIST v1.[Time Frame: Assessed every 8 weeks for 12 months, then every 12 weeks, up to 18 months]

> Defined as CR, PR, and SD as measured from first report of SD or better until disease progression or death from any cause, if occurring sooner than progression.

Phase 1 & Phase 2: Progression-free survival based on RECIST v1.1 and mRECIST v1.1[Time Frame: Assessed every 8 weeks for 12 months, then every 12 weeks, up to 18 months]

> Defined as the time from the start of combination therapy until the earliest date of disease progression or death due to any cause, if occurring sooner than progression.

Phase 1 & Phase 2: Overall survival[Time Frame: At 1 year, 2 years, and end of study, up to 24 months]

> Determined from the start of combination therapy until death due to any cause.

Phase 1 & Phase 2: Participants With Treatment-Emergent Adverse Events (TEAEs) [Safety and Tolerability][Time Frame: Screening through 60 days after end of treatment, up to 18 months]

> TEAEs defined as any untoward medical occurrence associated with the use of a drug in humans, whether or not considered drug related, that occurs after a subject provides informed consent.

Descriptive Information

Offical Title

A Phase 1/2 Study Exploring the Safety, Tolerability, and Efficacy of INCAGN01949 in Combination With Immune Therapies in Subjects With Advanced or Metastatic Malignancies

Brief Summary

The purpose of this study is to determine the safety, tolerability, and efficacy of INCAGN01949 when given in combination with immune therapies in participants with advanced or metastatic malignancies.

Study Type

Interventional

Study Phase

Phase 1/Phase 2

Condition

- Advanced or Metastatic Malignancies

Intervention

Drug: INCAGN01949

> In Phase 1 subjects will receive INCAGN01949 administered intravenously (IV) at the protocol-defined dose according to cohort enrollment.

Drug: Nivolumab

> Nivolumab will be administered IV at the protocol-defined dose according to assigned treatment group.

Drug: Ipilimumab

> Ipilimumab will be administered IV at the protocol-defined dose according to assigned treatment group.

Drug: INCAGN01949

> In Phase 1 subjects will receive INCAGN01949 administered intravenously (IV) at the protocol-defined dose according to cohort enrollment. In Phase 2, subjects will be administered IV study drug at the recommended dose from Phase 1.

Study Arms

Experimental: INCAGN01949 + Nivolumab
> INCAGN01949 combined with nivolumab.

Experimental: INCAGN01949 + Ipilimumab
> INCAGN01949 combined with ipilimumab.

Experimental: INCAGN01949 + Nivolumab + Ipilimumab
> INCAGN01949 combined with nivolumab and ipilimumab.

Recruitment Information

Recruitment Status

Recruiting

Estimated Enrollment

651

Completion Date

November 2021

Primary Completion Date

May 2021

Eligibility Criteria

Inclusion Criteria:

- Locally advanced or metastatic disease; locally advanced disease must not be amenable to resection with curative intent.
- Phase 1: Subjects with advanced or metastatic solid tumors.
- Phase 1: Subjects who have disease progression after treatment with available therapies.
- Phase 2: Subjects with advanced or metastatic urothelial carcinoma or RCC.
- Presence of measurable disease based on RECIST v1.1.
- Eastern Cooperative Oncology Group (ECOG) performance status 0 to 1.

Exclusion Criteria:

- Laboratory and medical history parameters not within the Protocol-defined range
- Receipt of anticancer medications or investigational drugs within protocol-defined intervals before the first administration of study drug.

- Has not recovered to ≤ Grade 1 from toxic effects of prior therapy.
- Active autoimmune disease.
- Known active central nervous system metastases and/or carcinomatous meningitis.
- Evidence of active, noninfectious pneumonitis or history of interstitial lung disease.
- Evidence of hepatitis B virus or hepatitis C virus infection or risk of reactivation.
- Known history of human immunodeficiency virus (HIV); HIV 1/2 antibodies.

Sex/Gender

All

Ages

18 Years to N/A

Accepts Healthy Volunteers

No

Contacts

Incyte Corporation Call Center (US)   1.855.463.3463   medinfo@incyte.com

Incyte Corporation Call Center (ex-US)   +800 00027423   globalmedinfo@incyte.com

A Study of SC-007 in Subjects With Advanced Cancer

Study ID:

NCT03253185

Sponsor:

AbbVie

Information provided by (Responsible Party):

AbbVie (AbbVie)

Tracking Information

First Submitted Date

August 14, 2017

Start Date

September 13, 2017

Primary Completion Date

September 1, 2020

Last Update Posted Date

February 2, 2018

Current Primary Outcome Measures

Number of participants with dose-limiting toxicities (DLTs)[Time Frame: Minimum first cycle of dosing (Up to 21 days)]

DLTs graded according to the National Cancer Institute's Common Terminology Criteria for Adverse Events (NCI CTCAE) version 4.03.

Current Secondary Outcome Measures

Clinical Benefit Rate (CBR)[Time Frame: Approximately 4 years]

CBR is defined as the proportion of participants with an objective response or stable disease (CR+PR+SD).

Progression Free Survival (PFS)[Time Frame: Approximately 4 years]

PFS time is defined as the time from the participant's first dose of study drug (Day 1) to either the participant's disease progression or death due to any cause.

Observed plasma concentrations at trough (Ctrough) of SC-007[Time Frame: Approximately 1 year]

Observed plasma concentrations at trough of SC-007

Incidence of Anti-therapeutic Antibodies (ATAs) against SC-007[Time Frame: Approximately 4 years]

Incidence of ATAs against SC-007

Overall Survival (OS)[Time Frame: Approximately 4 years]

OS is defined as the time from the participant's first dose date to death due to any cause.

Terminal half life (T1/2) of SC-007[Time Frame: Approximately 1 year]

Terminal half life of SC-007

Objective Response Rate (ORR)[Time Frame: Approximately 4 years]

ORR is defined as the proportion of participants with complete response or partial response (CR+PR)

Duration of Response (DOR)[Time Frame: Approximately 4 years]

DOR is defined as the time from the participant's initial objective response (CR or PR) to study drug therapy, to disease progression or death due to any cause, whichever occurs first.

Time to Cmax (Tmax) of SC-007[Time Frame: Approximately 1 year]

Time to Cmax of SC-007

Area under the plasma concentration-time curve within a dosing interval (AUC) of SC-007[Time Frame: Approximately 1 year]

Area under the plasma concentration-time curve within a dosing interval of SC-007

QTcF Change from Baseline[Time Frame: Up to 9 weeks based on 3 cycles of dosing (21-day cycles)]

QT interval measurement corrected by Fridericia's formula (QTcF)

Maximum observed serum concentration (Cmax) of SC-007[Time Frame: Approximately 1 year]

Maximum observed serum concentration of SC-007

Descriptive Information

▦ Offical Title

An Open Label Study of SC-007 in Subjects With Advanced Cancer

▦ Brief Summary

This is a multicenter, open-label, Phase 1 study in participants with colorectal cancer (CRC) or gastric cancer to study the safety and tolerability of SC-007 and consists of Part A (dose regimen finding) in participants with CRC followed by Part A in participants with gastric cancer. Part B (dose expansion) will enroll participants into separate disease specific cohorts of CRC or gastric cancer.

▦ Study Type

Interventional

▦ Study Phase

Phase 1

▦ Condition

- Colorectal Cancer (CRC)
- Gastric Cancer

▦ Intervention

Drug: SC-007

intravenous

▦ Study Arms

Experimental: SC-007

SC-007 intravenous (IV) (various doses and dose regimens)

Recruitment Information

▦ Recruitment Status

Recruiting

▦ Estimated Enrollment

146

▦ Completion Date

July 28, 2021

▦ Primary Completion Date

September 1, 2020

▦ Eligibility Criteria

Inclusion Criteria:

- Histologically or cytologically confirmed advanced metastatic or unresectable advanced colorectal cancer (CRC) or gastric cancer that is relapsed, refractory, or progressive after:
- CRC: at least 2 prior systemic regimens in the metastatic setting, and as appropriate in patients whose tumors are microsatellite instability-high (MSI-H), pembrolizumab as well.
- Gastric cancer (including gastric and EGJ cancers): at least 2 prior systemic regimens in adjuvant, advanced, or metastatic setting and, as appropriate, a human epidermal growth factor receptor 2 (HER2) targeted agent.
- Eastern Cooperative Oncology Group (ECOG) performance status of 0 or 1

- Adequate hematologic, hepatic, and renal function.

Exclusion Criteria:

- Any significant medical condition that, in the opinion of the investigator or sponsor, may place the participant at undue risk from the study.
- Has electrocardiogram (ECG) abnormalities that make QT interval corrected (QTc) evaluation difficult.
- Prior exposure to a pyrrolobenzodiazepine or indolinobenzodiazepine based drug.

▦ Sex/Gender

All

▦ Ages

18 Years to N/A

▦ Accepts Healthy Volunteers

Accepts Healthy Volunteers

▦ Contacts

ABBVIE CALL CENTER   847.283.8955   abbvieclinicaltrials@abbvie.com

Lidocaine for Oxaliplatin-induced Neuropathy

Study ID:

NCT03254394

Sponsor:

Washington University School of Medicine

Information provided by (Responsible Party):

Washington University School of Medicine (Washington University School of Medicine)

Tracking Information

▦ First Submitted Date

August 9, 2017

▦ Primary Completion Date

December 1, 2018

▦ Start Date

September 15, 2017

▦ Last Update Posted Date

October 3, 2017

▦ Current Primary Outcome Measures

Intensity of oxaliplatin-induced cold hypersensitivity[Time Frame: 12 weeks]

The intensity of cold hypersensitivity, assessed on a 0-10 scale, upon holding a pre--cooled (~8°C) metal cylinder, will serve as primary outcome measure. Comparison between intervention (lidocaine) and placebo after 6 cycles of oxaliplatin.

▦ Current Secondary Outcome Measures

Occurence of Grade 2+ peripheral Neuropathy[Time Frame: 12 weeks]

The occurrence of Grade 2+ peripheral neuropathy , measured by NCI-CTC Peripheral Neuropathy Grading, compared between arms after 6 cycles of oxaliplatin.

CIPN score on EORTC QLQ-CIPN20[Time Frame: 12 weeks and 34-36 weeks]

Change in CIPN score (on EORTC QLQ-CIPN20 tool) over time until last follow-up

Sensory changes on QST[Time Frame: 6 weeks, 12 weeks, 34-36 weeks.]

The magnitude of sensory disturbances on quantitative sensory testing (QST) (change from baseline to last follow-up.

Changes in NPSI.[Time Frame: 6 weeks, 12 weeks, 34-36 weeks]

Changes in NPSI descriptors of neuropathic pain over time from baseline to last follow-up.

The cumulative dose of oxaliplatin[Time Frame: 24 weeks]

The cumulative dose of oxaliplatin received over the course (up to 12 cycles) of mFOLFOX6.

Progression-free survival[Time Frame: 2 years]

Two-year progression-free survival determined by medical record review.

Overall survival[Time Frame: 2 years]

Two-year overall survival determined by medical record review.

Descriptive Information

▨ Offical Title

Intravenous Lidocaine for Preventing Painful Oxaliplatin-induced Peripheral Neuropathy (OIPN)

▨ Brief Summary

Oxaliplatin-induced neuropathy is a major dose-limiting side effect in patients with colorectal cancer treated with the FOLFOX chemotherapy regimen. Hypersensitivity to cold is the sensory hallmark of oxaliplatin-induced neuropathy, and it can predict the development of long-term neuropathy. In this study, the investigators aim to determine whether intravenous lidocaine can prevent oxaliplatin-induced cold hypersensitivity.

▨ Detailed Description

Colorectal cancer is the third leading cause of cancer death in the United States, with an estimated incidence of 130.000 cases per year. Oxaliplatin is the first-line chemotherapy regimen for gastro-intestinal cancers. Despite its efficacy, oxaliplatin causes peripheral neuropathy in 72% of the treated patients. Acute oxaliplatin-induced peripheral neuropathy [OIPN] is the most common dose-limiting side effect of oxaliplatin and characterized by profound cold allodynia in the extremities. In about 21% of the patients acute OIPN exacerbates into chronic neuropathic pain, which is treatment resistant to currently approved drugs, pointing towards a great need to identify an effective strategy in preventing OIPN. Recent literature suggests that certain methods of assessing sensory nerve function in neuropathic pain patients may provide a prediction to an individual analgesic response; however, no placebo-controlled studies have been performed with the primary goal of identifying treatment response predictors in preventing OIPN.

In this pilot study we will both determine the tolerability and the efficacy of intravenous Lidocaine, for preventing oxaliplatin-induced cold hypersensitivity in the setting of mFOLFOX6 chemotherapy for advanced colorectal cancer.

The proposed study will be conducted in two phases. The tolerability phase is an open-label study to determine the tolerable dose regimen of IV lidocaine in patients with advanced colorectal cancer receiving oxaliplatin chemotherapy. The efficacy pilot phase is a randomized, double-blinded, controlled study comparing the outcomes between IV lidocaine versus placebo in the same setting of colorectal cancer. Consented subjects will attend a screening visit and six intervention visits, during which they will undergo sensory testing and receive intravenous lidocaine or placebo infusion. Cold hypersensitivity and spontaneous pain will be assessed at baseline, daily for 12 weeks and at follow-up visits. At enrollment, each patient will be assigned a study number, which will match a previously prepared computer-generated list of randomization numbers to determine the interventions lidocaine or placebo. The participants and all other study personnel will be blinded to the treatment allocation.

▨ Study Type

Interventional

▨ Study Phase

Phase 1/Phase 2

▨ Condition

- Neuropathy, Painful
- Chemotherapy-induced Peripheral Neuropathy
- Colorectal Cancer

▨ Intervention

Drug: Lidocaine Hydrochloride

> Intravenous lidocaine will be dosed as a brief 1 mg/kg infusion (based on Ideal Body Weight (IBW)) over 10 minutes, followed by a 0.04 mg/kg/min infusion over additional 120 minutes, resulting in a total dose of 5.8 mg/kg IBW.

> If this dose is tolerable in four consecutive sessions of mFOLFOX6 in six or more of the eight patients in the tolerability phase, we will initiate the randomized efficacy pilot study.

Drug: Placebo

Dextrose 5% in water will be administered as active comparator.

Drug: FOLFOX regimen

Each cycle (repeated every 14 days):

Oxaliplatin 85mg/m2 IV over 2h, Leucovorin 400 mg/m2 IV over 2h, 5-FU 400mg/m2 IV bolus, followed by a 1200mg/m2/day continuous infusion for 2 days.

Other Names:

mFOLFOX6

▨ Study Arms

Placebo Comparator: Placebo + FOLFOX

> Intravenous infusion of D5W solution over a 130 minute period.

> FOLFOX:

Oxaliplatin 85mg/m2 IV over 2h, Leucovorin 400 mg/m2 IV over 2h, 5-FU 400mg/m2 IV bolus, followed by a 1200mg/m2/day continuous infusion for 2 days.

Active Comparator: Lidocaine + FOLFOX

Intravenous infusion of lidocaine hydrochloride solution in D5W over a 130 minute period.

FOLFOX:

Oxaliplatin 85mg/m2 IV over 2h, Leucovorin 400 mg/m2 IV over 2h, 5-FU 400mg/m2 IV bolus, followed by a 1200mg/m2/day continuous infusion for 2 days.

▨ Publications

(Includes publications given by the data provider as well as publications identified by ClinicalTrials.gov Identifier (NCT Number) in Medline.)Seretny M, Currie GL, Sena ES, Ramnarine S, Grant R, MacLeod MR, Colvin LA, Fallon M. Incidence, prevalence, and predictors of chemotherapy-induced peripheral neuropathy: A systematic review and meta-analysis. Pain. 2014 Dec;155(12):2461-70. doi: 10.1016/j.pain.2014.09.020. Epub 2014 Sep 23. Review. (https://www.ncbi.nlm.nih.gov/pubmed/25261162)

Attal N, Rouaud J, Brasseur L, Chauvin M, Bouhassira D. Systemic lidocaine in pain due to peripheral nerve injury and predictors of response. Neurology. 2004 Jan 27;62(2):218-25. (https://www.ncbi.nlm.nih.gov/pubmed/14745057)

Attal N, Gaudé V, Brasseur L, Dupuy M, Guirimand F, Parker F, Bouhassira D. Intravenous lidocaine in central pain: a double-blind, placebo-controlled, psychophysical study. Neurology. 2000 Feb 8;54(3):564-74. (https://www.ncbi.nlm.nih.gov/pubmed/10680784)

Recruitment Information

▨ Recruitment Status

Recruiting

▨ Estimated Enrollment

38

▨ Completion Date

June 1, 2019

▨ Primary Completion Date

December 1, 2018

▨ Eligibility Criteria

Inclusion Criteria:

- Stage III and IV colorectal cancer.
- Scheduled for oxaliplatin treatment in mFOLFOX6-based chemotherapy regimen.
- Able to understand and willing to sign an IRB-approved written informed consent document.

Exclusion Criteria:

- Renal insufficiency (defined as calculated Creatinine clearance < 30mL/min)
- Moderate to severe liver failure (defined as ALT or AST > 3 times upper limit of normal if no liver metastases are present; ALT or AST > 5 times upper limit of normal if liver metastases are present).
- Presence of brain metastases.
- Patients with currently uncontrolled cardiac arrhythmias (non-sinus rhythm).
- Patients with history of arrhythmias under pharmacological/pacemaker control will be allowed, except if receiving antiarrhythmic medication listed in "contra-indicated medications".
- Contraindication or allergy to intravenous lidocaine.
- Pre-existing symmetric peripheral painful neuropathy.
- Treated with chemotherapy within the past 12 months.
- Pregnancy or breastfeeding
- Currently treated with any of the following contraindicated medications: Saquinavir, Lopinavir, Amprenavir, Atazanavir, Delavirdine, Mexiletine (and other types of sodium-channel blocker antiarrhythmics), Phenytoin, Carbamazepine, Oxcarbazepine, Lamotrigine, Amiodarone, Dronedarone, Dihydroergotamine, Cimetidine

▨ Sex/Gender

All

▨ Ages

18 Years to N/A

▨ Accepts Healthy Volunteers

No

▨ Contacts

Simon Haroutounian, PhD   314 286 1715   haroutos@anest.wustl.edu

Karen Frey, BS   314 454 5980   freyk@anest.wustl.edu

A Study to Evaluate eFT508 Alone and in Combination With Avelumab in Subjects With MSS Colorectal Cancer

Study ID:

NCT03258398

Sponsor:

Effector Therapeutics

Information provided by (Responsible Party):

Effector Therapeutics (Effector Therapeutics)

Tracking Information

▥ **First Submitted Date**

August 21, 2017

▥ **Start Date**

September 13, 2017

▥ **Primary Completion Date**

May 2018

▥ **Last Update Posted Date**

December 13, 2017

▥ **Current Primary Outcome Measures**

Part 1: Proportion of subjects with a dose limiting toxicity (DLT) during the first treatment cycle[Time Frame: 28 days]
Part 2: Overall Response Rate[Time Frame: 8-16 weeks]

the proportion of subjects whose best overall response is a complete or partial response

Descriptive Information

▥ **Offical Title**

A Phase 2, Open-Label, Randomized, Non-Comparative Study With Preliminary Dose Finding to Evaluate eFT508 Monotherapy or eFT508 in Combination With Avelumab in Subjects With Microsatellite Stable Relapsed or Refractory Colorectal Cancer

▥ **Brief Summary**

This is a Phase 2, open-label, 2-part, multicenter study in subjects with MSS relapsed/refractory colorectal cancer. The primary objective of Part 1 is to evaluate the safety and tolerability of escalating doses of eFT508 in combination with a fixed dose of avelumab to determine the maximum tolerated dose (MTD) of eFT508 and to select a recommended dose for Part 2. The primary objective of Part 2 is to evaluate antitumor activity of eFT508 at the recommended dose in combination with avelumab or eFT508 monotherapy. Parts 1 and 2 will also evaluate pharmacokinetics (PK) and pharmacodynamics.

▥ **Study Type**

Interventional

▥ **Study Phase**

Phase 2

▥ **Condition**

- Microsatellite Stable Relapsed or Refractory Colorectal Cancer

▥ **Intervention**

Drug: eFT508

eFT508 will be taken orally (PO) twice a day (bid).

Drug: Avelumab

Avelumab 10 mg/kg will be administered intravenously (IV) on Day 1 and once every 2 weeks (q2wk) thereafter

▥ **Study Arms**

Experimental: Part 1: eFT508 plus avelumab dose finding Arm
subjects will receive eFT508 in combination with a fixed dose of avelumab

Experimental: Part 2: eFT508 plus avelumab
subjects will receive eFT508 in combination with a fixed dose of avelumab

Experimental: Part 2: eFT508 alone
subjects will receive eFT508 alone

Recruitment Information

Recruitment Status

Recruiting

Completion Date

November 2018

Estimated Enrollment

70

Primary Completion Date

May 2018

Eligibility Criteria

Inclusion Criteria:

- ECOG performance status of 0, 1, or 2
- Pathologically documented diagnosis of colorectal adenocarcinoma.
- Progressed on or intolerant of at least 2 prior cancer therapy regimens administered for metastatic disease.
- Completion of all previous therapy (including surgery, radiotherapy, chemotherapy, immunotherapy, or investigational therapy) for the treatment of cancer ≥3 weeks before the start of study therapy.
- Part 2 only: Presence of radiographically measurable disease (defined as the presence of ≥1 lesion that measures ≥10 mm [≥15 mm for lymph nodes]). Measurable disease that was previously radiated is only permitted if progressing.
- Agrees to undergo a pretreatment and a post-treatment biopsy.
- Microsatellite stable disease determined by IHC and/or polymerase chain reaction (PCR).
- Adequate bone marrow function
- Adequate hepatic function
- Adequate renal function
- Normal coagulation profile
- Negative antiviral serology
- Female subjects of childbearing potential must not be pregnant or breastfeeding
- Willingness to use protocol-recommended methods of contraception or to abstain from heterosexual intercourse from start of therapy until at lest 30 days after the last dose of study therapy
- Life expectancy of ≥3 months.

Exclusion Criteria:

- History of another malignancy except for adequately treated local basal cell or squamous cell carcinoma of the skin; in situ cervical or breast carcinoma; adequately treated, papillary, noninvasive bladder cancer; other adequately treated Stage 1 or 2 cancers currently in complete remission, or any other cancer that has been in complete remission for ≥2 years.
- Known symptomatic brain metastases requiring ≥10 mg/day of prednisolone (or its equivalent).
- Significant cardiovascular disease.
- Significant screening ECG abnormalities.
- Active autoimmune disease that might deteriorate when receiving an immunostimulatory agent.
- Known history of colitis, inflammatory bowel disease, pneumonitis, or pulmonary fibrosis.
- Ongoing risk for bleeding due to active peptic ulcer disease or bleeding diathesis.
- Evidence of an ongoing systemic bacterial, fungal, or viral infection.
- Any condition that may impact the subject's ability to swallow oral medications.
- Major surgery within 4 weeks before the start of study therapy.
- Prior solid organ or bone marrow progenitor cell transplantation.
- Prior therapy with any known inhibitor of MNK-1 or MNK-2.
- Prior therapy with any of the following: PD-1, PD-L1, CTLA4 antibody, or any other drug targeting T cell checkpoint pathways.
- Prior high dose chemotherapy requiring stem cell rescue.
- Intolerance to or prior severe (≥Grade 3) allergic or anaphylactic reaction to infused antibodies or infused therapeutic proteins.
- Vaccination within 4 weeks of the first dose of avelumab and while on study.
- Ongoing immunosuppressive therapy.
- Use of a strong inhibitor or inducer of cytochrome P450 3A4 (CYP3A4) within 7 days prior to the start of study therapy or expected requirement for use of a strong CYP3A4 inhibitor or inducer during study therapy.
- Previously received investigational product in a clinical trial within 30 days or within 5 elimination half lives (whichever is longer) prior to the start of study therapy, or is planning to take part in another clinical trial while participating in this study.
- Has any illness, medical condition, organ system dysfunction, or social situation, including mental illness or substance abuse, deemed by the Investigator to be likely to interfere with a subject's ability to sign informed consent, adversely affect the subject's ability to cooperate and participate in the study, or compromise the interpretation of study results

Sex/Gender

All

Combination of TATE and PD-1 Inhibitor in Liver Cancer

Study ID:

NCT03259867

Sponsor:

Teclison Ltd.

Information provided by (Responsible Party):

Teclison Ltd. (Teclison Ltd.)

Tracking Information

■ **First Submitted Date**

August 16, 2017

■ **Start Date**

July 1, 2017

■ **Current Primary Outcome Measures**

Response rate[Time Frame: up to 24 months]
Objective response rate in non-TATE treated lesion

■ **Current Secondary Outcome Measures**

Overall Response rate[Time Frame: up to 24 months]
All tumor lesions

Duration of Response[Time Frame: up to 24 months]
All tumor lesions

Progression Free Survival[Time Frame: up to 24 months]
From randomization to disease progression or death

Overall survival[Time Frame: through study completion, an average of 3 years]
From randomization to death

■ **Primary Completion Date**

March 30, 2019

■ **Last Update Posted Date**

August 24, 2017

Descriptive Information

■ **Offical Title**

Phase IIA Single-Arm Study of Treatment of Patients With Advanced Liver Cancer With a Combination of TATE (Transarterial Tirapazamine Embolization) Followed by an Anti-PD-1 Monoclonal Antibody

■ **Brief Summary**

This is a single center, open-label phase IIA study that investigates the preliminary efficacy of TATE treatment of liver cancer followed by a PD-1 checkpoint inhibitor (either nivolumab or pembrolizumab). At least two cohorts will be enrolled, one for patients with hepatocellular carcinoma (HCC) and the other with metastatic colorectal cancer (mCRC).

■ **Detailed Description**

The goal of the study is to investigate whether tumor necrosis induced by TATE treatment can boost anti-tumor immunity and enhance the therapeutic efficacy of immune checkpoint inhibitor. Patients with advanced HCC or metastatic CRC with liver lesions will be enrolled in the study. Liver lesions will be treated with up to 4 TATE treatments for optimal debulking, which also serve as a vaccination process toward tumor. Lesion not treated with TATE will be used for monitoring the response toward a PD-1 inhibitor (either Nivolumab or Pembrolizumab per investigator decision). If a patient subsequently develops an "escape" to the PD-1 inhibitor, patient can have another 2 TATE treatments of the escaped tumor lesion. Dosing of the PD-1 inhibitor is per standard FDA-approved dosing schedule and continues until progressive disease. The efficacy will be assessed by the response rate (RR) using RECIST and irRC for the non-TATE treated lesion, and compared with the historic RR of the PD-1 inhibitor in HCC (~16%) and mCRC (almost 0% for those without mismatch repair defect).

Study Type

Interventional

Study Phase

Phase 2

Condition

- Carcinoma
- Hepatocellular
- Colorectal Neoplasms

Intervention

Drug: Opdivo Injectable Product or Keytruda Injectable Product

a PD-1 immune check inhibitor per Investigator decision

Combination Product: Trans-arterial tirapazamine embolization

Embolization with Lipiodol and Gelfoam

Study Arms

Experimental: Hepatocellular carcinoma

PD-1 inhibitor (either Opdivo 240 mg Q2W IV or Keytruda 200 mg Q3W IV) starts at day 1, and continues until progression.

TATE treatment starts at day 8 for debulking up to 4 cycles. If escape lesion appears, two more TATE treatments can be given. Tirapazamine dose at 35 mg flat dose given before embolization.

Experimental: Colorectal cancer

PD-1 inhibitor (either Opdivo 240 mg Q2W IV or Keytruda 200 mg Q3W IV) starts at day 1, and continues until progression.

TATE treatment starts at day 8 for debulking up to 4 cycles. If escape lesion appears, two more TATE treatments can be given. Tirapazamine dose at 35 mg flat dose given before embolization.

Recruitment Information

Recruitment Status

Recruiting

Estimated Enrollment

40

Completion Date

October 1, 2020

Primary Completion Date

March 30, 2019

Eligibility Criteria

Inclusion Criteria:

1. Patients with either a confirmed diagnosis of (1) metastatic colorectal cancer in liver based on histopathology of either a prior resection of primary lesion or a biopsied liver metastatic lesion, or (2) advanced HCC (BCLC-stage C) with a characteristic 3 or 4-phase CT or dynamic contrast enhanced MRI finding showing arterial uptake followed by "washout" of contrast in the venous-delayed phases per American Association for the Study of Liver Disease (AASLD) criteria.

2. Patients between ages 18 and 80

3. If HCC patients, they should have progressive disease (PD) on, intolerant of, or refusing, sorafenib. If mCRC, they should have received at least one regimen of 5-fluouracil based systemic chemotherapy such as FOLFOX, FOLFIRI, CAPOX, or XELOX, with or without a VEGF or EGFR receptor inhibitor.

4. Patients with at least two liver tumor lesions with at least one with a diameter of 2 cm or bigger, which is amendable for (super-)selective TATE as the target lesion. Alternatively, patients with one intra-hepatic lesion of 2 cm or bigger and exhapetic lesion(s) are also acceptable.

5. ECOG score 2 or less

6. Child-Pugh scores 5-7

7. Patients should have measurable disease by contrast CT or contrast-enhanced MRI.

8. All prior therapy must be at least 4 weeks prior to enrollment and free from treatment-related toxicity.

9. Patients have normal organ function: Hemoglobin ≥ 8.5 gm/dL, Platelets ≥ 50,000 /µL, Creatinine ≤ 2 mg/dL, AST and ALT < 10 X upper normal limit of the current institution; bilirubin < 3.0 mg/dL

10. Patients are able to understand and willing to sign the informed consent.

11. Men and women of child-bearing age need to commit to using two methods of contraception simultaneously to avoid

pregnancy.

Exclusion Criteria:

1. Patients who have had a liver or any organ transplantation

2. Patients who take any immune or bone marrow suppressive agents including any systemic corticosteroid that exceed an equivalent of 10 mg prednisone per day within 2 weeks from the study treatment. Inhalation or topical steroids are allowed.

3. Patients who have received any checkpoint inhibitor, including ipilimumab, nivolumab, pembrolizumab or others.

4. Patients who have major medical problems such as severe cardiac, pulmonary (COPD requiring constant oxygen), or non-healing ulceration.

5. Patients with a history of autoimmune disease (e.g., rheumatoid arthritis, Addison's syndrome, multiple sclerosis, uveitis, systemic lupus erythematosus or Wegener's granulomatosis). Patients with vitiligo or alopecia are allowed. Patients with Graves disease or psoriasis not requiring systemic treatment within the past 2 years are allowed.

6. Patients who have any clinical evidence of hypoxia with O2 saturation less than 92% on room air.

7. Patients with evidence of significant arterial insufficiency or microangiopathy in any organ due to any reason, which could lead to distal extremity hypoxia, as evidenced by any gangrenous change in distal limbs or requiring resection for this reason.

8. Patients with major gastrointestinal bleeding in the prior 2 months of enrollment.

9. Patients who are pregnant or lactating.

10. Patients with QTc interval > 480 msec or those known to have congenital long QTc syndrome.

11. Patients who have received live, attenuated vaccine within 28 days prior to the first dose of PD-1 inhibitor.

Sex/Gender

All

Ages

18 Years to 80 Years

Accepts Healthy Volunteers

No

Contacts

Jennifer Berg   714-456-7687   jdberg@uci.edu

A Study to Evaluate the Safety, Tolerability, and Activity of TAK-931 in Participants With Metastatic Pancreatic Cancer or Metastatic Colorectal Cancer

Study ID:

NCT03261947

Sponsor:

Millennium Pharmaceuticals, Inc.

Information provided by (Responsible Party):

Takeda (Millennium Pharmaceuticals, Inc.)

Tracking Information

First Submitted Date

August 23, 2017

Start Date

October 25, 2017

Primary Completion Date

February 22, 2019

Last Update Posted Date

January 23, 2018

Current Primary Outcome Measures

Percentage of Participants with Dose Limiting Toxicities (DLTs) in Western Safety Cohort[Time Frame: Baseline up to 1 year]

DLT includes: Non-febrile Grade 4 neutropenia, Febrile neutropenia: Grade ≥3 neutropenia, Grade 4 thrombocytopenia, grade ≥3 thrombocytopenia of any duration accompanied by grade 2 bleeding or requiring transfusion, delay in the initiation of cycle 2 by more than 14 days due to a lack of adequate recovery of treatment-related hematological or nonhematologic toxicities, grade 2 ejection fraction decreased by echocardiogram (ECHO) or multiple gated acquisition (MUGA) scan, Grade 4 laboratory abnormalities, other grade 2 nonhematologic toxicities that are considered by the investigator to be related to study drug and dose-limiting, participants receiving <50% of doses (<7 doses) of the planned TAK-931 dosing in cycle 1 due to study drug-related AEs, grade ≥3 nonhematologic toxicity with the few exceptions: Grade 3 arthralgia/ myalgia, fatigue, laboratory abnormalities, nausea and/or emesis or diarrhea.

Percentage of Participants with Treatment Emergent Adverse Events (TEAEs), Serious Adverse Events (SAEs), TEAEs Leading to Dose Modifications and TEAEs Leading to Treatment Discontinuation in Western Safety Cohort[Time Frame: Baseline up to 1 year]

An AE is defined as any untoward medical occurrence in a clinical investigation participant administered a drug; it does not necessarily have to have a causal relationship with this treatment. A TEAE is defined as an adverse event with an onset that occurs after receiving study drug. A SAE is any untoward medical occurrence or effect that at any dose results in death, is life-threatening, requires inpatient hospitalization or prolongation of existing hospitalization, results in persistent or significant disability / incapacity, is a congenital anomaly / birth defect or is medically important due to other reasons than the above mentioned criteria.

Disease Control Rate (DCR)[Time Frame: Baseline up to 1 year]

DCR is defined as percentage of participants with complete response (CR), partial response (PR) plus stable disease (SD) ≥6 weeks from treatment initiation. Response and progression is evaluated in this study using the Response Evaluation Criteria in Solid Tumors (RECIST) V 1.1 for lesions: CR is defined as disappearance of all lesions. PR is defined as at least a 30% decrease in the sum of the longest diameter (LD) of lesions, taking as reference the baseline sum LD. Progressive disease (PD) is defined as at least a 20% increase in the sum of the LD of lesions, taking as reference the smallest sum LD recorded since the treatment started or the appearance of one or more new lesions Stable disease (SD) is defined as neither sufficient shrinkage to qualify for PR nor sufficient increase to qualify for PD, taking as reference the smallest sum LD since the treatment started.

Current Secondary Outcome Measures

Cmax: Maximum Observed Plasma Concentration for TAK-931[Time Frame: Days 1 and 8 pre-dose and at multiple timepoints (up to 24 hours) post-dose]

Tmax: Time to Reach the Maximum Plasma Concentration (Cmax) for TAK-931[Time Frame: Days 1 and 8 pre-dose and at multiple timepoints (up to 24 hours) post-dose]

AUC(0-24): Area Under the Plasma Concentration-Time Curve From Time 0 to 24 Hours Postdose for TAK-931[Time Frame: Days 1 and 8 pre-dose and at multiple timepoints (up to 24 hours) post-dose]

AUClast: Area Under the Plasma Concentration-Time Curve From Time 0 to the Time of the Last Quantifiable Concentration for TAK-931[Time Frame: Days 1 and 8 pre-dose and at multiple timepoints (up to 24 hours) post-dose]

CLr: Renal Clearance of TAK-931[Time Frame: Day 1 pre-dose and at multiple timepoints (up to 24 hours) post-dose]

CLr is a measure of apparent clearance of the drug from the urine. The clearance is the rate at which waste substances are cleared from the blood.

t1/2z: Terminal disposition phase half-life[Time Frame: Day 8 pre-dose and at multiple timepoints (up to 24 hours) post-dose]

CLss/F: Steady-state Apparent Oral Clearance[Time Frame: Day 8 pre-dose and at multiple timepoints (up to 24 hours) post-dose]

CL/F is apparent clearance of the drug from the plasma, calculated as the drug dose divided by AUC expressed in liters/hour (L/hr).

Rac(AUC): Accumulation Ratio Based on AUC Over the Dosing Interval (AUCτ)[Time Frame: Day 8 pre-dose and at multiple timepoints (up to 24 hours) post-dose]

Overall Response Rate (Complete Response [CR] and Partial response [PR])[Time Frame: Baseline up to 1 year]

Overall Response rate is defined as the sum of percentage of participants with complete response rate and partial response rate. Response and progression was evaluated in this study Per RECIST V1.1 where CR is defined as disappearance of all lesions, PR is defined as at least a 30% decrease in the sum of the LD of lesions, taking as reference the baseline sum LD. PD is defined as at least a 20% increase in the sum of the LD of lesions, taking as reference the smallest sum LD recorded since the treatment started or the appearance of one or more new lesions.

Duration of Response (DOR)[Time Frame: Baseline up to 1 year]

DOR is defined as the time from the date of first documentation of a CR or PR to the date of first documentation of tumor progression. Per RECIST V1.1, CR is defined as disappearance of all lesions, PR is defined as at least a 30% decrease in the sum of the LD of lesions, taking as reference the baseline sum LD. PD is defined as at least a 20% increase in the sum of the LD of lesions, taking as reference the smallest sum LD recorded since the treatment started or the appearance of one or more new lesions.

Progression Free Survival (PFS)[Time Frame: From randomization until disease progression or death whichever occurs first (up to 1 year)]

PFS is defined as time from start of study treatment to first documentation of disease progression. Per RECIST V1.1, PD is defined as at least a 20% increase in the sum of the LD of lesions, taking as reference the smallest sum LD recorded since the treatment started or the appearance of one or more new lesions.

Overall Survival (OS)[Time Frame: Baseline up to 1 year]

OS is the time from start of study treatment to date of death due to any cause.

Percentage of Participants with TEAEs in the Tumor-Specific Cohorts[Time Frame: Baseline up to 1 year]

Percentage of participants with Grade ≥3 TEAEs, SAEs, TEAEs leading to treatment discontinuation or dose modifications, and clinically significant changes in laboratory values and vital sign measurements in the tumor-specific cohorts will be reported. An AE is defined as any untoward medical occurrence in a clinical investigation participant administered a drug; it does not necessarily have to have a causal relationship with this treatment. A TEAE is defined as an adverse event with an onset that occurs after receiving study drug. A SAE is any untoward medical occurrence or effect that at any dose results in death, is life-threatening, requires inpatient hospitalization or prolongation of existing hospitalization, results in persistent or significant disability / incapacity, is a congenital anomaly / birth defect or is medically important due to other reasons than the above mentioned criteria.

Descriptive Information

▦ Offical Title

An Open-Label, Phase 2, Parallel Arm Study to Evaluate the Safety, Tolerability, and Activity of TAK-931 Single Agent in Patients With Metastatic Pancreatic Cancer or Metastatic Colorectal Cancer

▦ Brief Summary

The purpose of this study is to confirm the safety and tolerability of TAK-931 in a cohort of Western participants with metastatic solid tumors and to evaluate the anti-tumor activity of TAK-931 in participants with metastatic pancreatic cancer and colorectal cancer (CRC).

▦ Detailed Description

The drug being tested in this study is called TAK-931. TAK-931 blocks the function of a specific protein in the body called CDC7 kinase. TAK-931 is being tested in participants with metastatic pancreatic cancer or metastatic colorectal cancer plus a cohort of US patients with metastatic cancer with no other standard therapeutic alternative. This study will look at safety, tolerability and pharmacokinetics of TAK-931 in people who take TAK-931.

The study will enroll approximately 88 patients. Participants will be enrolled in 3 cohorts: 1) Western safety cohort to be enrolled in the US only which will include non-Japanese participants who have metastatic solid tumors with no standard therapeutic alternative, 2) Participants with metastatic pancreatic cancer 3) Participants with metastatic colorectal cancer. All participants will receive:

• TAK-931 50 mg

All participants will be asked to take one capsule at the same time each day throughout the study.

This multi-center trial will be conducted in United States and Japan. The overall time to participate in this study is approximately 24 months. Participants will make multiple visits to the clinic, and participants in both Western cohort and disease specific cohort will be followed-up for up to 12 weeks for progression-free survival. Once disease progression is confirmed, participants in disease-specific cohort will be followed for overall survival for up to 12 weeks after last dose of study drug.

▦ Study Type

Interventional

▦ Study Phase

Phase 2

▦ Condition

• Metastatic Pancreatic Cancer
• Colorectal Cancer

▦ Intervention

Drug: TAK-931

    TAK-931 capsules.

▦ Study Arms

Experimental: TAK-931

    TAK-931 50 mg, capsules, orally, once daily for 14 days, followed by 7-day washout period, in 21-day cycles until disease progression or unacceptable treatment-related toxicity (Up to 1 year).

Recruitment Information

▦ Recruitment Status

Recruiting

▦ Estimated Enrollment

88

▦ Eligibility Criteria

Inclusion Criteria:

▦ Completion Date

February 22, 2019

▦ Primary Completion Date

February 22, 2019

1. Adult male or female patients aged ≥20 years (Japan) or ≥18 years (US).

2. Eastern Cooperative Oncology Group (ECOG) performance status of 0-1

3. Has pathologically confirmed metastatic pancreatic adenocarcinoma that has progressed after, at least, a first line of standard systemic chemotherapy for the metastatic disease, OR participants with pathologically confirmed metastatic adenocarcinoma of the colon or rectum who have progressed to at least 2 lines of standard systemic chemotherapy for the metastatic disease.

4. For the Western safety cohort only: participants with locally advanced or metastatic solid tumor for whom no standard treatment with an established survival benefit is available or if the participant refuses other standard therapy.

5. For disease-specific cohort participants: measurable disease per RECIST v. 1.1

6. Left ventricular ejection fraction >50% as measured by echocardiogram (ECHO) or multiple gated acquisition (MUGA) scan within 4 weeks before receiving the first dose of study drug.

7. Recovered to Grade 1 or baseline from all toxic effects of previous therapy (except alopecia or neuropathy).

8. Suitable venous access for the study-required blood sampling.

9. For the Western safety cohort only: willingness to undergo serial skin tissue biopsies.

10. For disease-specific cohort participants: Must have an archival (banked) tumor sample or agree to have a new (fresh) tumor biopsy during the screening period. If a new tumor sample is needed, the disease should be accessible for a nonsignificant risk biopsy procedure (those occurring outside the brain, lung/mediastinum, and pancreas, or obtained with endoscopic procedures not extending beyond the stomach or bowel). For participants in the Western safety cohort, this biopsy is optional.

Exclusion Criteria:

1. Participants who require continuous use of proton pump inhibitors (PPIs) or histamine-2 (H2) receptor antagonists and participants who are taking PPIs within 5 days before the first dose of study drug.

2. Treatment with clinically significant enzyme inducers, such as phenytoin, carbamazepine, phenobarbital, rifampin, rifabutin, rifapentine, or Saint John's wort within 14 days before the first dose of study drug.

3. Treatment with any systemic anticancer treatment (including investigational products) within 30 days or 5 half-lives, whichever is shorter, before the first dose of study drug.

4. History of any of the following within the last 3 months before administration of the first dose of study drug:

- Ischemic myocardial event including angina requiring therapy and artery revascularization procedures, myocardial infarction, and unstable symptomatic ischemic heart disease.
- Ischemic cerebrovascular event, including transient ischemic attack and artery, revascularization procedures.
- Significant, uncontrolled cardiac arrhythmia (including atrial flutter/fibrillation, ventricular fibrillation, or ventricular tachycardia).
- Current use of rate control drugs for arrhythmias or to control cardiac frequency (including β-blockers [e.g., metoprolol], acetylcholine, digoxin, and nondihydropyridine calcium channel blockers [e.g., diltiazem and verapamil]). Patients will not be excluded if these drugs are used for other indications other than arrhythmia control.
- Placement of a pacemaker for control of cardiac rhythm.
- New York Heart Association Class II to IV heart failure.
- Any other cardiac condition that, in the opinion of the investigator, could pose an additional risk for participation in the study (e.g., pericardial effusion or restrictive cardiomyopathy).
- Baseline prolongation of the QT interval corrected for HR using Fridericia's formula (QTcF; e.g., repeated demonstration of QTcF interval >480 ms, history of congenital long QT syndrome, or torsades de pointes).

5. Participants with any of the following blood pressure (BP) conditions:

- History of orthostatic hypotension or syncope that required medical intervention.
- Orthostatic hypotension is defined as a 20-mmHg decrease in systolic BP and/or a 10-mmHg decrease in diastolic BP within 2 to 5 minutes of quiet standing immediately after 5 minutes of supine rest.
- Postural orthostatic tachycardia syndrome or postural tachycardia syndrome (defined as an increase in HR of >30 beats per minute over baseline after 10 minutes of quiet standing).
- Hypertension that is unstable or not controlled by medication.

6. History of uncontrolled brain metastasis unless:

- Previously treated with surgery, whole-brain radiation, or stereotactic radiosurgery, and
- Stable disease (SD) for ≥30 days, without steroid use (or stable steroid dose established for ≥14 days before the first dose of TAK-931).

7. Known history of human immunodeficiency virus infection.

8. Known hepatitis B virus (HBV) surface antigen seropositive or detectable hepatitis C virus (HCV) infection viral load. Note: Participants who have positive HBV core antibody or HBV surface antigen antibody can be enrolled but must have an undetectable HBV viral load.

9. Prior treatment with radiation therapy involving ≥25% of the hematopoietically active bone marrow within 3 months before the first dose of study drug.

10. Western Safety Cohort Only: Participants with Japanese heredity.

11. Colorectal cancer (CRC) Cohort Only: Participants with known microsatellite instability-high (MSI-H) genotype.

- ▣ **Sex/Gender**

  All

- ▣ **Ages**

  18 Years to N/A

- ▣ **Accepts Healthy Volunteers**

  No

- ▣ **Contacts**

  Takeda Study Registration Call Center   +1-844-662-8532   globaloncologymedinfo@takeda.com

Novel PET/CT Imaging Biomarkers of CB-839 in Combination With Panitumumab and Irinotecan in Patients With Metastatic and Refractory RAS Wildtype Colorectal Cancer

Study ID:

NCT03263429

Sponsor:

Vanderbilt-Ingram Cancer Center

Information provided by (Responsible Party):

Vanderbilt-Ingram Cancer Center (Vanderbilt-Ingram Cancer Center)

Tracking Information

- ▣ **First Submitted Date**

  August 23, 2017

- ▣ **Start Date**

  August 23, 2017

- ▣ **Primary Completion Date**

  September 2020

- ▣ **Last Update Posted Date**

  September 14, 2017

- ▣ **Current Primary Outcome Measures**

  Maximum tolerated dose (Phase I) B-839 in combination with panitumumab and irinotecan hydrochloride[Time Frame: Up to 12 months]

  The maximum tolerated dose will be determined

  Response rate (Phase II)[Time Frame: Up to 12 months]

  Will use Simon's optimal 2-stage design to monitor efficacy in this trial.

  Recommended phase 2 dose of CB-839 in combination with panitumumab and irinotecan hydrochloride (Phase I)[Time Frame: Up to 12 months.]

  The recommended phase 2 dose will be determined.

- ▣ **Current Secondary Outcome Measures**

  Disease control rate[Time Frame: Up to 12 months]

  The disease control rate will be evaluated.

  Maximum Standardized Uptake Value (SUVmax) of fluorine F 18 L-glutamate derivative BAY94-9392 (18F-FSPG) uptake (Phase II)[Time Frame: Up to 8 weeks]

  evaluate the relationship between 18F-FSPG uptake at baseline and change in tumor size at the time of objective response assessment using a standard linear regression analysis. The slope will describe the shape of the relationship between SUVmax and change in tumor size, while the coefficient of determination ($R2$) describes the strength of the relationship between the two measures. A similar linear regression analysis will be conducted to quantify the relationship between the change in SUVmax as measured from baseline to after one cycle of therapy and change in tumor size.

  Plasma exosomal content (phase II)[Time Frame: Up to 12 months]

  Plasma exosomal content will be assessed at pre-treatment, after one cycle of treatment, and at disease progression.

Progression free survival (phase II)[Time Frame: Up to 12 months]

will use Cox proportional hazards model to estimate the association between PET SUVmax and OS.

Overall Survival[Time Frame: Up to 12 months]

will use Cox proportional hazards model to estimate the association between PET SUVmax and OS.

Descriptive Information

Offical Title

Phase I/II Study to Evaluate the Safety, Efficacy, and Novel PET/CT Imaging Biomarkers of CB-839 in Combination With Panitumumab and Irinotecan in Patients With Metastatic and Refractory RAS Wildtype Colorectal Cancer

Brief Summary

This phase I/II trial studies the best dose and side effects of glutaminase inhibitor CB-839 and how well it works with panitumumab and irinotecan hydrochloride in treating patients with RAS wildtype colorectal cancer that has spread to other places in the body and does not respond to treatment. Glutaminase inhibitor CB-839 may stop the growth of tumor cells by blocking some of the enzymes needed for cell growth. Monoclonal antibodies, such as panitumumab, may interfere with the ability of tumor cells to grow and spread. Drugs used in chemotherapy, such as irinotecan hydrochloride, work in different ways to stop the growth of tumor cells, either by killing the cells, by stopping them from dividing, or by stopping them from spreading. Giving glutaminase inhibitor CB-839 with panitumumab and irinotecan hydrochloride may work better in treating patients with colorectal cancer.

Detailed Description

Objectives:

Primary Objective of Phase I:

• Determine the safety and tolerability of CB-839 in combination with panitumumab and irinotecan.

Primary Objective of Phase II:

• Determine the efficacy of CB-839 in combination with panitumumab and irinotecan as measured by the response rate (RR) in patients with previously EGFR treated RAS wildtype colorectal adenocarcinoma.

Secondary Objectives of Phase II:

OUTLINE: This is a dose-escalation study of glutaminase inhibitor CB-839.

Patients receive glutaminase inhibitor CB-839 orally (PO) twice daily (BID) on days 1-28, panitumumab intravenously (IV) over 60-90 minutes on days 1 and 15, and irinotecan hydrochloride IV over 90 minutes on day 1 and 15. Courses repeat every 28 days in the absence of disease progression or unacceptable toxicity.

After completion of study treatment, patients are followed up at 28 days and then every 3 months for up to 1 year.

• Determine the disease control rate (DCR), progression-free survival (PFS), and overall survival (OS).

• **Perform the following correlative studies (in the Phase II component):**

• Correlate radiological features of preand post-treatment 18F-FSPG PET/CT with clinical outcome and biological correlates (plasma glutamate levels, exosomes)

• Quantify exosomal content in the plasma.

Study Type

Interventional

Study Phase

Phase 1/Phase 2

Condition

• Colorectal Cancer
• Metastatic Colorectal Cancer
• RAS Wild Type Colorectal Cancer
• Refractory Colorectal Cancer

Intervention

Drug: Glutaminase Inhibitor CB-839

Given by mouth

Biological: Panitumumab

Given by vein

Drug: Irinotecan Hydrochloride

Given by vein

Other: Laboratory Biomarker Analysis

Correlative studies

Other: Pharmacological Study
Correlative studies

Device: Imaging with 18F-FSPG PET/CT scans
During phase II at baseline and day 28 of cycle 1

Study Arms

Experimental: Panitumumab/Irinotecan/CB-839
CB-839 in a pill form taken by mouth two times a day

Panitumumab given through a vein over 60 or 90 minutes on day 1 and 15 of each 28-day cycle

Irinotecan given through a vein over 90 minutes on Day 1 and 15 of each 28-day cycle

18F-FSPG PET/CT scans (during phase II) at baseline and day 28 of cycle 1

Recruitment Information

Recruitment Status
Recruiting

Estimated Enrollment
40

Completion Date
August 2021

Primary Completion Date
September 2020

Eligibility Criteria

Inclusion Criteria:
- Signed and dated written informed consent.
- Histologically or cytologically-confirmed diagnosis of metastatic KRAS wildtype colorectal cancer (CRC).
- Eastern Cooperative Oncology Group (ECOG) performance status of 0 or 1.
- In Dose Escalation, patients must have had at least one prior line of chemotherapy for advanced disease or progressed within 6 months of adjuvant therapy (prior chemotherapy and/or anti-EGFR therapy is permitted).

In Dose Expansion, patients must have received prior anti-EGFR therapy.
- At least one measureable lesion as defined by RECIST 1.1 which can be followed by CT or MRI.
- Adequate organ function including:
- Absolute neutrophil count (ANC) ≥ 1,500/μL
- Platelets ≥ 100,000/μL
- Serum albumin ≥ 3.0 g/dL
- Serum creatinine ≤ 2 mg/dL, or calculated creatinine clearance > 50 mL/min (per the Cockcroft-Gault formula)
- Total bilirubin ≤ 1.5 times upper limit of normal (ULN)
- Aspartate transaminase (AST) and Alanine Aminotransferase (ALT) ≤ 5.0 x ULN.
- Women of childbearing potential must have a negative serum pregnancy test within 14 days prior to receiving first dose of protocol-indicated treatment; and additionally agree to use at least 2 methods of acceptable contraception or abstain from heterosexual intercourse from the time of signing consent, and until 2 months after patient's last dose of protocol-indicated treatment.

Women of childbearing potential are defined as those not surgically sterile or not post-menopausal (i.e. if a female patient has not had a bilateral tubal ligation, a bilateral oophorectomy, or a complete hysterectomy; or has not been amenorrheic for 12 months in the absence of an alternative medical cause, then patient will be considered a female of childbearing potential). Postmenopausal status in females under 55 years of age should be confirmed with a serum follicle-stimulating hormone (FSH) level within laboratory reference range for postmenopausal women.

Men able to father children who are sexually active with WOCBP must agree to use at least 2 methods of acceptable contraception (Appendix 4) from the time of signing consent and until 2 months after patient's last dose of protocol-indicated treatment.

Men able to father children are defined as those who are not surgically sterile (i.e. patient has not had a vasectomy).

Exclusion Criteria:
, Within 28 days before first dose of protocol-indicated treatment:
- Anti-cancer treatment including chemotherapy, radiation, hormonal therapy, targeted therapy, immunotherapy, or biological therapy.
- Major surgery requiring general anesthesia. (Note: within this time frame, placement of a central line or portacath is acceptable and does not exclude.)
- Receipt of an investigational agent.
. Within 14 days before first dose of protocol-indicated treatment:

- Active uncontrolled infection. Patients with infection under active treatment and controlled with antibiotics initiated at least 14 days prior to initiation of protocol-indicated treatment are not excluded (e.g. urinary tract infection controlled with antibiotics).
- Known Grade 4 toxicity probably or definitely attributed to past irinotecan treatment.
- Active inflammatory bowel disease, other bowel disease causing chronic diarrhea (defined as > 4 loose stools per day), or bowel obstruction.
- History of interstitial pneumonitis or pulmonary fibrosis, or evidence of interstitial pneumonitis or pulmonary fibrosis on baseline chest CT scan.
- Unable to receive oral medication.
- Central nervous system metastasis, unless asymptomatic or previously treated and stable; and no evidence of CNS progression for at least 30 days prior to initiating protocol-indicated treatment. Anticonvulsant and/or corticosteroid therapy will be allowed if patient is on a stable or decreasing dose of such treatment for at least 30 days prior to initiating protocol-indicated treatment.
- Patients with known Gilbert's disease.
- Patient is pregnant or breastfeeding.
- Current or previous malignant disease (other than colorectal cancer) within the last 5 years; with the exception of the following if considered curatively treated: non-melanoma skin cancer(s), carcinoma in situ of the cervix, and ductal carcinoma in situ. Subjects with another active malignancy requiring concurrent anti-cancer intervention are excluded. (Note the following does not exclude: effectively treated malignancy that has been in remission for more than 5 years and is considered to be cured AND no additional anti-cancer therapy is ongoing and required during the study period.)
- Known positive test for Human Immunodeficiency Virus (HIV), Acquired Immunodeficiency Syndrome (AIDS), Hepatitis A, Hepatitis B, Hepatitis C, or Cytomegalovirus (CMV).
- Known psychiatric condition, social circumstance, or other medical condition reasonably judged by the patient's study physician to unacceptably increase the risk of study participation; or to prohibit the understanding or rendering of informed consent or anticipated compliance with scheduled visits, treatment schedule, laboratory tests and other study requirements.

Sex/Gender

All

Ages

18 Years to N/A

Accepts Healthy Volunteers

No

Contacts

Clinical Trials Information Program   800-811-8480   cip@vanderbilt.edu

Study of Binimetinib + Nivolumab Plus or Minus Ipilimumab in Patients With Previously Treated Microsatellite-stable (MSS) Metastatic Colorectal Cancer With RAS Mutation

Study ID:
NCT03271047

Sponsor:
Array BioPharma

Information provided by (Responsible Party):
Array BioPharma (Array BioPharma)

Tracking Information

First Submitted Date
August 31, 2017

Start Date
October 4, 2017

Primary Completion Date
August 2018

Last Update Posted Date
December 15, 2017

547

Current Primary Outcome Measures

(Phase 1b) Incidence of dose-limiting toxicities (DLTs) resulting from binimetinib in combination with nivolumab[Time Frame: Duration of each treatment cycle, 28 days]

(Phase 1b) Incidence of dose-limiting toxicities (DLTs) resulting from binimetinib in combination with nivolumab plus ipilimumab[Time Frame: Duration of each treatment cycle, 28 days]

(Phase 2) Objective Response Rate (ORR)[Time Frame: Duration of each treatment cycle, 28 days]

Current Secondary Outcome Measures

(Phase 1b) Objective Response Rate (ORR)[Time Frame: Duration of each treatment cycle, 28 days]

(Phase 1b and Phase 2) Duration of Response (DOR)[Time Frame: Duration of each treatment cycle, 28 days]

(Phase 1b and Phase 2) Rate of complete response (CR)[Time Frame: Duration of each treatment cycle, 28 days]

(Phase 1b and Phase 2) Incidence and severity of adverse events (AEs)[Time Frame: Duration of each treatment cycle, 28 days]

(Phase 1b and Phase 2) Sparse plasma concentrations for binimetinib[Time Frame: Duration of each treatment cycle, 28 days]

Descriptive Information

Offical Title

An Open-label Phase 1b/2 Study of Binimetinib Administered in Combination With Nivolumab or Nivolumab Plus Ipilimumab in Patients With Previously Treated Microsatellite-stable (MSS) Metastatic Colorectal Cancer With RAS Mutation

Brief Summary

This is a multicenter, open-label, Phase 1B/2 study to evaluate the safety and assess the preliminary anti-tumor activity of binimetinib administered in combination with nivolumab or nivolumab + ipilimumab in adult patients with advanced metastatic colorectal cancer (mCRC) with microsatellite stable (MSS) disease and presence of a RAS mutation that have received at least one prior line of therapy and no more than 2 prior lines of therapy. The study contains a Phase 1b period to determine the maximum tolerated dose (MTD) and recommended Phase 2 dose (RP2D) and schedule of binimetinib followed by a randomized Phase 2 period to assess the efficacy of the combinations.

Study Type

Interventional

Study Phase

Phase 1/Phase 2

Condition

- MSS
- RAS-mutant Colorectal Cancer

Intervention

Drug: binimetinib

Orally, twice daily.

Drug: nivolumab

Intravenously (IV) every 4 weeks (Q4W)

Drug: ipilimumab

intravenously (IV) every 8 weeks (Q8W)

Study Arms

Experimental: Phase 1b / Arm 1A
binimetinib + nivolumab

Experimental: Phase 1b / Arm 1B
binimetinib + nivolumab + ipilimumab

Experimental: Phase 2 / Arm 2A
binimetinib + nivolumab

Experimental: Phase 2 / Arm 2B
binimetinib + nivolumab + ipilimumab

Recruitment Information

Recruitment Status

Recruiting

Completion Date

January 2020

Estimated Enrollment

90

Primary Completion Date

August 2018

Eligibility Criteria

Key Inclusion Criteria

- Measurable, histologically/cytologically confirmed metastatic colorectal cancer (mCRC).
- Able to provide a sufficient amount of representative tumor specimen for central laboratory testing of RAS mutation status and microsatellite stable (MSS).
- If a fresh tissue sample is provided, a blood sample is required.
- Metastatic colorectal cancer (mCRC) categorized as microsatellite stable (MSS) by polymerase chain reaction (PCR) per local assay at any time prior to Screening or by the central laboratory.
- RAS mutation per local assay at any time prior to Screening or by the central laboratory.
- Have received at least 1 prior line of therapy and meets at least one of the following criteria:
- were unable to tolerate the prior first-line regimen
- experienced disease progression during or after prior first-line regimen for metastatic disease
- progressed during or within 3 months of completing adjuvant chemotherapy. Note: Generally, treatments that are separated by an event of progression are considered different regimens.
- Have received no more than 2 prior lines of therapy (maintenance therapy given in the metastatic setting will not be considered a separate regimen). Generally, treatments that are separated by an event of progression are considered different regimens.
- Adequate bone marrow, cardiac, kidney and liver function
- Able to take oral medications
- Eastern Cooperative Oncology Group (ECOG) performance status (PS) of 0 or 1.
- Female patients are either postmenopausal for at least 1 year, are surgically sterile for at least 6 weeks, or must agree to take appropriate precautions to avoid pregnancy from screening through follow-up if of child-bearing potential
- Non-sterile male patients who are sexually active with female partners of childbearing potential must agree to follow instructions for acceptable or highly effective method(s) of contraception for the duration of study treatment and for 7 months after the last dose of study treatment with nivolumab

Key Exclusion Criteria

- Prior treatment with any MEK inhibitor, an anti-PD-1, anti-PD-L1, anti-PD-L2, anti-CD137, or anti-CTLA-4 antibody, or any other antibody or drug specifically targeting T-cell co-stimulation or checkpoint pathways.
- Any untreated central nervous system (CNS) lesion.
- Patients with an active, known or suspected autoimmune disease. Patients with type I diabetes mellitus, hypothyroidism only requiring hormone replacement, skin disorders (such as vitiligo, psoriasis, or alopecia) not requiring systemic treatment, or conditions not expected to recur in the absence of an external trigger are permitted to enroll.
- Known history of retinal vein occlusion (RVO).
- Known history of Gilbert's syndrome.
- Pregnant or breastfeeding females.
- Treatment with systemic immunosuppressive medications (including but not limited to prednisone, cyclophosphamide, azathioprine, methotrexate, thalidomide, and anti-tumor necrosis factor [anti-TNF] agents) within 2 weeks prior to first day of study treatment:
- History of thromboembolic or cerebrovascular events ≤ 6 months prior to starting study treatment, including transient ischemic attacks, cerebrovascular accidents, deep vein thrombosis or pulmonary emboli.
- Uncontrolled hypertension defined as persistent systolic blood pressure ≥ 150 mmHg or diastolic blood pressure ≥ 100 mmHg despite current therapy.
- Concurrent neuromuscular disorder that is associated with the potential of elevated creatine kinase (CK) (e.g., inflammatory myopathies, muscular dystrophy, amyotrophic lateral sclerosis, spinal muscular atrophy).
- History or current evidence of retinal vein occlusion (RVO) or current risk factors for RVO (e.g., uncontrolled glaucoma or ocular hypertension, history of hyperviscosity or hypercoagulability syndromes).
- Known history of positive test for human immunodeficiency virus (HIV) or known acquired immunodeficiency syndrome (AIDS). NOTE: Testing for HIV must be performed at sites where mandated locally.
- Any positive test for hepatitis B virus or hepatitis C virus indicating acute or chronic infection, and/or detectable virus.

Sex/Gender

All

- ◾ **Ages**

  18 Years to N/A

- ◾ **Accepts Healthy Volunteers**

  No

- ◾ **Contacts**

  Array BioPharma, Inc   303-381-6604   clinicaltrials@arraybiopharma.com

Glutamine PET Imaging Colorectal Cancer

Study ID:

NCT03275974

Sponsor:

Vanderbilt-Ingram Cancer Center

Information provided by (Responsible Party):

Vanderbilt-Ingram Cancer Center (Vanderbilt-Ingram Cancer Center)

Tracking Information

- ◾ **First Submitted Date**

  August 30, 2017

- ◾ **Start Date**

  October 17, 2017

- ◾ **Current Primary Outcome Measures**

  Pet imaging[Time Frame: Up to 4 years]
  Assessed in terms of Standardized Uptake Values (SUVs)

  Gene expression[Time Frame: Up to 4 years]
  Measured in terms of copy number

- ◾ **Primary Completion Date**

  November 2021

- ◾ **Last Update Posted Date**

  November 14, 2017

- ◾ **Current Secondary Outcome Measures**

  Change in tumor size (e.g., long-axis diameter, tumor volume)[Time Frame: Up to 24 months]
  Change in tumor size will be derived from standard-of-care computed tomography or magnetic resonance imaging

  Plasma levels of Gln, Glu, cystine, and substrates and metabolites related to glutaminolysis and amino acid transport[Time Frame: Up to 24 months]
  Progression free survival[Time Frame: Up to 4 years]

  Overall survival[Time Frame: Up to 4 years]

Descriptive Information

- ◾ **Offical Title**

  Glutamine PET Imaging of Colorectal Cancer

- ◾ **Brief Summary**

  The clinical trial studies how well 11C-glutamine and 18F-FSPG positron emission tomography (PET) imaging works in detecting tumors in patients with metastatic colorectal cancer compared to standard imaging methods such as magnetic resonance imaging (MRI) or computed tomography (CT) scanning.

- ◾ **Detailed Description**

  PRIMARY OBJECTIVES:

  I. To establish and validate a 11C-glutamine (11C-Gln) and fluorine F 18 L-glutamate derivative BAY94-9392 (18F-FSPG) PET image guided gene signature to predict response to EGFR-targeted therapy in patients with advanced wild-type RAS colorectal cancer (CRC).

  OUTLINE:

  Patients receive 11C-glutamine intravenously (IV) and undergo PET imaging over 120 minutes. Beginning 2 hours to 7 days after 11C-glutamine PET, patients receive fluorine F 18 L-glutamate derivative BAY94-9392 IV and also undergo PET imaging over 120 minutes.

Study Type

Interventional

Study Phase

Early Phase 1

Condition

- RAS Wild Type
- Stage IV Colorectal Cancer
- Stage IVA Colorectal Cancer
- Stage IVB Colorectal Cancer

Intervention

Biological: Carbon C 11 Glutamine

Given by IV

Biological: Fluorine F 18 L-glutamate Derivative BAY94-9392

Given by IV

Procedure: Positron Emission Tomography

Undergo PET scan

Study Arms

Experimental: Treatment

Patients receive 11C-glutamine IV and undergo PET imaging over 120 minutes. Beginning 2 hours to 7 days after 11C-glutamine PET, patients receive fluorine F 18 L-glutamate derivative BAY94-9392 IV and also undergo PET imaging over 120 minutes.

Recruitment Information

Recruitment Status

Recruiting

Estimated Enrollment

30

Completion Date

November 2022

Primary Completion Date

November 2021

Eligibility Criteria

Inclusion Criteria:

- Pathologically or cytologically confirmed diagnosis of metastatic (stage IV) RAS wildtype CRC
- Eligible for anti-EGFR monoclonal antibody (mAb) therapy as standard-of-care (SOC), either as a single agent or in combination with approved irinotecan-containing regimens
- Archived tissue from the CRC primary tumor in sufficient amounts to allow advanced quantitative real time-polymerase chain reaction (qRT-PCR) analysis; specimen from metastatic sites are not required but highly preferred
- Documented results from (or scheduled to undergo) CT or MRI of the chest, abdomen and pelvis as a SOC procedure within 28 days of baseline investigational 11C-Gln PET/CT and 18F-FSPG PET/CT
- Measurable disease by Response Evaluation Criteria in Solid Tumors (RECIST) version (v)1.1
- At least one lesion measurable according to PET Response Criteria in Solid Tumors (PERCIST) v1.0: > 2 cm in diameter to avoid PET partial volume effects
- Ability to provide written informed consent in accordance with institutional policies

Exclusion Criteria:

- Any other current or previous malignancy within the past 5 years
- Previous EGFR-directed therapy
- Body weight >= 400 pounds or body habitus or disability that will not permit the imaging protocol to be performed
- Pregnant or lactating females

Sex/Gender

All

Ages

18 Years to N/A

A Study of RO7198457 (Personalized Cancer Vaccine [PCV]) as a Single Agent and in Combination With Atezolizumab in Participants With Locally Advanced or Metastatic Tumors

Study ID:

NCT03289962

Sponsor:

Genentech, Inc.

Information provided by (Responsible Party):

Genentech, Inc. (Genentech, Inc.)

Tracking Information

■ **First Submitted Date**

September 19, 2017

■ **Start Date**

December 30, 2017

■ **Primary Completion Date**

September 11, 2020

■ **Last Update Posted Date**

December 12, 2017

■ **Current Primary Outcome Measures**

Percentage of Participants with Dose-Limiting Toxicities (DLTs)[Time Frame: Phase 1a: Days 1 to 14 / Phase 1b: Days 1 to 21]
MTD/Recommended Phase 2 Dose (RP2D) of RO7198457[Time Frame: Phase 1a: Days 1 to 14 / Phase 1b: Days 1 to 21]

Percentage of Participants with Adverse Events (AEs) by Severity According to National Cancer Institute (NCI) Common Terminology Criteria for Adverse Events (CTCAE) Version 4.0[Time Frame: Baseline up to end of the study (up to approximately 3 years)]

Percentage of Participants with Immune-Mediated Adverse Events (imAEs) by Severity According to NCI CTCAE Version 4.0[Time Frame: Baseline up to end of the study (up to approximately 3 years)]

Percentage of Participants by Number of Treatment Cycles Received[Time Frame: Baseline up to end of the study (up to approximately 3 years)]

Dose Intensity of RO7198457[Time Frame: Baseline up to end of the study (up to approximately 3 years)]

■ **Current Secondary Outcome Measures**

Plasma Concentration of (R)-N,N,N-Trimethyl-2,3-Dioleyloxy-1-Propanaminium Chloride (DOTMA)[Time Frame: Pre-infusion (0 hour [hr]) until treatment discontinuation (up to approximately 3 years)]

Plasma Concentration of Ribonucleic Acid (RNA)[Time Frame: Pre-infusion (0 hr) until treatment discontinuation (up to approximately 3 years)]

Serum Concentration of Atezolizumab[Time Frame: Pre-infusion (0 hr) until 2 months post treatment discontinuation (up to approximately 3 years)]

Percentage of Participants with Induction of Antigen-Specific T-Cell Responses in Peripheral Blood[Time Frame: Pre-infusion (0 hr) until treatment discontinuation (up to approximately 3 years)]

Immune-Related Cytokine Levels[Time Frame: Pre-infusion (0 hr) until treatment discontinuation (up to approximately 3 years)]

Percentage of Participants with Objective Response of Complete Response (CR) or Partial Response (PR) According to Response Evaluation Criteria for Solid Tumors Version 1.1 (RECIST v1.1)[Time Frame: Baseline until 90 days after last dose or initiation of another systemic anti-cancer therapy, whichever occurs first (up to approximately 3 years)]

Duration of Response (DoR) According to RECIST v1.1[Time Frame: From first occurrence of a documented objective response (CR or PR) until disease progression or death due to any cause, whichever occurs first (up to approximately 3 years)]

Percentage of Participants with Objective Response of CR or PR According to Immune-Modified RECIST[Time Frame:

Baseline until 90 days after last dose or initiation of another systemic anti-cancer therapy, whichever occurs first (up to approximately 3 years)]

DoR According to Immune-Modified RECIST[Time Frame: From first occurrence of a documented objective response (CR or PR) until disease progression or death due to any cause, whichever occurs first (up to approximately 3 years)]

Progression-Free Survival (PFS) According to RECIST v1.1[Time Frame: Baseline until 90 days after last dose or initiation of another systemic anti-cancer therapy, whichever occurs first (up to approximately 3 years)]

Overall Survival (OS)[Time Frame: Baseline until 90 days after last dose or initiation of another systemic anti-cancer therapy, whichever occurs first (up to approximately 3 years)]

Percentage of Participants with Anti-Drug Antibodies (ADAs) to Atezolizumab[Time Frame: Pre-infusion (0 hr) until 2 months post treatment discontinuation (up to approximately 3 years)]

Descriptive Information

▥ Offical Title

A Phase 1a/1b Open-Label, Dose-Escalation Study of the Safety and Pharmacokinetics of RO7198457 as a Single Agent and in Combination With Atezolizumab in Patients With Locally Advanced or Metastatic Tumors

▥ Brief Summary

This is a Phase 1a/1b, open-label, multicenter, global, dose-escalation study designed to evaluate the safety, tolerability, immune response, and pharmacokinetics of RO7198457 as a single agent and in combination with atezolizumab (MPDL3280A, an engineered anti-programmed death-ligand 1 [anti-PD-L1] antibody).

▥ Study Type

Interventional

▥ Study Phase

Phase 1

▥ Condition

- Melanoma
- Non-Small Cell Lung Cancer
- Bladder Cancer
- Colorectal Cancer
- Triple Negative Breast Cancer
- Renal Cancer
- Head and Neck Cancer
- Other Solid Cancers

▥ Intervention

Drug: RO7198457

RO7198457 will be administered by intravenous (IV) infusion, in 21-day cycles.

Other Names:

PCV

Drug: Atezolizumab

Atezolizumab will be administered by IV infusion, in 21-day cycles.

Other Names:

Tecentriq

RO5541267

MPDL3280A

An engineered anti-PDL1 antibody

▥ Study Arms

Experimental: Phase 1a Dose-Escalation: RO7198457

Participants will receive RO7198457 at escalated dosages.

Experimental: Phase 1b Dose-Escalation: RO7198457 + Atezolizumab

Participants will receive RO7198457 at escalated dosages along with atezolizumab at a fixed dose of 1200 milligrams (mg).

Experimental: Phase 1b Exploration: RO7198457 + Atezolizumab

Non-small cell lung cancer (NSCLC) cancer immunotherapy (CIT)-treated participants will receive RO7198457 (at dosage lower than maximum tolerated dose [MTD] based on available safety data) along with atezolizumab at a fixed dose of 1200 mg.

Experimental: Phase 1b Expansion: RO7198457 + Atezolizumab

Participants with different indications as per inclusion criteria, will receive RO7198457 (at multiple dose levels below MTD based on available safety data) along with atezolizumab at a fixed dose of 1200 mg.

Experimental: Phase 1b Expansion: RO7198457 + Atezolizumab (Serial Biopsy)

Participants with selected tumor types who consent to optional serial biopsies will receive RO7198457 (at multiple dose levels below MTD based on available safety data) along with atezolizumab at a fixed dose of 1200 mg.

Recruitment Information

▓ Recruitment Status

Recruiting

▓ Estimated Enrollment

572

▓ Completion Date

September 11, 2020

▓ Primary Completion Date

September 11, 2020

▓ Eligibility Criteria

Inclusion Criteria:

- Eastern Cooperative Oncology Group (ECOG) performance status of 0 or 1
- Life expectancy greater than or equal to (>=12 weeks)
- Adequate hematologic and end-organ function
- Measured or calculated creatinine clearance >=50 milliliters per minute (mL/min) on the basis of the Cockcroft-Gault glomerular filtration rate estimation

Cancer-Specific Inclusion Criteria:

- Participants with histologic documentation of locally advanced, recurrent, or metastatic incurable malignancy that has progressed after at least one available standard therapy; or for whom standard therapy has proven to be ineffective or intolerable, or is considered inappropriate; or for whom a clinical trial of an investigational agent is a recognized standard of care
- Participants with confirmed availability of representative tumor specimens in formalin-fixed, paraffin-embedded (FFPE) blocks (preferred), or sectioned tissue
- Participants with measurable disease per RECIST v1.1

Additional Inclusion Criteria for Participants Who Backfill Cleared Cohorts of Phase 1a and Phase 1b:

- Backfill cohort enrollment may be limited to participants whose tumors have PD-L1 and/or different levels of cluster of differentiation 8 (CD8) expression, as defined by the Sponsor

Additional Inclusion Criteria for Participants in Each Indication-Specific Exploration/Expansion Cohort of Phase 1b:

- NSCLC Cohorts (CIT-Naïve): Participants with histologically confirmed incurable, advanced NSCLC not previously treated with CIT (investigational or approved), including anti-PD–L1/programmed death-1 (PD-1) and/or anti-cytotoxic T-lymphocyte-associated protein 4 (anti-CTLA–4), for whom a clinical trial of an investigational agent in combination with an anti-PD–L1 antibody is considered an acceptable treatment option, if CIT (including anti-PD–L1/PD-1 agents) is approved as treatment for NSCLC by local regulatory authorities
- NSCLC Cohort (CIT-Treated): Participants with histologically confirmed incurable, advanced NSCLC previously treated with CIT (investigational or approved) including anti-PD–L1/PD-1
- Triple negative breast cancer (TNBC) Cohort: Participants with histologically confirmed incurable, advanced estrogen receptor (ER)-negative, progesterone receptor-negative, and human epidermal growth factor receptor 2 (HER2)-negative adenocarcinoma of the breast (triple-negative)
- Colorectal cancer (CRC) Cohort: Participants with histologically confirmed incurable, advanced adenocarcinoma of the colon or rectum
- Head and neck squamous cell carcinoma (HNSCC) Cohort: Participants with histologically confirmed inoperable, locally advanced or metastatic, recurrent, or persistent HNSCC (oral cavity, oropharynx, hypopharnyx, or larynx) not amenable to curative therapy
- Urothelial carcinoma (UC) Cohort (CIT-Naïve): Participants with histologically confirmed incurable, advanced transitional cell carcinoma of the urothelium (including renal pelvis, ureters, urinary bladder, and urethra not previously treated with CIT (investigational or approved), including anti-PD–L1/PD-1 and/or anti-CTLA–4, for whom a clinical trial of an investigational agent in combination with an anti-PD–L1 antibody is considered an acceptable treatment option, if CIT (including anti-PD–L1/PD-1 agents) is approved as treatment for UC by local regulatory authorities
- UC Cohort (CIT-Treated): Participants with histologically confirmed incurable advanced transitional cell carcinoma of the urothelium (including renal pelvis, ureters, urinary bladder, and urethra) previously treated with CIT (investigational or approved) including anti-PD–L1/PD-1
- Renal cell carcinoma (RCC) Cohort: Participants with histologically confirmed incurable, advanced RCC with component of clear cell histology and/or component of sarcomatoid histology

Additional Inclusion Criteria for Participants in the Serial-Biopsy Expansion Cohort of Phase 1b:

- Participants must have one of the following tumor types: NSCLC, UC, HNSCC, TNBC, RCC, melanoma, cervical cancer, anal cancer, Merkel-cell carcinoma, microsatellite instability (MSI)-High tumors, squamous cell carcinoma of the skin, hepatocellular carcinoma (non-viral), and CRC including microsatellite stable (MSS) and MSI-Low
- Participants must have accessible lesion(s) that permit a total of two to three biopsies (pretreatment and on-treatment) or one biopsy (on-treatment, if archival tissue can be submitted in place of a pre-treatment biopsy) without unacceptable risk of a significant procedural complication

Exclusion Criteria:

- Known clinically significant liver disease, including active viral, alcoholic, or other hepatitis, cirrhosis, and inherited liver disease or current alcohol abuse
- Major surgical procedure within 28 days prior to Cycle 1, Day 1, or anticipation of need for a major surgical procedure during the course of the study
- Any other diseases, metabolic dysfunction, physical examination finding, and/or clinical laboratory finding giving reasonable suspicion of a disease or condition that contraindicates the use of an investigational drug or that may affect the interpretation of the results or may render the participant at high risk from treatment complications
- Previous splenectomy
- Known primary immunodeficiencies, either cellular (e.g., DiGeorge syndrome, T-negative severe combined immunodeficiency [SCID]) or combined T and B-cell immunodeficiencies (e.g., T and B-negative SCID, Wiskott Aldrich syndrome, ataxia telangiectasia, common variable immunodeficiency)
- Any medical condition or abnormality in clinical laboratory tests that, in the investigator's judgment, precludes the participant's safe participation in and completion of the study Cancer-Specific Exclusion Criteria
- Any anti-cancer therapy, whether investigational or approved, including chemotherapy, hormonal therapy, and/or radiotherapy, within 3 weeks prior to initiation of study treatment, with the exceptions as mentioned in the protocol
- Eligibility based on prior treatment with CIT depends on the mechanistic class of the drug and the cohort for which the participant is being considered, as described below. In addition, all criteria pertaining to adverse events attributed to prior cancer therapies must be met

All Cohorts (Dose-Escalation in Phase 1a and Dose-Escalation, Backfill, and Expansion in Phase 1b):

- Prior cancer vaccines are not allowed, with the exception as specified in protocol
- Prior treatment with cytokines is allowed provided that at least 6 weeks or 5 half-lives of the drug, whichever is shorter, have elapsed between the last dose and the proposed Cycle 1, Day 1
- Prior treatment with immune checkpoint inhibitors, immunomodulatory monoclonal antibody (mAbs), and/or mAb-derived therapies is allowed provided that at least 6 weeks have elapsed between the last dose and the proposed Cycle 1, Day 1, with the exceptions as specified in protocol

Dose-Exploration/Expansion Cohorts in Phase 1b:

- In the NSCLC CIT-Treated exploration cohort in Phase 1b, the most recent systemic treatment should have been anti-PD–L1/PD-1 as monotherapy or in combination
- In the NSCLC CIT-Naïve expansion cohort in Phase 1b, prior treatment with immune checkpoint inhibitors (such as anti-PD–L1/PD-1), immunomodulatory mAbs, and/or mAb-derived therapies is not allowed
- Prior treatment with immunomodulators, including toll-like receptor (TLR) agonists, inhibitors of indoleamine 2,3-dioxygenase (IDO)/ tryptophan-2,3-dioxygenase (TDO), or agonists of OX40, is allowed provided that at least 5 half-lives of the drug or a minimum of 3 weeks have elapsed between the last dose of the prior treatment and the proposed Cycle 1, Day 1, with the exception as specified in protocol
- Any history of an immune-related Grade 4 adverse event attributed to prior CIT (other than endocrinopathy managed with replacement therapy or asymptomatic elevation of serum amylase or lipase)
- Any history of an immune-related Grade 3 adverse event attributed to prior CIT (other than hypothyroidism managed with replacement therapy) that resulted in permanent discontinuation of the prior immunotherapeutic agent and/or occurred less than or equal to (<=) 6 months prior to Cycle 1 Day 1
- Adverse events from prior anti-cancer therapy that have not resolved to Grade <=1 except for alopecia, vitiligo, or endocrinopathy managed with replacement therapy
- All immune-related adverse events related to prior CIT (other than endocrinopathy managed with replacement therapy or stable vitiligo) must have resolved completely to baseline
- Primary central nervous system (CNS) malignancy, untreated CNS metastases, or active CNS metastases (progressing or requiring corticosteroids for symptomatic control)
- Leptomeningeal disease
- Uncontrolled tumor-related pain
- Uncontrolled pleural effusion, pericardial effusion, or ascites requiring recurrent drainage procedures
- Malignancies other than disease under study within 5 years prior to Cycle 1, Day 1, with the exception of those with a negligible risk of metastasis or death
- Uncontrolled hypercalcemia
- Participant has spinal cord compression not definitively treated with surgery and/or radiation or previously diagnosed and treated spinal cord compression without evidence that disease has been clinically stable for >=2 weeks prior to screening

Treatment-Specific Exclusion Criteria:

- History of autoimmune disease with caveats as specified in protocol
- Treatment with systemic immunosuppressive medications within 2 weeks prior to Cycle 1, Day 1
- History of idiopathic pulmonary fibrosis, pneumonitis, organizing pneumonia, or evidence of active pneumonitis on screening chest computed tomography (CT) scan
- Positive test for human immunodeficiency virus (HIV) infection
- Active hepatitis B, hepatitis C, or tuberculosis
- Severe infections within 4 weeks prior to Cycle 1, Day 1
- Recent infections not meeting the criteria for severe infections within 2 weeks prior to Cycle 1, Day 1
- Prior allogeneic bone marrow transplantation or prior solid organ transplantation
- Administration of a live, attenuated vaccine within 4 weeks before Cycle 1, Day 1 or anticipation that such a live attenuated vaccine will be required during the study
- Known hypersensitivity to the active substance or to any of the excipients in the vaccine
- Phase 1b and crossover only: History of severe allergic, anaphylactic, or other hypersensitivity reactions to chimeric or humanized antibodies or fusion proteins; Known hypersensitivity to Chinese Hamster Ovary (CHO)-cell products; Allergy or hypersensitivity to components of the atezolizumab formulation

Sex/Gender

All

Ages

18 Years to N/A

Accepts Healthy Volunteers

No

Contacts

Reference Study ID Number: GO39733 www.roche.com/about roche/roche worldwide.htm 888-662-6728 (U.S. and Canada) global-roche-genentech-trials@gene.com

Clinical Trial Evaluating the Safety and Response With PF-05082566, Cetuximab and Irinotecan in Patients With Advanced Colorectal Cancer

Study ID:

NCT03290937

Sponsor:

M.D. Anderson Cancer Center

Information provided by (Responsible Party):

M.D. Anderson Cancer Center (M.D. Anderson Cancer Center)

Tracking Information

First Submitted Date

September 20, 2017

Start Date

December 27, 2017

Primary Completion Date

December 2021

Last Update Posted Date

January 4, 2018

Current Primary Outcome Measures

Dose Limiting Toxicity (DLT) of Irinotecan with PF-05082566 and Cetuximab in Patients with Advanced Colorectal Cancer[Time Frame: 28 days]

DLT determined according to Common Terminology Criteria for Adverse Events (CTCAE) version 4.03.

Overall Response Rate (ORR) in Patients with Advanced Colorectal Cancer Who Are RAS-RAF Wild Type (WT) or RAS Mutant[Time Frame: Every 2 cycles up to 3 years]

ORR determined by irRECIST.

Current Secondary Outcome Measures

Evaluation of Pharmacodynamic (PD) Biomarkers[Time Frame: On Days 3, 4, 9, and 22 of Cycle 1, then on Day 15 of each Cycle up to 3 years]

Patient serum may be analyzed for activation markers such as: sCD137, TNF-α, IFN-γ, IL-10, IL-8, IL-6, IL-4, IL-2, IL-1, or IL-12.

Characterization of Serum Biomarkers Linked to Immunomodulation and Cytokine Release[Time Frame: Day 1 of each cycle up to 3 years]

Blood samples and peripheral blood mononuclear cells (PBMC) for biomarker analyses obtained for the escalation and expansion cohorts at screening then on Day 1 of each cycle to evaluate CD3, CD8, CD4, FoxP3, CD127, Ki67, Eomesodermin, KLRG1, CD14, CD33, HLA-DR, CD16, CD56, Granzyme B, CD68, PD-1, CD11c, sCD137, and 4-1BB.

Assess Markers of T Cell Phenotype[Time Frame: Day 1 of each cycle up to 3 years]

PD biomarkers assessed by flow cytometry and include changes of proliferation status in T cells via monitoring Ki-67 levels.

Assess Markers of NK Cell Phenotype[Time Frame: Day 1 of each cycle up to 3 years]

PD biomarkers assessed by flow cytometry and include changes of proliferation status in NK cells via monitoring Ki-67 levels.

Descriptive Information

Offical Title

Phase I Clinical Trial Evaluating the Safety and Response With PF-05082566, Cetuximab and Irinotecan in Patients With Advanced Colorectal Cancer

Brief Summary

Any time the words "you," "your," "I," or "me" appear, it is meant to apply to the potential participant.

The goal of this clinical research study is to find the highest tolerable dose of irinotecan that can be given in combination with PF-05082566 and cetuximab to patients with advanced colorectal cancer. Researchers also want to learn about possible side effects of the study drugs and if the study drug can help to control the disease.

This is an investigational study. PF-05082566 is not FDA approved or commercially available. It is currently being used for research purposes only. Cetuximab and irinotecan are FDA approved and commercially available to treat several types of cancers, including colorectal cancer. Their use in combination with PF-05082566 is investigational.

The study doctor can describe how the drugs are designed to work.

Up to 32 participants will be enrolled in this study. All will take part at MD Anderson.

Detailed Description

Study Groups:

If you are found to be eligible to take part in this study, you will be assigned to a dose level of irinotecan based on when you join this study. Up to 3 dose levels of irinotecan will be tested. Up to 6 participants will be enrolled at each dose level. The first group of participants will receive the lowest dose level. Each new group will receive a higher dose than the group before it, if no intolerable side effects were seen. This will continue until the highest tolerable dose of Irinotecan is found.

After the highest tolerable dose level of irinotecan is found, an additional 20 participants will be enrolled on the study and will receive this dose.

All participants will receive the same dose of cetuximab and PF-05082566.

Study Drug Administration:

You will receive irinotecan and cetuximab by vein on Days 1 and 15 of each 28-day cycle. The first time you receive cetuximab, it will be given over about 2 hours. If you tolerate it well, you will receive it over about 1 hour each time after that. Irinotecan will be given over about 90 minutes.

On Day 2 of each cycle, you will receive PF-05082566 by vein over about 1 hour.

You will also be given standard drugs to help decrease the risk of side effects. You may ask the study staff for information about how the drugs are given and their risks.

Length of Study:

You may continue receiving the study drugs for as long as your study doctor thinks it is in your best interest. You will no longer be able to take the study drugs if the disease gets worse, if intolerable side effects occur, or if you are unable to follow study directions.

Your participation on the study will be over after the end-of-study visit.

Study Visits:

On Day 1 of each Cycle:

- You will have a physical exam.
- Blood (about 1-2 tablespoons) will be drawn for routine tests and biomarker testing. If you can become pregnant, part of this sample will also be used for a pregnancy test.
- Urine will be collected for routine tests.

On Day 2 of each Cycle:

- Blood (about 1-2 tablespoons) will be drawn for pharmacodynamic (PD) testing. PD testing measures how the level of study drug in your body may affect the disease. At Cycle 1, this will be done before and 3 times over the 6 hours after the dose. At Cycles 2 and beyond, this will only be done before the dose.
- You will have an EKG before you receive the study drug.

On Days 3, 4, 9, and 22 of Cycle 1, blood (about 1-2 tablespoons) will be drawn for PD testing.

On Day 15 of each Cycle, blood (about 1-2 tablespoons) will be drawn for routine tests and PD testing.

If you had a core needle biopsy at screening, you will have another biopsy about 6-8 weeks after screening.

Every 8 weeks, you will have the same imaging scan(s) you had at screening.

End-of-Study Visit:

After you stop receiving the study drugs:

- You will have a physical exam.
- Blood (about 1-2 tablespoons) will be drawn for routine tests, PD testing, and biomarker testing.
- You will have the same imaging scan(s) you had at screening.

Follow-Up:

- Every 3 months (+/1 month) after the end-of-study visit, you will be called and asked about how you are doing and any other treatments you may be receiving. These calls should last about 10 minutes each time.

Study Type

Interventional

Study Phase

Phase 1

Condition

- Malignant Neoplasms of Digestive Organs
- Colorectal Cancer

Intervention

Drug: Irinotecan

Dose Escalation Starting Dose: 60 mg/m2 by vein on Days 1 and 15 of a 28 day cycle.

Dose Expansion Starting Dose: Maximum tolerated dose from Dose Escalation by vein on Days 1 and 15 of a 28 day cycle.

Other Names:

CPT-11

Camptosar

Drug: PF-05082566

Dose Escalation and Dose Expansion: 100 mg by vein on Day 2 of a 28 day cycle.

Other Names:

Utomilumab

Anti-CD137

Drug: Cetuximab

Dose Escalation and Dose Expansion: 500 mg/m2 by vein on Days 1 and 15 of a 28 day cycle.

Other Names:

C225

Erbitux

IMC-C225

MOAB C225

Study Arms

Experimental: Metastatic Wild Type (RAS-RAF) Colorectal Cancer Group

Dose Expansion: Participants receive Irinotecan at the maximum tolerated dose from Dose Escalation Phase.

Participants receive the same dose of Cetuximab and PF-05082566.

Participants continue receiving the study drugs for as long as study doctor thinks it is in participant's best interest.

Experimental: Mutated RAS Colorectal Cancer Group

Dose Expansion: Participants receive Irinotecan at the maximum tolerated dose from Dose Escalation Phase.

Participants receive the same dose of Cetuximab and PF-05082566.

Participants continue receiving the study drugs for as long as study doctor thinks it is in participant's best interest.

Experimental: Irinotecan + PF-05082566 + Cetuximab

Dose Escalation: Participants assigned to a dose level of Irinotecan based on when joining study. Up to 3 dose levels of Irinotecan tested. Up to 6 participants enrolled at each dose level. First group of participants receive the lowest dose level. Each new group receives a higher dose than the group before it, if no intolerable side effects were seen. This continues until the highest tolerable dose of Irinotecan is found.

Participants receive the same dose of Cetuximab and PF-05082566.

Recruitment Information

Recruitment Status

Recruiting

Estimated Enrollment

32

Completion Date

December 2021

Primary Completion Date

December 2021

Eligibility Criteria

Inclusion Criteria:

1. Patients must have histologically and or cytologically confirmed metastatic colorectal cancer

2. Age 16 years or older.

3. Patients must have a wild type or mutated RAS tumor status known prior to enrollment

4. Metastatic colorectal cancer patients have progressed following at least one line of 5-FU-based chemotherapy.

5. Eastern Cooperative Oncology Group (ECOG) performance status of 0 to 2.

6. Patients must have measurable disease per irRECIST criteria for part 2 (dose expansion).

7. Adequate bone marrow function, defined as ANC $\geq$ 1.0 x 10^9/L ($\geq$ 1,000/uL), platelet count $\geq$ 75 x 10^9/L ($\geq$ 75000/µL), and hemoglobin $\geq$ 8.0 g/dL ($\geq$ 5.0 mmol/L). Patients must be transfusion independent (i.e., no blood product transfusions for a period of at least 14 days prior to screening).

8. Adequate Renal Function, including serum creatinine < 2 x upper limit of normal (ULN) or estimated creatinine clearance > 30 ml/min as calculated using the method standard for the institution.

9. Adequate Liver Function, including: a) Total serum bilirubin < 1.5 x ULN, unless the patient has documented Gilbert syndrome; b) Aspartate and Alanine Aminotransferase (AST and ALT) < 3 x ULN

10. Adequate Cardiac Function, as measured by left ventricular ejection fraction (LVEF) that is greater than 40%, or the absence of New York Heart Association (NYHA) classification of greater than stage II congestive heart failure.

11. Resolved acute effects of any prior therapy to baseline severity or Grade < /= 2 CTCAE v. 4.03 except for AEs not constituting a safety risk by investigator judgment.

12. Serum or urine pregnancy test (for females of childbearing potential) negative at screening and at the baseline visit (before the patient may receive the investigational product).

- 13. Male and female patients of childbearing potential and at risk for pregnancy must agree to use two highly effective methods of contraception throughout the study and for at least 90 days after the last dose of assigned treatment. Female patients who are not of childbearing potential (permanently sterilized or postmenopausal; i.e., meet at least one of the following criteria): Have undergone a documented hysterectomy and/or bilateral oophorectomy; or Have medically confirmed ovarian failure; or Achieved postmenopausal status, defined as follows: cessation of regular menses for at least 12 consecutive months with no alternative pathological or physiological cause; status may be confirmed by having a serum follicle stimulating hormone (FSH) level within the laboratory's reference range for postmenopausal women

14. High microsatellite instability (MSI-H) colorectal cancer patients must have received an approved PD-1 targeted agent prior to enrolling in this trial.

15. Evidence of a personally signed and dated informed consent document indicating that the patient has been informed of all pertinent aspects of the study

16. Willingness and ability to comply with the study scheduled visits, treatment plans, laboratory tests and other procedures.

Exclusion Criteria:

1. Patients with known symptomatic brain metastases requiring steroids. Patients with previously diagnosed brain metastases are eligible if they are asymptomatic or have completed their treatment and have recovered from the acute effects of radiation therapy or surgery prior to the start of study medication, have discontinued corticosteroid treatment for these metastases for at least 4 weeks and are neurologically stable

2. Patient has had any treatment specific for tumor control within 3 weeks of dosing, or for investigational drugs and cytotoxic agents, within 5 half-lives or 3 weeks, whichever is shorter

3. Patients receiving any medications or substances that are strong inhibitors or inducers of CYP3A4 complex. Lists including medications and substances known or with the potential to interact with the CYP3A4 isoenzymes

4. Prior therapy with a compound of the same mechanism as PF-05082566 (immunomodulation of 4-1BB).

5. Major surgery within 28 days of starting study treatment.

6. Radiation therapy within 14 days of starting study treatment

7. Autoimmune disorders (e.g., Crohn's Disease, rheumatoid arthritis, scleroderma, systemic lupus erythematosus) and other diseases that compromise or impair the immune system except patients who have grade 1 psoriasis (in remission or controlled with topical steroids) or mild degree of autoimmune thyroiditis that are controlled with medications

8. Active and clinically significant bacterial, fungal or viral infection including hepatitis B (HBV), hepatitis C (HCV), known human immunodeficiency virus (HIV) or acquired immunodeficiency syndrome (AIDS)-related illness (HIV testing is not required)

9. Unstable or serious concurrent medical conditions in the previous 6 months, eg, pancreatitis, severe/unstable angina, prolonged QT interval corrected by Fridericia's formula(QTcF) > 470 msec (calculated as average of triplicate readings, taken no greater than 2 minutes apart, and no history of Torsades de Pointes or symptomatic QTc abnormality), symptomatic congestive heart failure, myocardial infarction and/or pulmonary hypertension, ongoing maintenance therapy for life-threatening ventricular arrhythmia, stroke, and uncontrolled major seizure disorder

10. Concurrent active malignancy other than non-melanoma skin cancer or carcinoma in situ of the cervix

11. Patients who are pregnant or breastfeeding

12. Patients with intolerance to or who have had a severe allergic or anaphylactic reaction to antibodies or infused therapeutic proteins, or patients who have had a severe allergic or anaphylactic reaction to any of the substances included in the study drug (including excipients).

13. Other severe acute or chronic medical or psychiatric condition, including recent (within the past year) or active suicidal ideation or behavior, or laboratory abnormality that may increase the risk associated with study participation or investigational product administration or may interfere with the interpretation of study results and, in the judgment of the investigator, would make the patient inappropriate for entry into this study.

■ Sex/Gender

All

■ Ages

16 Years to N/A

■ Accepts Healthy Volunteers

No

■ Contacts

David S. Hong, MD   713-563-1930   CR   Study   Registration@mdanderson.org

A Phase 1/2 Study of INCB001158 in Combination With Chemotherapy in Subjects With Solid Tumors

Study ID:
NCT03314935

Sponsor:
Incyte Corporation

Information provided by (Responsible Party):
Incyte Corporation (Incyte Corporation)

Tracking Information

■ First Submitted Date

October 16, 2017

■ Start Date

November 20, 2017

■ Primary Completion Date

March 25, 2020

■ Last Update Posted Date

December 22, 2017

■ Current Primary Outcome Measures

Phase 1: Participants with treatment-emergent adverse events (TEAE)[Time Frame: 28 days]

TEAE is defined as any adverse event either reported for the first time or worsening of a pre-existing event after first dose of study drug.

Phase 2: Objective response rate[Time Frame: Every 8 weeks for duration of study participation which is estimated to be 18 months.]

Defined as the percentage of subjects having a complete response (CR) or partial response (PR) per Response Evaluation Criteria in Solid Tumors (RECIST) v1.1.

▣ Current Secondary Outcome Measures

Phase 2: Participants with TEAEs[Time Frame: Screening through 90 days after end of treatment, up to 21 months.]

TEAE is defined as any adverse event either reported for the first time or worsening of a pre-existing event after first dose of study drug.

Phase 1: Objective response rate[Time Frame: Every 8 weeks for duration of study participation, up to 18 months.]

Defined as the percentage of subjects having a CR or PR per RECIST v1.1.

Duration of response[Time Frame: Every 8 weeks for duration of study participation, up to 18 months.]

Defined as the time from earliest date of CR or PR (per RECIST v1.1) until the earliest date of disease progression or death due to any cause, if occurring sooner than disease progression.

Disease control rate[Time Frame: Every 8 weeks for duration of study participation, up to 18 months.]

Defined as the percentage of subjects having CR, PR, or stable disease for at least 8 weeks (per RECIST v1.1).

Progression-free survival[Time Frame: Every 8 weeks for duration of study participation, up to 18 months]

Defined as the time from date of first dose of study drug until the earliest date of disease progression (per RECIST v1.1) or death due to any cause, if occurring sooner than progression.

Descriptive Information

▣ Offical Title

A Phase 1/2 Study to Evaluate the Safety, Tolerability, and Efficacy of INCB001158 in Combination With Chemotherapy, in Subjects With Advanced or Metastatic Solid Tumors

▣ Brief Summary

The purpose of this open-label nonrandomized Phase 1/2 study is to evaluate INCB001158 in combination with chemotherapy in participants with advanced/metastatic solid tumors.

▣ Study Type

Interventional

▣ Study Phase

Phase 1/Phase 2

▣ Condition

- Advanced or Metastatic Solid Tumors
- Advanced or Metastatic Microsatellite Stable Colorectal Cancer (MSS-CRC)
- Advanced or Metastatic Biliary Tract Cancer (BTC)
- Advanced or Metastatic Gastroesophageal Cancer (GC)
- Advanced or Metastatic Endometrial Cancer
- Recurrent Ovarian Carcinoma

▣ Intervention

Drug: INCB001158

Phase 1: INCB001158 administered orally twice daily at the protocol-defined dose. Phase 2: INCB001158 administered orally twice daily at the recommended dose from Phase 1.

Other Names:

Arginase inhibitor

Drug: Oxaliplatin

Oxaliplatin administered intravenously at the protocol-defined dose and schedule.

Drug: Leucovorin

Leucovorin at the protocol-defined dose and regimen.

Drug: 5-Fluorouracil

5-Fluorouracil at the protocol-defined dose and regimen.

Drug: Gemcitabine

Gemcitabine at the protocol-defined dose and regimen.

Drug: Cisplatin

Cisplatin at the protocol-defined dose and regimen.

Drug: Paclitaxel

Paclitaxel at the protocol-defined dose and regimen.

■ **Study Arms**

Experimental: Treatment Group A
 INCB001158 + FOLFOX

Experimental: Treatment Group B
 INCB001158 + gemcitabine/cisplatin

Experimental: Treatment Group C
 INCB001158 + paclitaxel

Recruitment Information

■ **Recruitment Status**

Recruiting

■ **Estimated Enrollment**

249

■ **Completion Date**

May 27, 2020

■ **Primary Completion Date**

March 25, 2020

■ **Eligibility Criteria**

Inclusion Criteria:

- Histologically or cytologically confirmed diagnosis of selected advanced or metastatic solid tumors.
- Presence of measurable disease per RECIST v1.1.
- Eastern Cooperative Oncology Group (ECOG) performance status of 0 or 1.
- Baseline archival tumor specimen available or willingness to undergo a pretreatment tumor biopsy to obtain the specimen.
- Resolution of treatment-related toxicities.
- Adequate hepatic, renal, cardiac, and hematologic function.
- Additional cohort-specific criteria may apply.

Exclusion Criteria:

- Subjects who participated in any other study in which receipt of an investigational study drug or device occurred within 28 days or 5 half-lives (whichever is longer) prior to first dose.
- Has received a prior monoclonal antibody within 4 weeks or 5 half-lives (whichever is shorter) before administration of study drug.
- Has had prior chemotherapy or targeted small molecule therapy within 2 weeks before administration of study treatment.
- Has received prior approved radiotherapy within 14 days of study therapy.
- Has had known additional malignancy that is progressing or requires active treatment, or history of other malignancy within 2 years of study entry.
- Has an active autoimmune disease that has required systemic treatment in past 2 years.
- Has an active infection requiring systemic therapy.
- Has known active CNS metastases and/or carcinomatous meningitis.
- Women who are pregnant or breastfeeding.

■ **Sex/Gender**

All

■ **Ages**

18 Years to N/A

■ **Accepts Healthy Volunteers**

No

■ **Contacts**

Incyte Corporation Call Center (US)   1.855.463.3463   medinfo@incyte.com
Incyte Corporation Call Center (ex-US)   +800 00027423   globalmedinfo@incyte.com

FATE-NK100 as Monotherapy and in Combination With Monoclonal Antibody in Subjects With Advanced Solid Tumors

Study ID:

NCT03319459

Sponsor:

Fate Therapeutics

Information provided by (Responsible Party):

Fate Therapeutics (Fate Therapeutics)

Tracking Information

First Submitted Date

October 19, 2017

Start Date

January 18, 2018

Primary Completion Date

March 2019

Last Update Posted Date

February 8, 2018

Current Primary Outcome Measures

Incidence of dose-limiting toxicity (DLT)[Time Frame: 28 days]
- The incidence of dose-limiting toxicity (DLT) within each dose cohort within the first 28 days after FATE-NK100 administration (ie, Day 1 through Day 29).

Current Secondary Outcome Measures

Objective-response rate (ORR)[Time Frame: 28 days, 57 days, 113 days, 169 days, 225 days, 281 days, 337 days, 393 days, 449 days, 505 days, 561 days, 617 days, 673 days and 729 days.]
- Objective-response rate (ORR): defined as the proportion of patients who achieve partial response (PR) or complete response (CR) per Response Evaluation Criteria in Solid Tumors (RECIST) 1.1 at any time on study.

FATE-NK100 persistence[Time Frame: 0 days, 1 day, 3 days, 5 days, 8 days, 10 days, 12 days, 15 days, 22 days, 29 days, 43 days, 57 days, 85 days, 113 days]
- Duration of FATE-NK100 persistence: defined as duration from Day 1 to undetectable levels of FATE-NK100 cells per uL blood.

Descriptive Information

Offical Title

FATE-NK100 as Monotherapy and in Combination With Monoclonal Antibody in Subjects With Advanced Solid Tumors

Brief Summary

This is a Phase 1, single-dose, open-label, dose-escalation study. The study will be conducted in three parts (i.e. regimens) in an outpatient setting as follows:
- Regimen A: FATE-NK100 as a monotherapy in subjects with advanced solid tumor malignancies.
- Regimen B: FATE-NK100 in combination with trastuzumab in subjects with human epidermal growth factor receptor 2 positive (HER2+) advanced breast cancer, HER2+ advanced gastric cancer or other advanced HER2+ solid tumors.
- Regimen C: FATE-NK100 in combination with cetuximab in subjects with advanced colorectal cancer (CRC) or head and neck squamous cell cancer (HNSCC), or other epidermal growth factor receptor 1 positive (EGFR1+) advanced solid tumors.

Study Type

Interventional

Study Phase

Phase 1

Condition

- HER2 Positive Gastric Cancer
- Colorectal Cancer
- Head and Neck Squamous Cell Carcinoma
- EGFR Positive Solid Tumor

- Advanced Solid Tumors
- HER2-positive Breast Cancer
- Hepatocellular Carcinoma
- Small Cell Lung Cancer
- Renal Cell Carcinoma
- Pancreas Cancer

▨ Intervention

Drug: FATE-NK100

FATE-NK100 is a donor-derived NK cell product comprised of ex vivo activated effector cells with enhanced anti-tumor activity

Drug: Cetuximab

Epidermal growth factor receptor inhibitor antineoplastic agent

Other Names:

Erbitux

Drug: Trastuzumab

HER2/neu receptor inhibitor

Other Names:

Herceptin

▨ Study Arms

Experimental: Regimen A

FATE-NK100 as a monotherapy in subjects with advanced solid tumor malignancies.

Experimental: Regimen B

FATE-NK100 in combination with trastuzumab in subjects with human epidermal growth factor receptor 2 positive (HER2+) advanced breast cancer, HER2+ advanced gastric cancer or other advanced HER2+ solid tumors.

Experimental: Regimen C

Regimen C: FATE-NK100 in combination with cetuximab in subjects with advanced colorectal cancer (CRC) or head and neck squamous cell cancer (HNSCC), or other epidermal growth factor receptor 1 positive (EGFR1+) advanced solid tumors.

▨ Publications

(Includes publications given by the data provider as well as publications identified by ClinicalTrials.gov Identifier (NCT Number) in Medline.)Cichocki F, Valamehr B, Bjordahl R, Zhang B, Rezner B, Rogers P, Gaidarova S, Moreno S, Tuininga K, Dougherty P, McCullar V, Howard P, Sarhan D, Taras E, Schlums H, Abbot S, Shoemaker D, Bryceson YT, Blazar BR, Wolchko S, Cooley S, Miller JS. GSK3 Inhibition Drives Maturation of NK Cells and Enhances Their Antitumor Activity. Cancer Res. 2017 Oct 15;77(20):5664-5675. doi: 10.1158/0008-5472.CAN-17-0799. Epub 2017 Aug 8. (https://www.ncbi.nlm.nih.gov/pubmed/28790065)

Recruitment Information

▨ **Recruitment Status**

Recruiting

▨ **Completion Date**

March 2020

▨ **Estimated Enrollment**

100

▨ **Primary Completion Date**

March 2019

▨ **Eligibility Criteria**

Inclusion Criteria:

1. Regimen A only (monotherapy): Subjects with advanced metastatic solid tumors

2. Regimen B only (combination with trastuzumab): Subjects with advanced metastatic HER2+ solid tumors

3. Regimen C only (combination with cetuximab): Subjects with advanced metastatic EGFR+ solid tumors

4. Available related donor who is CMV+ and HLA-haploidentical or better but not fully HLA-matched

5. Presence of measurable disease by RECIST 1.1

6. Life expectancy of at least 3 months.

7. Provision of signed and dated informed consent form (ICF).

8. Stated willingness to comply with study procedures and duration.

Exclusion Criteria:

1. Females of reproductive potential that are pregnant or lactating, and males or females not willing to use a highly effective form

of contraception from Screening through the end of the study.

2. Eastern Cooperative Oncology Group (ECOG) performance status >2.

3. Evidence of insufficient organ function as determined by the protocol.

4. Receipt of any biological therapy, chemotherapy, or radiation within 1 week of the Screening Visit and at least 3 weeks prior to Day 1, except for patients receiving maintenance trastuzumab.

5. Have central nervous system disease (CNS) as follows:

1. Dose Escalation Cohorts: Active CNS disease, including history of CNS metastases.

2. MTD/MFD Expansion Cohorts: CNS disease, including history of CNS metastases, that was not stable during the last 6 months.

6. Myocardial infarction (MI) within 6 months of Screening Visit.

7. Severe asthma.

8. Currently receiving or likely to require systemic immunosuppressive therapy from Day -7 to Day 29.

9. Uncontrolled infections.

10. Presence of any medical or social issues that are likely to interfere with study conduct, or may cause increased risk to subject.

Sex/Gender

All

Ages

18 Years to 75 Years

Accepts Healthy Volunteers

No

Contacts

Sara Weymer   858-875-1800   clinical@fatetherapeutics.com
Meenal Patel   858-875-1800

A Study of CDX-1140 in Patients With Advanced Solid Tumors

Study ID:

NCT03329950

Sponsor:

Celldex Therapeutics

Information provided by (Responsible Party):

Celldex Therapeutics (Celldex Therapeutics)

Tracking Information

First Submitted Date

October 23, 2017

Start Date

December 1, 2017

Primary Completion Date

July 2020

Last Update Posted Date

December 19, 2017

Current Primary Outcome Measures

Safety and Tolerability of CDX1140-01 as assessed by CTCAE v4.0[Time Frame: Within 28 days after first dose]

The rates of drug-related adverse events, serious drug-related adverse events, dose-limiting toxicities, laboratory test abnormalities, and maximum tolerated dose will be determined.

Descriptive Information

Offical Title

A Phase 1 Study of CDX-1140, a Fully Human Agonist Anti-CD40 Monoclonal Antibody, in Patients With Advanced Solid Tumors

▧ Brief Summary

This is a study to determine the maximum tolerated dose (MTD) for CDX-1140 and to further evaluate its tolerability and efficacy in expansion cohorts once the MTD is determined.

▧ Detailed Description

CDX-1140 is a fully human monoclonal antibody that binds to a cell receptor called CD40 found on certain cells to activate the immune system which may promote anti-tumor effects.

This study will determine the MTD of CDX-1140 while also evaluating the safety, tolerability and efficacy of CDX-1140.

Eligible patients that enroll to the dose-escalation portion of the study will be assigned to one of several levels of CDX-1140. The first part of the study will test the safety profile of CDX-1140 and determine which dose(s) of CDX-1140 will be studied in the expansion portion of the study.

Up to 105 patients will be enrolled. All patients enrolled in the study will be closely monitored to determine if there is a response to the treatment as well as for any side effects that may occur.

▧ Study Type

Interventional

▧ Study Phase

Phase 1

▧ Condition

- Melanoma
- Non-small Cell Lung Cancer
- Breast Cancer
- Gastric Cancer
- Renal Cell Carcinoma
- Ovarian Cancer
- Cholangiocarcinoma
- Bladder Urothelial Carcinoma
- Pancreatic Adenocarcinoma
- Colorectal Cancer
- Esophageal Cancer
- Hepatic Cancer
- Head and Neck Cancer

▧ Intervention

Drug: CDX-1140

CDX-1140 will be administered every 4 weeks.

▧ Study Arms

Experimental: CDX-1140

Dose-escalation phase: Eligible patients will receive treatments, based on cohort assigned, in 4 week cycles until progression or intolerance.

Expansion phase: To further study the safety, tolerability, and efficacy of CDX-1140. Patients enrolled in the expansion phase of the study will receive CDX-1140 at the dose level(s) chosen during the escalation phase.

Recruitment Information

▧ Recruitment Status

Recruiting

▧ Estimated Enrollment

105

▧ Completion Date

December 2020

▧ Primary Completion Date

July 2020

▧ Eligibility Criteria

Inclusion Criteria:

1. Histologically confirmed diagnosis of one of the following cancers: melanoma (including mucosal and/or ocular), bladder/urothelial, non-small cell lung cancer, pancreatic adenocarcinoma, breast, colorectal, gastric, esophageal, renal cell, hepatic, ovarian, head and neck, and cholangiocarcinoma

2. Receipt of all standard therapies for the tumor type:

1. Must have had all standard approved and unapproved therapies as deemed appropriate by the treating physician.

2. Patients are not required to have all approved therapies in a drug class (e.g., patients with kidney cancer do not need all tyrosine kinase inhibitors, patients with melanoma do not need all approved checkpoint blockade inhibitors)

3. Patients who refuse standard therapy are excluded from the study

3. Measurable disease.

4. Life expectancy ≥ 12 weeks.

5. If of childbearing potential (male or female), agrees to practice an effective form of contraception during study treatment and for at least 6 months following last treatment.

6. Willingness to undergo a tumor biopsy prior to treatment.

7. Willingness to undergo a tumor biopsy while on study treatment.

Exclusion Criteria:

1. History of severe hypersensitivity reactions to other monoclonal antibodies.

2. Previous treatment with any anti-CD40 antibody.

3. Received any antibody targeting T-cell check point or co-stimulation pathways within 4 weeks, received any other monoclonal antibody within 4 weeks, and all other immunotherapy (tumor vaccine, cytokine, or growth factor) within 2 weeks prior to study treatment.

4. Chemotherapy within 21 days (6 weeks for nitrosoureas) or at least 5 half-lives (whichever is longer) prior to study treatment.

5. Received any kinase inhibitors within 2 weeks prior to study treatment.

6. Systemic radiation therapy within 4 weeks, prior focal radiotherapy within 2 weeks, or radiopharmaceuticals (strontium, samarium) within 8 weeks prior to study treatment.

7. Major surgery within 4 weeks prior to study treatment.

8. Use of immunosuppressive medications within 4 weeks or systemic corticosteroids within 2 weeks prior to study treatment.

9. Other prior malignancy, except for adequately treated basal or squamous cell skin cancer or in situ cancers. For all other cancers, the patient must be disease-free for at least 3 years to be allowed to enroll.

10. Active, untreated central nervous system metastases.

11. Active autoimmune disease or documented history of autoimmune disease.

12. Active infection requiring systemic therapy, known infection of HIV, Hepatitis B, or Hepatitis C.

13. Significant cardiovascular disease including Congestive Heart Failure or poorly controlled hypertension.

- **Sex/Gender**

  All

- **Ages**

  18 Years to N/A

- **Accepts Healthy Volunteers**

  No

- **Contacts**

  Celldex Therapeutics   844-723-9363   info@celldex.com

Pembrolizumab in Combination With Ibrutinib for Advanced, Refractory Colorectal Cancers

Study ID:
NCT03332498

Sponsor:
H. Lee Moffitt Cancer Center and Research Institute

Information provided by (Responsible Party):
H. Lee Moffitt Cancer Center and Research Institute (H. Lee Moffitt Cancer Center and Research Institute)

Tracking Information

- **First Submitted Date**

  November 2, 2017

- **Start Date**

  January 18, 2018

- **Primary Completion Date**

  February 2021

- **Last Update Posted Date**

  January 23, 2018

- Phase I Recommended Phase II Dose (RP2D)[Time Frame: 42 days post first dose]

  Standard 3+3 Design: The first cohort will enroll a minimum of 3 participants, according to a standard 3+3 design. If 0 out of the first 3 participants in the first cohort experience a dose-limiting toxicity (DLT), then dose escalation will continue as planned. If 1 out of the first 3 participants experience a DLT, then the cohort will be expanded to a total of 6 participants, and if no more than 1 out of 6 participants experiences a DLT in a given dose cohort, dose escalation will continue as planned. If ≥ 2 DLTs are observed in the first dose cohort, the principle investigator will discuss with Janssen on how to proceed. The DLT evaluation period will be defined as the time from the first dose of pembrolizumab and ibrutinib to 42 days after the first dose or if a participant experiences a DLT within this time period. A maximum of 2 cohorts is expected, making a total of approximately 12 evaluable participants during the dose escalation phase.

- Phase II Disease Control Rate at 4 Months[Time Frame: 4 months]

  Complete Response (CR) + Partial Response (PR) + Stable Disease (SD). Tumor response by Response Evaluation Criteria in Solid Tumors (RECIST) 1.1 and RECIST based immune-related response criteria (irRC).

Descriptive Information

■ Offical Title

A Phase I/II Study of Pembrolizumab in Combination With Ibrutinib for Advanced, Refractory Colorectal Cancers

■ Brief Summary

The purpose of this study is to determine the safety and tolerability, describe the dose-limiting toxicities (DLTs), and determine the maximum tolerated dose (MTD) (or the highest protocol-defined dose level in the absence of establishing an MTD) of ibrutinib in combination with pembrolizumab in participants with advanced, refractory colorectal cancers.

■ Detailed Description

On this study, one treatment cycle equals 21 days. On the first day of each study treatment cycle, 200 milligrams of pembrolizumab will be given through an IV (intravenously) for about thirty minutes. In addition, participants will begin taking the ibrutinib capsules every day starting on cycle 1, day 1. Participants will have a follow-up visit every 3 weeks, on about the first day of each cycle with laboratories drawn to make sure that the study drugs are not causing any side effects. In addition, participants will have a computed tomography (CT) scan every 6 to 7 weeks to determine whether your cancer is getting better or worse.

■ Study Type

Interventional

■ Study Phase

Phase 1/Phase 2

■ Condition

- Colon Cancer
- Colorectal Cancer
- Colorectal Carcinoma
- Colon Disease

■ Intervention

Drug: Pembrolizumab

  200 milligrams of pembrolizumab will be given through an IV (intravenously) for about thirty minutes. Pembrolizumab is an anti-PD1 that functions by inhibiting checkpoint inhibition and reversing T cell suppression.

Other Names:

  Keytruda®

Drug: Ibrutinib

  Ibrutinib oral capsules every day starting on cycle 1, day 1. Ibrutinib is primarily a BTK inhibitor which has been approved for the treatment of several hematologic malignancies.

Other Names:

  Imbruvica®

■ Study Arms

Experimental: Pembrolizumab and Ibrutinib

  Pembrolizumab intravenously (IV): 200 mg every 3 weeks (Q3W).

  Ibrutinib by mouth (PO): Phase I Dose Escalation at doses of 420 mg daily (cohort 0) and 560 mg daily (cohort 1);. Phase II treatment at Recommended Phase II dose.

Recruitment Information

Recruitment Status

Recruiting

Estimated Enrollment

42

Completion Date

February 2022

Primary Completion Date

February 2021

Eligibility Criteria

Inclusion Criteria:

- Histologically confirmed diagnosis of colorectal adenocarcinoma.
- Measurable or non-measurable disease by Response Evaluation Criteria in Solid Tumors (RECIST) 1.1. Stage IV or recurrent disease is required.
- Participants must have received and progressed through or become intolerant to fluoropyrimidine, irinotecan, oxaliplatin, and bevacizumab. If RAS wild type, participants should have received and progressed or become intolerant to the above as well as cetuximab or panitumumab containing therapies. Prior therapy with Regorafenib and/or TAS 102 is allowed.
- Eastern Cooperative Oncology Group (ECOG) Performance Score 0 or 1.
- Estimated life expectancy > 3 months.
- **Adequate bone marrow, liver and renal function as assessed by the following:**
- Hemoglobin > 8.0 g/dl
- Absolute neutrophil count (ANC) > 1,000/mm^3 independent of growth factor support
- Platelet count > 100,000/mm^3
- Total bilirubin < 1.5 times upper limit of normal (ULN) unless bilirubin rise is due to Gilbert's syndrome or of non-hepatic origin
- AST, ALT and Alkaline Phosphatase ≤2.5 times the ULN (≤5 x ULN for potential participants with liver involvement)
- Creatinine clearance ≥ 30 ml/min
- Must not have had chemotherapy, major surgery, monoclonal antibody therapy or experimental therapy within the 21 days prior to the start of ibrutinib administration
- Women of childbearing potential must have a negative serum or urine pregnancy test performed within 7 days prior to the start of study drug. Post-menopausal women and surgically sterilized women are not required to undergo a pregnancy test.
- Men and women of childbearing potential must agree to use adequate contraception beginning at the signing of the informed consent form (ICF) until at least 4 months for both females and males after the last dose of study drug. The definition of adequate contraception will be based on the judgment of the principal investigator or a designated associate.
- Must agree to not donate sperm (males) or eggs (females) during and up to 120 days after the last dose of study treatment.
- Must be able to understand and be willing to sign the written informed consent form. A signed informed consent form must be appropriately obtained prior to the conduct of any trial-specific procedure. Must be willing and able to comply with scheduled visits, treatment schedule, laboratory testing, and other study requirements.

Exclusion Criteria:

- Active central nervous system (CNS) metastases. If CNS metastases are treated and patients are at neurologic baseline for at least 2 weeks prior to enrollment, they will be eligible but will need a Brain MRI prior to enrollment. Must be off corticosteroids or on a dose of less than 10mg per day.
- Active, known or suspected autoimmune disease. Patients with vitiligo, type I diabetes mellitus, residual hypothyroidism due to autoimmune thyroiditis only requiring hormone replacement, or conditions not expected to recur in the absence of an external trigger are permitted to enroll.
- A condition requiring systemic treatment with either corticosteroids (>10 mg daily prednisone equivalent) or other immunosuppressive medications within 14 days of enrollment. Inhaled or topical steroids, and adrenal replacement steroid doses > 10 mg daily prednisone equivalent, are permitted in the absence of active autoimmune disease.
- Prior therapy with anti-PD-1, anti-PD-L1, anti-PD-L2, anti-CD137, or anti-CTLA-4 antibody (including ipilimumab or any other antibody or drug specifically targeting T-cell costimulation or checkpoint pathways).
- Prior therapy with ibrutinib or other BTK inhibitors.
- Previous or concurrent cancer within 3 years prior to treatment start EXCEPT for curatively treated cervical cancer in situ, non-melanoma skin cancer, superficial bladder tumors [Ta (non-invasive tumor), Tis (carcinoma in situ) and T1 (tumor invades lamina propria)].
- Known history of human immunodeficiency virus (HIV) infection or acquired immunodeficiency syndrome (AIDS).
- Serologic status reflecting active hepatitis B or C infection. Patients who are hepatitis B core antibody positive and who are antigen negative, will need to have a negative PCR result prior to enrollment. Those who are hepatitis B antigen positive or PCR positive, will be excluded.
- Child Pugh B or C cirrhosis. Patients with Child Pugh A cirrhosis will be excluded from the dose escalation portion of the trial but can be included in the dose expansion portion of the trial with one dose reduction from the established dose.
- History of severe hypersensitivity reactions to other monoclonal antibodies.
- Substance abuse, medical, psychological or social conditions that may interfere with participation in the study or evaluation of

the study results.

- History or concurrent condition of interstitial lung disease of any grade or severely impaired pulmonary function.
- Unresolved toxicity higher than CTCAE grade 1 attributed to any prior therapy or procedure, excluding alopecia.
- Clinically significant cardiovascular disease such as uncontrolled or symptomatic arrhythmia, congestive heart failure, any Class 3 or 4 cardiac disease as defined by the New York Heart Association Functional Classification, or history of myocardial infarction within 6 months prior to first dose with study drug.
- Unable to swallow capsules or disease significantly affecting gastrointestinal function and/or inhibiting small intestine absorption such as; malabsorption syndrome, resection of the small bowel, or poorly controlled inflammatory bowel disease affecting the small intestine.
- Requires anticoagulation with warfarin or equivalent vitamin K antagonists (e.g., phenprocoumon).
- Requires treatment with a strong CYP3A4/5 and/or CYP2D6 inhibitor.
- History of stroke or intracranial hemorrhage within 6 months prior to enrollment.
- Any illness or medical conditions that are unstable or could jeopardize the safety of the participant and his/her compliance in the study.
- Major surgery or a wound that has not fully healed within 4 weeks of enrollment.
- Vaccinated with live, attenuated vaccines within 4 weeks of enrollment.
- History of (non-infectious) pneumonitis that required steroids or current pneumonitis within 6 months.

Sex/Gender

All

Ages

18 Years to N/A

Accepts Healthy Volunteers

No

S1613, Trastuzumab and Pertuzumab or Cetuximab and Irinotecan Hydrochloride in Treating Patients With Locally Advanced or Metastatic HER2/Neu Amplified Colorectal Cancer That Cannot Be Removed by Surgery

Study ID:

NCT03365882

Sponsor:

Southwest Oncology Group

Information provided by (Responsible Party):

Southwest Oncology Group (Southwest Oncology Group)

Tracking Information

First Submitted Date

October 2, 2017

Start Date

October 9, 2017

Primary Completion Date

February 1, 2019

Last Update Posted Date

January 4, 2018

Current Primary Outcome Measures

Progression-free survival (PFS)[Time Frame: From date of registration to date of first documentation of progression or symptomatic deterioration, or death due to any cause, assessed up to 3 years]

Analysis of PFS will be conducted using the stratified log rank test upon the observation of 115 PFS events. PFS among patients who register to Arm 3 will be summarized using descriptive statistics.

Current Secondary Outcome Measures

Incidence of adverse events[Time Frame: Up to 3 years]

Evaluated according to National Cancer Institute Common Terminology Criteria for Adverse Events version 4.0.

Overall response rate (ORR)[Time Frame: Up to 3 years]

ORR including confirmed complete and partial responses per Response Evaluation Criteria in Solid Tumors 1.1 will be compared using using the Cochran-Mantel-Haenszel test. ORR among patients who register to Arm 3 will be summarized using descriptive statistics.

Overall survival (OS)[Time Frame: From date of registration to date of death due to any cause, assessed up to 3 years]

Distributions of OS in each arm will be estimated using the method of Kaplan-Meier and compared using the stratified log-rank test. OS among patients who register to Arm 3 will be summarized using descriptive statistics.

Descriptive Information

▨ Offical Title

S1613, A Randomized Phase II Study of Trastuzumab and Pertuzumab (TP) Compared to Cetuximab and Irinotecan (CETIRI) in Advanced/Metastatic Colorectal Cancer (mCRC) With HER-2 Amplification

▨ Brief Summary

This randomized phase II trial studies how well trastuzumab and pertuzumab work compared to cetuximab and irinotecan hydrochloride in treating patients with HER2/neu amplified colorectal cancer that has spread from where it started to other places in the body and cannot be removed by surgery. Monoclonal antibodies, such as trastuzumab and pertuzumab, may interfere with the ability of tumor cells to grow and spread. Drugs used in chemotherapy, such as cetuximab and irinotecan hydrochloride, work in different ways to stop the growth of tumor cells, either by killing the cells, by stopping them from dividing, or by stopping them from spreading. Giving trastuzumab and pertuzumab may work better compared to cetuximab and irinotecan hydrochloride in treating patients with colorectal cancer.

▨ Detailed Description

PRIMARY OBJECTIVES:

I. To evaluate the efficacy of trastuzumab and pertuzumab (TP) (Arm 1) in HER-2 amplified metastatic colorectal cancer (mCRC) by comparing progression-free survival (PFS) on TP compared to control arm (Arm 2) of cetuximab and irinotecan hydrochloride (irinotecan) (CETIRI).

SECONDARY OBJECTIVES:

I. To evaluate the overall response rate (ORR), including confirmed complete and partial response per Response Evaluation Criteria in Solid Tumors (RECIST) 1.1, in treatment Arms 1 and 2.

II. To evaluate the overall survival (OS) in treatment Arms 1 and 2. III. To evaluate the safety and toxicity of TP compared to CETIRI.

TERTIARY OBJECTIVES:

I. To estimate the rates of PFS, OS, and ORR in patients who crossover to TP (Arm 3) after disease progression on CETIRI.

II. To bank images for future retrospective analysis. III. To evaluate if HER-2/centromeric probe (CEP17) signal ratio and HER-2 gene copy number (GCN) are predictive of clinical efficacy for patients receiving TP versus CETIRI.

IV. To bank tissue and blood samples for other future correlative studies from patients enrolled on the study.

OUTLINE: Patients with HER2 gene amplification are randomized to 1 of 2 arms.

ARM I: Patients receive pertuzumab intravenously (IV) over 30-60 minutes and trastuzumab IV over 30-120 minutes on day 1. Courses repeat every 21 days in the absence of disease progression or unacceptable toxicity.

ARM II: Patients receive cetuximab IV over 60-120 minutes and irinotecan hydrochloride IV over 90 minutes on day 1. Courses repeat every 14 days in the absence of disease progression or unacceptable toxicity. Patients with documented disease progression may optionally crossover to Arm I.

After completion of study treatment, patients are followed up for 3 years.

▨ Study Type

Interventional

▨ Study Phase

Phase 2

▨ Condition

- Colon Adenocarcinoma
- ERBB2 Gene Amplification
- Rectal Adenocarcinoma
- Recurrent Colon Carcinoma
- Recurrent Rectal Carcinoma
- Stage III Colon Cancer AJCC v7
- Stage III Rectal Cancer AJCC v7
- Stage IIIA Colon Cancer AJCC v7
- Stage IIIA Rectal Cancer AJCC v7

- Stage IIIB Colon Cancer AJCC v7
- Stage IIIB Rectal Cancer AJCC v7
- Stage IIIC Colon Cancer AJCC v7
- Stage IIIC Rectal Cancer AJCC v7
- Stage IV Colon Cancer AJCC v7
- Stage IV Rectal Cancer AJCC v7
- Stage IVA Colon Cancer AJCC v7
- Stage IVA Rectal Cancer AJCC v7
- Stage IVB Colon Cancer AJCC v7
- Stage IVB Rectal Cancer AJCC v7

Intervention

Biological: Cetuximab
   Given IV

Other Names:
   Chimeric Anti-EGFR Monoclonal Antibody

   Chimeric MoAb C225

   Chimeric Monoclonal Antibody C225

   Erbitux

   IMC-C225

Drug: Irinotecan Hydrochloride
   Given IV

Other Names:
   Campto

   Camptosar

   Camptothecin 11

   Camptothecin-11

   CPT 11

   CPT-11

   Irinomedac

   U-101440E

Other: Laboratory Biomarker Analysis
   Correlative studies

Biological: Pertuzumab
   Given IV

Other Names:
   2C4

   2C4 Antibody

   MoAb 2C4

   Monoclonal Antibody 2C4

   Perjeta

   rhuMAb2C4

   RO4368451

Biological: Trastuzumab
   Given IV

Other Names:
   ABP 980

   Anti-c-ERB-2

Anti-c-erbB2 Monoclonal Antibody

Anti-ERB-2

Anti-erbB-2

Anti-erbB2 Monoclonal Antibody

Anti-HER2/c-erbB2 Monoclonal Antibody

Anti-p185-HER2

c-erb-2 Monoclonal Antibody

HER2 Monoclonal Antibody

Herceptin

Herceptin Biosimilar PF-05280014

Herceptin Trastuzumab Biosimilar PF-05280014

MoAb HER2

Monoclonal Antibody c-erb-2

Monoclonal Antibody HER2

PF-05280014

rhuMAb HER2

RO0452317

Trastuzumab Biosimilar ABP 980

Trastuzumab Biosimilar PF-05280014

Device: HER-2 testing

Central testing of HER-2 for eligibility

▦ Study Arms

Experimental: Arm I (pertuzumab, trastuzumab)

Patients receive pertuzumab IV over 30-60 minutes and trastuzumab IV over 30-120 minutes on day 1. Courses repeat every 21 days in the absence of disease progression or unacceptable toxicity.

Experimental: Arm II (cetuximab, irinotecan hydrochloride)

Patients receive cetuximab IV over 60-120 minutes and irinotecan hydrochloride IV over 90 minutes on day 1. Courses repeat every 14 days in the absence of disease progression or unacceptable toxicity. Patients with documented disease progression may optionally crossover to Arm I.

Recruitment Information

▦ Recruitment Status

Recruiting

▦ Estimated Enrollment

130

▦ Completion Date

June 15, 2023

▦ Primary Completion Date

February 1, 2019

▦ Eligibility Criteria

Inclusion Criteria:

- STEP 1 INITIAL REGISTRATION: HER2 TESTING
- Patients must have histologically or cytologically documented adenocarcinoma of the colon or rectum that is metastatic or locally advanced and unresectable
- Mutation results:
- All patients must have molecular testing performed in a Clinical Laboratory Improvement Act (CLIA) certified lab which includes which includes KRAS and NRAS gene and exon 15 of BRAF gene (BRAF V600E mutation); patients with any known activating mutation in exon 2 [codons 12 and 13], exon 3 [codons 59 and 61] and exon 4 [codons 117 and 146]) of KRAS/NRAS genes and in exon 15 (BRAFV600E mutation) of BRAF gene are not eligible
- Patients must not have been treated with any of the following prior to step 1 initial registration:
- Cetuximab, panitumumab, or any other monoclonal antibody against EGFR or inhibitor of EGFR
- HER-2 targeting for treatment of colorectal cancer; patients who have received prior trastuzumab or pertuzumab for other indications such as prior history of adjuvant or neoadjuvant breast cancer treatment prior to the development of advanced colorectal cancer are eligible

- Patients must not have had history of severe toxicity and intolerance to or hypersensitivity to irinotecan or any other study drug; patients must not have had a severe infusion-related reaction during any prior therapy with pertuzumab or trastuzumab
- Patients must have tumor slides available for submission for HER-2 testing; HER-2 testing must be completed by the central lab prior to step 2 randomization
- Patients must be informed of the investigational nature of this study and must sign and give informed consent in accordance with institutional and federal guidelines; for step 1 initial registration, the appropriate consent form is the step 1 consent form
- As a part of the OPEN registration process the treating institution's identity is provided in order to ensure that the current (within 365 days) date of institutional review board approval for this study has been entered in the system
- STEP 2 RANDOMIZATION
- Patients must have HER-2 amplification as determined by central testing (3+ or 2+ by immunohistochemistry and HER-2 gene amplification by in situ hybridization with a ratio of HER-2 gene signals to centromere 17 signals >= 2.0)
- Patients must have measurable disease that is metastatic or locally advanced and unresectable; imaging used to assess all disease per RECIST 1.1 must have been completed within 28 days prior to step 2 randomization; all disease must be assessed and documented on the Baseline Tumor Assessment Form
- Patients must have had at least one prior regimen of systemic chemotherapy for metastatic or locally advanced, unresectable disease; patients must have progressed following the most recent therapy; prior treatment with irinotecan is allowed; for patients that received adjuvant chemotherapy: prior treatment for metastatic disease is not required for patient who experienced disease recurrence during or within 6 months of completion of adjuvant chemotherapy; if the patient received one line of adjuvant treatment and had disease recurrence after 6 months of completing chemotherapy, patients will only be eligible after failing one additional line of chemotherapy used to treat the metastatic or locally advanced, unresectable disease; patients who have received >= 3 lines of systemic chemotherapy for metastatic or locally advanced, unresectable disease are not eligible
- Patients must have completed prior chemotherapy, immunotherapy, or radiation therapy at least 14 days prior to step 2 randomization and all toxicity must be resolved to Common Terminology Criteria for Adverse Events (CTCAE) version (v)4.0 grade 1 (with the exception of CTCAE v4.0 grade 2 neuropathy) prior to step 2 randomization
- Brain metastases are allowed if they have been adequately treated with radiotherapy or surgery and stable for at least 30 days prior to step 2 randomization; eligible patients must be neurologically asymptomatic and without corticosteroid treatment for at least 7 days prior to step 2 randomization
- Patients must have a Zubrod performance status of 0 or 1
- Patients must have a complete physical examination and medical history within 28 days prior to step 2 randomization
- Absolute neutrophil count (ANC) >= 1,500/mcL
- Platelets >= 75,000/mcL
- Hemoglobin >= 9 g/dL
- Aspartate aminotransferase (AST) and alanine aminotransferase (ALT) both =< 5 x institutional upper limit of normal (IULN)
- Bilirubin =< 1.5 mg/dL
- Calculated creatinine clearance > 30 ml/min within 14 days prior to step 2 randomization
- Patients who have had an echocardiogram performed within 6 months prior to step 2 randomization must have ventricular ejection fraction (left ventricular ejection fraction [LVEF]) >= 50% or >= within normal limits for the institution
- Patients must not have an uncontrolled intercurrent illness including, but not limited to diabetes, hypertension, severe infection, severe malnutrition, unstable angina, class III-IV New York Heart Association (NYHA) congestive heart failure, ventricular arrhythmias, active ischemic heart disease, or myocardial infarction within 6 months prior to step 2 randomization
- Patients must not have any known previous or concurrent condition suggesting susceptibility to hypersensitivity or allergic reactions, including, but not limited to: known hypersensitivity to any of the study treatments or to excipients of recombinant human or humanized antibodies; patients with mild or seasonal allergies may be included after discussion with the study chairs
- Patients must not be planning treatment with other systemic anti-cancer agents (e.g., chemotherapy, hormonal therapy, immunotherapy) or other treatments not part of protocol-specified anti-cancer therapy including concurrent investigational agents of any type
- No prior malignancy is allowed except for adequately treated basal cell or squamous cell skin cancer, in situ cervical cancer, ductal carcinoma in situ, other low grade lesions such as incidental appendix carcinoid, or any other cancer from which the patient has been disease and treatment free for two years; prostate cancer patients on active surveillance are eligible
- Patients must not be pregnant or nursing; females of child-bearing potential must have a negative serum pregnancy test within 7 days prior to registration; women/men of reproductive potential must have agreed to use an effective contraceptive method while on study and for at least 7 months after the last dose of study treatment; a woman is considered to be of "reproductive potential" if she has had menses at any time in the preceding 12 consecutive months; in addition to routine contraceptive methods, "effective contraception" also includes heterosexual celibacy and surgery intended to prevent pregnancy (or with a side-effect of pregnancy prevention) defined as a hysterectomy, bilateral oophorectomy or bilateral tubal ligation; however, if at any point a previously celibate patient chooses to become heterosexually active during the time period for use of contraceptive measures outlined in the protocol, he/she is responsible for beginning contraceptive measures
- Patients must be given the opportunity to consent to the optional submission of tissue for future research
- STEP 2 RANDOMIZATION: As a part of the Oncology Patient Enrollment Network (OPEN) registration process the treating institution's identity is provided in order to ensure that the current (within 365 days) date of institutional review board approval for this study has been entered in the system
- STEP 3 CROSSOVER REGISTRATION (OPTIONAL): Patients must have documented disease progression while on CETIRI

(Arm 2) on this protocol; the Follow-up Tumor Assessment Form documenting disease progression must be submitted to Southwest Oncology Group (SWOG) prior to step 3 crossover registration; registration to step 3 crossover must be within 28 days of discontinuation of CETIRI protocol treatment; patients going off treatment for any other reason are not eligible

- STEP 3 CROSSOVER REGISTRATION (OPTIONAL): Patients must have a Zubrod performance status of 0 or 1
- STEP 3 CROSSOVER REGISTRATION (OPTIONAL): ANC >= 1,500/mcL
- STEP 3 CROSSOVER REGISTRATION (OPTIONAL): Platelets >= 75,000/mcL
- STEP 3 CROSSOVER REGISTRATION (OPTIONAL): Hemoglobin >= 9 g/dL
- STEP 3 CROSSOVER REGISTRATION (OPTIONAL): AST and ALT both =< 5 x institutional upper limit of normal (IULN)
- STEP 3 CROSSOVER REGISTRATION (OPTIONAL): Bilirubin =< 1.5 mg/dL
- STEP 3 CROSSOVER REGISTRATION (OPTIONAL): Calculated creatinine clearance > 30 ml/min within 14 days prior to step 3 crossover registration
- STEP 3 CROSSOVER REGISTRATION (OPTIONAL): Patients must have left ventricular ejection fraction (LVEF) >= 50% or >= lower limit of normal for the institution by echocardiogram within 14 days prior to step 3 crossover registration
- STEP 3 CROSSOVER REGISTRATION (OPTIONAL): Patients must have a magnesium, potassium, calcium, sodium, bicarbonate, and chloride performed within 14 days prior to step 3 crossover registration
- STEP 3 CROSSOVER REGISTRATION (OPTIONAL): Patients must be informed of the investigational nature of this study and must sign and give written informed consent in accordance with institutional and federal guidelines; the appropriate consent form for this registration is the step 2 consent form
- STEP 3 CROSSOVER REGISTRATION (OPTIONAL): As a part of the OPEN registration process the treating institution's identity is provided in order to ensure that the current (within 365 days) date of institutional review board approval for this study has been entered in the system

Sex/Gender

All

Ages

18 Years to N/A

Accepts Healthy Volunteers

No

Contacts

Danae Campos   2106148808   dcampos@swog.org
Dana Sparks   2106148808   dsparks@swog.org

TAS102 in Combination With NAL-IRI in Advanced GI Cancers

Study ID:

NCT03368963

Sponsor:

Emory University

Information provided by (Responsible Party):

Emory University (Emory University)

Tracking Information

First Submitted Date

December 6, 2017

Start Date

January 30, 2018

Primary Completion Date

February 29, 2020

Last Update Posted Date

February 5, 2018

Current Primary Outcome Measures

Incidence of adverse events of trifluridine/tipiracil hydrochloride combination agent TAS-102 in combination with nanoliposomal irinotecan[Time Frame: Up to 3 years after end of treatment]

Assessed using Common Terminology Criteria for Adverse Events version 4.0.

Overall response rate based on modified Response Evaluation Criteria in Solid Tumors (RECIST) version 1.1[Time Frame: Up to 3 years after end of treatment]

Defined as the proportion of patients who achieved a complete response (complete response: disappearance of all target tumors) or a partial response (partial response: ≥ 30% decrease in the sum of the longest diameters of target tumors).

▦ Current Secondary Outcome Measures

Progression free survival[Time Frame: Up to 3 years after end of treatment]
Will be evaluated.

Response duration[Time Frame: From initial response until documented tumor progression, assessed up to 3 years]
Will be estimated by Kaplan-Meier method. P values will be two-sided with significance level of .05.

Response rate[Time Frame: Up to 3 years after end of treatment]
Response assessment will be done according to RECIST 1.1 criteria. A repeat imaging scan of the same modality and technique will be repeated after 4 weeks for confirmation of response.

Descriptive Information

▦ Offical Title

A Phase I/II Study of Trifluridine/Tipiracil (TAS102) in Combination With Nanoliposomal Irinotecan (NAL-IRI) in Advanced GI Cancers

▦ Brief Summary

This phase I/II trial studies the best dose and how well trifluridine/tipiracil hydrochloride combination agent TAS-102 (TAS-102) and nanoliposomal irinotecan work in treating patients with gastrointestinal cancers that have spread to other places in the body or cannot be removed by surgery. Drugs used in the chemotherapy, such as trifluridine/tipiracil hydrochloride combination agent TAS-102 and nanoliposomal irinotecan, work in different ways to stop the growth of tumor cells, either by killing the cells, by stopping them from dividing, or by stopping them from spreading.

▦ Detailed Description

PRIMARY OBJECTIVES:

I. Determine the recommended phase II dose for the combination of TAS-102 and nanoliposomal irinotecan (nanoliposomal [nal]-IRI). (Phase I)

II. Evaluate the activity of the combination of TAS102 and nal-IRI in previously treated patients with metastatic colorectal cancer and pancreatic cancer. (Phase II)

SECONDARY OBJECTIVES:

I. Define the toxicity profile of the combination of TAS-102 and nal-IRI.

II. Evaluate the response duration, progression free, and overall survival of the combination of TAS-102 and nal-IRI in previously treated patients with metastatic colorectal cancer and pancreatic cancer.

OUTLINE: This is a phase I, dose-escalation study followed by a phase II study.

Patients receive nanoliposomal irinotecan intravenously (IV) over 90 minutes on day 1 and trifluridine/tipiracil hydrochloride combination agent TAS-102 orally (PO) twice daily (BID) on days 1-5. Courses repeat every 2 weeks in the absence of disease progression or unacceptable toxicity.

After completion of study treatment, patients are followed up for 30 days and then every 8 or 12 weeks thereafter.

▦ Study Type

Interventional

▦ Study Phase

Phase 1/Phase 2

▦ Condition

- Colorectal Adenocarcinoma
- Gastric Adenocarcinoma
- Metastatic Pancreatic Adenocarcinoma
- Non-Resectable Cholangiocarcinoma
- Stage IV Colorectal Cancer
- Stage IV Gastric Cancer
- Stage IV Pancreatic Cancer
- Stage IVA Colorectal Cancer
- Stage IVB Colorectal Cancer
- Unresectable Pancreatic Carcinoma

▦ Intervention

Drug: Nanoliposomal Irinotecan

Given IV

Other Names:

Irinotecan Liposome

Onivyde

PEP02

Camptosar

Liposomal Irinotecan

Drug: Trifluridine and Tipiracil Hydrochloride
Given PO

Other Names:

Lonsurf

TAS-102

Trifluridine/Tipiracil

■ Study Arms

Experimental: Treatment (Nal-IRI, TAS-102)

Patients receive nanoliposomal irinotecan IV over 90 minutes on day 1 and combination of trifluridine and tipiracil hydrochloride combination agent TAS-102 PO BID on days 1-5. Courses repeat every 2 weeks in the absence of disease progression or unacceptable toxicity.

Recruitment Information

■ **Recruitment Status**

Recruiting

■ **Estimated Enrollment**

64

■ **Completion Date**

February 29, 2020

■ **Primary Completion Date**

February 29, 2020

■ **Eligibility Criteria**

Inclusion Criteria:

- Subjects must have histologic or cytological confirmation of a malignancy that is advanced (metastatic and/or unresectable) with measurable disease per Response Evaluation Criteria in Solid Tumors (RECIST) version (v)1.1
- In the dose escalation phase, the trial will be open for patients with stage IV or locally advanced unresectable gastrointestinal adenocarcinomas (gastric, cholangiocarcinoma, pancreatic, colorectal) who have failed at least one prior therapy; subjects must have received, and then progressed or been intolerant to, at least 1 standard treatment regimen in the advanced or metastatic setting
- In the dose expansion phase, Arm A will be open for 25 patients with pancreatic adenocarcinoma; patients must have histologic diagnosis and either locally advanced unresectable or metastatic disease and have not received prior irinotecan; patients must have received at least one prior line of standard treatment for locally advanced or metastatic disease
- In dose expansion phase, Arm B will be open for 25 patients with colorectal adenocarcinoma; patients must have histologic diagnosis and metastatic disease and have not received prior irinotecan; patients must have received at least one prior line of standard treatment for locally advanced or metastatic disease
- Eastern Cooperative Oncology Group (ECOG) performance status (PS) 0-1
- Adequate organ function
- Recovered from the effects of any prior surgery, radiotherapy or other antineoplastic therapy

Exclusion Criteria:

- History of any second malignancy in the last 5 years; subjects with prior history of in-situ cancer or basal or squamous cell skin cancer are eligible; subjects with other malignancies are eligible if they have been continuously disease free for at least 5 years
- Severe arterial thromboembolic events (myocardial infarction, unstable angina pectoris, stroke) less than 6 months before inclusion
- New York Heart Association (NYHA) class III or IV congestive heart failure, ventricular arrhythmias or uncontrolled blood pressure
- Known hypersensitivity to any of the components of nal-IRI, other liposomal products, fluoropyrimidines or leucovorin
- Investigational therapy administered within 4 weeks, or within a time interval less than at least 5 half-lives of the investigational agent, whichever is longer, prior to the first scheduled day of dosing in this study
- Known active central nervous system (CNS) metastases and/or carcinomatous meningitis; subjects with previously treated brain metastases may participate provided they are stable (without evidence of progression by imaging for at least four weeks

prior to the first dose of trial treatment and any neurologic symptoms have returned to baseline), have no evidence of new or enlarging brain metastases, and are not using steroids for at least 7 days prior to trial treatment; this exception does not include carcinomatous meningitis which is excluded regardless of clinical stability

- Known history of human immunodeficiency virus (HIV) (HIV 1/2 antibodies)
- Inability to take oral medications
- Homozygous for the UGT1A1

28 allele (UGT1A1 7/7 genotype) or heterozygotes for UGT1A1

28 (UGT1A11 7/6 genotype) only for the phase I part

- Patients who are not appropriate candidates for participation in this clinical study for any other reason as deemed by the investigator
- Patients with history of positive dihydropyrimidine dehydrogenase (DPD) deficiency

Other protocol defined inclusion/exclusion criteria could apply

▦ Sex/Gender

All

▦ Ages

18 Years to N/A

▦ Accepts Healthy Volunteers

No

▦ Contacts

Olatunji B. Alese, MD   404-778-2670   olatunji.alese@emory.edu

VX15/2503 and Immunotherapy in Resectable Pancreatic and Colorectal Cancer

Study ID:

NCT03373188

Sponsor:

Emory University

Information provided by (Responsible Party):

Emory University (Emory University)

Tracking Information

▦ First Submitted Date

December 11, 2017

▦ Start Date

December 15, 2017

▦ Primary Completion Date

December 31, 2022

▦ Last Update Posted Date

December 28, 2017

▦ Current Primary Outcome Measures

Evaluate treatment effects of the study drugs on tumor CD8+ T cell infiltration between the treatment groups.[Time Frame: Up to 4 years from date of last treatment dose]

CD8+ T cells in tumor samples will be identified by immunohistochemistry and immunofluorescence staining, and we will quantitate the percentage and staining of the cells in the pancreatic and liver tissue with Integrated Cellular Imaging.

▦ Current Secondary Outcome Measures

Incidence of adverse events according to National Cancer Institute Common Terminology Criteria for Adverse Events scale version 4.0[Time Frame: Up to 4 years from the date of last treatment dose]

Summary statistics will be presented for all safety analyses. Toxicities will be presented as worst toxicity per patient and will be reported as percent toxicity. Adverse events will be classified using MedDRA System Organ Classes and Preferred Terms.

Descriptive Information

▦ Offical Title

Phase I Integrated Biomarker Trial of VX15/2503 in Combination With Ipilimumab or Nivolumab in Patients With Pancreatic and Colorectal Cancer

Brief Summary

This randomized phase I trial studies how well anti-SEMA4D monoclonal antibody VX15/2503 with or without ipilimumab or nivolumab work in treating patients with stage I-III pancreatic cancer that can be removed by surgery or stage IV colorectal cancer that has spread to the liver and can be removed by surgery. Monoclonal antibodies, such as anti-SEMA4D monoclonal antibody VX15/2503, ipilimumab, and nivolumab, may interfere with the ability of tumor cells to grow and spread.

Detailed Description

PRIMARY OBJECTIVE:

To evaluate the effect of the anti-SEMA4D monoclonal antibody VX15/2503 (VX15/2503) alone and VX15/2503 in combination with immune checkpoint inhibitors, ipilimumab or nivolumab, on the immune profile in the tumor microenvironment and in peripheral blood.

SECONDARY OBJECTIVE:

To extend the previously reported safety profile of single agent VX15/2503 to the combination of VX15/2503 and immune checkpoint inhibitors, ipilimumab or nivolumab, in patients with pancreatic and colorectal cancer.

OUTLINE:

Patients are randomized to 1 of 4 arms.

ARM I: Patients undergo surgery.

ARM II: Patients receive anti-SEMA4D monoclonal antibody VX15/2503 intravenously (IV) over 60 minutes on day 1. Patients then proceed to surgery 22-36 days after drug administration.

ARM III: Patients receive anti-SEMA4D monoclonal antibody VX15/2503 IV over 60 minutes and ipilimumab IV over 90 minutes on day 1. Patients then proceed to surgery 22-36 days after drug administration.

ARM IV: Patients receive anti-SEMA4D monoclonal antibody VX15/2503 IV over 60 minutes and nivolumab IV over 60 minutes on day 1. Patients then proceed to surgery 22-36 days after drug administration.

After completion of study treatment, patients are followed up at 90 days and then every 12 weeks thereafter.

Study Type

Interventional

Study Phase

Phase 1

Condition

- Colon Carcinoma Metastatic in the Liver
- Colorectal Adenocarcinoma
- Pancreatic Adenocarcinoma
- Resectable Pancreatic Carcinoma
- Stage I Pancreatic Cancer
- Stage IA Pancreatic Cancer
- Stage IB Pancreatic Cancer
- Stage II Pancreatic Cancer
- Stage IIA Pancreatic Cancer
- Stage IIB Pancreatic Cancer
- Stage III Pancreatic Cancer
- Stage IV Colorectal Cancer
- Stage IVA Colorectal Cancer
- Stage IVB Colorectal Cancer

Intervention

Biological: Anti-SEMA4D Monoclonal Antibody VX15/2503

    Given IV

Other Names:

    moAb VX15/2503

    VX15/2503

    Biological: Ipilimumab

    Given IV

Other Names:

    BMS-734016

MDX-010

MDX-CTLA4

Yervoy

Biological: Nivolumab

Given IV

Other Names:
BMS-936558

MDX-1106

NIVO

ONO-4538

Opdivo

Procedure: Surgery

Undergo therapeutic conventional surgery

Study Arms

Active Comparator: Arm I (surgery)

Patients undergo surgery.

Experimental: Arm II (VX15/2503, surgery)

Patients receive anti-SEMA4D monoclonal antibody VX15/2503 IV over 60 minutes on day 1. Beginning 22-36 days after administration, patients undergo surgery.

Experimental: Arm III (VX15/2503, ipilimumab, surgery)

Patients receive anti-SEMA4D monoclonal antibody VX15/2503 IV over 60 minutes and ipilimumab IV over 90 minutes on day 1. Beginning 22-36 days after administration, patients undergo surgery.

Experimental: Arm IV (VX15/2503, nivolumab, surgery)

Patients receive anti-SEMA4D monoclonal antibody VX15/2503 IV over 60 minutes and nivolumab IV over 60 minutes on day 1. Beginning 22-36 days after administration, patients undergo surgery.

Recruitment Information

Recruitment Status

Recruiting

Estimated Enrollment

32

Completion Date

December 31, 2022

Primary Completion Date

December 31, 2022

Eligibility Criteria

Inclusion Criteria:

- For patients with pancreatic cancer:
- Stage I-III cytologically or histologically-proven pancreatic adenocarcinoma
- Cancer confirmed to be surgically resectable, with surgery evaluation with planned resection
- No prior lines of therapy
- For patients with metastatic colorectal cancer:
- Stage IV histologically-proven colorectal adenocarcinoma
- Liver metastasis confirmed to be surgically resectable, with surgery evaluation and planned resection; may have minimal extrahepatic disease that is determined to be resectable
- Tumor must be confirmed to be microsatellite stable (MSS); if not already reported at a Clinical Laboratory Improvement Act (CLIA)-certified laboratory, we will be able to perform this at Emory University
- No prior immunotherapy
- No cancer treatment 2 weeks prior to day 1 of treatment
- Eastern Cooperative Oncology Group (ECOG) performance status 0 or 1
- Absolute neutrophil count ≥ 1,500 cells/μL
- Platelets ≥ 100,000/μL
- Hemoglobin ≥ 9.0 g/dL (may receive packed red blood cell [prbc] transfusion)
- Total bilirubin ≤ 1.5 x the upper limit of normal (ULN)

- Aspartate aminotransferase (AST) and alanine aminotransferase (ALT) ≤ 2.5 x ULN
- Albumin ≥ 3.0 g/dL
- Serum creatinine ≤ 1.5 x ULN
- Calculated creatinine clearance of ≥ 50 mL/min
- International normalized ratio (INR) ≤ 1.5; anticoagulation is allowed only with low molecular weight heparin (LMWH); patient receiving LMW heparin on stable therapeutic dose for more than 2 weeks or with factor Xa level < 1.1 U/mL are allowed on the trial
- Willingness and ability to comply with scheduled visits, treatment plans, laboratory tests, and other study procedures
- Ability to understand and willingness to sign a written informed consent document
- Female subjects of childbearing potential must agree to use adequate contraception (e.g., hormonal or barrier method of birth control; abstinence) for the duration of study treatment and 3 months after completion
- Male subjects must agree to use adequate contraception (e.g., condoms; abstinence) for the duration of study treatment and 3 months after completion
- Female subjects of childbearing age must have a negative serum pregnancy test at study entry

Exclusion Criteria:

- Poor venous access for study drug administration
- Determined not to be a surgical candidate due to medical co-morbidities
- Treatment with chronic immunosuppressants (e.g., cyclosporine following transplantation)
- Prior organ allograft or allogeneic bone marrow transplantation
- Subjects with any active autoimmune disease or history of known or suspected autoimmune disease except for subjects with vitiligo, resolved childhood asthma/atopy, type I diabetes mellitus, residual hypothyroidism, psoriasis not requiring systemic treatment, or conditions not expected to recur in the absence of an external trigger are permitted to enroll
- Subjects with a condition requiring systemic treatment with either corticosteroids (> 10 mg daily prednisone equivalents) or other immunosuppressive medications within 14 days of study drug administration; inhaled or topical steroids and adrenal replacement doses > 10 mg daily prednisone equivalents are permitted in the absence of active autoimmune disease
- Women who are pregnant or lactating
- Uncontrolled intercurrent illness including, but not limited to, human immunodeficiency virus (HIV)-positive subjects receiving combination antiretroviral therapy, ongoing or active infection, symptomatic congestive heart failure (New York Heart Association [NYHA] class III or IV), unstable angina pectoris, ventricular arrhythmia, or psychiatric illness/social situations that would limit compliance with study requirements
- Other medications, or severe acute/chronic medical or psychiatric condition, or laboratory abnormality that may increase the risk associated with study participation or study drug administration, or may interfere with the interpretation of study results, and in the judgment of the investigator would make the subject inappropriate for entry into this study
- Clinical evidence of bleeding diathesis or coagulopathy
- Patients with prior malignancies, including pelvic cancer, are eligible if they have been disease free for > 5 years; patients with prior in situ carcinomas are eligible provided there was complete removal
- Active bacterial or fungal infections requiring systemic treatment within 7 days of treatment
- Use of other investigational drugs (drugs not marked for any indication) within 28 days or at least 5 half-lives (whichever is longer) before study drug administration
- History of severe hypersensitivity reactions to other monoclonal antibodies
- Non-oncology vaccines within 28 days prior to or after any dose of ipilimumab

Sex/Gender

All

Ages

18 Years to N/A

Accepts Healthy Volunteers

No

Contacts

Christina Wu, MD   404-778-2670   christina.wu@emoryhealthcare.org

An Investigational Immuno-therapy Study Of Nivolumab In Combination With Trametinib With Or Without Ipilimumab In Patients With Previously Treated Cancer of the Colon or Rectum That Has Spread

Study ID:

NCT03377361

Sponsor:

Bristol-Myers Squibb

Information provided by (Responsible Party):

Bristol-Myers Squibb (Bristol-Myers Squibb)

Tracking Information

▥ **First Submitted Date**

December 14, 2017

▥ **Start Date**

January 22, 2018

▥ **Current Primary Outcome Measures**

Number of Adverse Events (AEs)[Time Frame: Approximately 40 months]
  Number of Serious Adverse Events (SAEs)[Time Frame: Approximately 40 months]

  Objective response rate (ORR)[Time Frame: Approximately 20 months]

▥ **Primary Completion Date**

September 26, 2021

▥ **Last Update Posted Date**

February 6, 2018

▥ **Current Secondary Outcome Measures**

Disease control rate (DCR)[Time Frame: Approximately 20 months]
  Duration of response (DoR)[Time Frame: Approximately 20 months]

  Time to response (TTR)[Time Frame: Approximately 20 months]

  Progression free survival (PFS)[Time Frame: Approximately 20 months]

  Overall survival (OS)[Time Frame: Approximately 40 months]

Descriptive Information

▥ **Offical Title**

A Study Of Nivolumab In Combination With Trametinib With Or Without Ipilimumab In Participants With Previously Treated Metastatic Colorectal Cancers

▥ **Brief Summary**

The purpose of this study is to investigate treatment with Nivolumab in combination with Trametinib with or without Ipilimumab in patients with previously treated cancer of the colon or rectum that has spread.

▥ **Study Type**

Interventional

▥ **Study Phase**

Phase 1/Phase 2

▥ **Condition**

- Colorectal Cancer
- Colorectal Tumors
- Colorectal Carcinoma
- Colorectal Neoplasm

▥ **Intervention**

Biological: Nivolumab
  specified dose on specified days

Other Names:

  Opdivo

  BMS-936558

  Drug: Trametinib

  specified dose on specified days

Other Names:

  Mekinist

  Biological: Ipilimumab

  specified dose on specified days

Other Names:

  Yervoy

  BMS-734016

▦ Study Arms

Experimental: Previously Treated Metastatic Colorectal Cancer Doublet
  Treatment of mCRC participants

Experimental: Previously Treated Metastatic Colorectal Cancer Triplet
  Treatment of mCRC participants

Recruitment Information

▦ Recruitment Status

Recruiting

▦ Estimated Enrollment

345

▦ Completion Date

November 29, 2022

▦ Primary Completion Date

September 26, 2021

▦ Eligibility Criteria

For more information regarding Bristol-Myers Squibb Clinical Trial participation, please visit www.BMSStudyConnect.com

Inclusion Criteria:

- Must have previously treated metastatic colorectal cancer
- Must have RAS mutation and microsatellite stability status results as part of medical history
- Must agree to provide archival or newly obtained tumor tissue sample prior to the start of treatment in this study
- Eastern Cooperative Oncology Group (ECOG) performance status of ≤1
- Ability to swallow pills or capsules
- Adequate organ functions
- Ability to comply with study visits, treatment, procedures, PK and PD sample collection, and required study follow-up

Exclusion Criteria:

- BRAF V600 mutant colorectal cancer
- Active brain metastases or leptomeningeal metastases
- Active, known or suspected autoimmune disease
- Histology other than adenocarcinoma
- Participants with a condition requiring systemic treatment with either corticosteroids (> 10 mg daily prednisone equivalents) or other immunosuppressive medications within 14 days of study treatment administration
- History of interstitial lung disease or pneumonitis
- Prior treatment with immune checkpoint inhibitors and MEK inhibitors
- History of allergy to study treatments or any of its components of the study arm that participant is enrolling

Sex/Gender

All

▦ Ages

18 Years to N/A

▦ Accepts Healthy Volunteers

No

■ **Contacts**

Recruiting sites have contact information. Please contact the sites directly. If there is no contact information,   please email: Clinical.Trials@bms.com

First line of the email MUST contain NCT # and Site #.

Multi-Targeted Recombinant Ad5 (CEA/MUC1/Brachyury) Based Immunotherapy Vaccine Regimen in People With Advanced Cancer

Study ID:

NCT03384316

Sponsor:

National Cancer Institute (NCI)

Information provided by (Responsible Party):

National Institutes of Health Clinical Center (CC) (National Cancer Institute (NCI))

Tracking Information

■ **First Submitted Date**

December 23, 2017

■ **Start Date**

January 31, 2018

■ **Current Primary Outcome Measures**

Safety[Time Frame: 30 days after treatment]
List of adverse event frequency

Recommended phase 2 dose[Time Frame: 2 years]
Recommended phase 2 dose

■ **Primary Completion Date**

January 1, 2020

■ **Last Update Posted Date**

February 5, 2018

■ **Current Secondary Outcome Measures**

Objective response rate (ORR)[Time Frame: At tumor progression]
Proportion of patients whose tumors shrunk after therapy

Disease control rate (DCR)[Time Frame: 6 months]
Proportion of patients with confirmed response or SD lasting for at least 6 months

Duration of response[Time Frame: At progression]
Time from the measurement criteria are met for CR or PR until the first date that recurrent or PD

Progression-free survival (PFS)[Time Frame: At progression]
Median amount of time subject survives without disease progression after treatment

Overall survival (OS)[Time Frame: Death]
Median amount of time subject survives after therapy

Descriptive Information

■ **Offical Title**

Multi-Targeted Recombinant Ad5 (CEA/MUC1/Brachyury) Based Immunotherapy Vaccine Regimen in People With Advanced Cancer

■ **Brief Summary**

Background:

ETBX-011, ETBX-061, and ETBX-051 are cancer vaccines. Their goal is to teach the immune system to target and kill cancer cells. The vaccines target 3 proteins found in many types of cancer. Researchers think targeting all 3 proteins in unison will have the best results.

Objective:

To test the safety of combining ETBX-011, ETBX-061, and ETBX-051 and their effects on the immune system.

Eligibility:

People ages 18 and older with advanced cancer that has not responded to standard therapies

Design:

Participants will be screened with:

Medical history / Physical exam

Blood, urine, and heart tests

Scan: They will lie in a machine that takes pictures of the body.

Participants will receive the 3 vaccines through 3 shots under the skin every 3 weeks for 3 doses, then every 8 weeks for up to 1 year. They will have blood and urine tests at each vaccine visit. They will have scans and other measurements of their tumor after 9 weeks and then at their vaccine visits every 8 weeks.

Participants will keep a diary of symptoms at the injection site.

Participants will have a visit 90 days after their final treatment. This will include a physical exam and blood and urine tests. If they have any ongoing side effects, they will be followed until these end or are not changing.

After this visit, they will be called every 3 months for the first year, every 6 months for the next 2 years, then every 12 months for another 2 years to see how they are doing.

Participants will have the option to enroll in a long-term follow-up study.

Detailed Description

Background:

- The overall goal of the current project is to expand our immunotherapeutic approach for the treatment of advanced cancer employing a multi-targeted approach.
- Therapeutic cancer vaccines targeting overexpressed proteins offer a potential method to activate T cells against tumors.
- A novel adenovirus based vaccine targeting three (3) human tumor associated antigens (TAA), CEA, MUC1, and brachyury, respectively has demonstrated anti-tumor cytolytic T cell responses in pre-clinical animal models of cancer.

Objectives:

-To determine the overall safety and recommended phase 2 dose of a combination of three immunotherapeutic vaccines (ETBX-011/ETBX-061/ETBX-051), when administered subcutaneously (SC) to subjects with advanced solid tumors

Eligibility:

- Subjects age 18 and older with cytologically or histologically confirmed locally advanced or metastatic solid tumor malignancy who have completed or had disease progression on at least one prior line of disease-appropriate therapy or who are not candidates for therapy of proven efficacy for their disease.
- Subjects may have measurable or non-measurable but evaluable disease. Subjects with surgically resected metastatic disease at high risk of relapse are also eligible.
- ECOG performance status less than or equal to 1
- Adequate organ and bone marrow function
- Subjects with active autoimmune diseases requiring systemic treatment and subjects requiring systemic steroids (except for physiologic doses for steroid replacement) are not allowed

Design:

- This is a Phase I trial in subjects with advanced cancer. A combination of three therapeutic vaccines (ETBX-011, ETBX-51, EBX-61) using the same modified Adenovirus vector backbone, separately encoding three well-studied tumor-associated antigens will be assessed. The vaccine will be tested at a single dose level, and a dose de-escalation design (if required). The dose level of each vaccine tested will be 5×10^{11} VP. This dose has been found in prior phase 1 testing of Ad5 [E1-, E2b-]-CEA(6D) (ETBX-011) to be well tolerated (with no dose-limiting toxicities (DLTs) or related Serious adverse events (SAEs), and optimal for induction of immune responses. Each of the three vaccines will be administered subcutaneously (SC) at separate injection sites (proximal limb, preferably the thigh), every 3 weeks for 3 doses, then bi-monthly (every 8 week) boosts for up to a year.
- Up to six patients will be enrolled at Dose Level 1. If less than or equal to 1 of 6 patients experience a DLT, initiation of the dose expansion phase will occur. If greater than or equal to 2 of 6 experience DLT at Dose Level 1, then dose de-escalation will occur. Up to six patients will be enrolled at the lower dose level Dose Level -1 (1×10^{11} VP). If less than or equal to 1 of 6 patients experience a DLT, then the maximum tolerated (MTD) will be declared at this dose, and initiation of the dose expansion phase will occur. If greater than or equal to 2 of 6 experience DLT at Dose Level -1, then a protocol amendment may be written to evaluate a further dose de-escalation.
- A dose expansion phase of study will be enrolled after the MTD of the combination vaccine has been determined. An additional 4 subjects will be enrolled in the dose expansion component of the trial, for a total of 10 subjects at the MTD.

- **Study Type**

Interventional

Study Phase

Phase 1

Condition

- Neoplasms

- Prostate Cancer
- Lung Cancer
- Breast Cancer
- Colon Cancer

Intervention

Biological: ETBX-051; adenoviral brachyury vaccine

immunotherapeutic vaccine administered subcutaneously every 3 weeks for 3 doses, and then every 8 weeks for up to a year

Biological: ETBX-061; adenoviral MUC1 vaccine

immunotherapeutic vaccine administered subcutaneously every 3 weeks for 3 doses, and then every 8 weeks for up to a year

Biological: ETBX-011; adenoviral CEA vaccine

immunotherapeutic vaccine administered subcutaneously every 3 weeks for 3 doses, and then every 8 weeks for up to a year

Study Arms

Experimental: 1-Dose De-Escalation
Dose De-Escalation

Experimental: 2-Dose Expansion
Dose Expansion

Publications

(Includes publications given by the data provider as well as publications identified by ClinicalTrials.gov Identifier (NCT Number) in Medline.)Balint JP, Gabitzsch ES, Rice A, Latchman Y, Xu Y, Messerschmidt GL, Chaudhry A, Morse MA, Jones FR. Extended evaluation of a phase 1/2 trial on dosing, safety, immunogenicity, and overall survival after immunizations with an advanced-generation Ad5 [E1-, E2b-]-CEA(6D) vaccine in late-stage colorectal cancer. Cancer Immunol Immunother. 2015 Aug;64(8):977-87. doi: 10.1007/s00262-015-1706-4. Epub 2015 May 9. (https://www.ncbi.nlm.nih.gov/pubmed/25956394)

Morse MA, Chaudhry A, Gabitzsch ES, Hobeika AC, Osada T, Clay TM, Amalfitano A, Burnett BK, Devi GR, Hsu DS, Xu Y, Balcaitis S, Dua R, Nguyen S, Balint JP Jr, Jones FR, Lyerly HK. Novel adenoviral vector induces T-cell responses despite anti-adenoviral neutralizing antibodies in colorectal cancer patients. Cancer Immunol Immunother. 2013 Aug;62(8):1293-301. doi: 10.1007/s00262-013-1400-3. Epub 2013 Apr 30. (https://www.ncbi.nlm.nih.gov/pubmed/23624851)

Gabitzsch ES, Tsang KY, Palena C, David JM, Fantini M, Kwilas A, Rice AE, Latchman Y, Hodge JW, Gulley JL, Madan RA, Heery CR, Balint JP Jr, Jones FR, Schlom J. The generation and analyses of a novel combination of recombinant adenovirus vaccines targeting three tumor antigens as an immunotherapeutic. Oncotarget. 2015 Oct 13;6(31):31344-59. doi: 10.18632/oncotarget.5181. (https://www.ncbi.nlm.nih.gov/pubmed/26374823)

Recruitment Information

Recruitment Status

Recruiting

Estimated Enrollment

32

Completion Date

September 1, 2020

Primary Completion Date

January 1, 2020

Eligibility Criteria

- **INCLUSION CRITERIA:**
- Age greater than or equal to 18 years (male and female).
- Ability to understand and provide signed informed consent that fulfills Institutional Review Board (IRB)'s guidelines.
- Subjects with cytologically or histologically confirmed locally advanced or metastatic solid tumor malignancy.
- Subjects must have completed or had disease progression on at least one prior line of disease-appropriate therapy or not be candidates for therapy of proven efficacy for their disease.
- Subjects may have measurable or non-measurable but evaluable. Subjects with surgically resected locally advanced or metastatic disease at high risk of relapse are also eligible.
- Eastern Cooperative Oncology Group (ECOG) performance status less than or equal to 1.
- Subjects who have received prior CEA, MUC1, and/or Brachyury-targeted immunotherapy (vaccine) are eligible for this trial if this treatment was discontinued at least 4 weeks prior to enrollment.
- Resolution of clinically significant side effects of prior chemotherapy, radiotherapy, immunotherapy or surgical procedures to NCI CTCAE Grade less than or equal to 1 or grade less than or equal to 2 for neuropathy.
- **Adequate hematologic function at screening, as follows:**
- Absolute neutrophil count (ANC) >= 1 x 10^9/L
- Hemoglobin >= 9 g/dL
- Platelets >= 75,000/mcL.

- Adequate renal and hepatic function at screening, as follows:
- Serum creatinine less than or equal to 1.5 x upper limit of normal (ULN) OR creatinine clearance (CrCl) >= 40 mL/min (if using the Cockcroft-Gault formula below):
- Female CrCl = ((140 age in years) x weight in kg x 0.85) / (72 x serum creatinine in mg/dL)
- Male CrCl = ((140 age in years) x weight in kg x 1.00)/ 1.00) / (72 x serum creatinine in mg/dL)
- Bilirubin less than or equal to 1.5 x ULN OR in subjects with Gilbert s syndrome, a total bilirubin less than or equal to 3.0 x ULN
- Alanine aminotransferase (ALT) and aspartate aminotransferase (AST) less than or equal to 2.5 x ULN, unless liver metastases are present, then values must be less than or equal to 3 x ULN)
- The effects of the combination ETBX-011, ETBX-051, ETBX-061 vaccine regimen on the developing human fetus are unknown. For this reason, female subjects of childbearing potential defined as any female who has experienced menarche and who has not undergone surgical sterilization (hysterectomy or bilateral oophorectomy or tubal ligation) or who is not postmenopausal (menopause being defined clinically as 12 months of amenorrhea in a woman over 45 in the absence of other biological or physiological causes) and male patients who are not surgically sterile (vasectomy etc.), must agree to use acceptable contraceptive methods for the duration of the study and for one month after the last vaccination. Acceptable forms of contraception include oral contraceptives, intrauterine device, condom or vaginal diaphragm plus spermicidal (gel/foam/cream/vaginal suppository), or total abstinence.
- Ability to attend required study visits and return for adequate follow up, as required by this protocol.

EXCLUSION CRITERIA:

- Pregnant and nursing women. Because there is an unknown but potential risk for adverse events in nursing infants secondary to treatment of the mother with combination ETBX-011, ETBX-051, ETBX-061, breastfeeding should be discontinued if the mother is treated with combination ETBX-011, ETBX-051, ETBX-061. These potential risks may also apply to other agents used in this study.
- There should be a minimum of 4 weeks from any prior investigational drug, chemotherapy, immunotherapy, with the exception of hormonal therapy for prostate and breast cancers, HER2-directed therapy for HER2+ breast or stomach cancer (3+ IHC or FISH+), drugs targeting EGFR, ALK or ROS1 in EGFR,ALK, ROS1-mutated lung cancer, respectively, or standard maintenance therapies for any solid tumor under the condition that subjects are on these therapies for at least two months before start of trial treatment.
- There should also be a minimum of 4 weeks from any prior radiotherapy except for palliative bone directed therapy.
- Known active brain or central nervous system metastasis (less than 1 month out from definitive radiotherapy or surgery), or seizures requiring anticonvulsant treatment, or clinically significant cerebrovascular accident or transient ischemic attack (<3 months).
- Subjects with active autoimmune disease requiring systemic immunosuppressive treatment within the past 4 weeks such as but not restricted to inflammatory bowel disease, systemic lupus erythematosus, ankylosing spondylitis, scleroderma, or multiple sclerosis. A history of autoimmune disease which is not active nor has required recent systemic immunosuppressive therapy (< 4 weeks prior to enrollment) is not reason for exclusion.
- Subjects with serious intercurrent chronic or acute illness, such as cardiac or pulmonary disease, hepatic disease, or other illness considered by the Investigator as high risk for investigational drug treatment.
- Subjects with clinically significant heart disease, such as congestive heart failure (class II, III, or IV defined by the New York Heart Association functional classification), history of unstable or poorly controlled angina, or history (< 1 year) of ventricular arrhythmia.
- Subjects with a medical or psychological impediment that would impair the ability of the subject to receive therapy per protocol or impact ability to comply with the protocol or protocol-required visits and procedures.
- History of second malignancy within 3 years prior to enrollment except for the following: adequately treated non-melanoma skin cancer, cervical carcinoma in situ, superficial bladder cancer or other localized malignancy after discussion with the medical monitor.
- Presence of a known active acute or chronic infection, including human immunodeficiency virus (HIV, as determined by enzyme-linked immunosorbent assay (ELISA) and confirmed by western blot) and hepatitis B and hepatitis C virus (HBV/HCV, as determined by HBsAg and hepatitis C serology).
- Subjects on systemic intravenous or oral corticosteroid therapy with the exception of physiologic doses of corticosteroids (less than or equal to the equivalent of prednisone 10 mg/day) or other immunosuppressives such as azathioprine or cyclosporin A are excluded on the basis of potential immune suppression. For these subjects these excluded treatments must be discontinued at least 2 weeks prior to enrollment for recent short course use (less than or equal to 14 days) or discontinued at least 4 weeks prior to enrollment for long term use (> 14 days). In addition, the use of corticosteroids as premedication for contrast-enhanced studies is allowed prior to enrollment and on study.
- Subjects with known allergy or hypersensitivity to any component of the investigational product will be excluded.
- Subjects with acute or chronic skin disorders that will interfere with injection into the skin of the extremities or subsequent assessment of potential skin reactions will be excluded.
- Subjects vaccinated with a live (attenuated) vaccine (e.g., FluMist(R)) or a killed (inactivated)/subunit vaccine (e.g., PNEUMOVAX(R), Fluzone(R)) within 28 days or 14 days, respectively, of the first planned dose of ETBX vaccine.

Sex/Gender

All

- **Ages**

  18 Years to 100 Years

- **Accepts Healthy Volunteers**

  No

- **Contacts**

  Alanvin D Orpia, R.N.   (240) 760-7972   alanvin.orpia@nih.gov

A Study of ASN007 in Patients With Advanced Solid Tumors

Study ID:

NCT03415126

Sponsor:

Asana BioSciences

Information provided by (Responsible Party):

Asana BioSciences (Asana BioSciences)

Tracking Information

- **First Submitted Date**

  January 15, 2018

- **Start Date**

  January 19, 2018

- **Primary Completion Date**

  May 2020

- **Last Update Posted Date**

  January 30, 2018

- **Current Primary Outcome Measures**

  Part A: Determine the maximum tolerated dose (MTD) of ASN007[Time Frame: First 21 days]

    The MTD will be determined by evaluating the number of subjects with treatment related dose limiting toxicity. This is the primary endpoint of Part A

  Part B: evaluate the overall response rate (number of Complete Responses + Partial Responses) in subjects receiving ASN007 for the treatment of metastatic melanoma, CRC, NSCLC, or pancreatic cancer.[Time Frame: First 6 months]

    This is the primary endpoint for Part B.

- **Current Secondary Outcome Measures**

  Calculate the pharmacokinetic area under the plasma concentration (AUC) of ASN007[Time Frame: First 21 days]

    Calculate the amount of ASN007 in the bloodstream

  Calculate the maximum plasma concentration (Cmax) at steady state.[Time Frame: First 21 days]

    Calculate the maximum amount of ASN007 in the bloodstream

  Calculate the terminal elimination rate (T 1/2).[Time Frame: First 21 days]

    Calculate how fast ASN002 leaves the body

Descriptive Information

- **Offical Title**

  A Phase 1, Open-Label, Dose-Finding Study Of ASN007 In Patients With Advanced Solid Tumors

- **Brief Summary**

  The study is divided into two parts. The first part of the study will test various doses of ASN007 to find out the highest safe dose to test in five specific groups. The second part of the study will test how well ASN007 can control cancer.

- **Detailed Description**

  Part A is a dose escalation study to determine a safe and tolerable dose of ASN007 for patients with advanced solid tumors. Part A will also describe how the body works on ASN007(pharmacokinetics) and the effects of ASN007 on the body (pharmacodynamics) of ASN007, through blood sampling and optional biopsies..

  Part B of the study will enroll patients with particular tumor types and genetic mutations for treatment at the Recommended Phase 2 Dose. Part B will enroll patients in five groups of fifteen patients each:

  Group 1: Patients with metastatic BRAF mutated melanoma Group 2: Patients with metastatic NRAS and HRAS mutated solid tumors Group 3: Patients with metastatic KRAS mutated colorectal cancer (CRC) Group 4: Patients with metastatic KRAS mutated non-small cell lung cancer (NSCLC) Group 5: Patients with metastatic pancreatic ductal adenocarcinoma (PDAC) Patients with melanoma will be required to have pre-dose and post-dose biopsies.

■ **Study Type**

Interventional

■ **Study Phase**

Phase 1

■ **Condition**

- Cancer
- Malignancy
- Neoplasia
- Neoplasm
- Neoplasm Metastasis
- Colon Cancer
- Colonic Neoplasms
- Colon Cancer Liver Metastasis
- Metastatic Cancer
- Metastatic Melanoma
- Metastatic Colon Cancer
- Metastatic Lung Cancer
- Non Small Cell Lung Cancer Metastatic
- Pancreatic Cancer
- Pancreas Cancer
- Pancreas Adenocarcinoma
- Pancreas Neoplasm
- Metastatic Nonsmall Cell Lung Cancer
- Metastatic Pancreatic Cancer

■ **Intervention**

Drug: ASN007: ascending doses

    Oral drug for the treatment of advanced solid tumors

    Drug: ASN007 RD

Oral drug for the treatment of advanced solid tumors

■ **Study Arms**

Experimental: ASN007 ascending doses

    Patients will receive escalating doses of ASN007 to identify the best dose.

Experimental: ASN007 RD: KRAS mutant Melanoma

    Patients with BRAF mutant metastatic melanoma will receive the recommended dose from Part A.

Experimental: ASN007 RD: NRAS mutant Melanoma

    Patients with NRAS and HRAS mutant solid tumors will receive the recommended dose from Part A.

Experimental: ASN007 RD: KRAS mutant metastatic CRC

    Patients with KRAS mutant CRC will receive the recommended dose from Part A

Experimental: ASN007 RD: KRAS mutant NSCLC

    Patients with KRAS mutant NSCLC will receive the recommended dose from Part A

Experimental: ASN007 RD: Metastatic Pancreatic Cancer

    Patients with pancreatic adenocarcinoma will receive the recommended dose from Part A

Recruitment Information

■ **Recruitment Status**

Recruiting

■ **Estimated Enrollment**

110

■ **Completion Date**

May 2020

■ **Primary Completion Date**

May 2020

■ **Eligibility Criteria**

Inclusion Criteria:

- Written informed consent obtained prior to any study-related procedure being performed;
- Male or non-pregnant, non-lactating female patient at least 18 years of age at the time of consent;
- Eastern Cooperative Oncology Group Performance Status 0-1 (Part A) and PS 0-2 (Part B)
- Histologically or cytologically confirmed
- advanced or metastatic solid tumor (Part A)
- Group 1: BRAF mutant melanoma (Part B)   Group 2: NRAS or HRAS mutant solid tumors(Part B)
- Group 3: KRAS mutant CRC.(Part B)   Group 4: KRAS mutant NSCLC (Part B)
- Group 5: Pancreatic Ductal Adenocarcinoma (Part B)
- Progressive disease after failure of or intolerant to all available standard systemic treatments that have shown a documented benefit in overall survival for their respective tumor type.
- Measurable or evaluable disease per RECIST v1.1
- Screening hematology values of the following:
- absolute neutrophil count ≥ 1000/μL,
- platelets ≥ 100,000/μL,
- hemoglobin ≥ 9 g/dL
- Screening chemistry values of the following:
- alanine aminotransferase (ALT) and aspartate transaminase (AST) ≤ 3.0 × upper limit of the normal (ULN),
- total bilirubin ≤ 1.5 × ULN,
- creatinine ≤ 1.5 × ULN,,
- albumin ≥ 2.8 g/dL.
- Screening heart function lab test
- creatinine kinase MB, troponin-I, and troponin-T within normal limits
- Subject is willing and able to comply with all protocol required visits and assessments, including biopsy if assigned.

Exclusion Criteria:

- Prior treatment with ASN007 or another ERK1/2 inhibitor
- Known hypersensitivity to ASN007 or its excipients;
- Part B: Prior treatment with a RAF or MEK pathway inhibitor, except BRAFmutant melanoma (Group 1)
- Prior chemotherapy, targeted therapy or monoclonal antibody therapy within 3 weeks of start of study treatment (Day1), or 5 half-lives, whichever is shorter.
- Concurrent or prior bone marrow factors (e.g. G-CSF, GM-CSF or erythropoietin) within 3 weeks prior to Day 1 of treatment.
- Febrile neutropenia or serious persistent infection within 2 weeks prior to Day 1 of treatment
- Failure to recover from major surgery or traumatic injury within 4 weeks or minor surgery within 2 weeks prior to Day 1 of treatment.
- History of or current evidence / risk of retinal vein occlusion (RVO) central serous retinopathy (CSR), or glaucoma with intraocular pressures ≥ 21 mmHg or other pre-existing ocular conditions that may put the patient at risk for ocular toxicities
- Known central nervous system (CNS) primary tumor, CNS metastases or carcinomatous meningitis (Part A). Patients may be enrolled with CNS metastasis in certain circumstances in Part B.
- Clinically significant heart disorders including an ejection fraction of < 50%
- Other serious uncontrolled conditions such as fungal, bacterial or viral infection; HIV, Hepatitis B or C, bleeding disorders, interstitial lung disease,

■ **Sex/Gender**

All

■ **Ages**

18 Years to N/A

■ **Accepts Healthy Volunteers**

No

■ **Contacts**

Study Manager   908-698-4973   penny.bristow@asanabio.com

Study Director   908-332-9119   sarper.toker@asanabio.com

www.ingramcontent.com/pod-product-compliance
Lightning Source LLC
Chambersburg PA
CBHW050617290326
41930CB00052B/3009